Obesity, Type 2 Diabetes and the Adipose Organ

Saverio Cinti

Obesity, Type 2 Diabetes and the Adipose Organ

A Pictorial Atlas from Research to Clinical Applications

Second Edition

Springer

Saverio Cinti MD
Professor of Anatomy, Director, Center of Obesity
University of Ancona (Politecnica delle Marche)
Ancona
Italy

First Edition published as "The Adipose Organ", ISBN 978-88-85030-32-7 © Kurtis 2009
ISBN 978-3-030-13249-1 ISBN 978-3-319-40522-3 (eBook)
https://doi.org/10.1007/978-3-319-40522-3

Softcover re-print of the Hardcover 2nd edition 2018

Printed on acid-free paper

This Springer imprint is published by Springer Nature
The registered company is Springer International Publishing AG
The registered company address is: Gewerbestrasse 11, 6330 Cham, Switzerland

To my wife, Emanuela; my kids, Alessandro, Francesca and Andrea Filippo; and my grandchild Leon Battista Jacopo.

Foreword

In this second edition of his atlas, Saverio Cinti contributes a large amount of new information on the anatomical distribution of the adipose organ and its structure, function, development, and clinical correlations. It is an unusual atlas, because it consists of over 500 micrographs, all obtained in Cinti's laboratory, that document the remarkable plasticity of the adipose organ, traditionally considered either a passive reservoir of energy or a heater for animals arousing from hibernation.

First and foremost, I am struck by the extraordinary quality of the illustrations: adipose tissue is not an easy material to process for microscopy, and, yet, this atlas is a rare example of superb technical proficiency. In an era in which unintelligible, stamp-size images dominate the literature, this book proves that good microscopy permits convincing visualization of function.

First among the numerous novelties of this new edition, Cinti confirms that fat, at the gross level, has the dignity of an organ, which manifests constant shape in both of its localizations, subcutaneous and visceral. Furthermore, new dissections show that in the mouse, visceral and subcutaneous fat are continuous with one another, thus further justifying their classification as an organ.

The adipose organ, in turn, consists of two adipose tissues, white and brown. New, careful microscopic analysis of the junction between white fat and brown fat shows images highly suggestive of the transformation of white into brown adipocytes, including the presence of unilocular fat cells that express UCP1, a marker typical of brown fat. Furthermore, several early experiments in the past had suggested that in the mouse, the two components, white and brown, could reversibly transdifferentiate into one another in response to changes in environmental stimuli. Chronic exposure to cold drives transformation of white into brown fat, and the reverse takes place upon exposure to warm temperature or to a long-lasting positive energy balance. Interestingly, even in human patients affected by pheochromocytoma, the neoplasia promotes white-to-brown transdifferentiation. Indeed, subsequent studies based on lineage tracing technique confirmed the white-brown-white plasticity.

The new edition also describes in greater detail the reversible transdifferentiation of white adipocytes into alveolar cells of the mammary gland during pregnancy, lactation, and involution. Both lineage tracing and experiments of transplantation show that labeled, mature, white adipocytes are incorporated into the murine mammary gland. In this context, Cinti defines a new type of fat cell, the pink adipocyte, which appears during pregnancy and lactation and defines the alveolar cells derived from white adipocytes.

A further novelty presented in this new edition concerns both lineage tracing and electron microscopic evidence supporting the developmental origin of adipose cells from vascular endothelium and perivascular pericytes.

Finally, the atlas illustrates all the findings, both structural and immunocytochemical, that interconnect obesity with type 2 diabetes mellitus: in both obese mice and obese humans, mainly visceral adipocytes die as a result of an adipocyte hypertrophy-linked inflammasome activation. This causes a chronic, low-grade inflammatory process responsible for insulin resistance and subsequent type 2 diabetes.

As a whole, this atlas is a real tour de force, containing the most accurate, complete, and aesthetically pleasing description of the structure and function of the adipose organ, as seen with the light and the electron microscopes, in both rodents and humans, from development to adulthood, in health and disease. At the core of the dynamic versatility of adipocytes is their property to reversibly differentiate from white to brown as a result of cold, brown to white following warm acclimation, and, finally, from white to pink in pregnancy and lactation. This opens new therapeutic perspectives in the fields of metabolic and neoplastic diseases.

The reader will marvel at both the biological interest of the adipose organ and the unique, single-minded focus of the book's author.

Department of Neurobiology
Harvard Medical School
Boston, MA, USA

Elio Raviola

Preface

Obesity and its associated disorders, often included in the metabolic syndrome, are reaching global epidemic proportions, and most physicians are involved in their treatment in spite of a scarce knowledge of the underlying physiopathologic processes. The first step toward the treatment of an illness is a deep knowledge of the normal anatomy of the sick organ. The sick organ of metabolic syndrome is the adipose organ. Anatomy defines an organ as a dissectible structure composed of at least two different tissues cooperating to achieve a common finalistic goal. In the last 40 years, the work of my group focused on describing the adipose organ of adult animals and humans during development and under different physiologic and pathologic conditions.

Our studies showed that mammals are provided with a large unitary structure composed of three different tissues (white, brown, and pink fat) cooperating to distribute energy for the maintenance of short- and long-term homeostasis.

This large unitary structure occupies the subcutaneous and visceral compartments of the body and satisfies three different functional needs for animal and species survival: thermogenesis (brown fat), fuel provision for cellular metabolism in the interval between meals (white fat), and energy provision for pup's survival through lactation (pink fat – alveolar glands that produce milk).

White, brown, and pink adipocytes are provided with a high capacity of transdifferentiation that allows a striking ability of the organ to adapt to specific conditions; thus, during chronic cold exposure, the adipose organ converts white into brown fat; during chronic positive energy balance periods, the organ converts brown into white fat; and during pregnancy and lactation, white and probably brown fat are converted into pink fat.

All the conversion phenomena are physiologic and reversible.

The obese organ has a specific histopathology that can explain the well-known link between obesity and insulin resistance and consequent type 2 diabetes.

The anatomy of this organ during development and under several physiologic and pathologic conditions in animals and humans is shown in this book with different morphologic techniques: from dissections to show the gross anatomy to light microscopy with different immunohistochemistry techniques and to scanning and transmission electron microscopy.

Finally, some lineage tracing data of white-pink-white and pink-brown are shown together with those showing developmental aspects of adipocytes in murine embryos.

Ancona, Italy — Saverio Cinti

Acknowledgments

I am deeply grateful to my "mentors" Professors Francesco Osculati, Elio Raviola, and Manlio Caucci for their invaluable suggestions and their support in these last 40 years of scientific activity in this field.

My heartfelt thanks go to my competent and dedicated lab collaborators, in particular: for gross anatomy, to M. Cristina Zingaretti, Rita de Matteis, and Antonio Giordano; for light microscopy, to M. Cristina Zingaretti, Rita de Matteis, Antonio Giordano, Enzo Ceresi, Mariella Marelli, and Ilenia Severi; for transmission electron microscopy, to Antonio Giordano, Manrico Morroni, Giorgio Barbatelli, Mariella Marelli, and M. Cristina Zingaretti; for immunohistochemistry, to M. Cristina Zingaretti, Antonio Giordano, Mario Castellucci, Daniela Marzioni, Pina Ciarmela, Ilenia Severi, Rita de Matteis, Enzo Ceresi, Raffaella Cancello, and Immacolata Murano; for immunoelectron microscopy, to Enzo Ceresi; for scanning microscopy, to Andrea Sbarbati, Paolo Bernardi, and Plinio Ferrara; for freeze-fracturing, to Plinio Ferrara; for in situ hybridization, to Raffaella Cancello; for molecular studies, to Antonio Giordano, Jessica Perugini, and Arianna Smorlesi; for fetal studies, to Monica Banita and Andrea Frontini; and for lineage tracing studies, to Antonio Giordano, Andrea Frontini, and M. Cristina Zingaretti.

I am also grateful to all collaborators in Europe, USA, Brazil, and Russia who allowed me to understand several aspects of adipose organ anatomy taking advantage from the study of genetically modified mice and rare human aspects and diseases involving adipose tissues.

Professor Alessandro Riva (University of Cagliari, Italy) took for us some of the SEM pictures with the osmium maceration technique.

Finally, I wish to particularly thank Maria Cristina Zingaretti for her instrumental contribution to most of the technical work of all my studies and for the final editing of this book.

Contents

1 Gross Anatomy

S. Cinti, *Obesity, Type 2 Diabetes and the Adipose Organ*, https://doi.org/10.1007/978-3-319-40522-3_1

1.1 Gross Anatomy

PLATE 1.1

The Adipose Organ

The adipose organ is composed of several depots. They are located in three main anatomical areas: skin (dermal), subcutis (anterior and posterior), and trunk (mediastinal, mesenteric, perirenal, perigonadal, peri-bladder, and retroperitoneal).
These depots, dissected from an adult C57BL mouse, are shown in this plate.
In this mouse strain, about 60% of the weight of the organ is represented by the two subcutaneous depots.
The bulk of the anterior subcutaneous depot is located in the dorsal position, with a central portion in the interscapular region and several symmetric projections reaching the cervical, axillary, and subscapular areas. All fat areas contained in the trunk should be considered as composed of visceral adipocytes for three main anatomical reasons: (1) tight contact with the viscera, (2) smaller size (compared with subcutaneous adipocytes), and (3) less expandability (compared with subcutaneous adipocytes) (see Chap. 9). The deep cervical and the axillary areas (i.e., those surrounding carotid and subclavian-axillary arteries) should also be considered visceral areas of the neck and axilla. As a matter of fact, they are both in tight contact with the viscera: pharynx, larynx, thyroid and parathyroid glands and vessels in the neck, and lymph nodes and vessels in the axillae. Furthermore deep connective fasciae anatomically separate these two sites from the subcutaneous fat.
The posterior subcutaneous depot is mainly located in ventral position, in the inguinal fold, with dorsolumbar, inguinal, and gluteal portions. Peritoneal sheets usually bound the visceral depots.
In adult animals acclimated at 20 °C, most of the organ appears white-colored. However, the interscapular, subscapular, and part of the cervical and axillary fat of the anterior subcutaneous depot, as well as some inguinal areas of the posterior subcutaneous depot and some of the mediastinal and perirenal visceral depots, appear brownish.

Suggested Reading

Hammar JA. Zur Kenntniss des Fettgewebes. Arch Mikroskop Anat. 45: 512–74, 1895.

Rasmussen AT. The so-called hibernating gland. J Morphology. 38:147–207, 1923.

Wells HG. Adipose tissue a neglected subject. JAMA. 114:2177–284, 1940.

Cinti S. Adipose tissues and obesity. Ital J Anat Embryol. 104:37–51, 1999.

Cinti S. Anatomy of the adipose organ. Eat Weight Disord. 5:132–42, 2000.

Cinti S. The adipose organ: morphological perspectives of adipose tissues. Proc Nutr Soc. 60:319–28, 2001a.

Cinti S. The adipose organ: endocrine aspects and insights from transgenic models. Eat Weight Disord. 6:4–8, 2001b.

Cinti S. The adipose organ. Prostaglandins Leukot Essent Fatty Acids. 73:9–15, 2005.

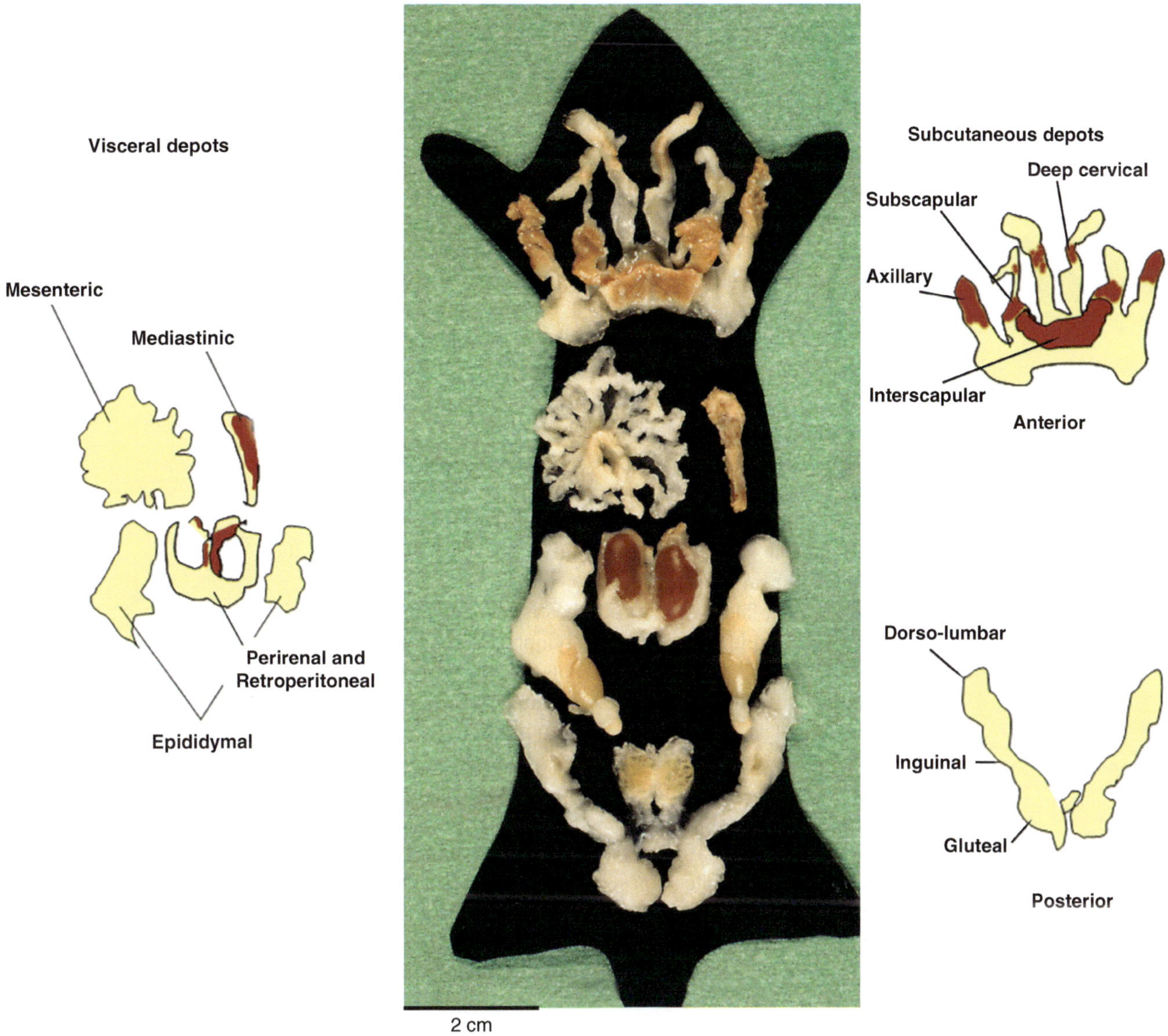

Plate 1.1 The adipose organ. Adult (20 weeks old) mouse C57/BL6 (B6) maintained at 20 °C. Kidneys, testes, and preputial glands were left for better orientation.

PLATE 1.2

Unitary Structure

Recent dissections revealed the anatomical continuity among all depots of the adipose organ, strongly supporting the concept that this organ is a unitary anatomic structure.

Mediastinal fat surrounding the aorta is in continuity with the anterior subcutaneous depot through the fat surrounding the subclavian arteries (see also the next plates). This last fat is in continuity with the cervical fat and axillary fat (see the previous plate) as parts of the anterior subcutaneous depot. Mediastinal fat is in continuity with the perirenal fat through the esophageal hiatus. All the visceral fat depots in the trunk are in continuity because perirenal fat is in continuity with the retroperitoneal, mesenteric, periovarian, parametrial (peri-gonadal in males), and peri-bladder fat. Peri-bladder fat is in continuity with the gluteal fat that is part of the posterior subcutaneous depot. Lateral fat projections join the anterior and posterior subcutaneous depots.

The only depot that is not in direct continuity with the rest of the organ is the omental depot. It is separated from the rest of the abdominal fat by the spleen that develops into the posterior peritoneal ligament joining the omentum to the posterior wall of the abdomen (dorsal mesogastrium).

Other relevant fats are present in the organs: bone marrow, parotid gland, parathyroid glands, thyroid, lymph nodes, heart, and skeletal muscles. In the legs two major depots are dissectible at the root of the thigh and in the popliteal fossa. Smaller depots are visible also in the deltoid and elbow areas in the anterior legs.

The anatomy definition for organ includes its dissectability and requires at least two different tissues, usually cooperating for a common finalistic role. The gross anatomy shows that the adipose organ presents two different colors corresponding to two different tissues: white for white adipose tissue and brown for brown adipose tissue. The two colors are well represented in both genders and both in visceral and subcutaneous parts of the organ. The common finalistic role of the adipose organ is mainly detailed in Chaps. 7, 8, and 11.

Suggested Reading

Giordano et al. in preparation.

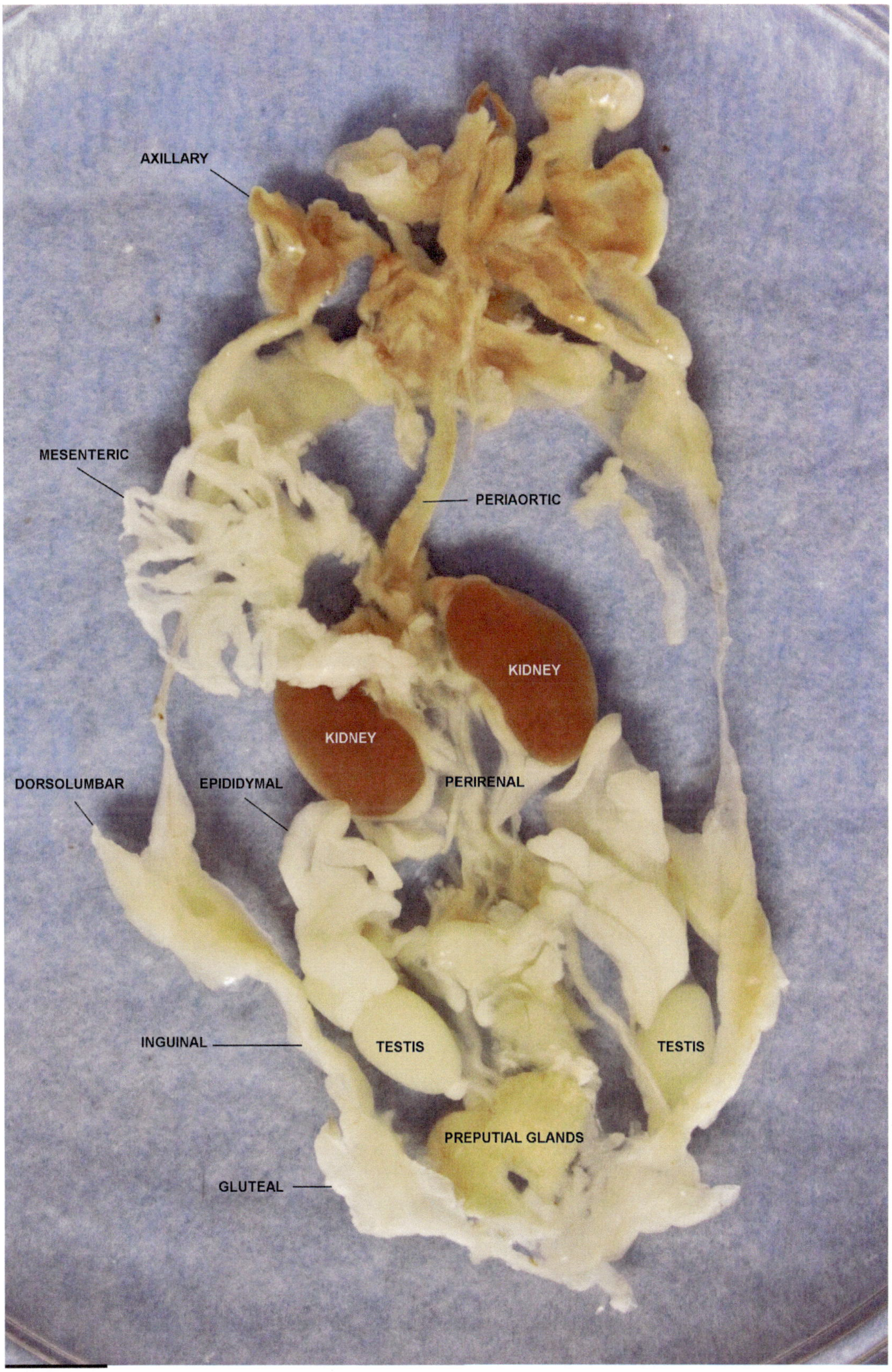

Plate 1.2 The adipose organ of young (7 weeks old) male B6 mouse, maintained at 24 °C. Kidneys, testes, and preputial glands were left for better orientation.

PLATE 1.3

Male and Female Adipose Organ

The distribution of the white and brown areas in the adipose organ of adult mice is similar in both genders. Most of the brown part is in the anterior part of the organ and mainly in the subcutaneous area. In particular the subcutaneous interscapular and subscapular areas as well as the visceral areas axillary and deep cervical (see also Plate 1.3) are brown and well visible even in these adult mice maintained at room temperature. In the trunk the brownish visceral fat is mainly visible in the mediastinal depot. Of note, the fat surrounding the subclavian vessels joining the mediastinal and subclavian areas is also brown.

Larger depots in females make the continuity between the abdominal and pelvic fat. The perirenal fat forming the bulk of the abdominal fat is continuous with the peri-gonadal fat that is in continuity with the parametrial fat that joins the pelvic peri-bladder fat. In males the fat surrounding the ureters ensures the continuity between the perirenal fat and pelvic fat.

Suggested Reading

Giordano et al. in preparation.

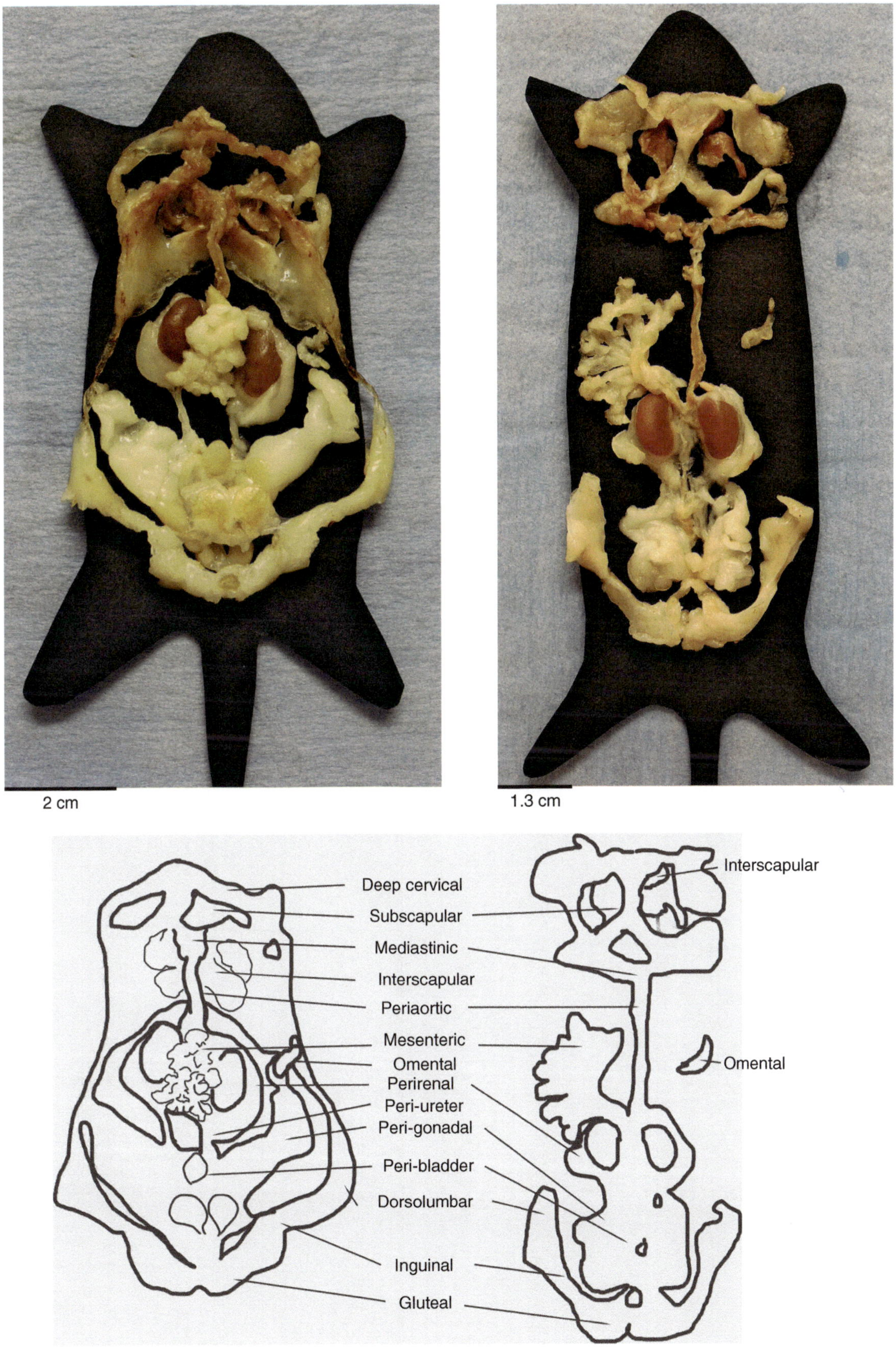

Plate 1.3 The adipose organ of adult (22 weeks old) male and female B6 mice, maintained at 24 °C. Kidneys, testes, and preputial glands were left for better orientation.

PLATE 1.4

Young Male Adipose Organ

In young animals the brown parts of the organ are more abundant. The color of the organ in the brown areas of adult mice organ is not so brown with a brownish tendency. This phenomenon corresponds to variability in cellular composition in the organ with age. We explored the interscapular area cellular composition in newborn and 1-, 3-, 5-, 7-, 13-, 26-, 52-, 78-, and 104-week-old Sprague Dawley rats maintained in standard laboratory conditions and found a progressive increase in the white fat component in this area with age. The right panel shows the interscapular and subscapular area after dislocation of the superficial layer of the subcutaneous anterior depot composed of white fat. With this dislocation all deep brown parts of the depot are evident.

Suggested Reading

Sbarbati A, et al. Rat interscapular brown adipose tissue at different ages: a morphometric study. Int J Obesity. 15:581–88, 1991.

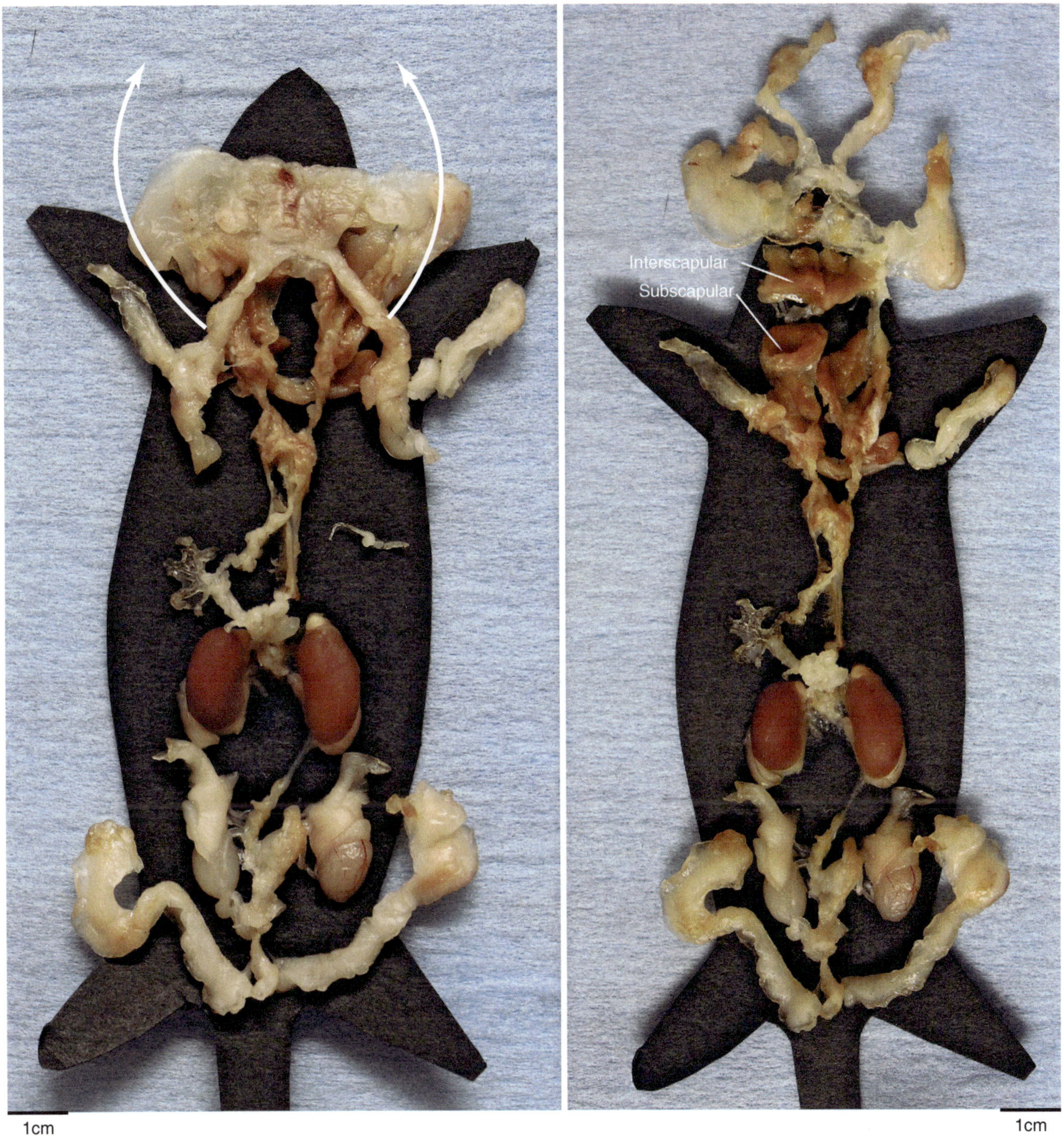

Plate 1.4 The adipose organ of young (4 weeks old) male B6 mouse, maintained at 24 °C. Kidneys and testes were left for better orientation.

PLATE 1.5

Young Female Adipose Organ

We performed extensive quantitative measurements of the white and brown components of the adipose organ of female adult mice of two strains (B6 and Sv129) maintained at 28 °C.
We choose the female gender because in males the composition of the organ is greatly dependent on the animal's dominance.
The total number of adipocytes in the organ was calculated in about 175 million cells in Sv129 and 150 million cells in B6 mice. Interestingly, about 60% of all adipocytes were brown in the obesity- and type 2 (T2) diabetes-resistant mice Sv129 and only about 15% of all adipocytes in the obese- and T2 diabetes-prone strain B6.

Suggested Reading

Murano I, et al. The Adipose Organ of Sv129 mice contains a prevalence of brown adipocytes and shows plasticity after cold exposure. Adipocytes. 1:121–30, 2005.
Vitali A, et al. The adipose organ of obesity-prone C57BL/6J mice is composed of mixed white and brown adipocytes. J Lip Res. 53:619–29, 2012.

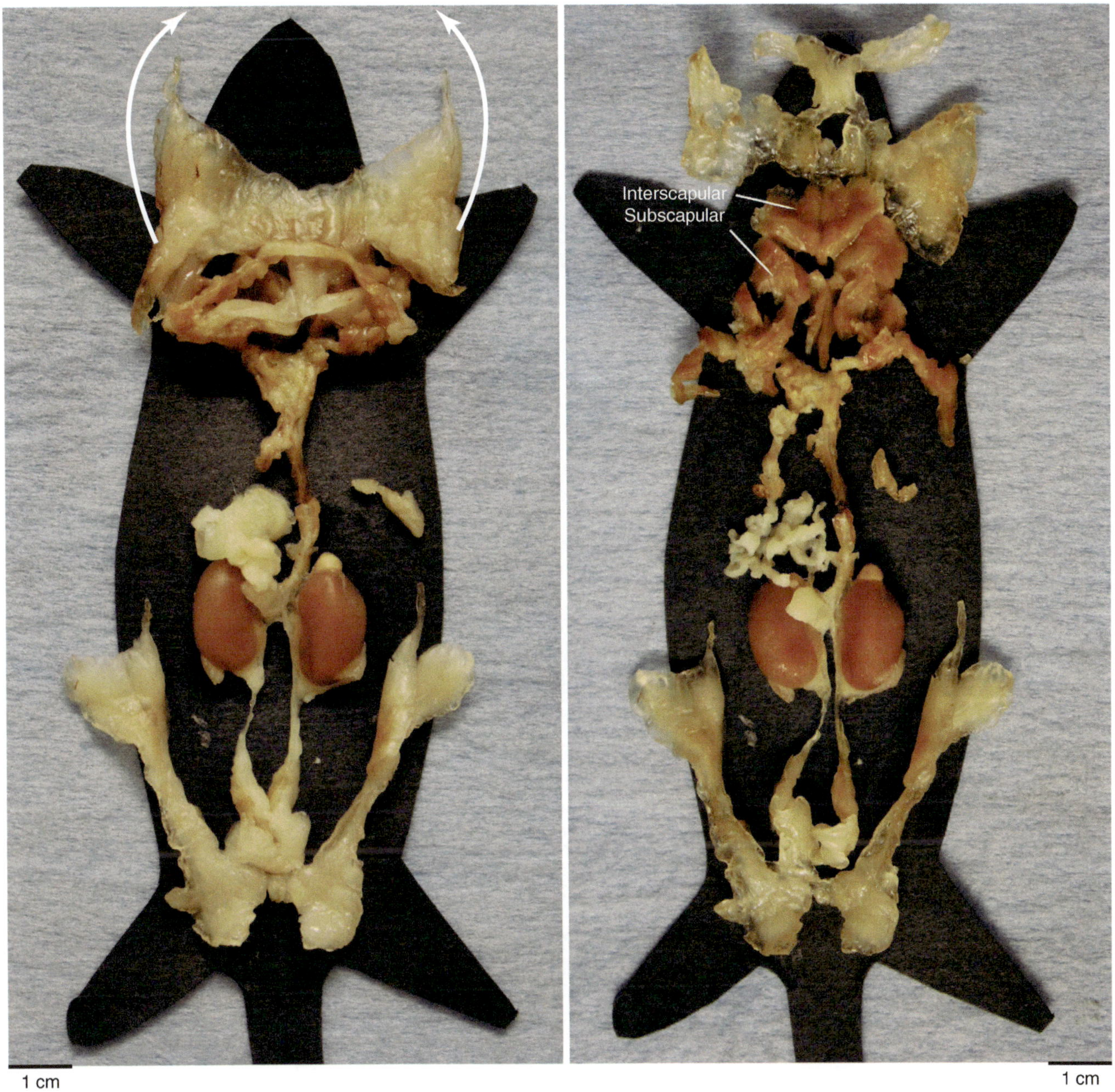

Plate 1.5 The adipose organ of young (4 weeks old) female B6 mouse, maintained at 24 °C. Kidneys were left for better orientation.

Murine Brown Adipose Tissue

2

S. Cinti, *Obesity, Type 2 Diabetes and the Adipose Organ*, https://doi.org/10.1007/978-3-319-40522-3_2

2.1 Murine Brown Adipose Tissue

PLATE 2.1

Brown Adipose Tissue Histology

The brownish areas of the adipose organ are constituted of brown adipose tissue (BAT). The lower right panel of this plate shows the color and gross appearance of white and brown fat. BAT is a lobular tissue in which the parenchymal cell is a multilocular roundish cell with a central nucleus, called brown adipocyte. The vacuoles are made up of triglycerides. These same molecules are stored in white adipocytes, which are mainly unilocular.

In the peripheral portion of a BAT lobule, usually, a strand of connective tissue separates BAT from white adipose tissue (WAT) (see schematic representation). Both multilocular brown adipocytes and unilocular white adipocytes are visible. Immunohistochemistry (IHC) is used to localize protein expression in situ. In this section (upper panel), processed for immunohistochemistry (IHC), brown adipocytes are positive for an anti-UCP1 antibody. UCP1 is a mitochondrial protein responsible for the uncoupling of respiration from ADP phosphorylation and therefore for the thermogenic activity of these cells. All brown adipocytes in the different areas and depots of the adipose organ are UCP1 immunoreactive. Our extensive immunohistochemistry studies showed that this protein is exclusively expressed by brown adipocytes. White adipocytes do not express UCP1 and are therefore unstained.

Most of the in situ techniques mentioned in this book (immunohistochemistry and in situ hybridization) were performed on paraffin-embedded fixed tissue, the method that, in our experience, offers the best cytological detail for localization studies.

Suggested Reading

Cannon B, et al. Exclusive occurrence of thermogenin antigen in brown adipose tissue. FEBS Letters. 150:129–32, 1982.

Himms-Hagen J. Brown adipose tissue thermogenesis: interdisciplinary studies, FASEB J. 4:2890–989, 1990.

Sbarbati A, et al. Rat interscapular brown adipose tissue at different ages: a morphometric study. Int J Obes. 15:581–7, 1991.

Ricquier D, et al. Molecular studies of the uncoupling protein FASEB J. 5:2237–42, 1991.

Osculati F, et al. The correlation between magnetic resonance imaging and ultrastructural patterns of brown adipose tissue. J Submicrosc Cytol Pathol. 23:167–74, 1991.

Klingenberg M, Huand SG. Structure and function of the uncoupling protein from brown adipose tissue. BBA. 1415:271–96, 1999.

Cinti S, et al. Morphologic techniques for the study of brown adipose tissue and white adipose tissue. Methods Mol Biol. 155:21–51, 2001.

Frontini A, et al. Thymus uncoupling protein 1 is exclusive to typical brown adipocytes and is not found in thymocytes. J Histochem Cytochem. 55:183–9, 2007.

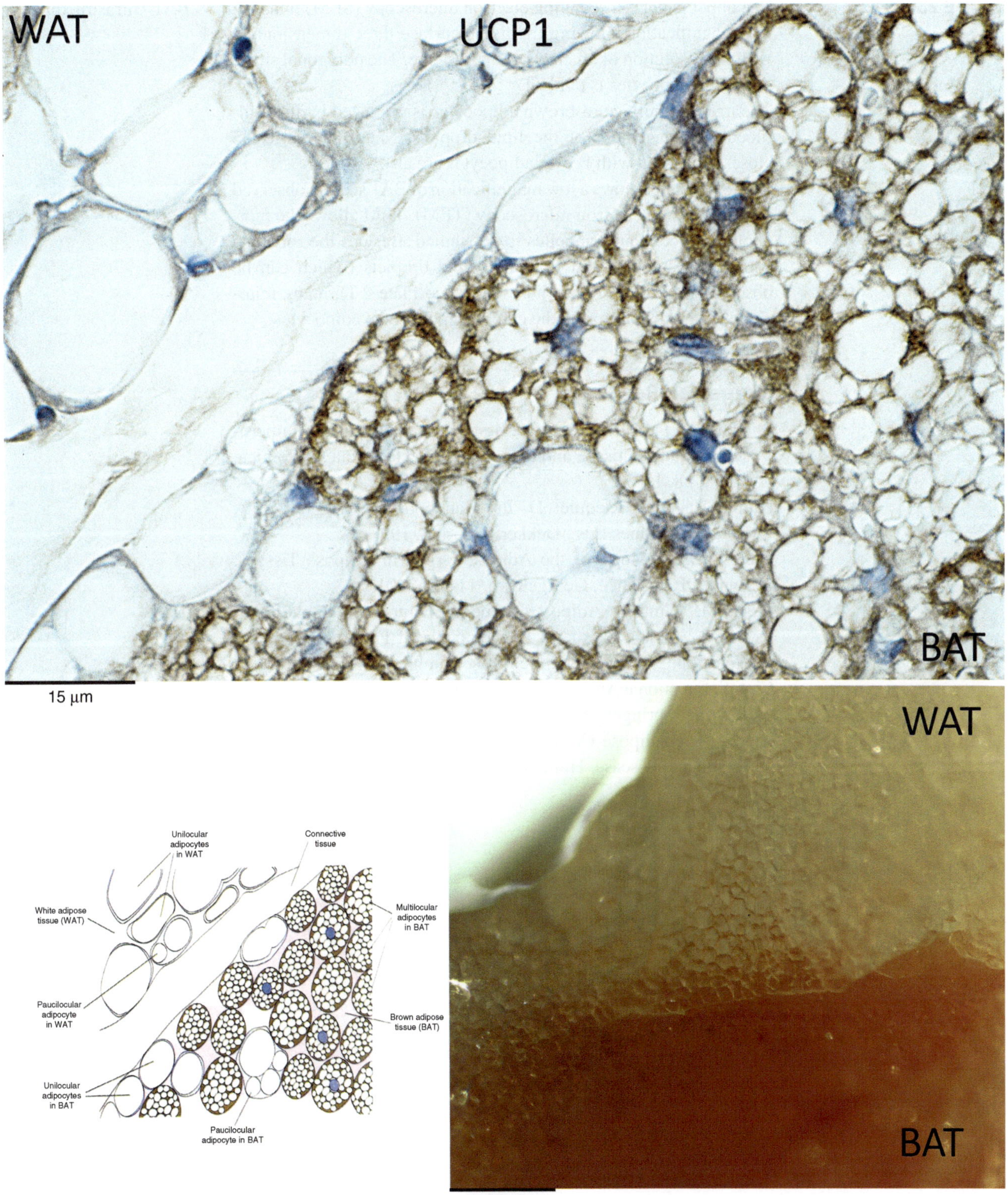

Plate 2.1 Rat anterior subcutaneous fat. Multilocular brown adipocytes expressing UCP1. Unilocular UCP1-negative adipocytes are also visible. LM. IHC: UCP1 ab (1:8,000)

PLATE 2.2

BAT Ultrastructure

The upper panel is a scanning electron microscopy (SEM) image at low magnification showing the tissue surface three-dimensionally with the resolution of an electron microscope. The polygonal shape of brown adipocytes is evident.

The irregular surface of brown adipocytes is produced by the multilocular arrangement of the lipid droplets. Many capillaries in close association with brown adipocytes are also visible.

The lower panel shows a low magnification of BAT section observed by transmission electron microscopy (TEM). TEM allows the morphology of cellular organelles to be studied. Besides the roundish and central nucleus and the small lipid droplets (which can be observed also at the light microscope; see Plate 2.1), many mitochondria are also found in the cytoplasm of brown adipocytes.

Suggested Reading

Sbarbati A, et al. Brown adipose tissue: a scanning electron microscopic study of tissue and cultured adipocytes. Acta Anatomica. 128:84–8, 1987.

Himms-Hagen J, Ricquier D. In "Handbook of Obesity" Bray, Boucherd, James Eds., Dekker, 415–441, 1998.

Cinti S. Morphology of the Adipose Organ in Adipose Tissues, Landes Bioscience, Georgetown, 11–26, 2001.

Stock MJ, Cinti S. Adipose Tissue. Structure and Function of Brown Adipose Tissue in Encyclopedia of Food Sciences and Nutrition, 2nd ed. Academic Press, Cambridge, 29–34, 2003.

Cinti S. Functional Anatomy of the Adipose Organ in Cachexia and Wasting. Springer, New York, 3–22, 2006.

Cinti S. The Adipose Organ in Adipose Tissue and Adipokines in Health and Disease. Humana Press, New York, 3–20, 2007.

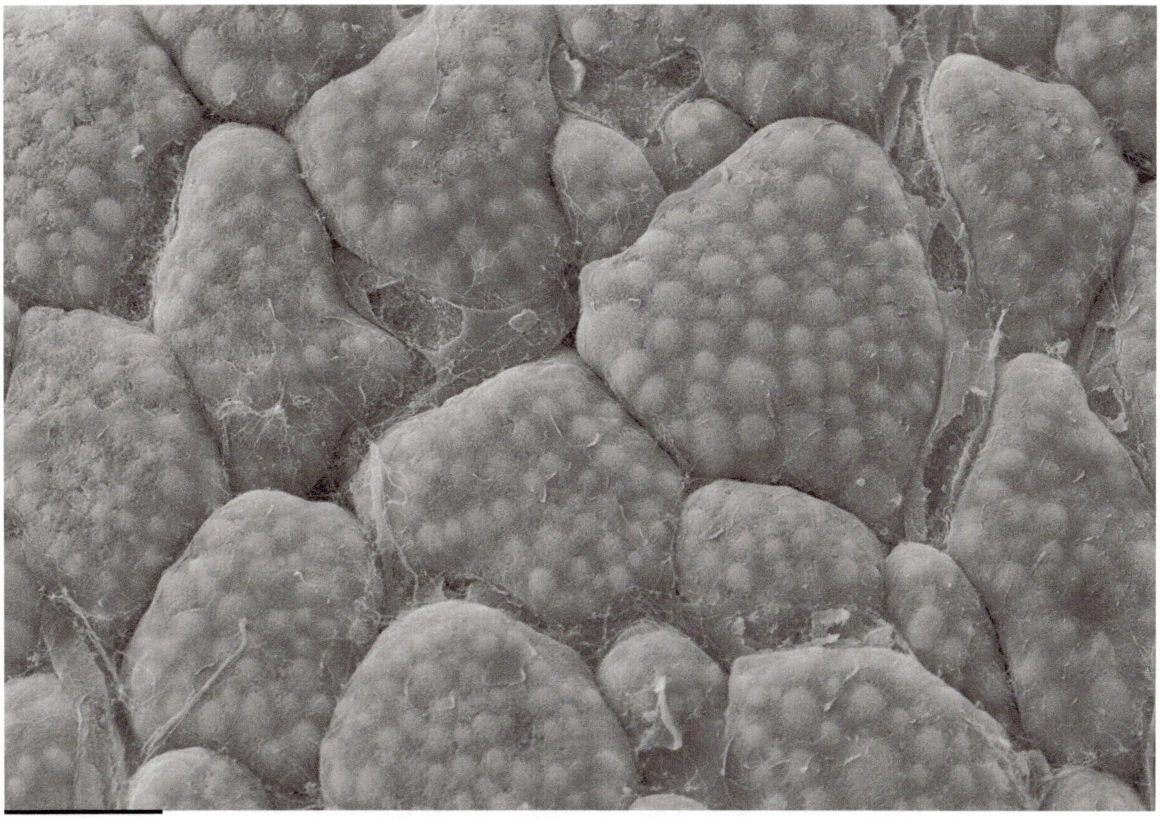

10 µm

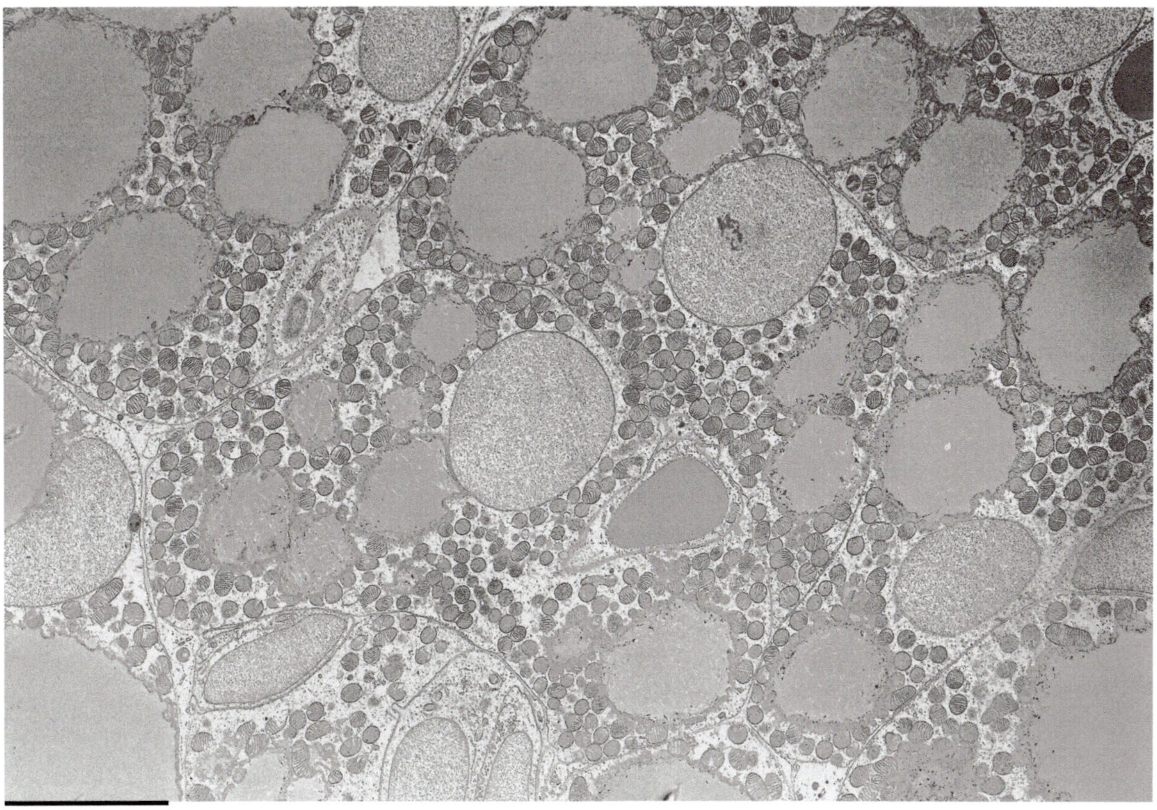

5 µm

Plate 2.2 Ultrastructure of mouse and rat interscapular brown adipose tissue (IBAT). *Upper*: SEM (mouse). *Lower*: TEM (rat)

PLATE 2.3

Brown Mitochondria

The most abundant organelle found in the cytoplasm of brown adipocytes is the mitochondrion. The cytoplasm surrounding the lipid droplets is almost entirely occupied by mitochondria. BAT mitochondria have a distinctive morphology: they are spherical and larger than those of other cell types and show numerous cristae (typical BAT mitochondria). Most cristae are laminar and can extend across the full width of the organelle.

BAT organelles can be observed at SEM using a modified OsO_4 maceration method, which allows cytoplasmic organelles and the internal and external sides of the plasmalemma to be visualized (top and middle panels).

The bottom panels show the morphology of typical BAT mitochondria observed by TEM. Note the morphological changes of these mitochondria after acclimation of the animals at cold or warm conditions (see Plates 7.6–7.10 and 8.3–8.4, respectively, for comparison). These changes reflect their different thermogenic activity. The most activated mitochondria in mice and rats are found in the neonatal period (see Plate 12.6).

aP2-UCP1 transgenic mice display a hyperexpression of this protein in the adipose organ. The ultrastructure of hypertrophic mitochondria in interscapular BAT (IBAT) of these transgenic mice is shown in the bottom right panel. Compare with the normal morphology of BAT mitochondria shown in the bottom left panel (unpublished results in collaboration with Dr. Jan Kopecky Academy of Sciences of the Czech Republic, Prague).

Suggested Reading

Dyer RF. Morphological features of brown adipose cell maturation in vivo and in vitro. Am J Anat. 123:255–82, 1968.

Ricquier D, Kader JC. Mitochondrial protein alteration in active brown fat: a soidum dodecyl sulfate-polyacrylamide gel electrophoretic study. Biochem Biophys Res Commun. 73:577–83, 1976.

Nicholls DG. Brown adipose tissue mitochondria. BBA. 549:1–29, 1979.

Cinti S, et al. Immunoelectron microscopical identification of the uncoupling protein in brown adipose tissue mitochondria. Biol Cell. 3:359–62, 1989.

Nedergaard J, Cannon B. In "Molecular mechanisms in bioenergetics", Ernster Ed., Elsevier, 385–429, 1992.

Riva A, et al. The application of the OsO_4 maceration method to the study of human bioptic material. A procedure avoiding freeze-fracture. Microsc Res Tech. 26:526–27, 1993.

Cannon B, Nedergaard J. Brown adipose tissue: function and physiological significance. J Physiol Rev 84:277–359, 2004.

Kopecky J, et al. Expression of the mitochondrial uncoupling protein gene from the aP2 gene promoter prevents genetic obesity. J Clin Invest. 96:2914–23, 1995.

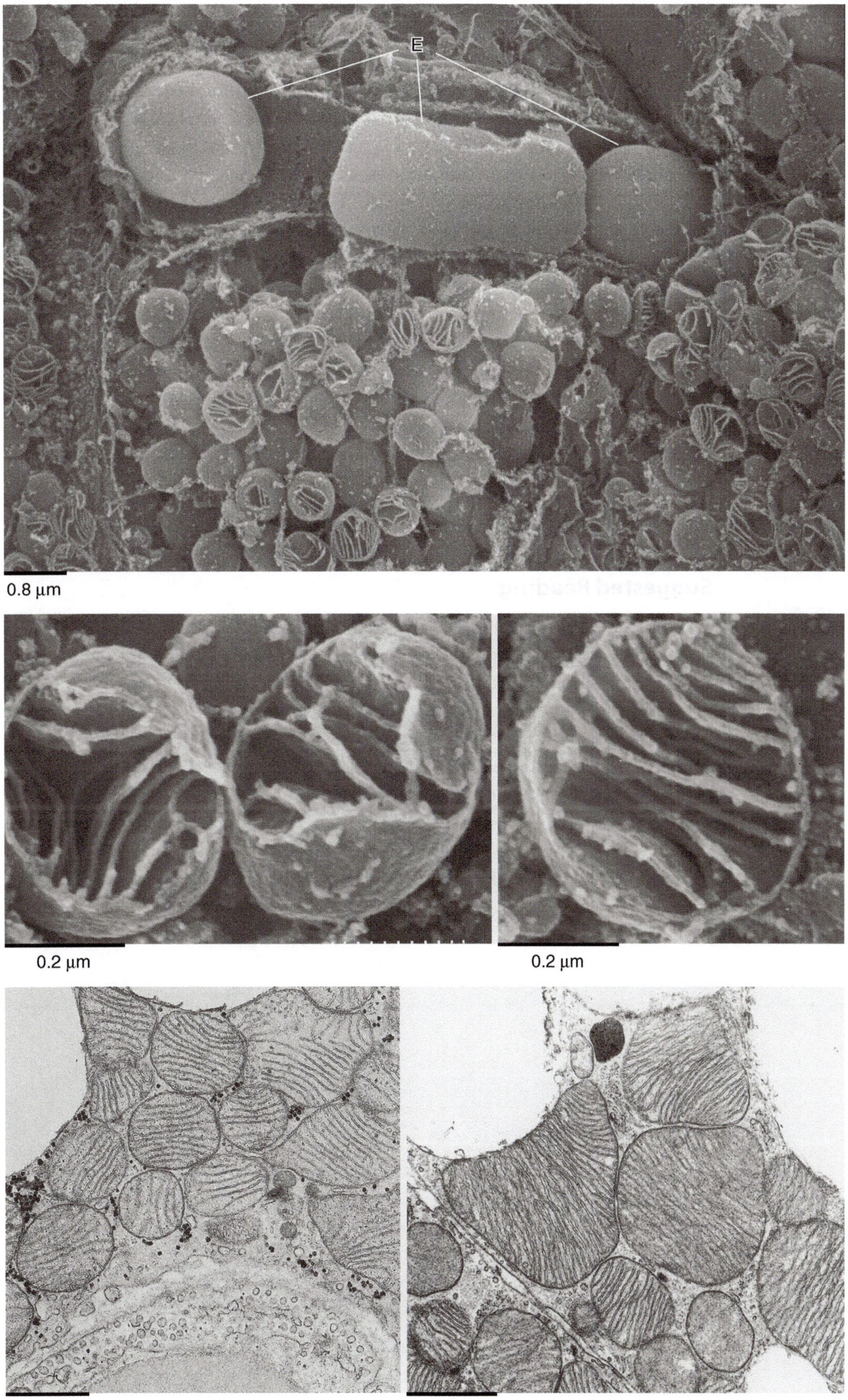

Plate 2.3 Mouse BAT. SEM (*top* and *middle panels*). A capillary containing three erythrocytes (E) is also visible. TEM (*bottom panels*)

PLATE 2.4

UCP1-KO Mitochondria

Mice lacking UCP1 are cold sensitive and suffer from a reduced diet-induced thermogenesis.

The ultrastructure of mitochondria in brown adipocytes of UCP1-KO mice is quite different from that observed in wild-type mice. The general morphology of the UCP1-KO mitochondria is quite variable, as shown in the bottom panel (compare with normal mitochondria in the upper panel; both panels from mice maintained at 24 °C). Most of the mitochondria in the UCP1-KO mice were large with an irregular shape. Only a few of the internal cristae were laminar, but they were irregularly disposed compared with those in wild-type mitochondria. Some of the laminar cristae were arranged to form whirl-like structures. Most of the cristae had a vermicular rambling shape. (These data are unpublished and were obtained in collaboration with Professor Barbara Cannon and Professor Jan Nedergaard (University of Stockholm) and Professor Antonio Giordano (University of Ancona).)

Also the absence of the mitochondrial transcription factor A (TFAM) specifically in adipocytes of the adipose organ results in mitochondria with an altered ultrastructure.

Suggested Reading

Enerback S, et al. Mice lacking mitochondrial uncoupling protein are cold-sensitive but not obese. Nature. 387:90–4, 1997.

Liu X, et al. Paradoxical resistance to diet-induced obesity in UCP1-deficient mice. J Clin Invest. 111:399–407, 2003.

Feldman HM, et al. UCP1 ablation induces obesity and abolishes diet-induced thermogenesis in mice exempt from thermal stress by living at thermoneutrality. Cell Metab. 9:203–9, 2008.

Vernochet C, et al. Adipose-specific deletion of TFAM increases mitochondrial oxidation and protects mice against obesity and insulin resistance. Cell Metab. 16:765–76, 2012.

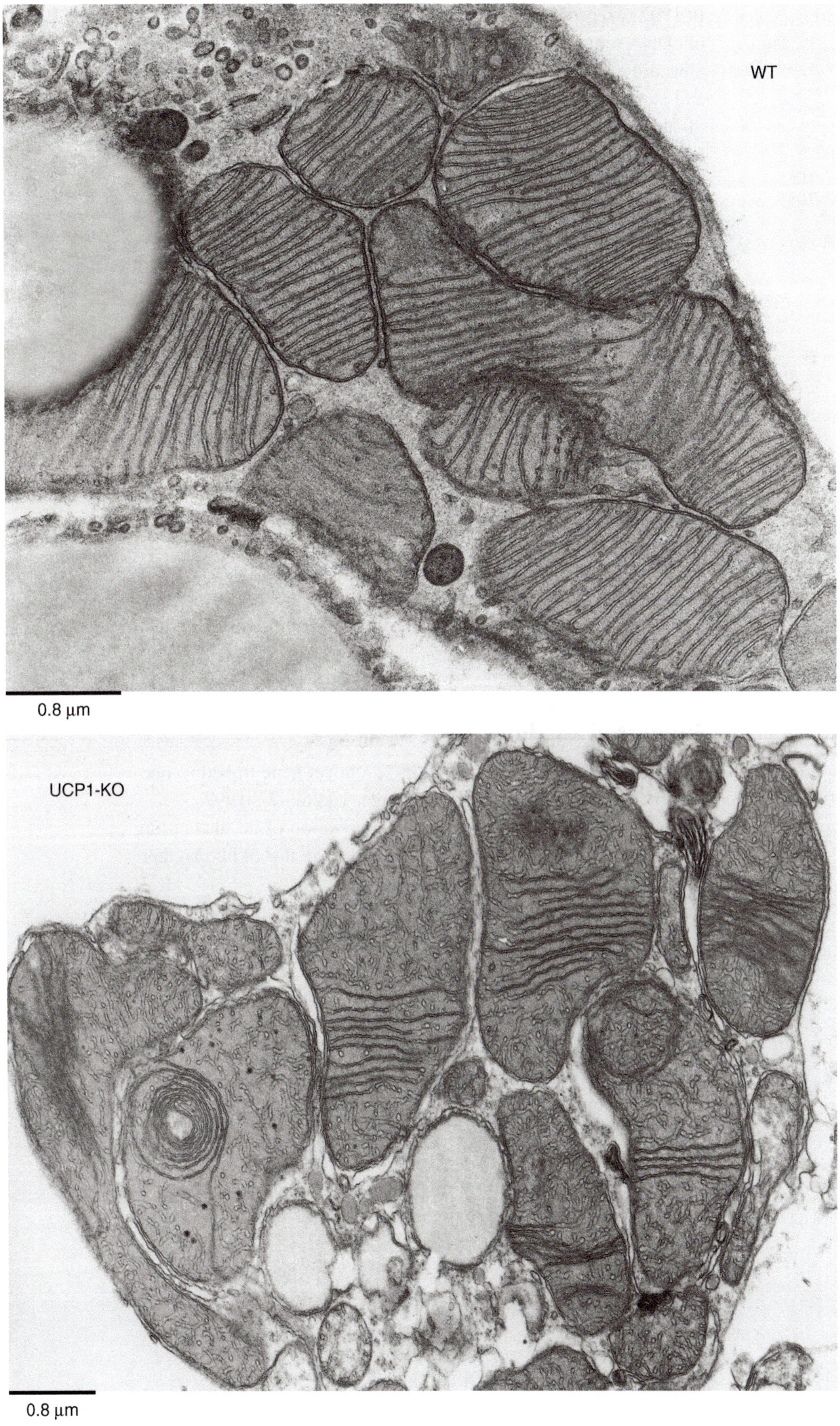

Plate 2.4 Mitochondria of brown adipocytes from interscapular IBAT of adult wild-type (*upper*) and UCP1-KO (*lower*) mice. TEM

PLATE 2.5

UCP3-KO Mitochondria

In 1997 two proteins similar to UCP1 were discovered on the basis of cDNA sequences and denominated UCP2 and UCP3. These proteins are expressed in many organs (UCP2) and mainly in skeletal and cardiac muscles (UCP3) besides brown adipose tissue. Gain-of-function and loss-of-function experiments quickly demonstrated a series of interesting functions for these uncoupling proteins, but none strictly linked to thermogenesis as UCP1.

We explored the morphology of mitochondria of both mice lacking UCP2 or UCP3 (unpublished data in collaboration with Dr. Brad Lowell, Harvard University, Boston). The ultrastructure was not different from that of control mice, but UCP3-KO mitochondria of cold-acclimated mice (upper panel) showed lamellar whorl (LW) structures similar to those found inside the cytoplasm of slimming adipocytes in fasted mice. These lamellar whorls are more evident when a special cytochemical method is used (tannic acid technique; see Plates 10.9–10.13). Lamellar whorls are thought to represent fatty acids mobilized from triacylglycerides and moving toward the blood vessels during functional conditions inducing lipolysis. In cold-exposed UCP3-KO mice, these lamellar whorls inside the mitochondria could be due to fatty acid accumulation due to the lack of UCP3 as a transporter. It has been hypothesized that this protein acts as fatty acid transporter from mitochondria when fatty acid oxidation predominates such as during cold exposure in brown adipose tissue.

Suggested Reading

Fleury C, et al. Uncoupling protein-2: a novel gene linked to obesity and hyperinsulinemia. Nat Genet. 15:269–72, 1997.

Gimeno RE, et al. Cloning and characterization of an uncoupling protein homolog: a potential molecular mediator of human thermogenesis. Diabetes. 46:900–6, 1997.

Boss O, et al Uncoupling protein-3: a new member of the mitochondrial carrier family with tissue-specific expression FEBS Lett. 408:39–42, 1997.

Solanes G, et al The human uncoupling protein-3 gene. Genomic structure, chromosomal localization, and genetic basis for short and long form transcripts. J Biol Chem. 272:25433–36, 1997.

Gong DW, et al. Uncoupling protein-3 is a mediator of thermogenesis regulated by thyroid hormone, beta3-adrenergic agonists, and leptin. J Biol Chem. 272:24129–32, 1997.

Himms-Hagen J, Harper ME. Physiological role of UCP3 may be export of fatty acids from mitochondria when fatty acid oxidation predominates: an hypothesis. Exp Biol Med. 226:78–84, 2001.

Giralt M, Villarroya F. Mitochondrial uncoupling and the regulation of glucose homeostasis. Curr Diabetes Rev. 2016.

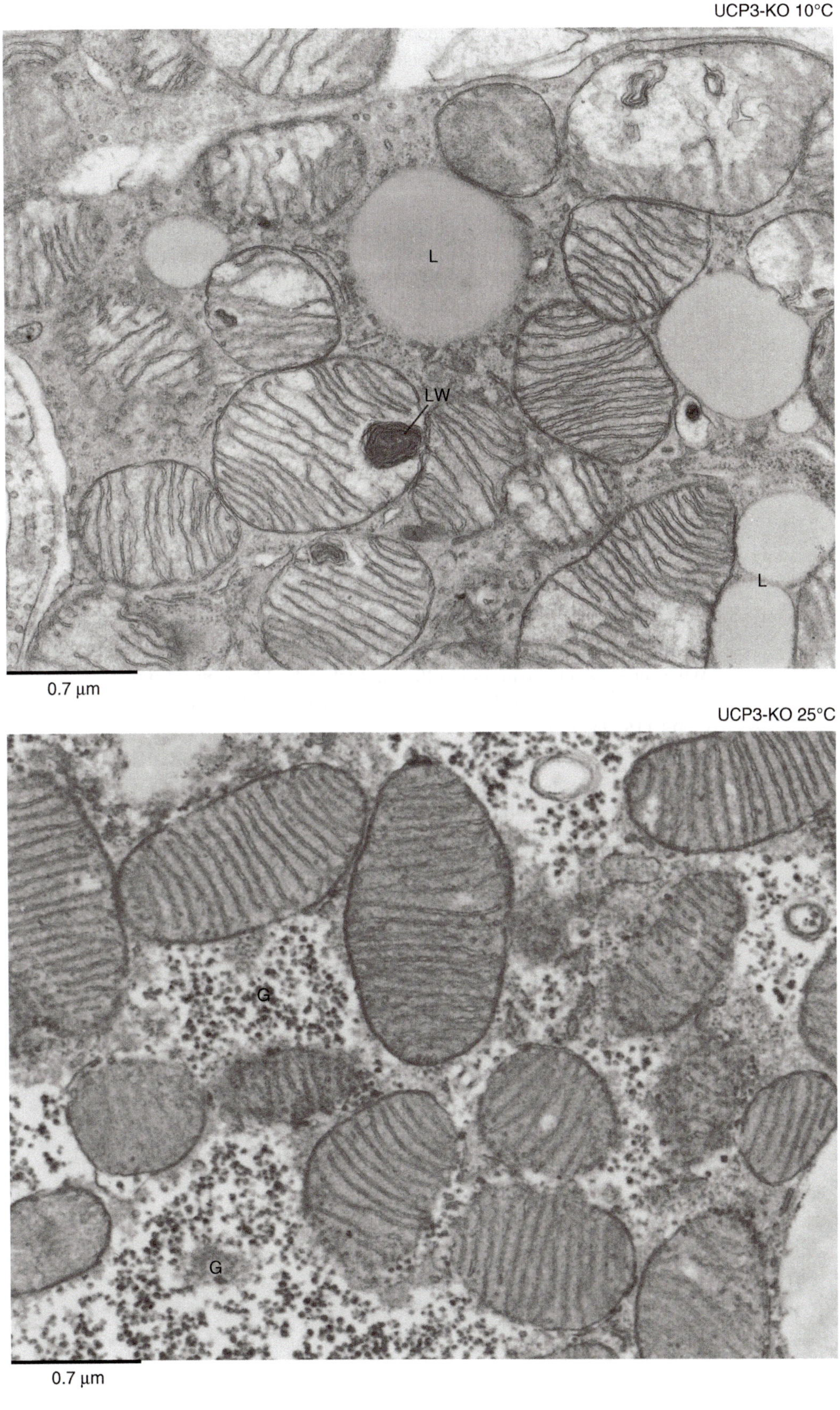

Plate 2.5 Mitochondria of brown adipocytes from IBAT of adult UCP3-KO mice maintained at 10 °C (*upper panel*) or 25 °C (*lower panel*). G: glycogen, L: lipid droplet (some indicated). TEM

PLATE 2.6

Mitochondria in Muscle Cells

Mitochondria of brown adipocytes have a characteristic morphology that allows distinguishing them from any other mitochondria in other tissues. The cells with mitochondria most similar to those in BAT are myocytes in the skeletal muscles and heart. Interestingly these cells share with brown adipocytes the expression of the important "brown characteristic" gene PGC1α. This plate shows the similarities in the morphology between these mitochondria and those in BAT.

The general shape of mitochondria in myocytes is more pleomorphic than that of brown mitochondria, and even when they assume a spherical shape (i.e., more similar to brown mitochondria, such as those presented in this plate), they show a clear different morphology in the shape of cristae. Only rarely, cristae of myocyte mitochondria are really laminar (i.e., traverse the entire width of the organelle, joining the two sides of the mitochondrion). This is the main distinctive feature of mitochondria in brown adipocytes (brown mitochondria), and it is easily visible by comparing mitochondria in the top and bottom panels (mitochondria of myocytes from the skeletal muscle and heart, respectively) with the brown mitochondria presented in the middle panel.

Suggested Reading

Fawcett DW. The Cell, 2nd ed. Sauders WB, Philadelphia, 1981.

Wu Z, et al. Mechanisms controlling mitochondrial biogenesis and respiration through the thermogenic coactivator PGC-1. Cell. 98:115–24, 1999.

Arany Z, et al. Transcriptional coactivator PGC-1α controls the energy state and contractile function of cardiac muscle. Cell Metab. 1:259–71, 2005.

Hao Q, et al. ADD1/SREBP1c activates the PGC1-alpha promoter in brown adipocytes. Biochim Biophys Acta. 1801:421–9, 2010.

Vianna CR, et al. Hypomorphic mutation of PGC-1beta causes mitochondrial dysfunction and liver insulin resistance. Cell Metab. 4:453–64, 2006.

Haemmerle G, et al. ATGL-mediated fat catabolism regulates cardiac mitochondrial function via PPAR-α and PGC-1. Nat Med. 17:1076–85, 2011.

Maraldi N, Tacchetti C. Istologia Medica. Edi Ermes, Milan, 2016.

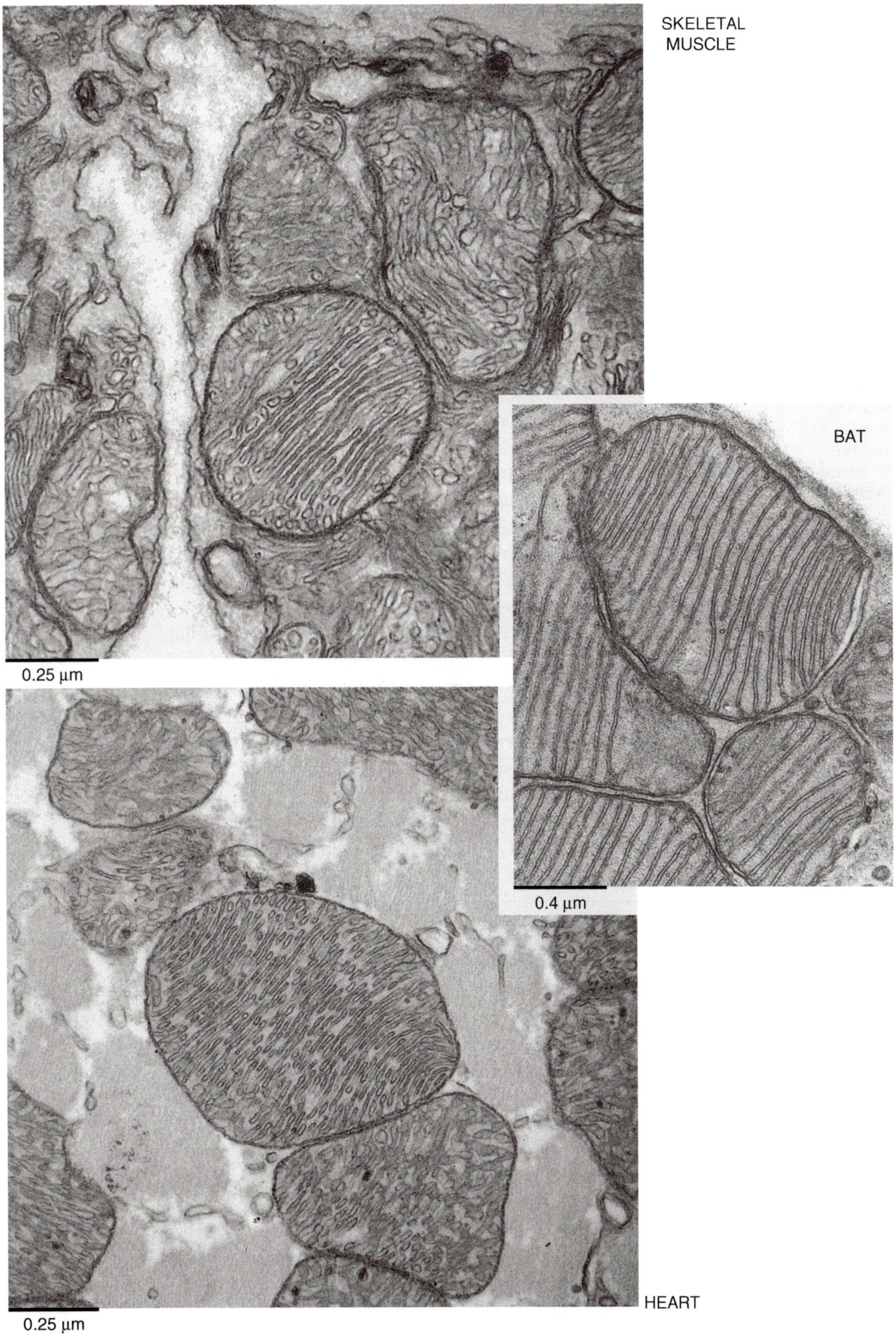

Plate 2.6 Mitochondria from skeletal muscle (quadriceps, *top panel*, in coll with Prof. Enzo Nisoli University of Milan), heart (*bottom panel*, in coll with Prof.ssa Maria Grano University of Bari), and IBAT (*middle panel*) of normal adult mice. TEM

PLATE 2.7

Granules

The endocrine role of BAT is well established and recently supported also by transplantation experiments. Endocrine glands store hormones in specific organelles called secretory granules. The general features of these membrane-coated organelles are (1) equal size, (2) regular shape, and (3) dislocation in several compartments of the cell including the Golgi complex area and periphery of the cytoplasm near the plasma membrane.

The size of endocrine granules is variable and in relationship to the type of hormone stored, but the range of size is quite restricted and usually between 100 and 500 nm.

In this plate membrane-bound structures with the ultrastructural features of endocrine secretory granules are shown in a brown adipocyte (arrows). Note the medium electron density of the granule content that allows to distinguish them from peroxisomes that are quite frequently observed in brown adipocytes (see Plate 7.6). The size of endocrine granules in brown adipocytes is quite constant around 120–150 nm.

The framed area in the upper panel is enlarged in the lower panel.

The content of these endocrine granules in brown adipocytes is not known and needs immunogold staining studies (see Plate 7.9), but considering the well-established endocrine role of brown adipocytes, several secretory products are candidates to be present in these granules (T3, prostaglandins, angiotensinogen, betatrophin, IL-1 and IL-6, insulin-like growth factor 1, vascular endothelial growth factor-A, fibroblast growth factors 2 and 21, retinol-binding protein-4, bone morphogenetic protein 8b, lipocalin prostaglandin D synthase).

Interestingly, a recent paper showed that brown adipocytes are enriched with a secreted enzyme (peptidase M20 domain containing 1, PM20D1) that catalyzes the condensation of fatty acids to generate N-acyl amino acids. N-Acyl amino acids bind to mitochondria inducing their UCP1-independent uncoupling.

Suggested Reading

Stanford KI, et al. Brown adipose tissue regulates glucose homeostasis and insulin sensitivity. J Clin Invest. 123:215–23, 2013.

Liu X, et al. Brown adipose tissue transplantation improves whole-body energy metabolism. Cell Res. 23:851–54, 2013.

Villarroya J, et al. An endocrine role for brown adipose tissue? Am J Physiol End Metab. 305: E567–72, 2013.

Villarroya F, Giralt M. The beneficial effects of brown fat transplantation: further evidence of an endocrine role of brown adipose tissue. Endocrinology.156:2368–70, 2015.

Giralt M, et al. Adipokines and the endocrine role of adipose tissues. Handb Exp Pharmacol. 233:265–82, 2016.

Long JZ, et al. The secreted enzyme PM20D1 regulates lipidated amino acid uncouplers of mitochondria. Cell. pii:S0092-8674(16)30675–4. 2016.

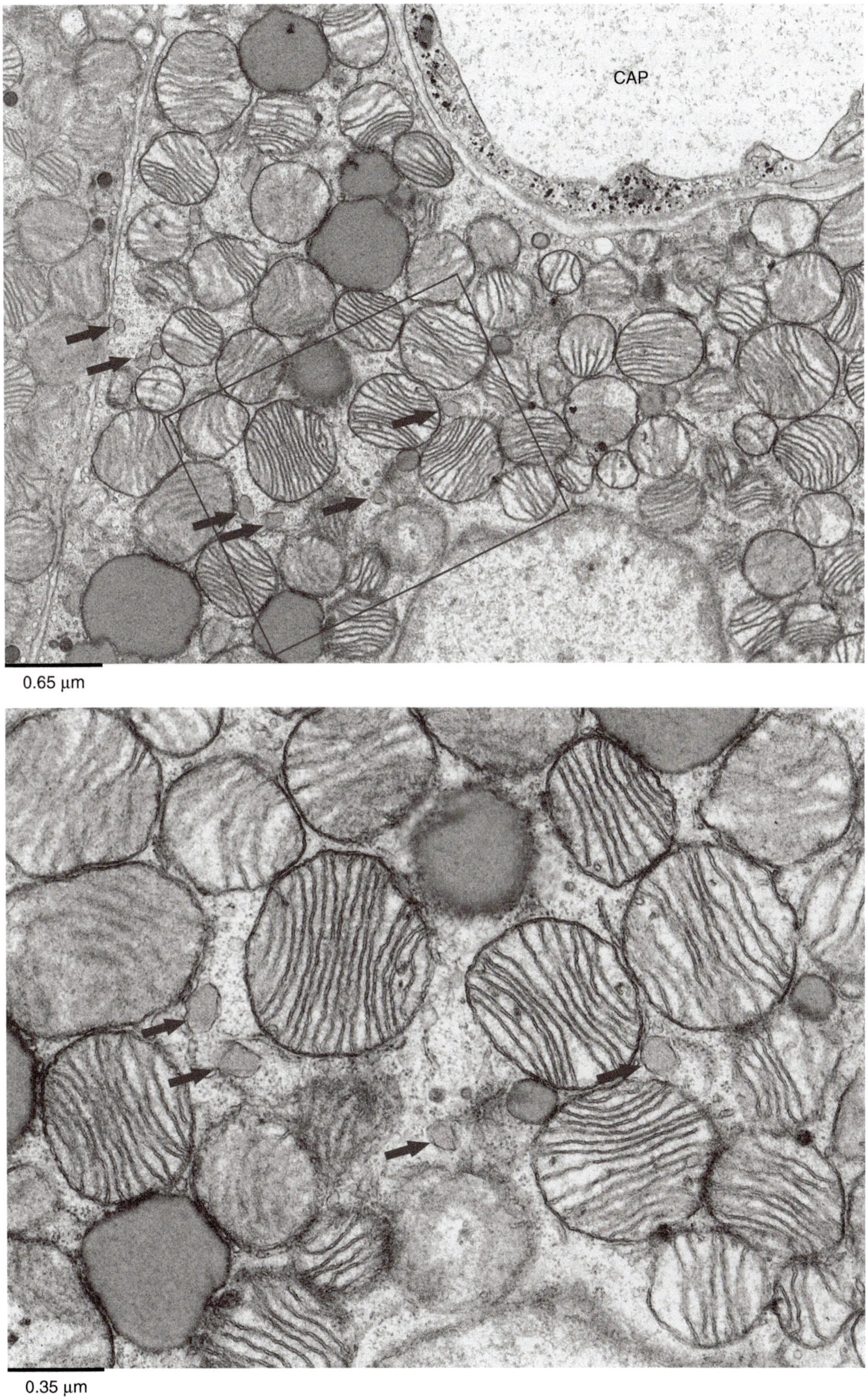

Plate 2.7 IBAT from a newborn rat. Endocrine-like secretory granules in the cytoplasm of a *brown* adipocyte. CAP, capillary. TEM

PLATE 2.8

Golgi Complex

The Golgi complex or apparatus is an organelle present in nearly all eukaryotic cells. Its main function is related to secretory activities of the cells. In most cells the Golgi complex is located near the nucleus. In brown adipocytes we observed it frequently at the periphery of the cell. Near Golgi complex peroxisomes, multivesicular bodies and secretory granules are found.

In this plate two examples of the Golgi complex are shown in two brown adipocytes (arrows). In the upper panel the Golgi complex is surrounded by several peroxisomes (P).

Suggested Reading

Fawcett DW. The Cell, 2nd ed. Sauders WB, Philadelphia, 1981.
Maraldi N, Tacchetti C. Istologia Medica. Edi Ermes, Milan, 2016.

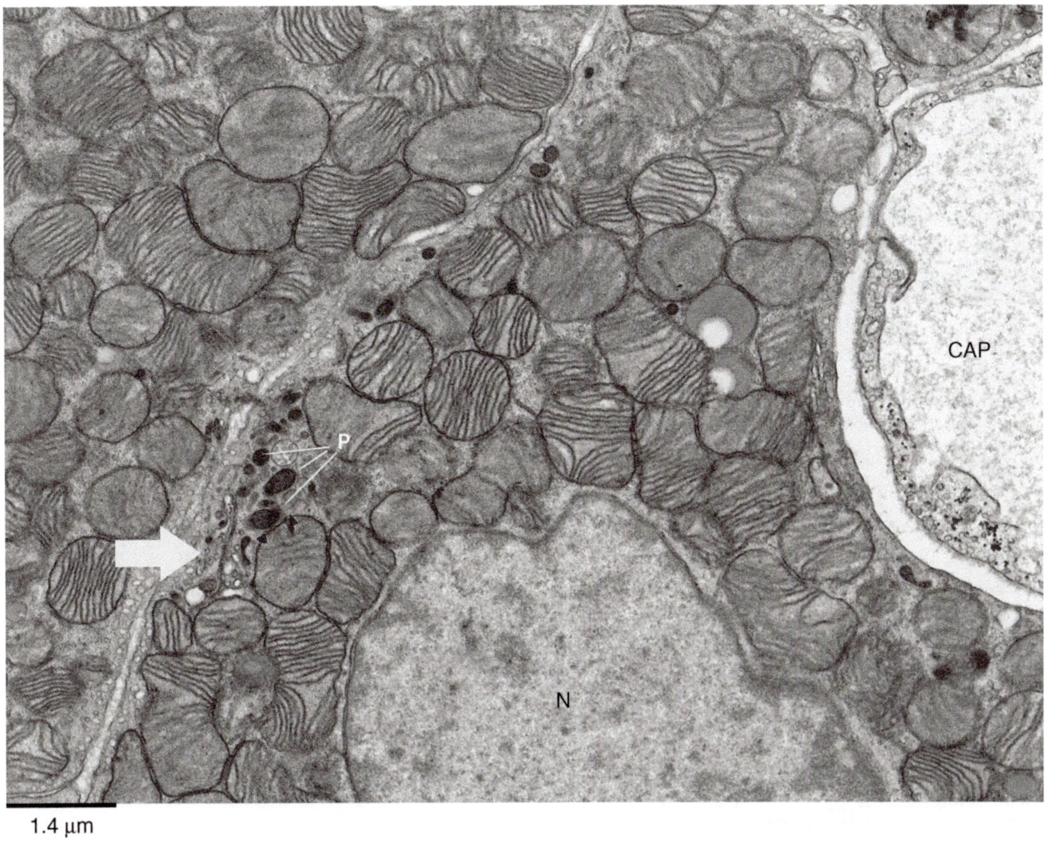

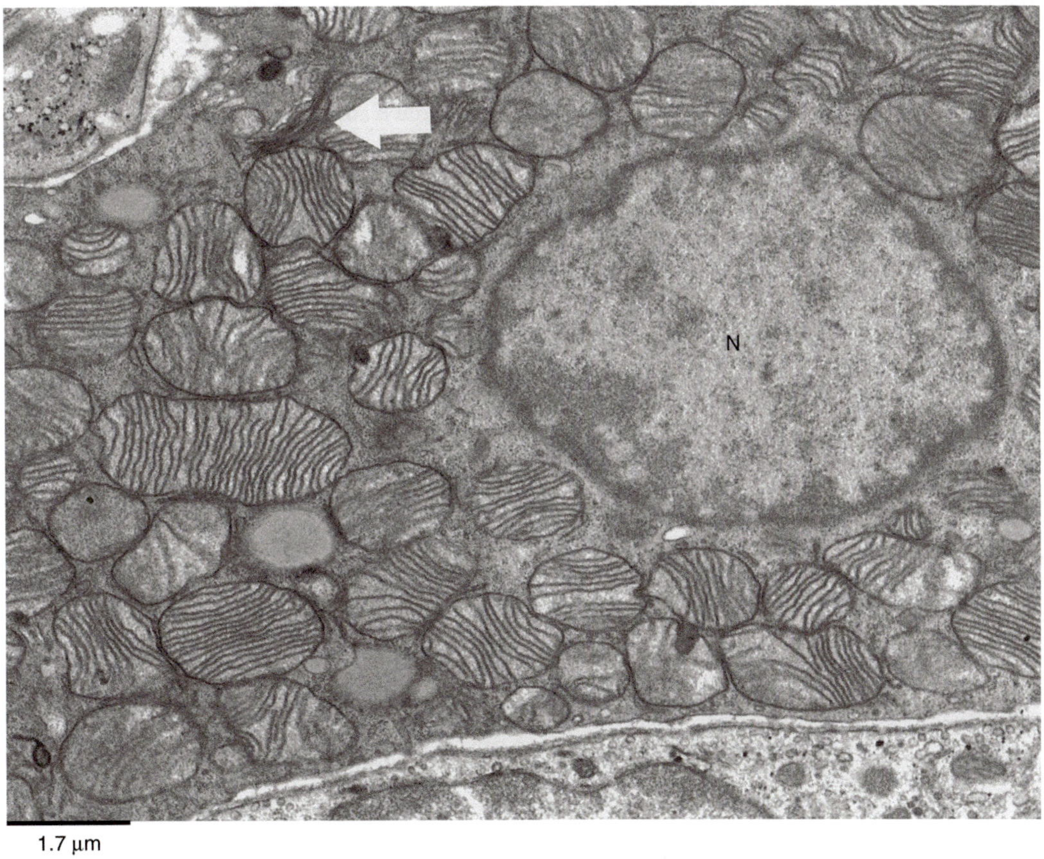

Plate 2.8 IBAT from a newborn rat. Golgi complex of brown adipocytes in the peripheral part of the cell. N, nucleus of adipocyte. Cap, capillary. TEM

PLATE 2.9

Interstitial Cells

Besides brown adipocytes, BAT contains many other cell types. It has been calculated that parenchymal cells of BAT (brown adipocytes) account for about 60–70% of the cellular composition of the tissue, thus vascular, nervous, and interstitial cells form 30–40%.
The most frequent interstitial cells found in BAT are shown in this and the next plates.
Fibroblast-like cells in close association with capillaries are often present.
The main organelle of true fibroblasts is the rough endoplasmic reticulum (RER), which occupies most of the cytoplasm. Note that the cell shown in the upper panel has three distinctive features, which are uncommon in true fibroblasts: glycogen (G), external lamina (EL), and interdigitations with endothelial cells (arrows). Its general ultrastructure is that of a well-differentiated cell, suggesting the possibility of a distinctive cell type (see also the next plate).
The cell shown in the lower panel has the classic fibroblast ultrastructure. Thus, the main ultrastructural differences between endothelial-associated fibroblast-like cells and true fibroblasts reside in the relationship with endothelial cells, the presence of basal membrane, and glycogen that are features present only in this cell type. Further studies are needed to understand the functional role of this cell.

Suggested Reading

Hunt TE, Hunt EA. A radioautographic study of proliferation in brown fat of the rat after exposure to cold. Anat Rec. 157:537–45, 1967.

Gèloèn A, et al. In vivo differentiation of brown adipocytes in adult mice: an electron microscopic study. Am J Anat. 188:366–72, 1990.

Lee MJ, et al. Adipose tissue heterogeneity: implication of depot differences in adipose tissue for obesity complications. Mol Aspects Med. 34:1–11, 2013.

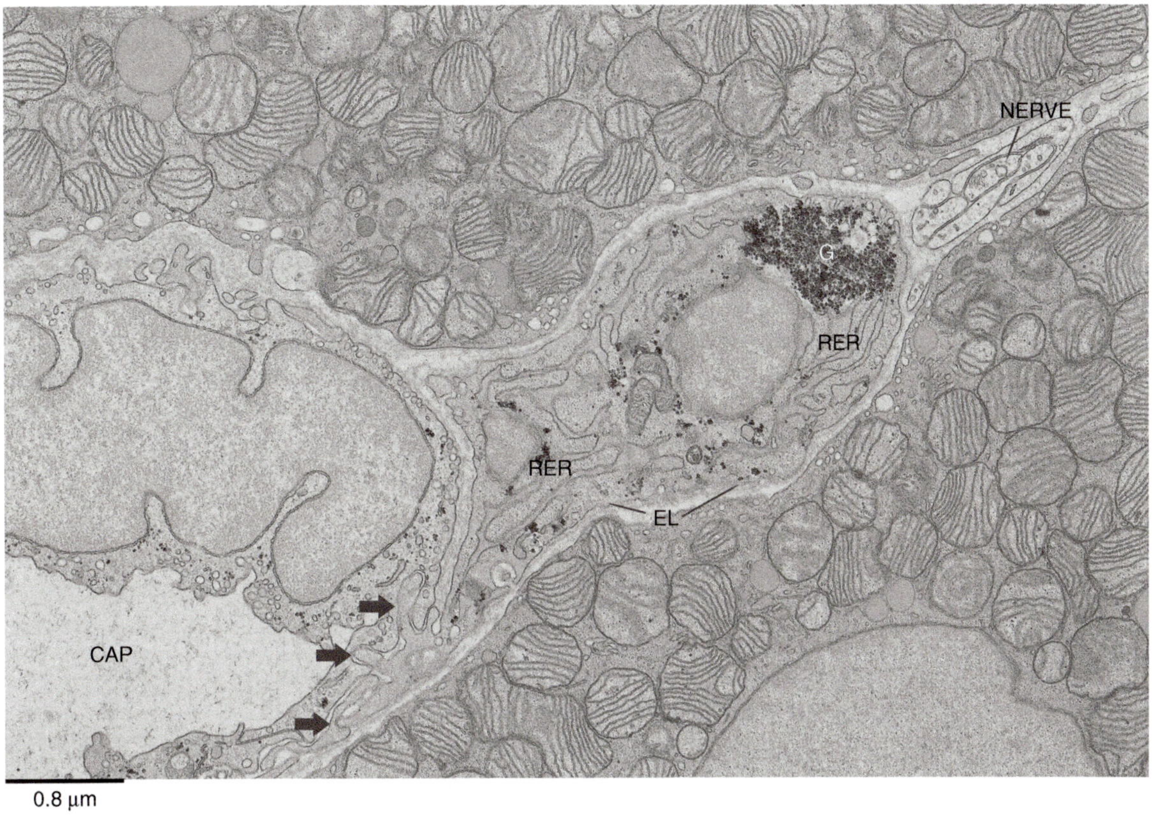

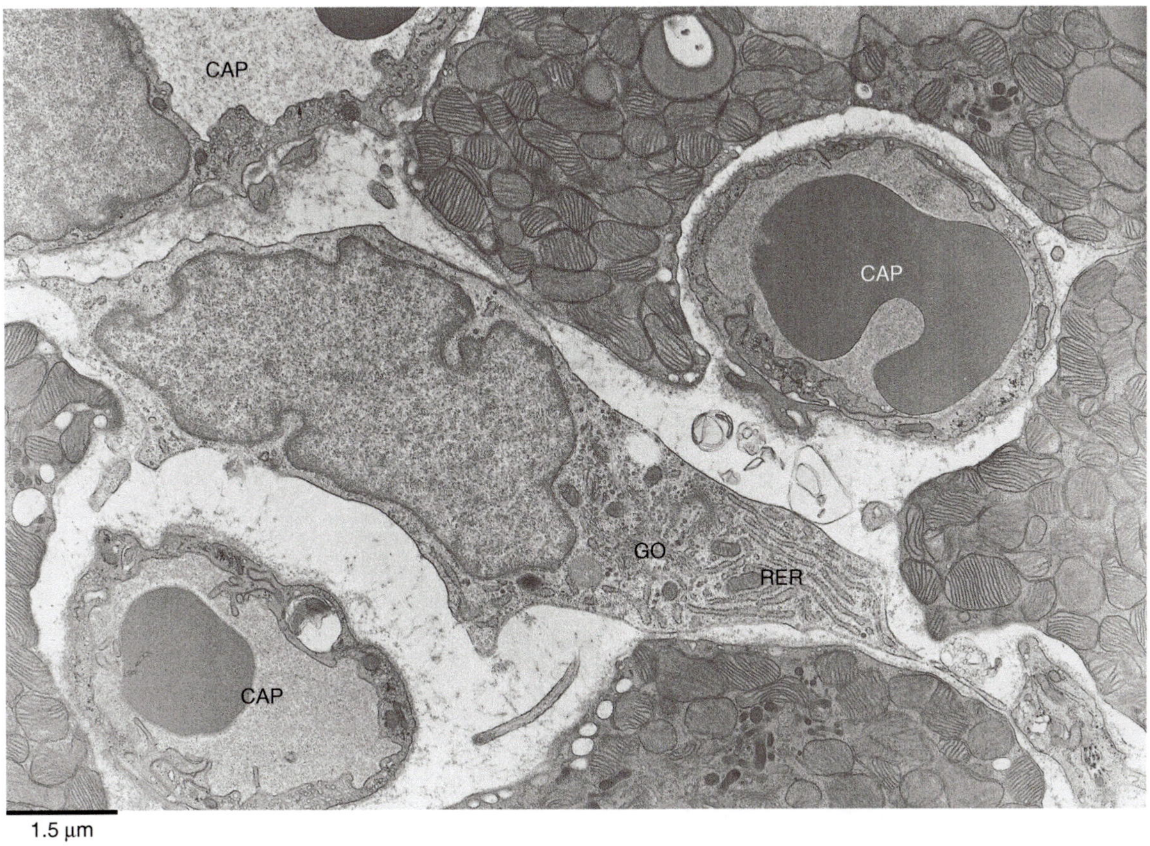

Plate 2.9 IBAT from a newborn rat. Endothelial-associated fibroblast-like cell in the perivascular interstitium (*upper panel*). Fibroblast in the perivascular interstitium (*lower panel*). CAP, capillary lumen. GO, Golgi complex. TEM

PLATE 2.10

Endothelial-Associated Fibroblast-Like Cells

In this plate two further examples of endothelial-associated fibroblast-like cells (EAFL cells) are shown. The general ultrastructure of this cell type indicates a well-differentiated phenotype. The cells associated with the vascular wall (CAP, capillary) are often indicated as possible adipoblasts or preadipocytes. Data on brown adipoblasts and preadipocytes are shown in Plates 2.26–2.28 of this chapter and in Plates 12.2–12.4. Here the direct comparison between an EAFL cell and a brown adipocyte precursor is shown. The ultrastructural differences are quite evident: EAFL cell – irregular nucleus with heterochromatin, abundant rough endoplasmic reticulum, small and few mitochondria, and interdigitations with endothelial cell; preadipocyte – regular roundish nucleus with euchromatin (general characteristic of poorly differentiated cells), abundant "pre-typical" mitochondria (see Plate 2.26 for explanation), and lipid droplets (L). A distinct basal membrane surrounds both cell types.

In the lower panels details of the most important characteristic of EAFL are shown: interdigitations with the endothelial cell. In the lower right panel, the enlargement of the framed area in the lower left panel is shown.

Altogether these morphologic data suggest that EAFL cells belong to a different lineage from that of adipocytes.

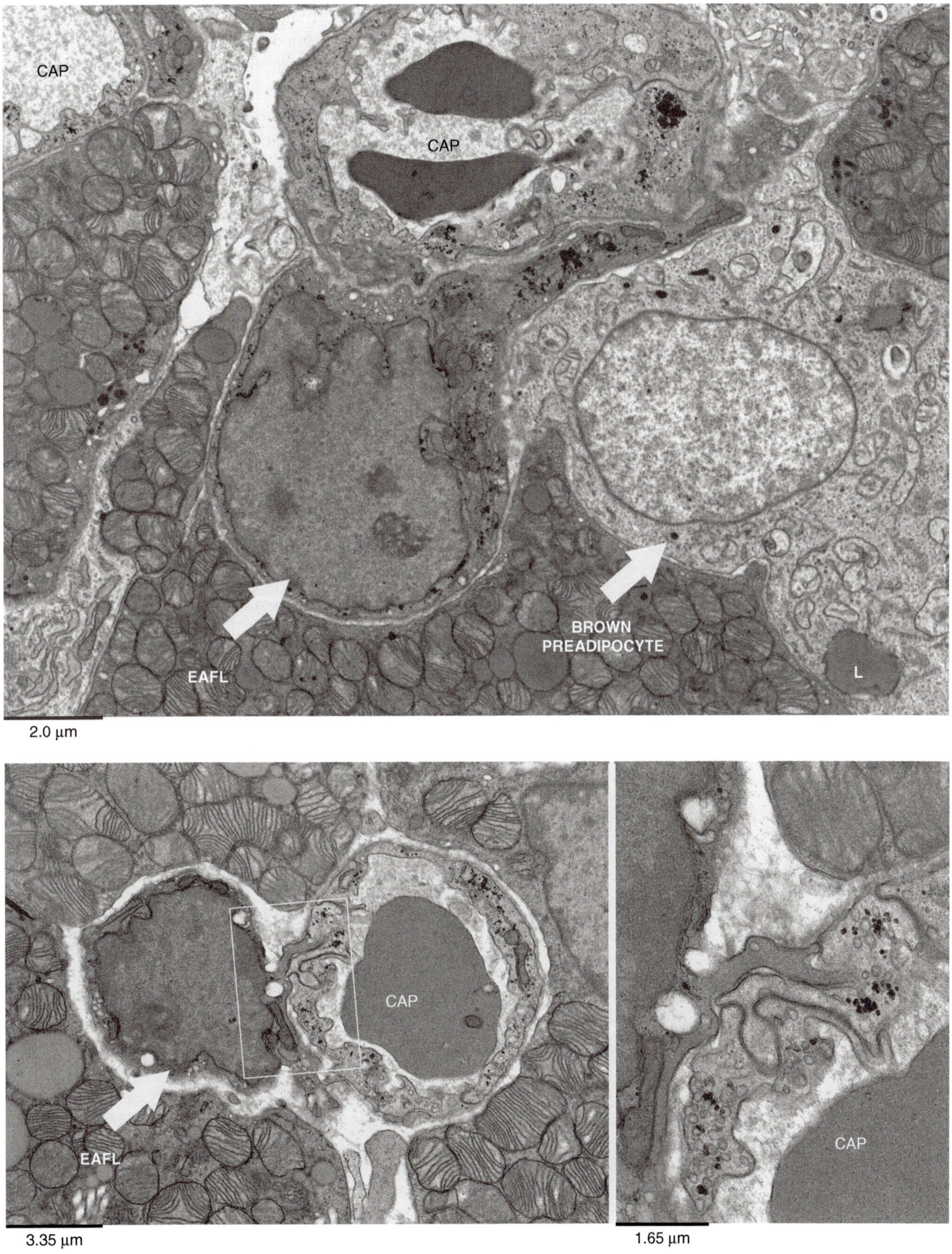

Plate 2.10 IBAT from a newborn rat. Endothelial-associated fibroblast-like (EAFL) cell and a brown preadipocyte (*upper panel*) are shown. Details of contact between EAFL and endothelial cell (*lower panels*). TEM

PLATE 2.11

Schwann Cells

In the peripheral nervous system, Schwann cells surround neural axons by their sheetlike cytoplasmic processes. Schwann cells are shown in this plate among BAT brown adipocytes. Their ultrastructure in this tissue is similar to that observed in other tissues, with an often indented nucleus and a cytoplasm with a well-developed Golgi complex, rough endoplasmic reticulum, and small mitochondria. A distinct basal membrane always surrounds Schwann cells. The axons are usually unmyelinated that is typical for axons of the sympathetic system, but sensory fibers are also present in brown adipose tissue (see also Plate 2.22).

Suggested Reading

Umahara Y. Light and electron microscopic studies on the brown adipose tissue in the bat. Arch Histol Jpn. 29:459–509, 1968.

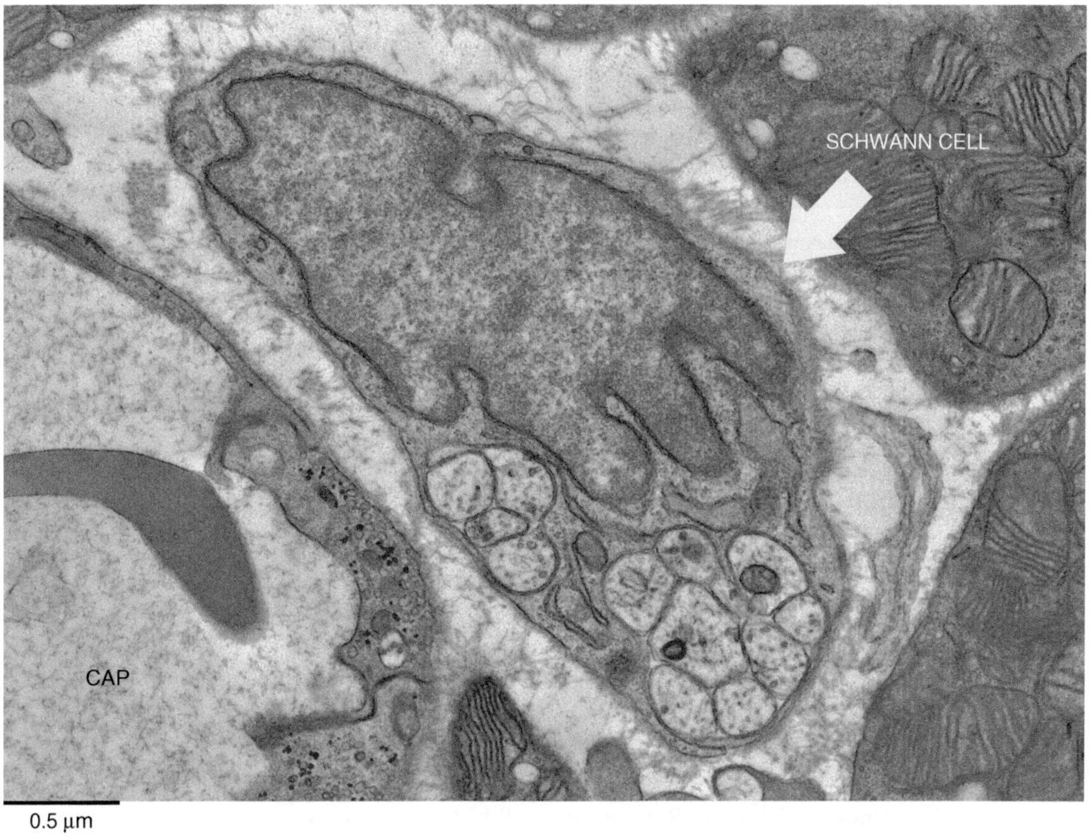

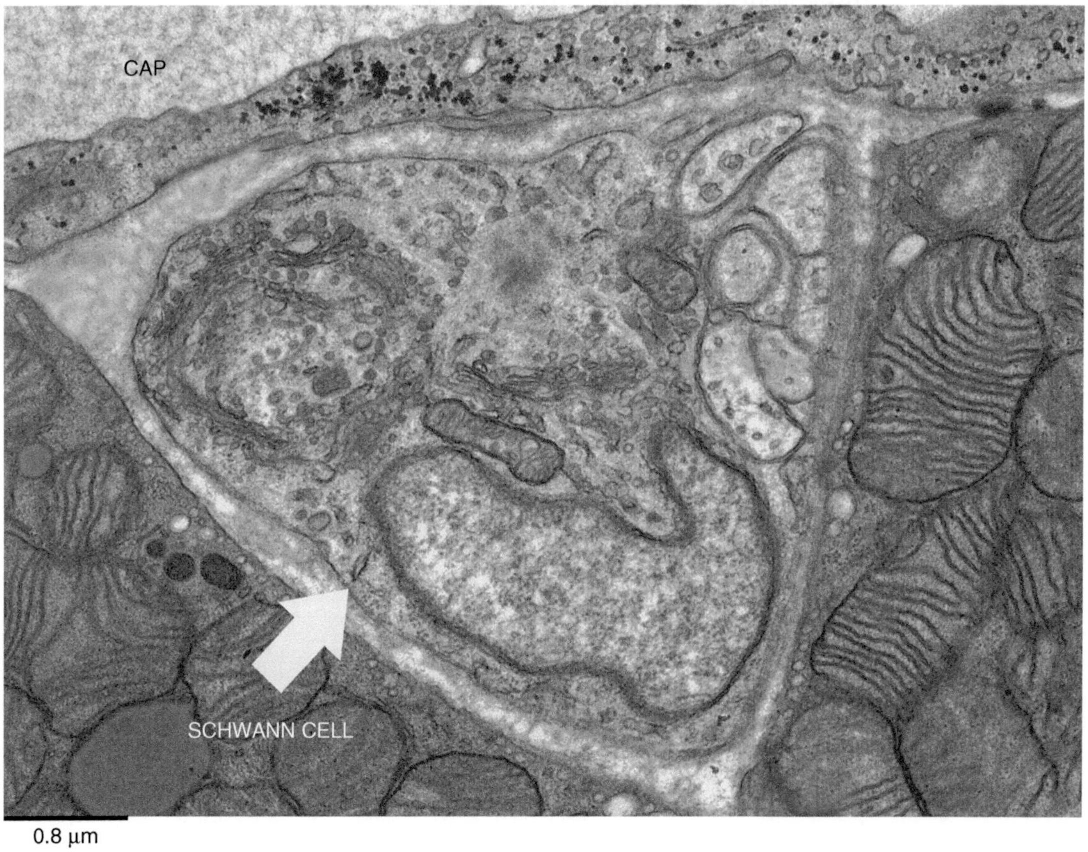

Plate 2.11 IBAT from a newborn rat. Schwann cells with unmyelinated axons in the pericapillary parenchyma. CAP, capillary. TEM

PLATE 2.12

Histiocytes and Mast Cells

Histiocytes and mast cells are regularly present in normal BAT of rats or mice maintained at room temperature. These cells have distinctive ultrastructural features that allow an easy identification by electron microscope.

Histiocytes (upper panel) have an indented heterochromatic nucleus and abundant but variable amount of cytoplasm rich in characteristic organelles. The most characteristic organelles visible in the cytoplasm of histiocytes are the well-developed Golgi complex and several primary and secondary lysosomes. Primary lysosomes are electron dense and extremely variable in size and shape (Ly, some indicated). An important feature of histiocytes is the extremely irregular cell boundary due to several cytoplasmic projections forming villi-like structures (small arrows). Many secondary lysosomes are visible in Plates 9.8–9.11 in histiocytes of white adipose tissue.

The contact with an adipoblast shown here could be in relationship with the recent observations that inflammatory cells could play a role in brown cell development (see also Plate 2.26).

Mast cells are usually located at the periphery of BAT lobules. Characteristic features of mast cells are the typical large electron-dense granules filling the cytoplasm (bottom panel).

Suggested Reading

Desautels M, et al. Role of mast cell histamine in brown adipose tissue thermogenic response to VMH stimulation. Am J Physiol. 266:R831–7, 1994.

Afzelius BA. In “Brown adipose tissue”, Lindberg Ed., Elsevier, 1–32, 1970.

Mory G, et al. Localization of serotonin and dopamine in the brown adipose tissue of the rat and their variations during cold exposure. Biol Cell. 48:159–66, 1983.

Rao RR, et al. Meteorin-like is a hormone that regulates immune-adipose interactions to increase beige fat thermogenesis. Cell. 6:1279–91, 2014.

Spencer M, et al. Pioglitazone treatment reduces adipose tissue inflammation through reduction of mast cell and macrophage number and by improving vascularity. PLoS One. 9(7):e102190, 2014.

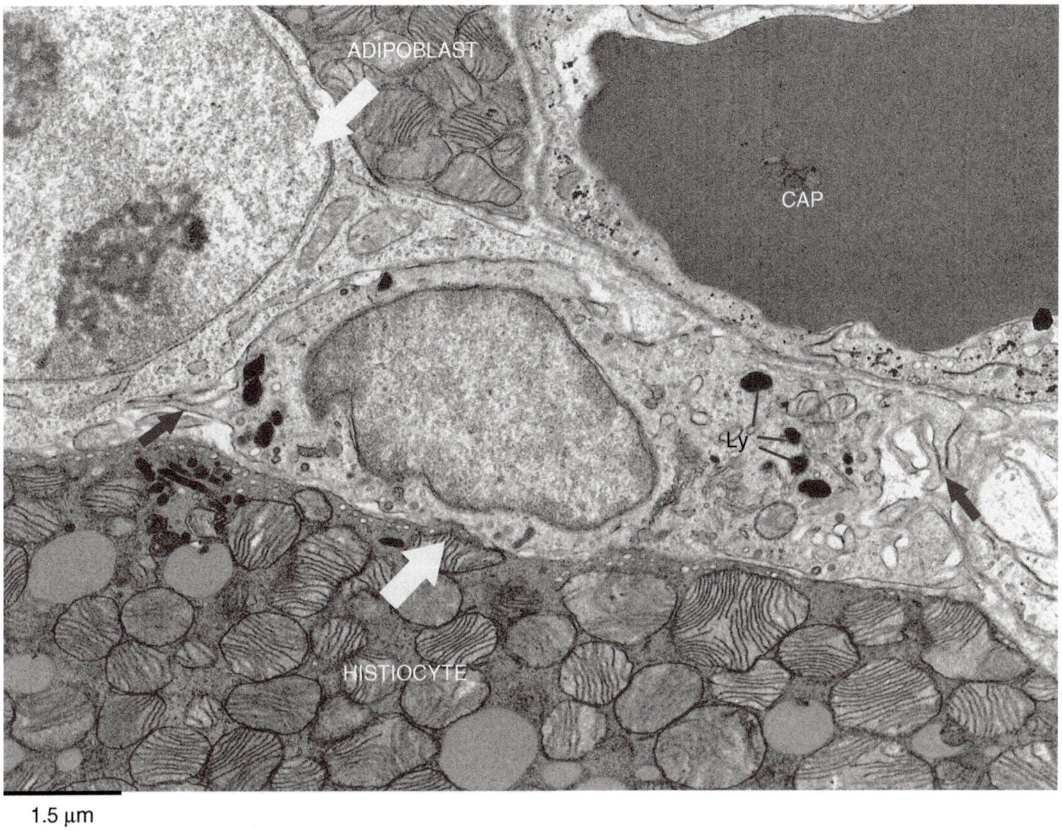

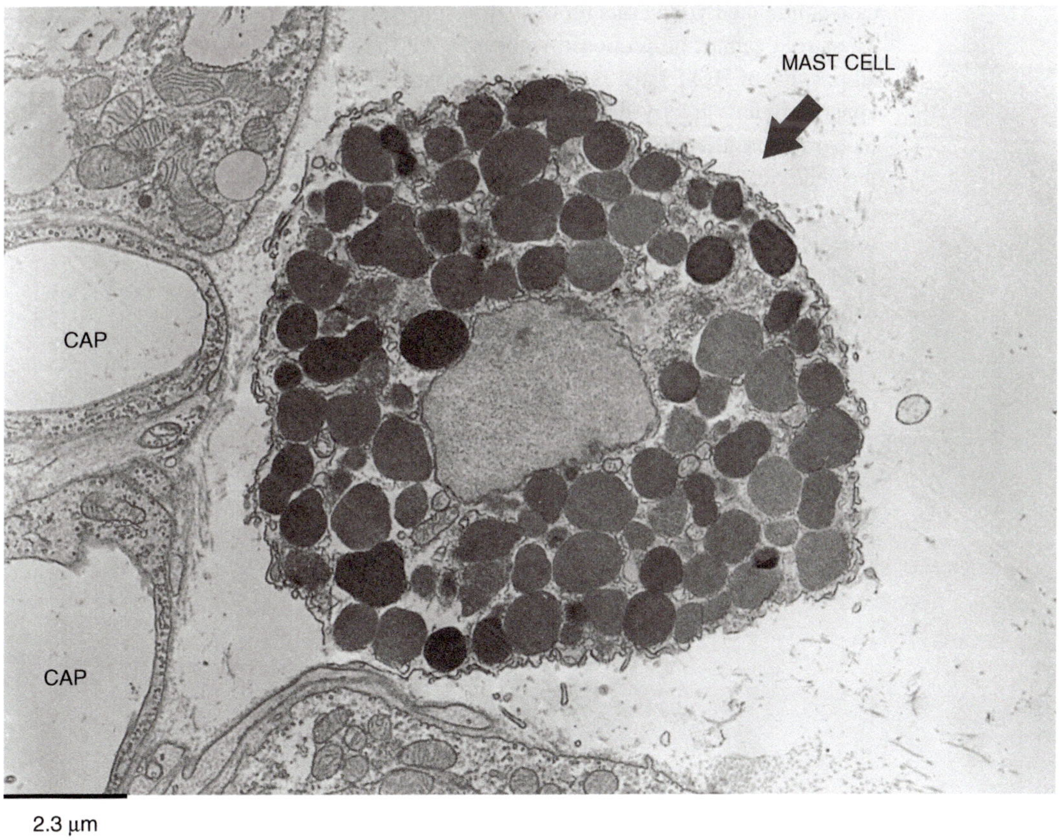

Plate 2.12 IBAT from a newborn rat. A histiocyte in close apposition to a preadipocyte (*upper panel*). A mast cell at the periphery of an IBAT lobule (*lower panel*). CAP, capillary. TEM

PLATE 2.13

Brown Adipocyte-Like Cell I

The electron microscope morphology of a classic brown adipocyte is quite characteristic and thoroughly shown in Plates 2.2–2.4, but cells similar to brown adipocytes with distinctive features can be detected in interscapular BAT of rats. Examples of these brown-like cells are shown in this and in the next plate. The main characteristic feature of this cell type is the nontypical morphology of their mitochondria. Interestingly, all other features of brown adipocytes, including multilocular lipids, central roundish nucleus, and abundance of mitochondria, are present.

This cell type is quite rare and probably UCP1 negative. This last sentence is supported by the experience of combining several experiments in which both TEM and immunohistochemistry were used to study IBAT under different experimental conditions (including KO and TG mice). In all cases in which mitochondrial morphology was nontypical at TEM than UCP1, immunohistochemistry resulted negative and vice versa. On the other hand, when brown adipocytes are less adrenergically stimulated (see Chaps. 8, 9, and 10, respectively; warm, obese, and fasting adipose organ), the ultrastructural morphology of mitochondria tends to become less typical toward completely atypical and similar to that found in white adipocytes and similar to that observed in these brown-like adipocytes presented here (compare with Plate 10.3).

Their exact frequency in BAT in relationship with a specific experimental condition is not known and should be studied in future experiments, but we observed these cells in newborn and adrenergically stimulated young rats (cold acclimated, next plate).

Their role cannot be proposed right now, but interestingly brown adipocytes of IBAT have been proved to have alterative functions apparently not directly linked with thermogenesis. As a matter of fact, trained adult rats with intense physical exercise do not increase the gene expression of UCP1 but clearly increase the expression of the proton-linked monocarboxylate transporter MCT-1 known to selectively transport lactate across the plasma membrane. Interestingly it has been recently shown that lactate induces FGF21 expression in adipocytes, and FGF21 regulates browning of white adipose tissue (see Plates 7.12–7.13).

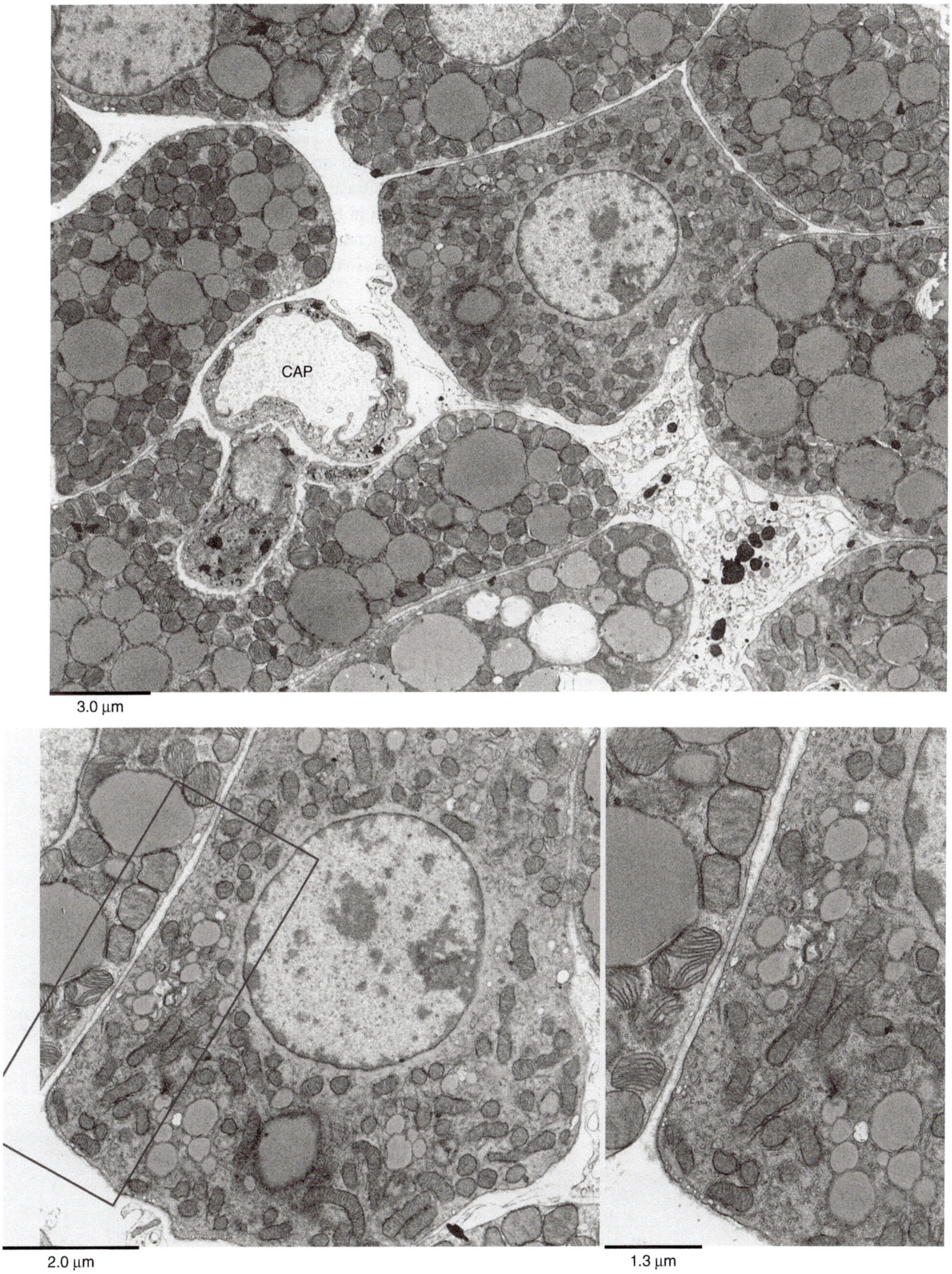

Plate 2.13 IBAT from a newborn rat. Brown adipocyte-like cell surrounded by classic brown adipocytes (*upper panel*). Enlargement of the brown adipocyte-like cell (*lower left panel*). Classic brown mitochondria (*left*) and nontypical mitochondria (*right*). Enlargement of the framed area in the *lower left panel* (*lower right panel*). CAP, capillary. TEM

PLATE 2.14

Brown Adipocyte-Like Cell II

In the previous plate, the brown-like adipocyte is shown for the first time. Here we show a second example of this rare cell mainly to demonstrate that this cell type is found also in cold-acclimated young rats and can bear substantially different amounts of lipid droplets. In the cell presented in Plate 2.13, lipid droplets are very small, and the cell is surrounded by the classic brown adipocytes.

In this plate the brown-like cell has larger lipid droplets and is located at the periphery of the fat lobule. The ultrastructure of mitochondria is identical to that in the cells shown in Plate 2.13, and a direct comparison with classic brown mitochondria is allowed in the lower panel (enlargement of the framed area in the upper panel).

Suggested Reading

De Matteis R, et al. Exercise as a new physiological stimulus for brown adipose tissue activity. Nutr Metab Cardiovasc Dis. 23:582–90, 2012.

Fisher FM, et al. FGF21 regulates PGC-1α and browning of white adipose tissues in adaptive thermogenesis. Genes Dev. 26:271–81, 2012.

Jeanson Y, et al. Lactate induces FGF21 expression in adipocytes through a p38-MAPK pathway. Biochem J. 473:685–92, 2016.

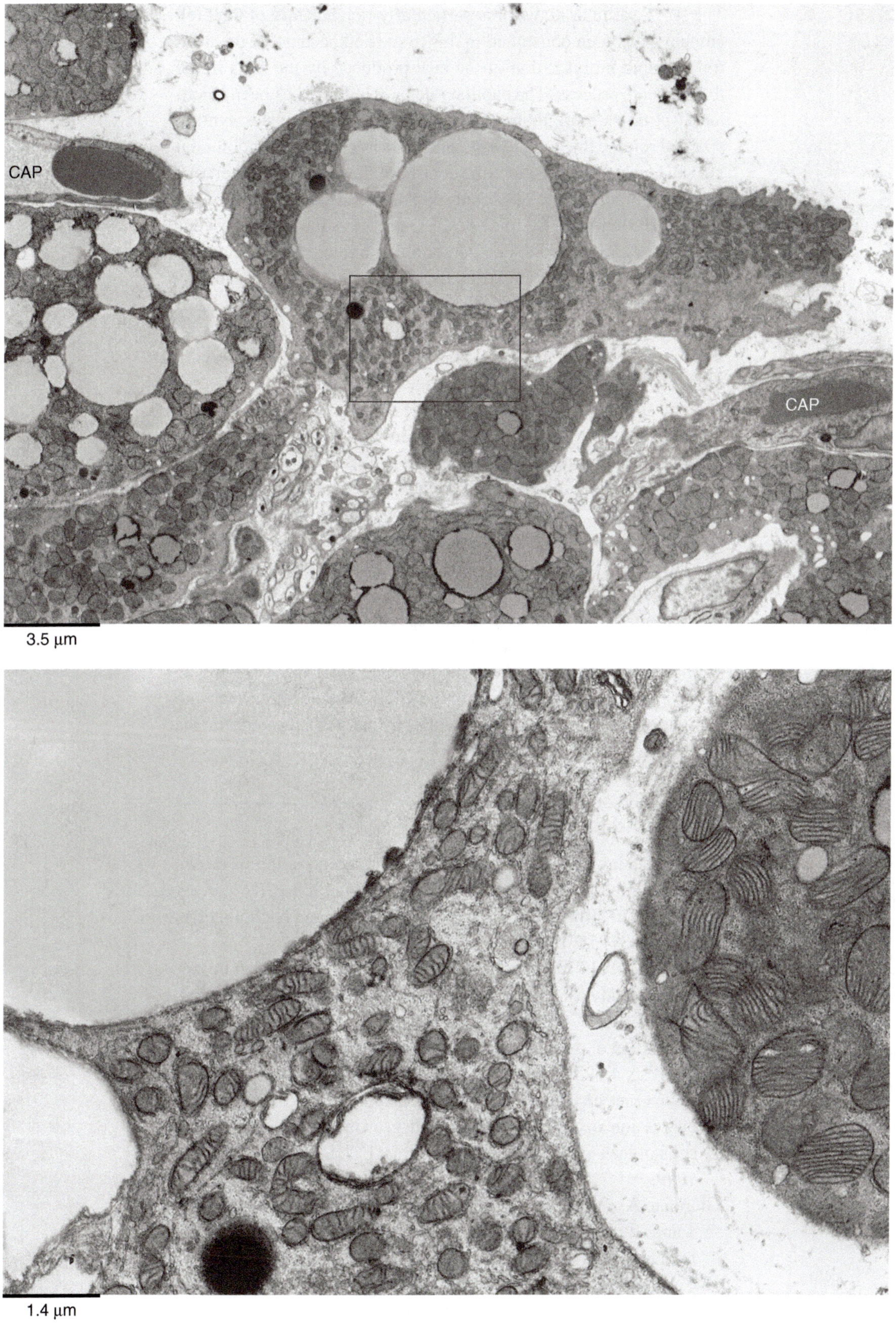

Plate 2.14 IBAT of young rat (4 weeks old) cold acclimated at 4 °C for 2 weeks. Brown adipocyte-like cell with abundant cytoplasmic lipids. CAP, capillary. TEM

PLATE 2.15

Blood Supply

The IBAT vascular network is particularly rich because of the high amount of oxygen consumed in this tissue and because of the need for the rapid mobilization of the heat produced by the cells in the thermogenic process. The capillary density in IBAT has been calculated six times more than that in WAT. Brown adipocytes synthesize and release the potent vasculogenic factor: vascular endothelial growth factor (VEGF) under the control of the sympathetic nervous system. Noradrenaline also controls the production of heme oxygenase (HO) by brown adipocytes. HO produces the potent gaseous vasodilator carbon monoxide. Carbon monoxide, like nitric oxide, is able to promote mitochondrial biogenesis in different organs.

The capillary network of an IBAT lobule (rat) is shown in a SEM low magnification (upper panel). It is a vascular cast obtained by injecting a resin into the aortic arch and by subsequently dissolving the tissue by sodium hypochlorite digestion.

An area similar to that indicated by the arrow in the upper left corner of the upper panel is enlarged in the bottom right panel. Hypochlorite digestion does not dissolve all cells, and the relationships between capillaries and residual adipocytes can sometimes still be observed. Note the absence of a clear multilocular organization of this adipocyte (compare with those shown in the upper panel of Plate 2.2). This is probably due to the fact that some adipocytes are unilocular at the peripheral part of BAT lobules (see Chap. 6), and the preserved adipocyte in this specimen probably belongs to that category (compare with Plate 6.3).

In the lower left panel, the light microscopy of an IBAT lobule (mouse) injected by Indian ink is shown. Ink-labeled arterioles and capillaries forming a dense network in line with the data in the upper panel of this plate are evident.

Suggested Reading

Rauch JC, Hayward JS. Topography and vascularization of brown fat in a hibernator. Can J Zool. 47:1315–23, 1969.

Foster DO. In "Brown adipose tissue", Trayhurn and Nicholls Eds., Arnold, 31–51, 1986.

Sbarbati A, et al. Brown adipose tissue: a scanning electron microscopic study of tissue and cultured adipocytes. Acta Anat. 128:84–8, 1987.

Hodde KC, et al. Advances in corrosion casting methods. Scanning Microsc. 4:693–704, 1990.

Tonello C, et al. Role of sympathetic activity in controlling the expression of vascular endothelial growth factor in brown fat cells of lean and genetically obese rats. FEBS Lett. 442:167–72, 1999.

Giordano A, et al. Expression and distribution of heme oxygenase-1 and -2 in rat brown adipose tissue: the modulatory role of the noradrenergic system. FEBS Lett. 487:171–5, 2000.

Xue Y, et al. Hypoxia-independent angiogenesis in adipose tissues during cold acclimation. Cell Metab. 9:99–109, 2009.

Suliman HB, Piantadosi CA. Mitochondrial quality control as a therapeutic target. Pharmacol Rev. 68:20–48, 2016.

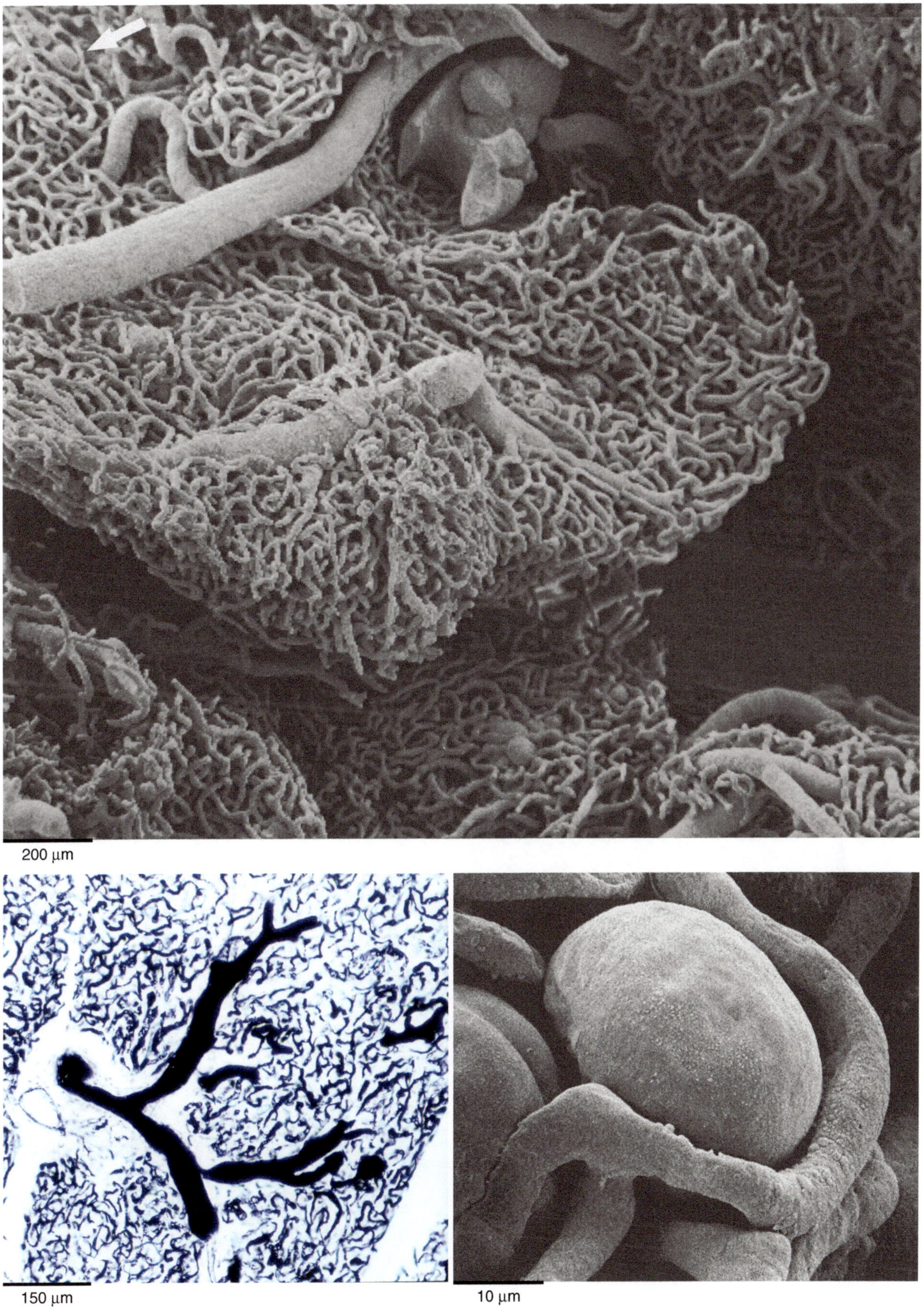

Plate 2.15 IBAT of young rat. Vascular cast showing a rich capillary network (*upper panel*). *Lower left*: Indian ink perfusion of IBAT in a young mouse. *Lower right*: capillary surrounding an adipocyte. From the same cast shown in the upper panel. SEM

PLATE 2.16

Arterioles

Arterioles 20–30 μm in diameter are often observed in the central portion of BAT lobules (see the previous plate). Their walls exhibit the usual three layers: intima, media, and adventitia.

The intima layer consists of thick endothelial cells lining the lumen; the media of a single layer of epithelioid muscle cells and the adventitia layer is bounded by periarteriolar thin, elongated cells. Numerous small nerves made up of unmyelinated fibers are always observed in the adventitia.

A precapillary arteriole is visible in the bottom panel. Note the absence of fully differentiated muscle cells (media), substituted by large pericytes or pericyte-like cells. Cytoplasmic projections of pericyte-like cells surround the entire vascular structure. Microfilaments characteristic of muscle cells of the media in arterioles (compare with muscle cells in the upper panel) are absent in the cytoplasm of pericyte-like cells. Their cytoplasm contains glycogen granules, rough endoplasmic reticulum, and small mitochondria. These cells are rich in pinocytotic vesicles and surrounded by a distinct basal membrane.

Suggested Reading

Rhodin JA. Fine structure of vascular walls in mammals with special reference to smooth muscle component. Physiol Rev S. 5:48–87, 1962.

Boerner-Patzelt D. Brown fat of the so-called hibernation gland in porcupines. Z Mikroskop Anat Forsch. 63:5, 1957.

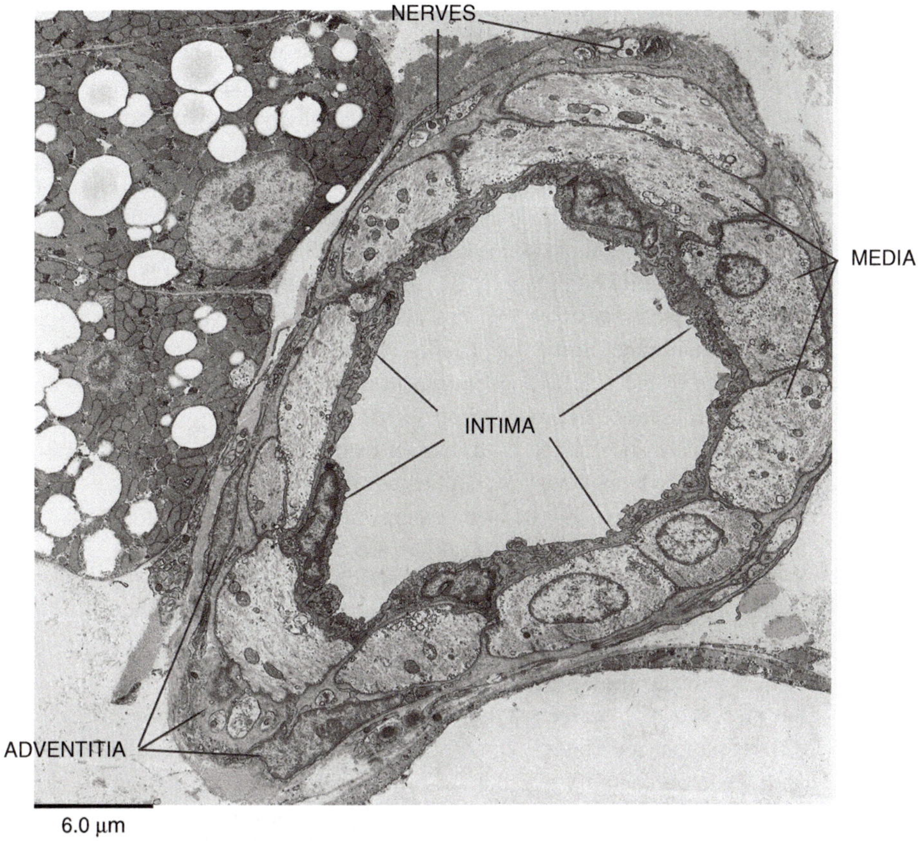

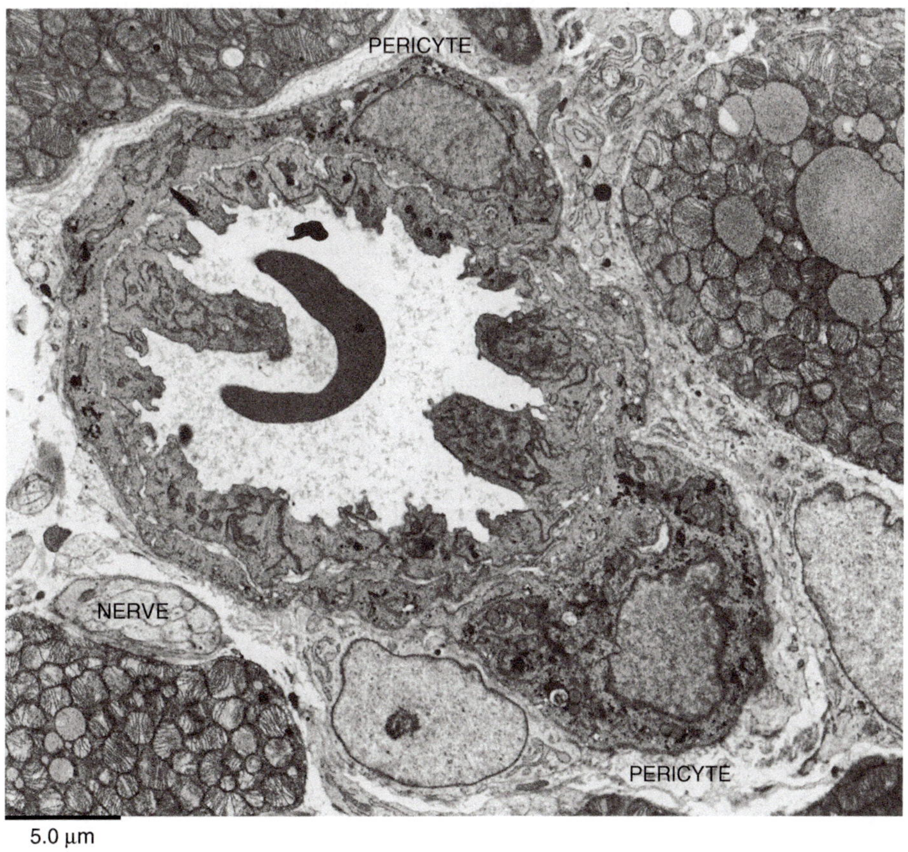

Plate 2.16 IBAT of adult (*upper*) and newborn (*lower*) rat. Intralobular arteriole (*upper panel*). Intralobular small precapillary arteriole. TEM

PLATE 2.17

Capillaries and Pericytes

BAT capillaries are lined with a special type of endothelial cells. Their ultrastructure may vary considerably even within the same specimen, some cells appearing very flattened (lower panels), with the lumen large enough to allow the passage of erythrocytes (see also Plates 2.2, 2.3, 2.9, and 2.10), and some appearing hypertrophic with the lumen reduced to a narrow fissure (Lu, upper panel) or completely closed. The plasticity of endothelial cells accounts for the quick regulation of local blood flow. Smooth (SER) and rough endoplasmic reticulum (RER) are often visible in endothelial cells. Pinocytotic vesicles (V) are abundant at the level of the plasma membrane lining the capillary lumen and the external boundaries of the cell. Mitochondria (m) are very small and very different from those of brown adipocytes (M).

Capillaries are surrounded by a distinct external lamina (or basal membrane), which often is duplicated to accommodate cells equipped with long and slender cytoplasmic projections (bottom panels). These cytoplasmic projections are often rich in glycogen that could represent an early sign of differentiation toward a preadipocyte. Details can be observed in the bottom right panel showing an enlargement of the framed area in the bottom left panel. Small arrows indicate the "preadipocyte" cytoplasmic projection. Note the presence of glycogen (Gly), i.e., an early sign of adipocyte differentiation (see Plates 2.26–2.29 for details). Interestingly, cells with immunoreactivity for markers of preadipocytes have been described as stellate cells when observed by confocal microscopy. In line with these data, the pericapillary projections described here could represent cytoplasmic projections of stellate cells.

Suggested Reading

Foster DO, Frydman ML. Measurements of blood flow with microspheres point to brown adipose tissue as the dominant site of the calorigenesis induced by noradrenaline. Can J Physiol Pharmacol. 56:110–22, 1978.

Foster DO, Frydman ML. Tissue distribution of cold-induced thermogenesis in conscious warm- or cold-acclimated rats reevaluated from changes in tissue blood flow: the dominant role of brown adipose tissue in the replacement of shivering by nonshivering thermogenesis. Can J Physiol Pharmacol. 57:257–70, 1979.

Lee YH, et al. In vivo identification of bipotential adipocyte progenitors recruited by β3-adrenoceptor activation and high-fat feeding. Cell Metab. 15:480–91, 2012.

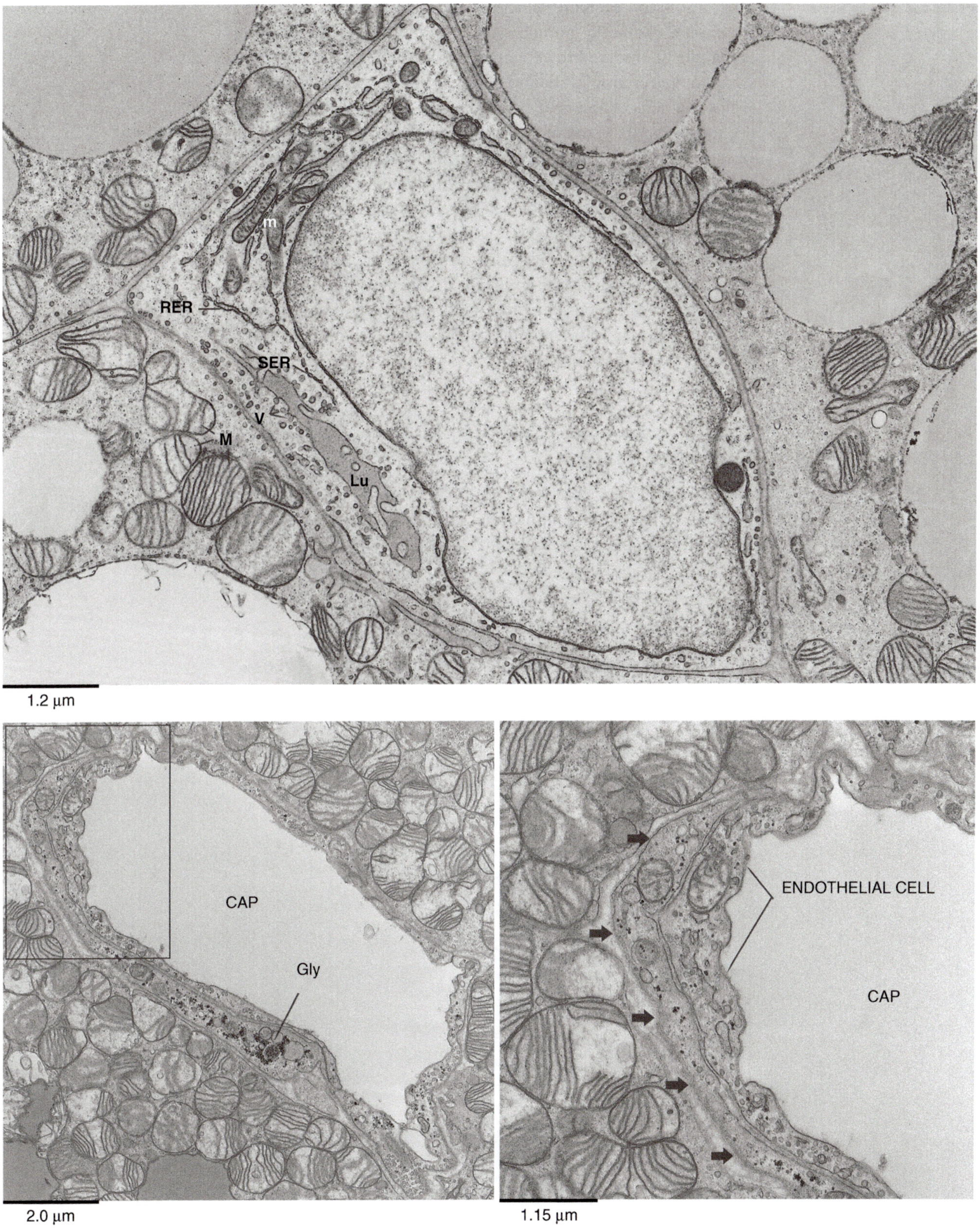

Plate 2.17 IBAT of young rat (*top*) and axillary BAT of newborn rat (*bottom*). Endothelial cells and peri-endothelial cytoplasmic projections. TEM

PLATE 2.18

Capillary Spherules

High-resolution scanning electron microscopy allows seeing 3D details not visible by normal scanning microscopy. We used this technique to observe brown adipose tissue treated with a modified osmium maceration technique that allows observing organelles inside the cells. The upper panel shows a low magnification of a sectioned capillary running among brown adipocytes. The cytoplasm of brown adipocyte, visible in the lower part of the upper panel, is full of typical mitochondria with laminar cristae. The wall of the endothelial cells is covered by very small spherules consistent with pinocytotic vesicles. The framed area is enlarged in the lower panel and shows elongated structures running among the pinocytotic spherules. These elongated structures are of unknown nature but could represent fused pinocytotic spherules (S, some indicated) similar to the smooth endoplasmic reticulum visible into the cytoplasm of endothelial cells (compare with SER in the top panel of Plate 2.17).

Suggested Reading

Riva A. et al. The application of the OsO_4 maceration method to the study of human bioptic material. A procedure avoiding freeze-fracture. Microsc Res Tech. 26:526–27, 1993.

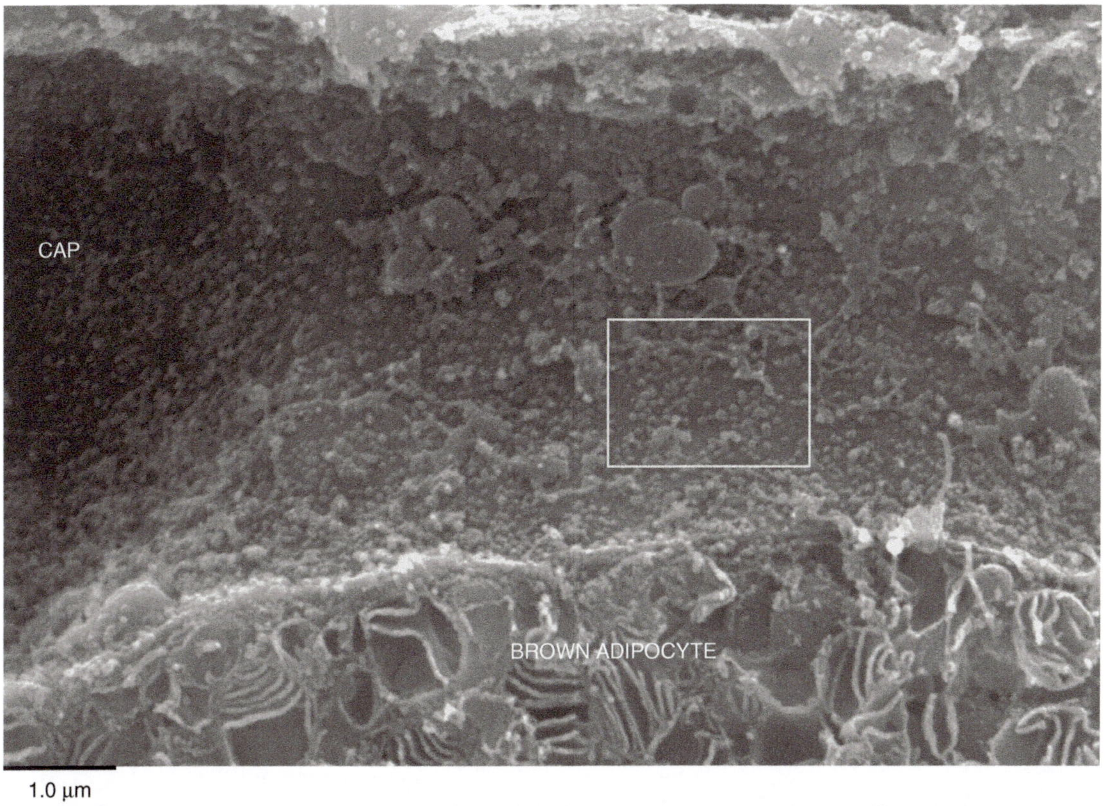

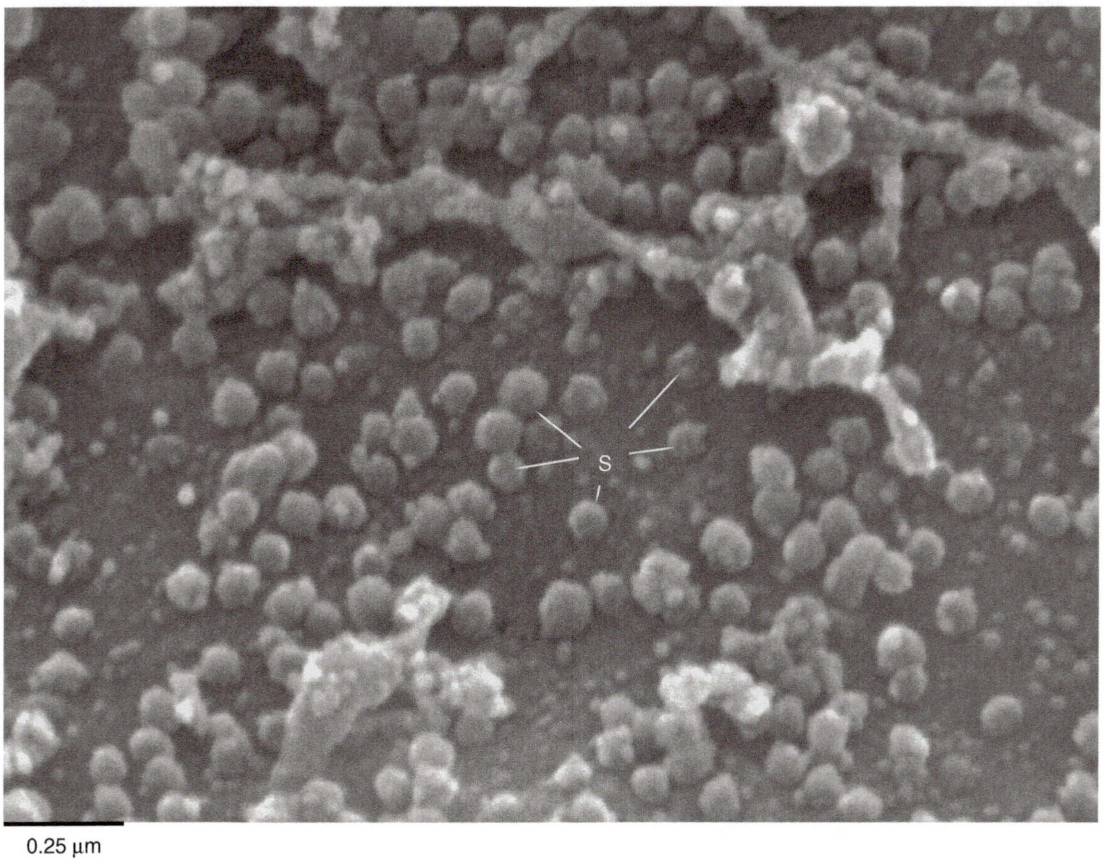

Plate 2.18 IBAT of cold-exposed mouse (6 °C for 24 h). A sectioned parenchymal capillary. Modified osmium maceration method. High-resolution SEM

PLATE 2.19

Nerves Gross Anatomy

BAT is richly innervated. Interscapular BAT (IBAT), in the anterior subcutaneous depot, is the most studied brown adipose tissue area in the adipose organ.

Five bilateral nerves coming from the intercostal region innervate IBAT. This plate shows the five nerves from the right intercostal region reaching the ventral portion of adult rat IBAT. IBAT has been pinched and folded back. The right scapula has been raised with a curved forceps, and a small piece of surgical cotton sheet has been placed under the nerves in order to evidence their topographic anatomy.

Suggested Reading

Sidman RL, Fawcett DW. The effect of peripheral nerve section on some metabolic responses of brown adipose tissue in mice. Anat Rec. 118:487–507, 1954.

Cottle WH. In "Brown adipose tissue", Lindberg. Ed., Elsevier, 155–78, 1970.

HEAD

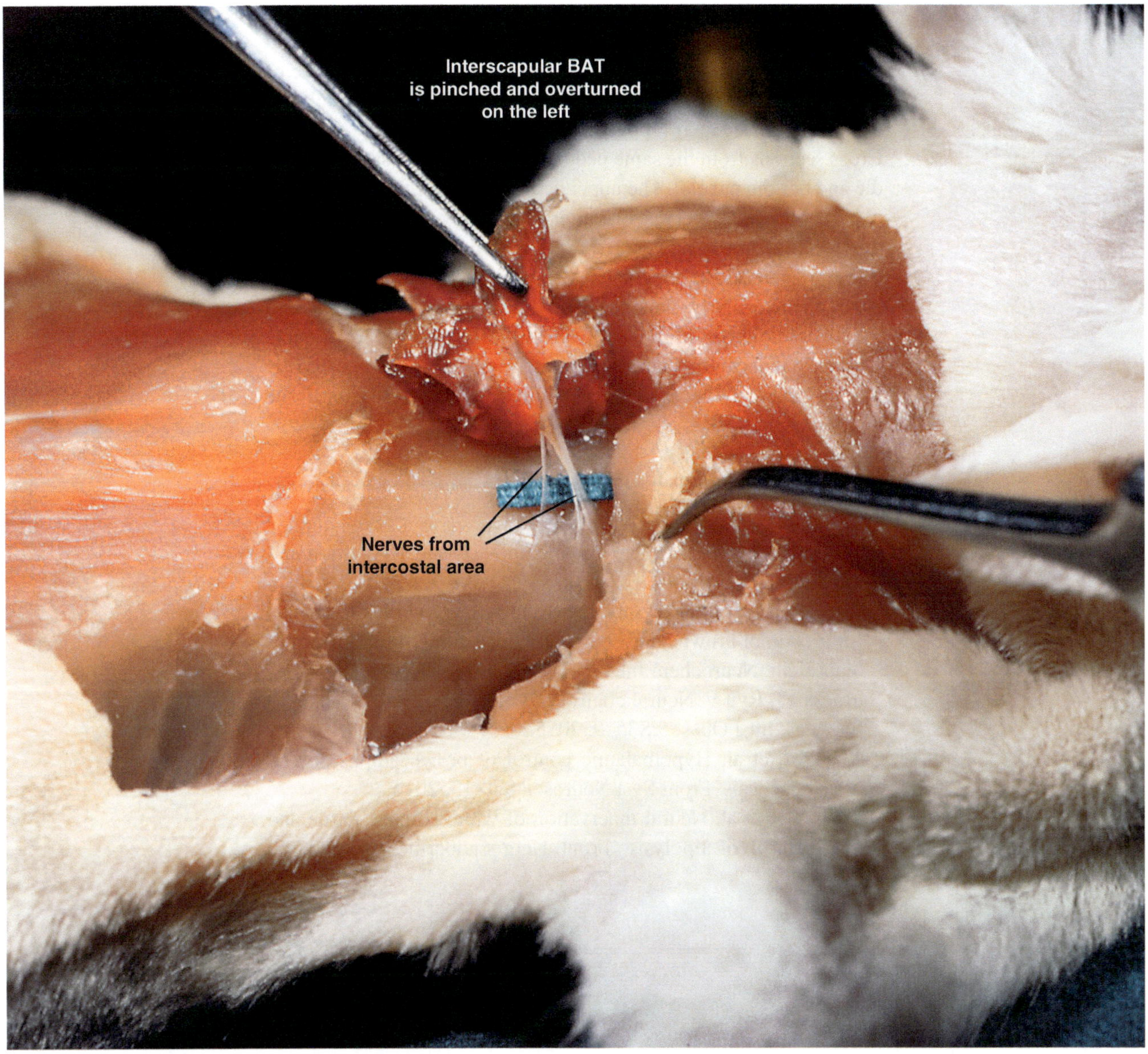

TAIL

Plate 2.19 Rat interscapular BAT (IBAT) nerves

PLATE 2.20

Nerve Histology

IBAT has two symmetric lateral peduncles that reach its lateral projections.

The plate shows the right portion of adult rat IBAT: the two lateral peduncles are dissected and easily recognizable. A small piece of blue surgical cotton sheet has been placed under the peduncles in order to evidence their topographic anatomy.

Cross sections from the same peduncles show their histology (middle and bottom panels). The upper peduncle (upper arrow in the top panel) contains six nerves, one artery, and one vein (middle panel). The lower peduncle (lower arrow) contains one artery and one vein (bottom panel). Both peduncles contain unilocular adipocytes. Note the irregularly flattened vein lumina and the regular and roundish lumina of arteries. The artery wall in the lower peduncle is thicker than that of the artery of the upper peduncle. Vascular lumina are empty because the animal has been perfused for tissue fixation.

Suggested Reading

Girardier L, Seydoux J. In "Brown adipose tissue", Trayhurn and Nicholls Eds., Arnold, 122–51, 1986.

Himms-Hagen J, et al. Sympathetic and sensory nerves in control of growth of brown adipose tissue: effects of denervation and of capsaicin. Neurochem Int.17:271–9, 1990.

Bartness TJ, Ryu V. Neural control of white, beige and brown adipocytes. Int J Obes. 5:S35–9. 2015.

Labbé SM, et al. Hypothalamic control of brown adipose tissue thermogenesis. Front Syst Neurosci. 9:1–13, 2015.

Bartness TJ, et al. Neural innervation of white adipose tissue and the control of lipolysis. Front Neuroendocrinol. 35:473–93, 2014.

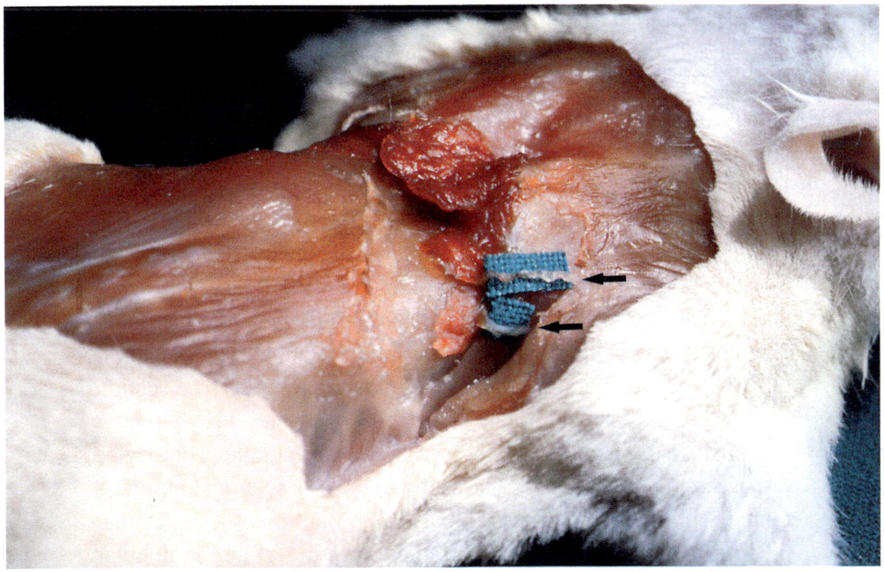

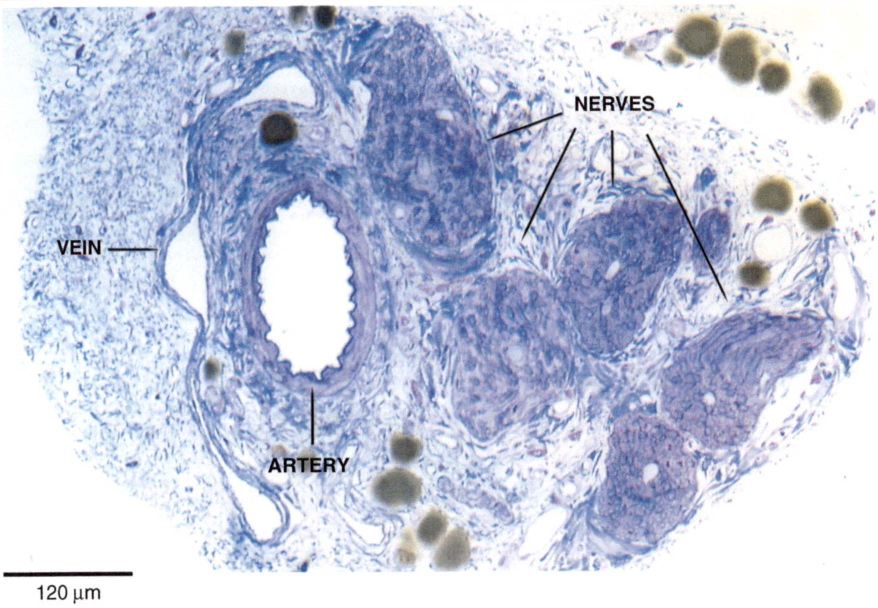

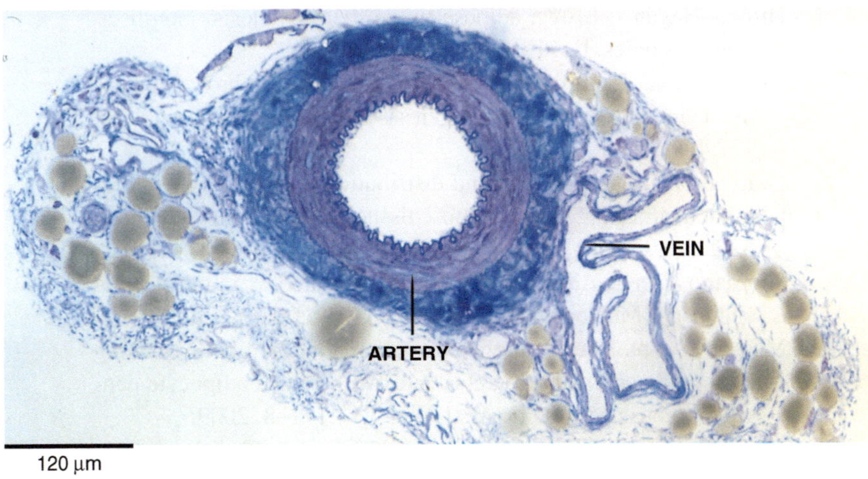

Plate 2.20 Adult rat. *Top*: nerves reach IBAT also through the upper lateral peduncle (*arrow*). *Middle* and *bottom*: histology of IBAT lateral peduncles. Toluidine blue-stained resin-embedded tissue. LM

PLATE 2.21

Nerves IHC

Some aspects of the complex IBAT innervation are shown in this plate. Two serial sections of some IBAT nerves are shown in the upper figures. The section on the left has been immunostained with an anti-tyrosine hydroxylase (TH) antibody (an enzyme found in noradrenergic fibers). On the right, the adjacent section has been immunostained with an anti-calcitonin gene-related peptide (CGRP) antibody (CGRP is usually found in sensitive fibers).
A comparison of the two sections shows that TH-immunoreactive noradrenergic fibers are mainly contained in small nerves (arrows) and CGRP-immunoreactive fibers mainly in large nerves (*).
The lower panels illustrate some features of parenchymal innervation (i.e., nerve fibers running among the adipocytes). The section on the left has been immunostained with an anti-TH antibody: TH-positive noradrenergic fibers can be seen among adipocytes (arrows, some indicated). The right figure—a section immunostained with an anti-neuropeptide Y (NPY) antibody—shows that NPY-positive fibers are present in the adventitia of an intralobular arteriole (arrows, some indicated). These fibers are also TH-positive.
Whereas BAT is richly provided with sympathetic noradrenergic nerves, it is believed to lack parasympathetic nerve supply. Indeed, in rodents the interscapular, cervical, and perirenal BAT depots are devoid of nerves containing acetylcholine, the predominant transmitter of postganglionic parasympathetic nerves. Interestingly, mediastinal BAT is the sole depot provided with putative parasympathetic cholinergic nerves at both the vascular and parenchymal levels. The cholinergic innervation of mediastinal BAT has been recently confirmed in humans.

Suggested Reading

Cannon B, et al. 'Neuropeptide tyrosine' (NPY) is co-stored with noradrenaline in vascular but not in parenchymal sympathetic nerves of brown adipose tissue. Exp Cell Res. 164:546–50, 1986.

Norman D, et al. Neuropeptides in interscapular and perirenal brown adipose tissue in the rat: a plurality of innervation. J Neurocytol. 17:305–11, 1988.

Himms-Hagen J. Brown adipose tissue thermogenesis: interdisciplinary studies. FASEB J. 4: 2890–98, 1990.

Nisoli E, et al. Expression of nerve growth factor in brown adipose tissue: implications for thermogenesis and obesity. Endocrinology. 137:495–503, 1996.

Giordano A, et al. Presence and distribution of cholinergic nerves in rat mediastinal brown adipose tissue. J Histochem Cytochem. 52:923–30, 2004.

Giordano A, et al. Adipose organ nerves revealed by immunohistochemistry. Methods Mol Biol. 456:83–95, 2008.

Murano I, et al. Noradrenergic parenchymal nerve fiber branching after cold acclimatisation correlates with brown adipocyte density in mouse adipose organ. J Anat. 214:171–8, 2009.

Possenti R, et al. Characterization of a novel peripheral pro-lipolytic mechanism in mice: role of VGF-derived peptide TLQP-21. Biochem J. 441:511–22, 2012.

Wei H, et al. A clinical approach to brown adipose tissue in the para-aortic area of the human thorax. PLoS One. 10:1–18, 2015.

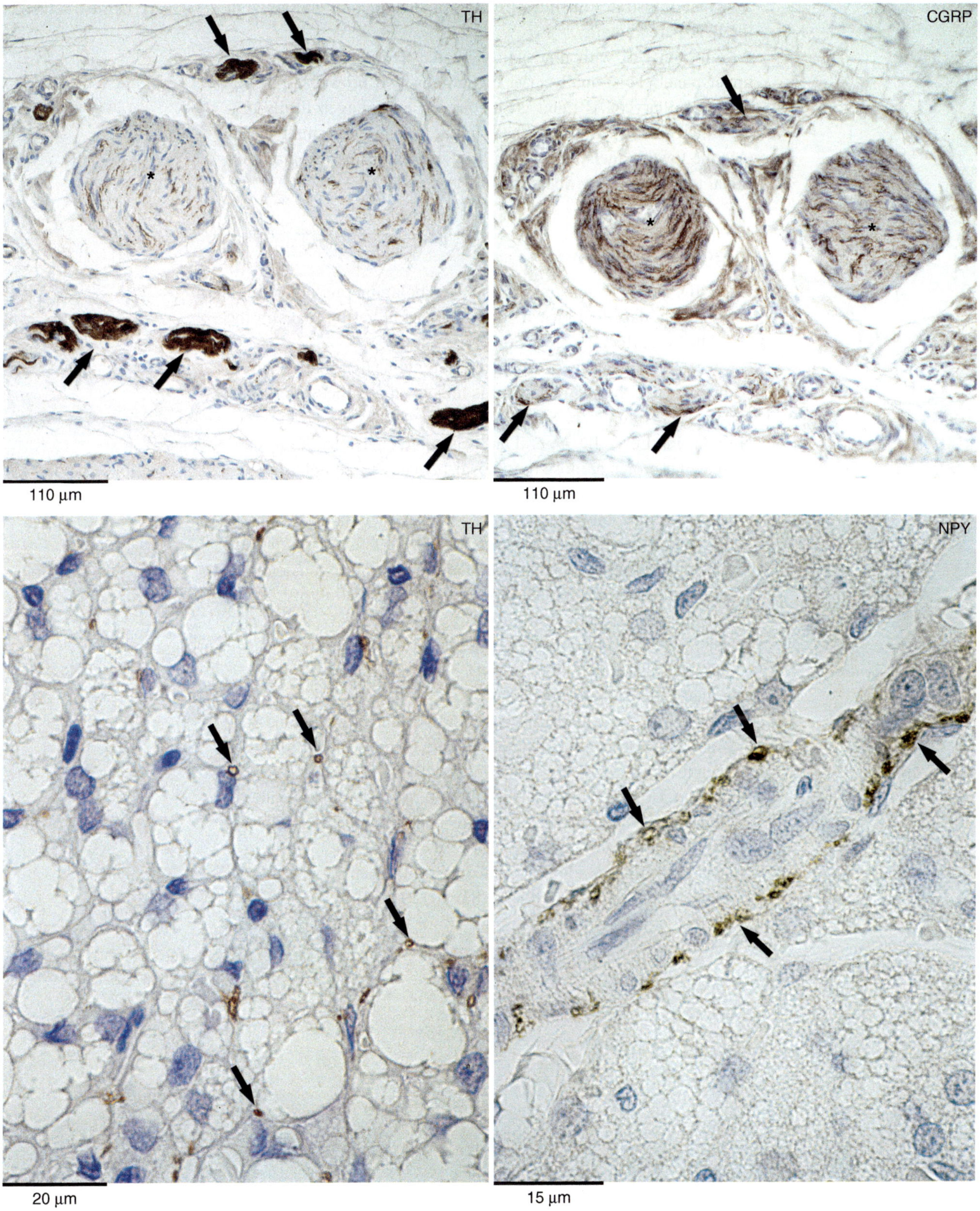

Plate 2.21 Adult rat IBAT. *Upper panels*: serial sections of IBAT nerves processed for immunohistochemistry (IHC). LM. IHC: TH ab (1:300), CGRP ab (1:2,000). *Lower left*: TH-immunoreactive fibers in the parenchyma. LM. IHC: TH ab (1:300). *Lower right*: NPY-immunoreactive fibers surrounding an arteriole. LM. IHC: NPY ab (1:600)

PLATE 2.22

Nerve Ultrastructure

This plate illustrates the ultrastructure of small nerves contained in the BAT parenchyma.

A Schwann cell with nine unmyelinated axons is shown in the upper panel. This small nerve lies among two brown adipocytes and a capillary (CAP) and is surrounded by collagen fibrils (C). Myelinated axons are occasionally found also in these small nerves (see the lower panels, arrows) in line with data supporting a functional role for sensory fibers in BAT.

Suggested Reading

Lever JD, et al. Demonstration of a catecholaminergic innervation in human perirenal brown adipose tissue at various ages in the adult. Anat Rec. 215:251–55, 1986.

Lever JD, et al. Neuropeptide and noradrenaline distributions in rat interscapular brown fat and in its intact and obstructed nerves of supply. J Auton Nerv Syst. 25:15–25, 1988.

Nnodim JO, Lever JD. Neural and vascular provisions of rat interscapular brown adipose tissue. Am J Anat. 182:283–93, 1988.

Mukherjee S, et al. A comparison of the effects of 6-hydroxydopamine and reserpine on noradrenergic and peptidergic nerves in rat brown adipose tissue. J Anat. 167:189–93,1989.

Shi H, et al. Sensory or sympathetic white adipose tissue denervation differentially affects depot growth and cellularity. Am J Physiol Regul Integr Comp Physiol. 288:R1028–37, 2005.

Bartness TJ, et al. Sympathetic and sensory innervation of brown adipose tissue. Int J Obes (Lond). 34(Suppl 1):S36–42, 2010.

Vaughan CH, Bartness TJ. Anterograde transneuronal viral tract tracing reveals central sensory circuits from brown fat and sensory denervation alters its thermogenic responses. Am J Physiol Regul Integr Comp Physiol. 302:R1049–58, 2012.

Vaughan CH, et al. Analysis and measurement of the sympathetic and sensory innervation of white and brown adipose tissue. Methods Enzymol. 537:199–225, 2014.

Ryu V, et al. Brown adipose tissue has sympathetic-sensory feedback circuits. J Neurosci. 35:2181–90, 2015.

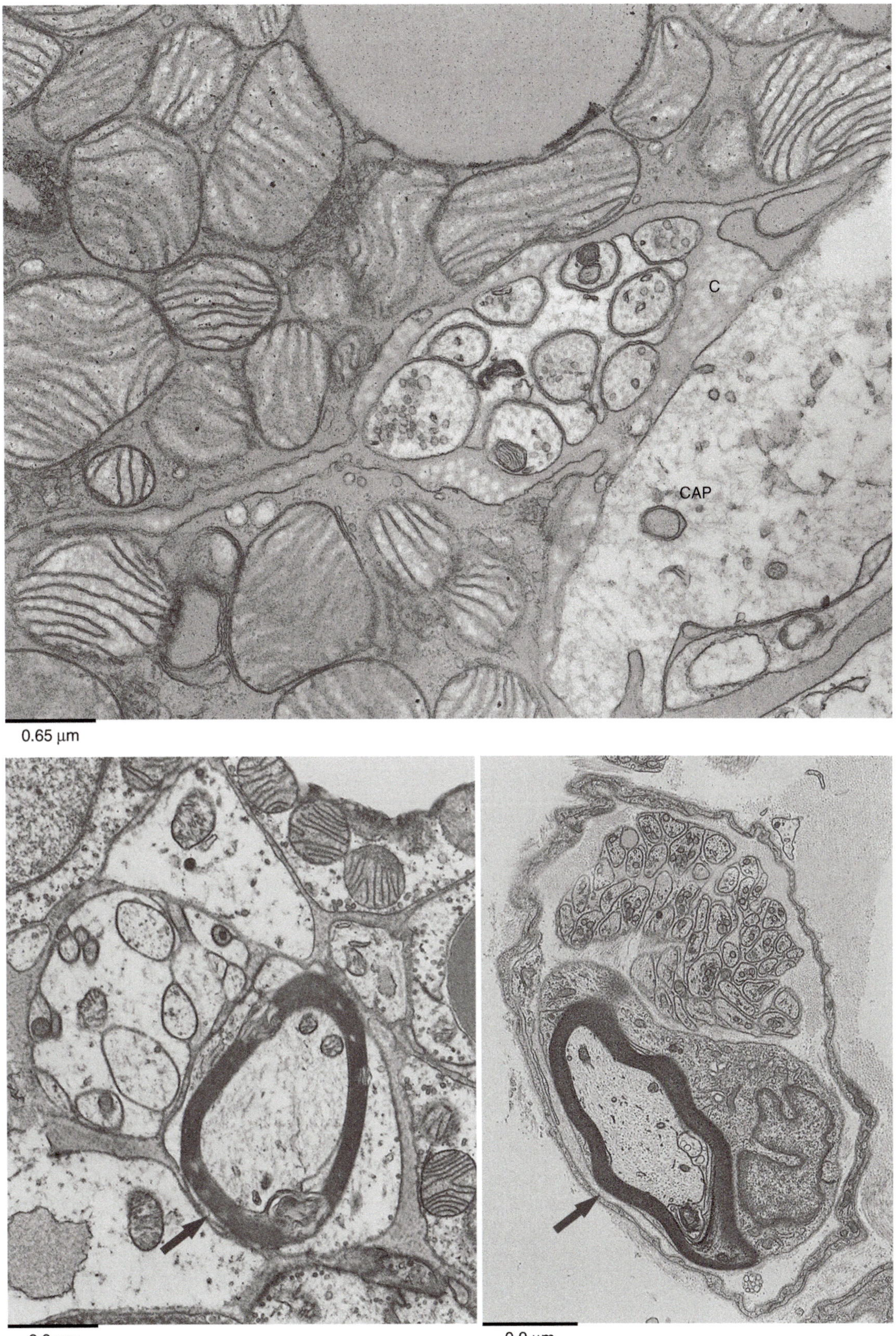

Plate 2.22 IBAT newborn (*upper*) and adult (*lower*) rat. *Upper*: Schwann cell with unmyelinated axons among two adipocytes and a capillary. *Lower*: small intraparenchymal nerves composed of unmyelinated and myelinated (*arrows*) fibers. TEM

PLATE 2.23

Nerve Endings

In BAT, synaptic nerve endings and nerve fiber varicosities are in direct contact with the plasma membrane of brown adipocytes. These structures contain numerous roundish or flattened, ostensibly empty, vesicles (SV) and are invaginated in brown adipocyte cytoplasmic foldings.

The plasma membrane in correspondence with synaptic nerve endings is usually of normal thickness and often rich in pinocytotic vesicles. In some occasions more than a single nerve ending seems to be in contact with a single adipocyte (see left middle and right bottom panels).

Suggested Reading

Bargmann W, et al. On the cells of the brown fatty tissue and their innervation. Z Zellforsch Mikroscop Anat. 85: 601–13, 1968.

Suter ER. The fine structure of brown adipose tissue. I. Cold-induced changes in the rat. J Ultrastruct Res. 26:216–41, 1969.

Mukherjee S, et al. A comparison of the effects of 6-hydroxydopamine and reserpine on noradrenergic and peptidergic nerves in rat brown adipose tissue. J Anat. 167:189–93, 1989.

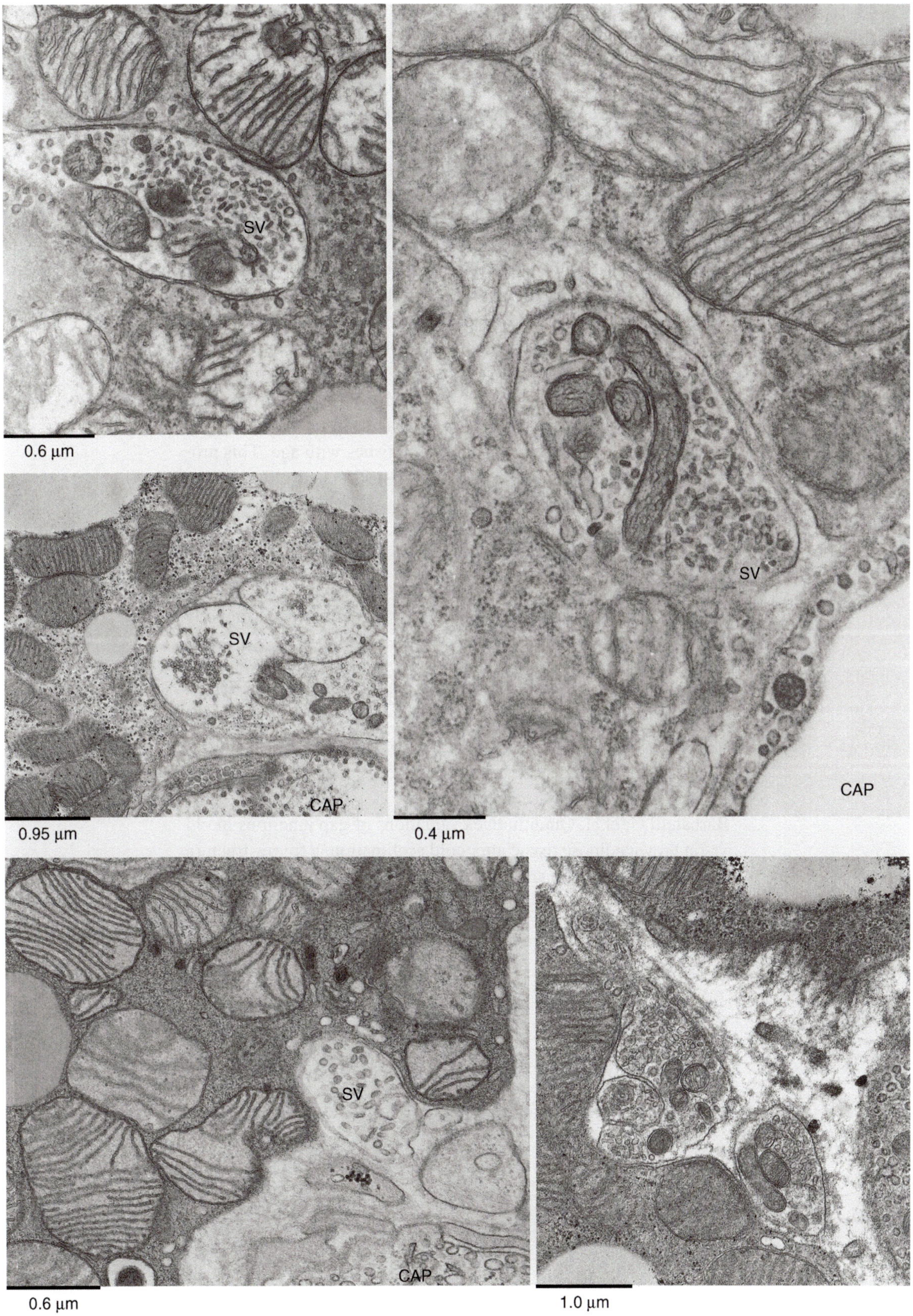

Plate 2.23 IBAT of mice (*top left* and *right* and *bottom right*) and rats (*middle* and *bottom left*). Nerve endings in direct contact with brown adipocytes. CAP, capillary. TEM

PLATE 2.24

Gap Junctions

Brown adipocytes are joined and electrically coupled by gap junctions. These can be seen by TEM with different techniques. The upper panel of this plate shows two gap junctions (arrows) between two brown adipocytes in a specimen processed for conventional TEM. The intercellular space is considerably narrowed in correspondence with the two gap junctions.

The same type of junction appears as a regular polygonal cluster of proteins with the freeze-fracture technique (lower panel). This method is based on the observation that a cooled knife cutting through a frozen tissue produces a fracture that passes through structurally weak paths within the frozen membranes, exposing the hydrophobic faces of inner and extracellular membranes. Metal (platinum) and carbon are evaporated on the fracture face. After removal of the tissue by the action of concentrated inorganic solvents, the metal-carbon replica is used for TEM observations.

The ultrastructure of the replica obtained from a freeze-fractured rat BAT sample is shown in the lower panel. In rat IBAT the gap junction area, but not their number, diminishes with age. This process is, however, reversible, and in cold-acclimated old rats, gap junction areas increase significantly.

Suggested Reading

Sheridan JD. Electrical coupling between fat cells in newt fat body and mouse brown fat. J Cell Biol. 50:795–803, 1971.

Schneider-Picard G, et al. Quantitative evaluation of gap junctions during development of the brown adipose tissue. J Lipid Res. 21:600–7, 1980.

Schneider-Picard G, et al. Quantitative evaluation of gap junctions in rat brown adipose tissue after cold acclimation. J Membrane Biol. 78:85–9, 1984.

Barbatelli G, et al. Quantitative evaluations of gap junctions in old rat brown adipose tissue after cold acclimation: a freeze-fracture and ultra-structural study Tiss. Cell. 26:667–76, 1994.

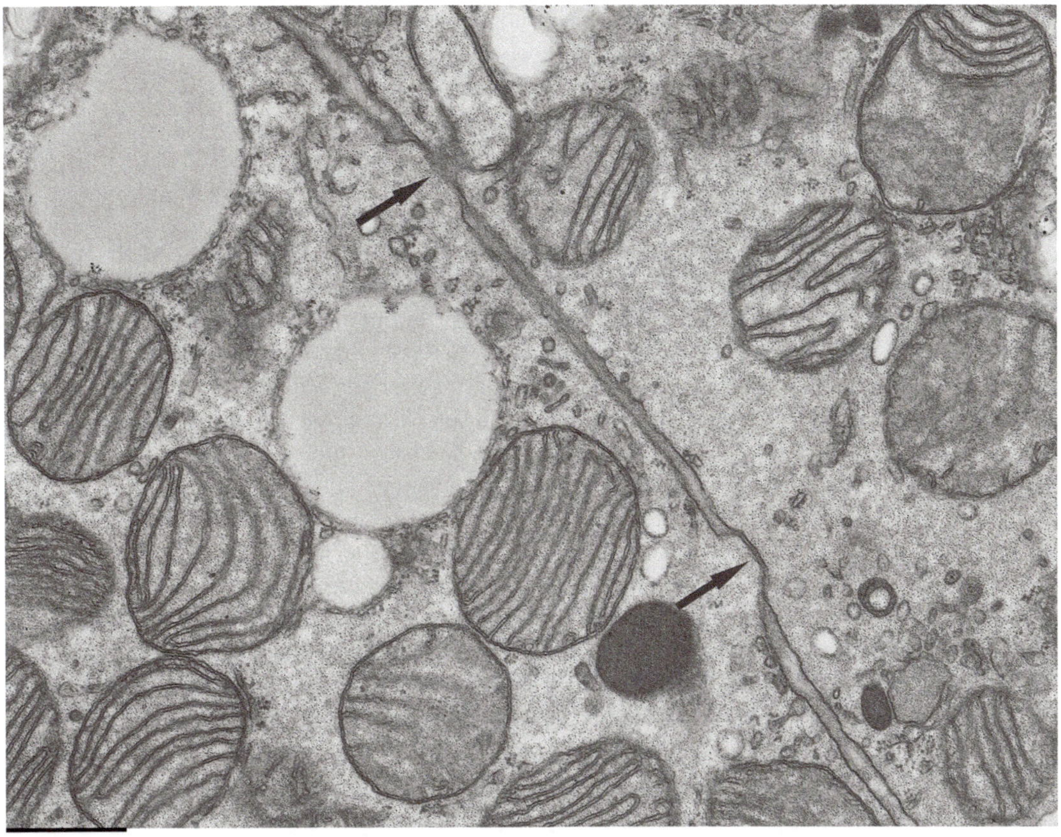

0.5 µm

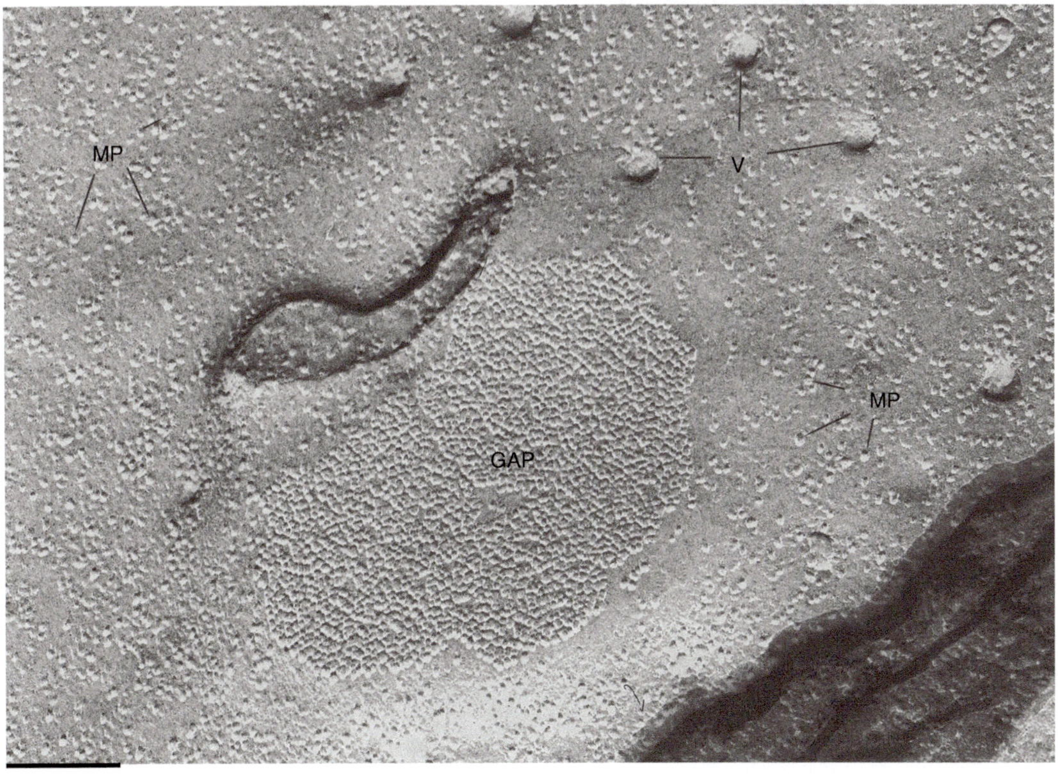

0.30 µm

Plate 2.24 IBAT of adult rats. *Upper*: gap junctions (*arrows*) between two adipocytes. TEM. *Lower*: gap junction (GAP) on the membrane of a brown adipocyte. V: pinocytotic vesicles (some indicated). MP: membrane proteins (some indicated). Freeze-fracture technique. TEM

PLATE 2.25

β-Less IBAT

All data on innervation of BAT outline the paramount importance of noradrenergic parenchymal fibers for its maintenance and functional thermogenic role. Brown adipocytes are mainly provided with β1 and β3 adrenergic receptors. β1 seems to play a role in adipocyte precursor differentiation, and β3 seems to be expressed only in mature adipocytes. β3 activation is the main functional stimulus for brown adipocytes.

Mice lacking all β-adrenergic receptors (β-less mice) show a dramatic change in morphology of interscapular brown adipocytes that become unilocular white-like adipocytes (lower panel). This morphologic alteration is accompanied by a reprogramming of these cells that express the most typical and important protein of white adipocytes: leptin that is never present in classic multilocular brown adipocytes, as proved by immunohistochemistry studies. Furthermore the most typical genes of brown phenotype in IBAT of these animals are strongly reduced. Interestingly, these animals with a reprogrammed BAT into a white-like adipose tissue, under high-fat diet, eating the same amount of food and performing the same physical exercise of controls became massively obese in few weeks. These data strongly support the idea that BAT activity is important to prevent obesity (see also Plate 7.12). In a recent study β-less mice under chronic stress reconstituted the IBAT normal morphology, thus suggesting alternative possibilities than β-receptor stimulation for normal IBAT activity.

Suggested Reading

Cinti S, et al. Immunohistochemical localization of leptin and uncoupling protein in white and brown adipose tissue. Endocrinology. 138:797–804, 1997.

Cancello R, et al. Leptin and UCP1 genes are reciprocally regulated in brown adipose tissue. Endocrinology. 139:4747–50, 1998.

Bronnikov G, et al. Beta-adrenergic, cAMP-mediated stimulation of proliferation of brown fat cells in primary culture. Mediation via beta 1 but not via beta 3 adrenoceptors. J Biol Chem. 267:2006–13, 1992.

Lowell BB, et al. Development of obesity in transgenic mice after genetic ablation of brown adipose tissue. Nature. 366:740–2, 1993.

Bachman ES, et al. betaAR signaling required for diet-induced thermogenesis and obesity resistance. Science. 297:843–5, 2002.

Razzoli M, et al. Stress-induced activation of brown adipose tissue prevents obesity in conditions of low adaptive thermogenesis. Mol Metab. 5:19–33, 2015.

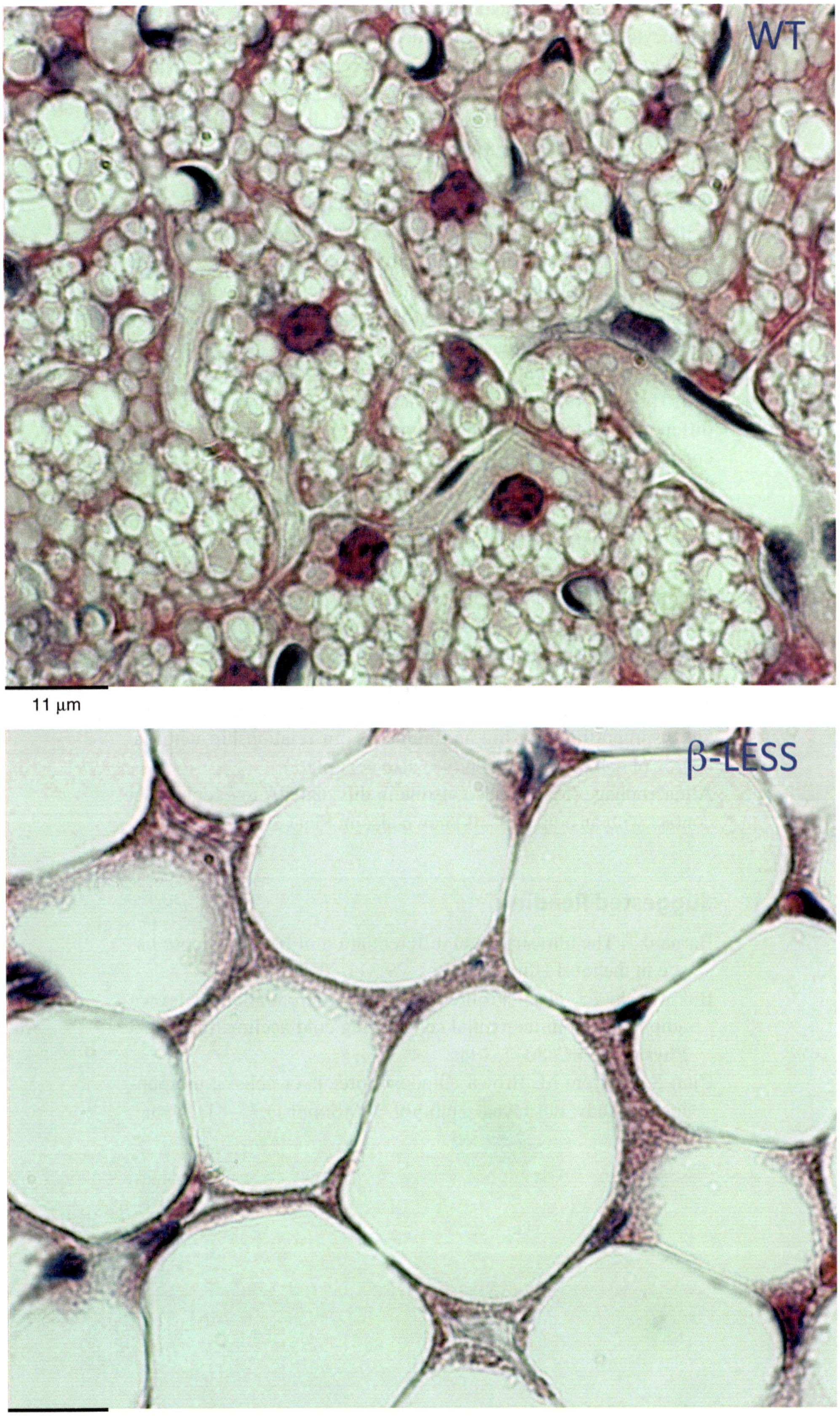

Plate 2.25 IBAT of adult wild-type (*upper*) and β-less mice (*lower*). LM, H&E staining

PLATE 2.26

Newborn Adipoblasts

In IBAT of newborn rats and mice, brown adipoblasts and brown adipocyte precursors are easily identified by electron microscopy. They have characteristic ultrastructural features, which allow distinguishing brown adipoblasts at an early stage of differentiation (this plate and the next plate), brown adipoblasts at a late stage of differentiation (Plate 2.28 upper panel), and brown adipocyte precursors (Plate 2.28 lower panel).

A 4-day-old rat IBAT is shown in this plate. In this tissue, blast cells are easily recognizable in close association with capillary (CAP) walls. The cell shown here can be identified as a blast cell by several morphologic characteristics: (1) the high nucleus/cytoplasm ratio, (2) the paucity of cytoplasmic organelles, and (3) the abundance of cytoplasmic ribosomes and polyribosomes. Characteristics 1 to 3 are all generic features of poorly developed cells (blasts). At the same time, there are features indicating early differentiation toward adipocyte lineage: (1) small clusters of glycogen (G) and (2) small lipid droplets (L).

These features indicate adipocyte differentiation only when they are found in blast cells.

Together with these characteristics of adipocyte lineage differentiation, this cell also shows features of brown adipocyte lineage differentiation: "pre-typical" mitochondria (m) (the biggest pre-typical mitochondrion is enlarged in the lower panel). We define as "pre-typical" mitochondria those mitochondria exhibiting some distinctive morphological aspects of typical mitochondria (see Plates 2.3–2.5) in poorly differentiated cells. "Pre-typical" mitochondria are disproportionately big and numerous in relationship with the degree of cell differentiation (see also next plate).

A macrophage (Mac) is also visible in this plate. A macrophage in contact with an adipoblast is shown also in Plate 2.12.

Suggested Reading

Barnard T. The ultrastructural differentiation of brown adipose tissue in the rat. J Ultrastruct Res. 29:311–22, 1969.

Bukowiecki LJ, et al. Proliferation and differentiation of brown adipocytes from interstitial cells during cold acclimation. Am J Physiol. 250:C880–7, 1986.

Cinti S, Morroni M. Brown adipocyte precursor cells: a morphological study. Ital J Anat Embryol. 100(Suppl 1):75–81, 1995.

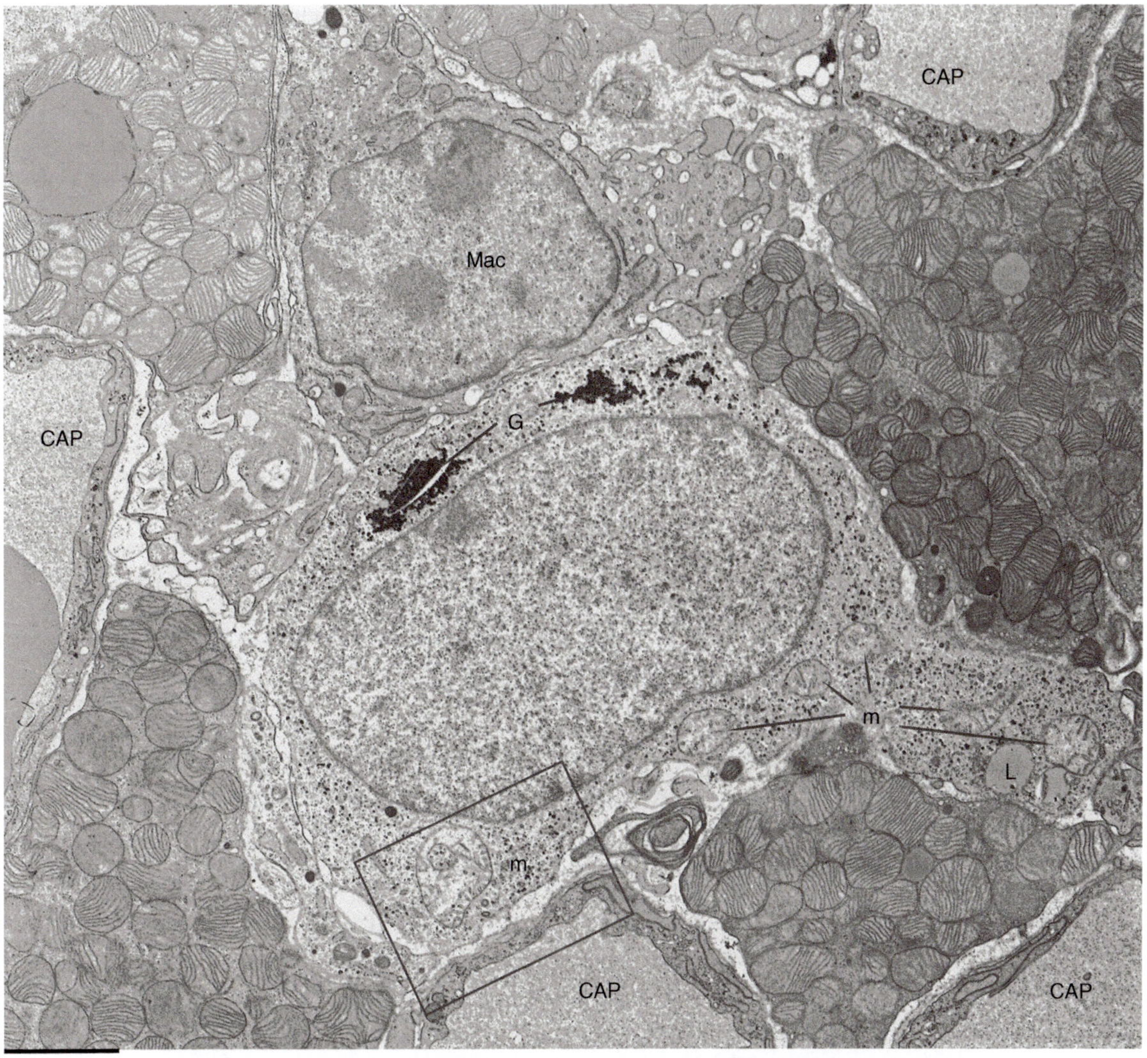

1.85 μm

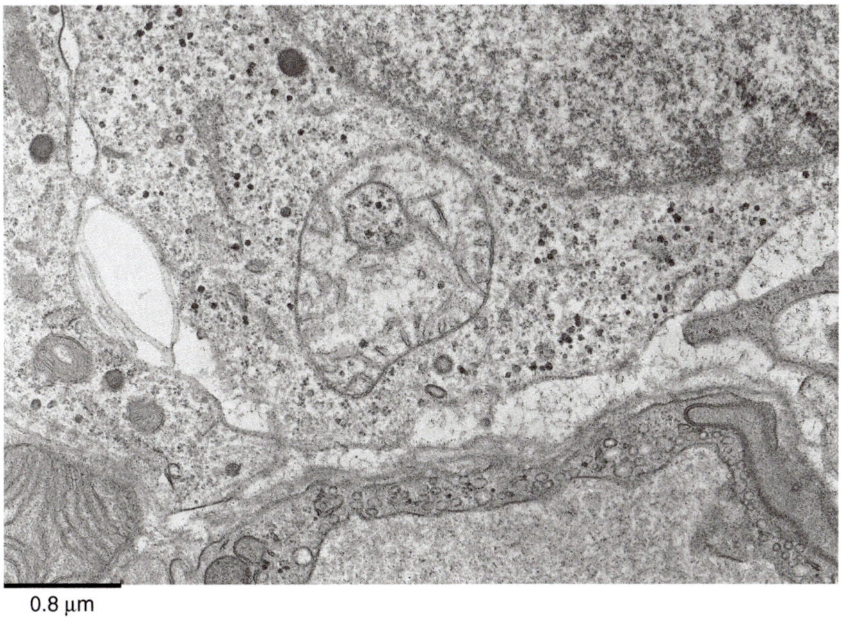

0.8 μm

Plate 2.26 IBAT of newborn rat. *Upper*: brown adipoblast at a very early stage of differentiation surrounded by mature brown adipocytes and in contact with a macrophage. *Lower*: enlargement of the framed area showing an example of "pre-typical" mitochondria. TEM

PLATE 2.27

Adult Adipoblasts

The distinctive morphological features of typical mitochondria shared by the organelles termed here as "pre-typical" (m) are size and number. Considering their stage of differentiation, the size and number of the mitochondria of these blast cells are obviously out of proportion and predict the importance of these organelles in the morphology and function in the mature brown adipocyte.

The blasts shown in this plate are from the IBAT of an adult rat acclimated at 4 °C for 3 days. The size of adipoblast mitochondria is similar to that of the mitochondria of the surrounding mature adipocytes. Therefore, the most remarkable difference between typical and "pre-typical" mitochondria (m) is the degree of development of the internal membrane (cristae). Note the large number of mitochondria in the blast cells and their typical general features of poorly differentiated cells: open nucleolus (Nu) and abundant cytoplasmic ribosomes and polyribosomes (*) together with an early sign of adipocyte differentiation, small lipid droplets (L) (framed area enlarged in the lower panel). All these features allow to consider these cells as brown adipoblasts at an early stage of differentiation.

Suggested Reading

Barnard T, Lindberg O. Ultrastructural changes in the chondriome during perinatal development in brown adipose tissue of rats. J Ultrastruct Res. 29:293–310, 1969.

Barnard T, Skála J. In "Brown adipose tissue", Lindberg Ed., Elsevier, 33–72, 1970.

Houstek J, et al. Differentiation of brown adipose tissue and biogenesis of thermogenic mitochondria in situ and in cell culture, BBA, 1018:243–47, 1990.

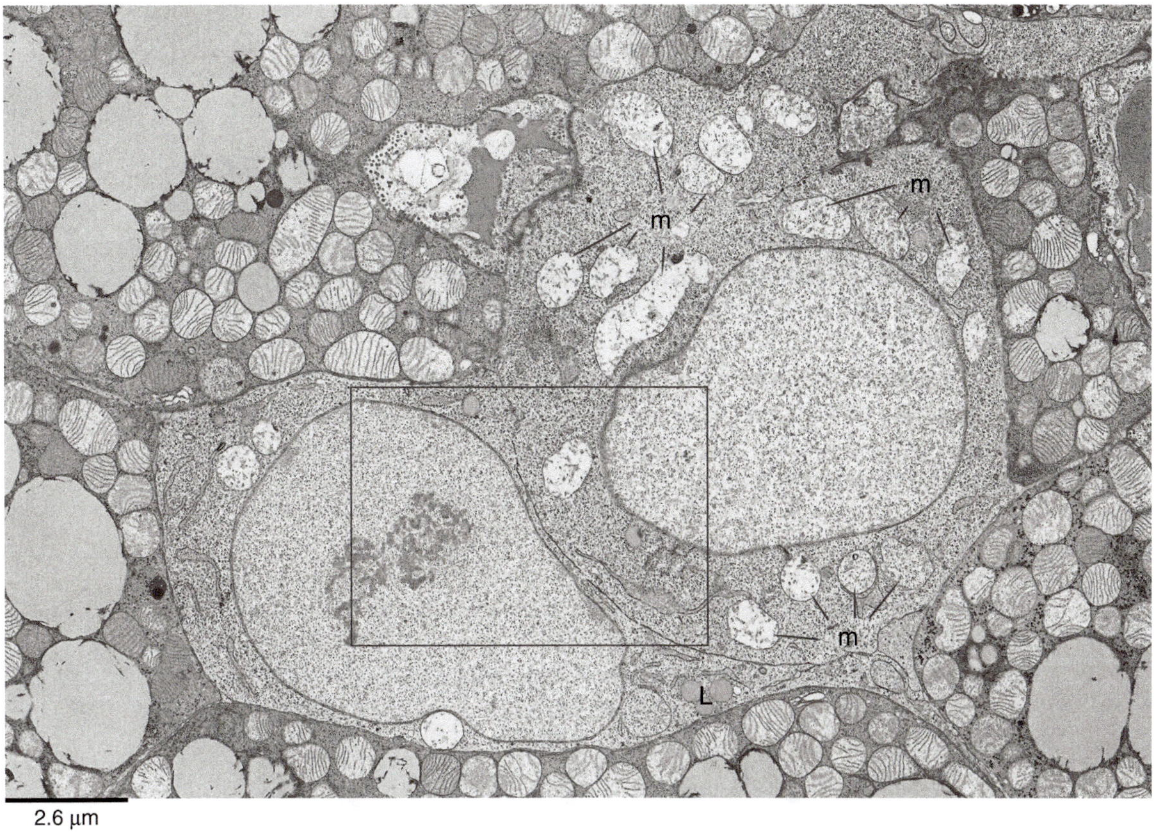

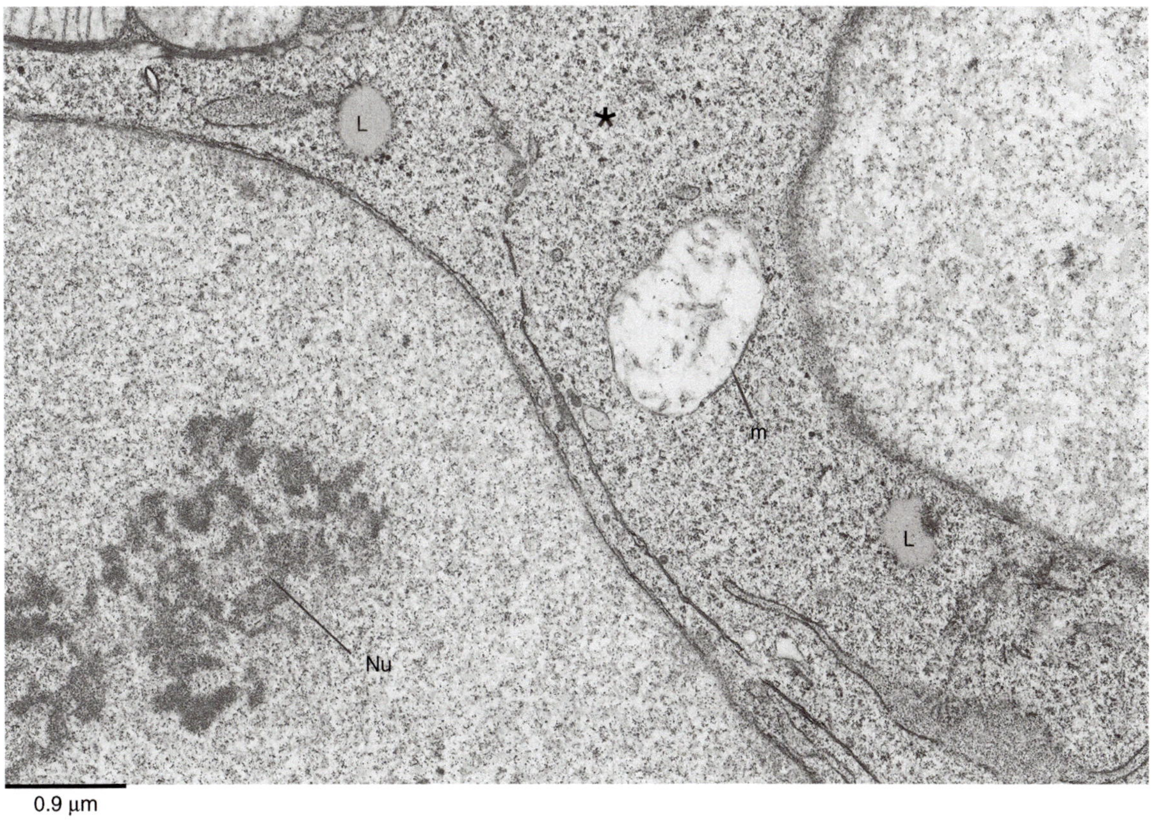

Plate 2.27 IBAT of cold-exposed (3 days at 4 °C) adult rat. *Upper*: two brown adipoblasts at a very early stage of differentiation among mature adipocytes. *Lower*: enlargement of the framed area. TEM

PLATE 2.28

Late Adipoblasts-Preadipocytes

The cells shown in this plate (IBAT of newborn rat) have a level of differentiation more advanced than that of blasts shown in previous Plates 2.26 and 2.27. Nevertheless, the general morphology of these cells is similar to those characterizing blast cells. We thus define these elements as adipoblasts at a late stage of differentiation.

Mitochondria (m, some indicated) are numerous and show more developed internal membranes (cristae). Usually a single droplet (L) represents the lipid storage (suggesting that the gene/s involved in the control of multilocularity is/are not yet activated). Note that the lipid droplets in the surrounding mature adipocytes are smaller than in the adipoblast.

In the lower panel a classic preadipocyte is shown. The ultrastructural differences between this cell and the above-described late adipoblasts are evident: (1) nucleus without an evident nucleolus, (2) less evidence for ribosomes and polyribosomes, (3) increased number of mitochondria, (4) increased number of cristae into mitochondria, (5) abundant "pseudo-holes" in mitochondria (see the next plate), (6) presence of matrix dense granules in mitochondria, (7) lipid storage more multilocular, and (8) abundant pinocytotic vesicles.

The possible schematic sequence suggested by these plates is:

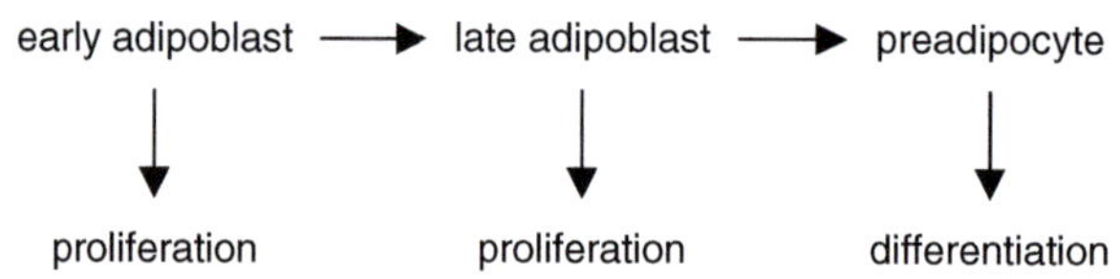

Suggested Reading

Napolitano L, Fawcett DW. The fine structure of brown adipose tissue in the newborn mouse and rat. J Biophys Biochem. Cytol. 4:685–92, 1958.

Girardier L. In "Mammalian Thermogenesis", Girardier and Stock Eds., Chapman, 50–98, 1983.

Nnodim JO, Lever JD. The pre- and postnatal development and ageing of interscapular brown adipose tissue in the rat. Anat Embryol. 173:215–23, 1985.

Nèchad M. In "Brown adipose tissue", Trayhurn and Nicholls Eds., Arnold, 1–30, 1986.

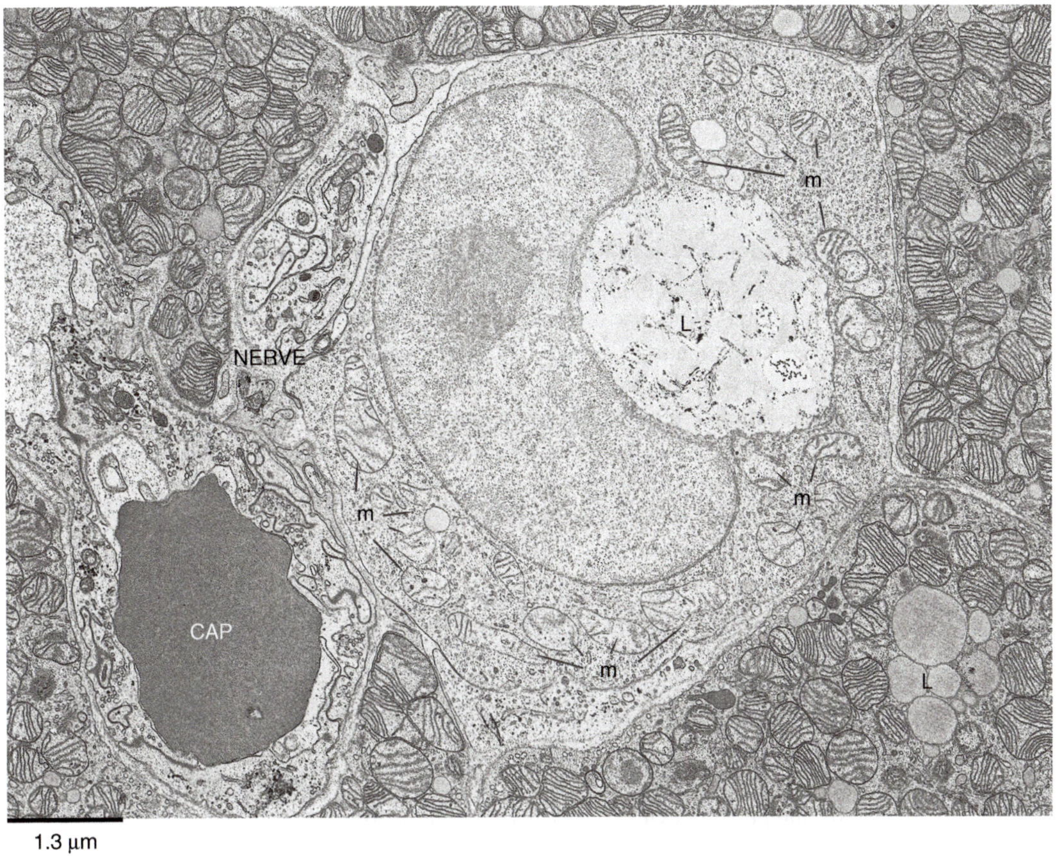

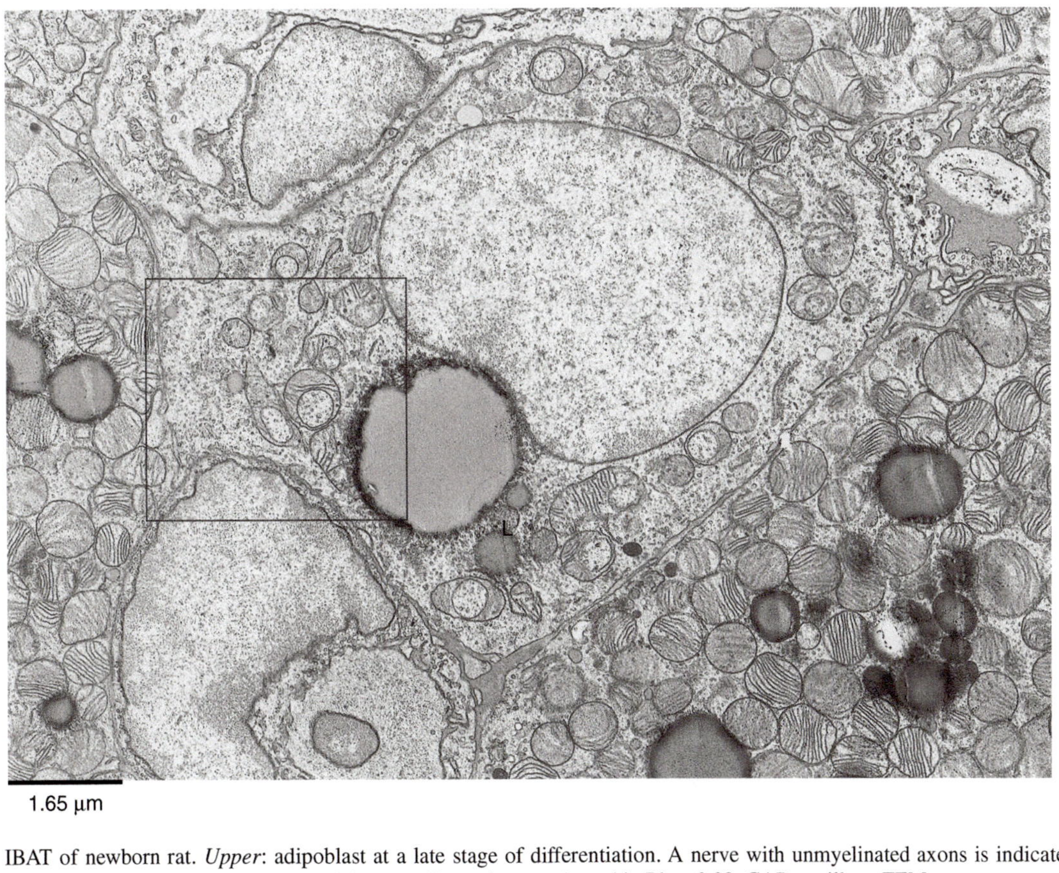

Plate 2.28 IBAT of newborn rat. *Upper*: adipoblast at a late stage of differentiation. A nerve with unmyelinated axons is indicated. *Lower*: a preadipocyte with classic distinctive ultrastructural features. Framed area enlarged in Plate 2.29. CAP, capillary. TEM

PLATE 2.29

Mitochondria of Preadipocytes

"Pre-typical" mitochondrial morphology in brown adipoblast and preadipocytes can vary as shown in previous Plates 2.26–2.28. In the present plate, two special features are shown. The panel (enlargement of the framed area in the lower panel of Plate 2.28) demonstrates the presence of pseudo-holes inside the "pre-typical" mitochondria. Pseudo-holes are due to the section plane intercepting the fold of irregular mitochondria. The double membrane of the mitochondrion demonstrates their "pseudo" nature; thus the content of the pseudo-hole is just a portion of the cytoplasm visible in this "window." Note also the presence of dense granules into the matrix of mitochondria (arrows). Dense granules are thought to be in relationship to the process of internal cristae development and are a typical feature of developing brown late adipoblasts and preadipocytes. Other features often detected in brown adipoblasts and preadipocytes are an external (or basal) membrane and numerous pinocytotic vesicles (V) at the plasma membrane.

In summary several intrinsic and extrinsic features allow a precise identification of brown adipoblasts and preadipocytes by ultrastructural features. The intrinsic features have been described in the previous plate and differ slightly between adipoblasts and preadipocytes. Among the extrinsic features are a distinct external (or basal) membrane and the close association with capillary walls. We never found cells with these ultrastructural features far more than few microns from the capillary wall. Often a nerve fiber is observed near adipoblasts and preadipocytes (see Plates 2.28 and 2.30).

Suggested Reading

Weinbach EC, Von Brand T. Formation, isolation and composition of dense granules from mitochondria. Biochim Biophys Acta. 148:256–66, 1967.

Pasquali-Ronchetti I, et al. On the nature of the dense matrix granules of normal mitochondria. J Cell Biol. 40:565–8, 1969.

Barnard T. Mitochondrial matrix granules, dense particles and the sequestration of calcium by mitochondria. Scan Electron Microsc. 1:419–33, 1981.

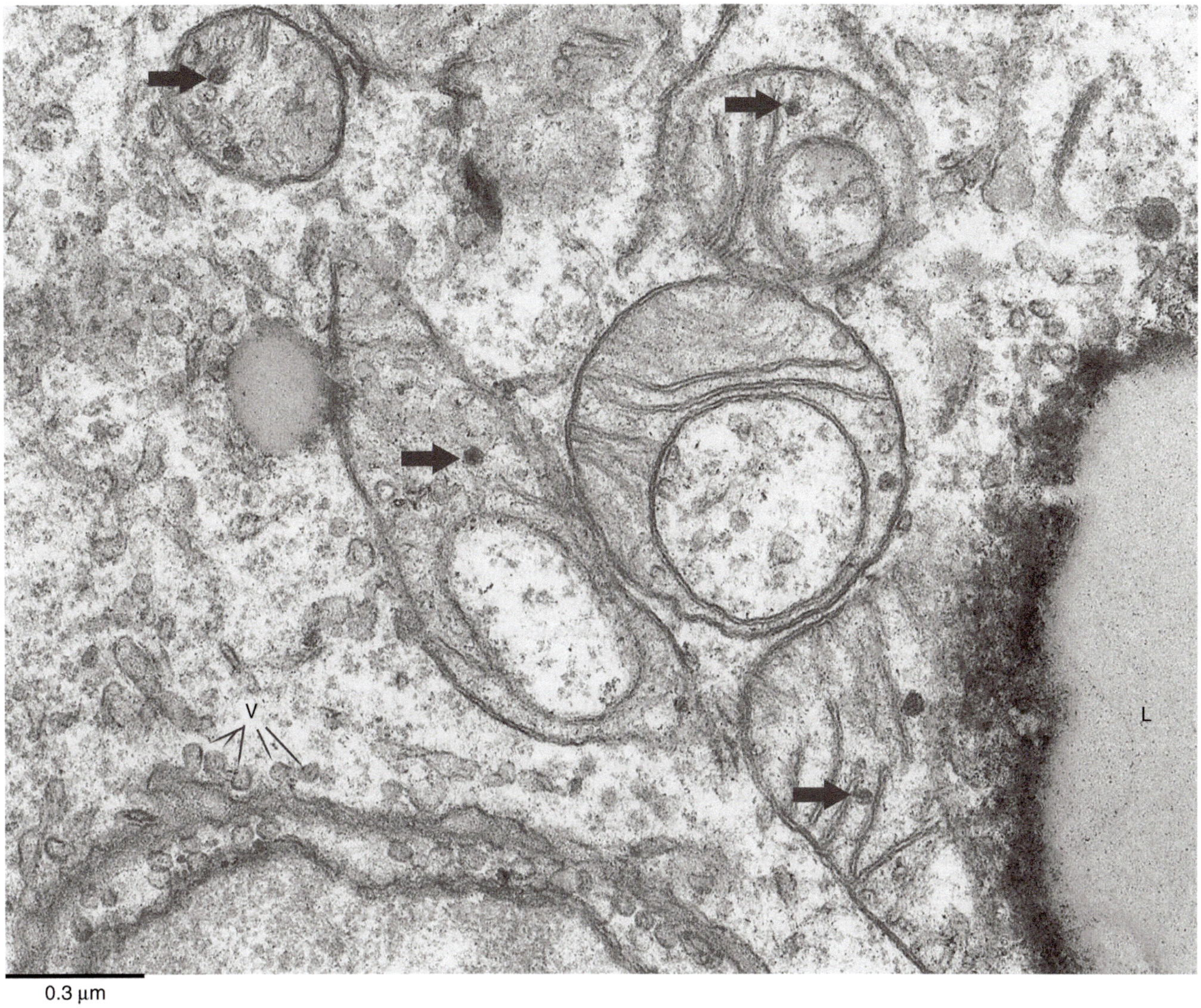

Plate 2.29 IBAT of newborn rat. Pleomorphic mitochondria with "pseudo-holes" and dense granules in the cytoplasm of a preadipocyte shown in Plate 2.28. L: lipid droplet. TEM

PLATE 2.30

Gap Junctions and Preadipocytes

We rarely observed gap junctions between brown preadipocytes and mature brown adipocytes in BAT of a newborn rat (framed area in the upper panel). The lower panel shows an enlargement of the framed area. The gap junction is indicated by arrows.

The functional role of these junctions is unknown. A paracrine-like role could be hypothesized considering the described general role for synchronized cell activities including secretion in glandular tissue. Paracrine factors such as FGF21, produced and secreted by brown adipocytes, could play a role in brown adipocyte differentiation. The gap junctions' physiologic role is usually referred as important for electrical coupling of brown adipocytes and never described hitherto between mature adipocytes and preadipocytes.

Note the difference between mitochondria of preadipocyte (lower left corner) and those in mature adipocyte (upper right corner) in the lower panel.

Note the close relationship between preadipocyte and a cell (*) whose ultrastructure does not allow a certain classification. The cytoplasm of this cell is rich in dilated rough endoplasmic reticulum (RER) suggesting that the phenotype is similar to that of endothelial-associated fibroblast-like cells but lacks the characteristic interdigitations with the endothelial cell in the capillary.

Suggested Reading

Michon L, et al. Involvement of gap junctional communication in secretion. Biochim Biophys Acta. 1719:82–101, 2005.

Burke S, et al. Adipocytes in both brown and white adipose tissue of adult mice are functionally connected via gap junctions: implications for Chagas disease. Microbes Infect. 6:893–901, 2014.

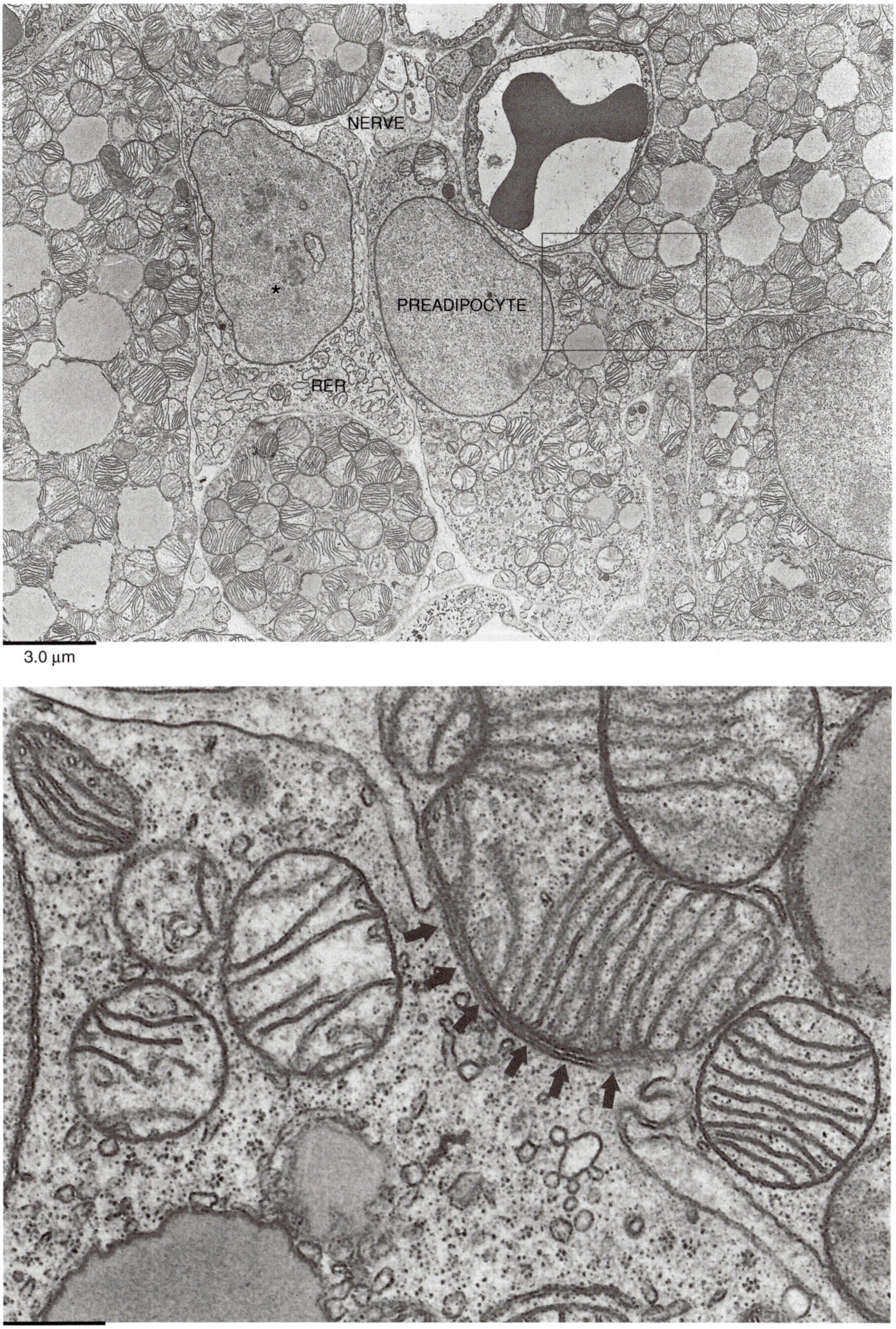

Plate 2.30 IBAT of newborn rat. Preadipocyte joined by a gap junction to a mature brown adipocyte. TEM

PLATE 2.31

β-Less Adipoblasts

In IBAT of newborn β-less mice, the morphology of adipoblasts and preadipocytes was identical to that of wild-type mice (compare the upper panel with lower panel of this plate). In these animals there was an abundance of glycogen particles (G, black-pointed areas of the cytoplasm). Our standard procedure for electron microscope specimen's preparations includes a post-fixation step made with osmium tetroxide-potassium ferrocyanide mixture that stains black glycogen. Note the abundance of mitochondria with well-developed internal cristae (insets are enlargements of framed areas) and numerous matrix dense granules. This level of differentiation is consistent with that of preadipocytes. The passage from the stage late adipoblast into that of preadipocytes is subtle and mainly indicated by the size of the cell and number and differentiation of mitochondria (indicated by the size and number of cristae). The lipid droplets' size and number are variable; in the preadipocytes shown in this plate, the lipid content is unusually scarce.

These data suggest that β-adrenergic receptors are dispensable for a normal development of brown precursors, but they are indispensable for the achievement and maintenance of typical mature brown adipocyte phenotype (see Plate 2.23) (our unpublished data in collaboration with Dr Brad Lowell, Harvard University).

Suggested Reading

Bachman ES, et al. betaAR signaling required for diet-induced thermogenesis and obesity resistance. Science. 297:843–5, 2002.

Razzoli M, et al. Stress-induced activation of brown adipose tissue prevents obesity in conditions of low adaptive thermogenesis. Mol Metab. 5:19–33, 2015.

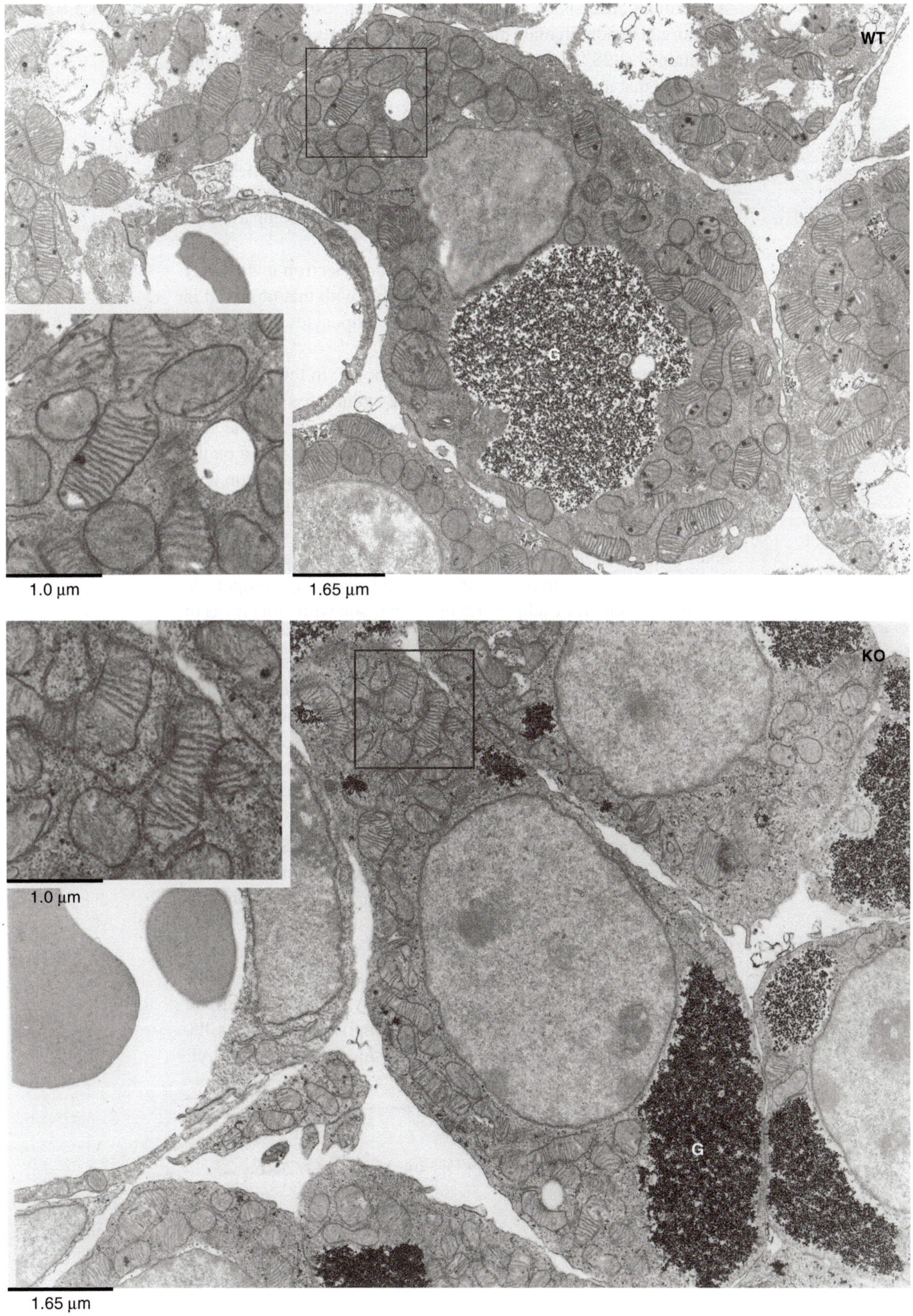

Plate 2.31 IBAT of newborn mice. *Upper*: preadipocyte from wild-type mouse. *Lower*: preadipocyte from β-less mouse. Insets: enlargements of the framed areas. TEM

PLATE 2.32

Visceral BAT LM and IHC

A thorough analysis of parenchymal cell composition of the adipose organ of adult female mice of different strains (Sv129 and B6) maintained at 28 °C (i.e., near thermoneutrality) for 10 days demonstrated that multilocular adipocytes immunoreactive for the thermogenic protein UCP1 were present in several subcutaneous and visceral areas of the adipose organ previously thought to be composed exclusively of white adipocytes. Thus, in warm-acclimated mice, brown adipocytes are part of the normal parenchymal composition of the adipose organ in all its anatomic compartments including subcutaneous and visceral depots.

The morphology, immunohistochemistry, and electron microscopy of visceral brown adipocytes are comparable with that observed in areas considered classic depot of brown adipocytes (IBAT) and thoroughly presented in previous plates.

In this plate mediastinal visceral BAT is shown. In the top panel a section of resin-embedded toluidine blue-stained tissue is shown. Note the classic multilocular morphology of the cells and the very high density of the capillary network (some indicated in red on the left half of the panel). In the bottom panel an immunoreaction with anti-UCP1 antibodies is shown. Most of the multilocular cells are positive as in the interscapular BAT (compare with Panel 2.1). Of note, in both strains, mediastinal BAT had the higher density of noradrenergic parenchymal nerve fibers and a very high proportion of brown versus white adipocytes in comparison with other areas of the organ.

In both strains the areas containing substantial amounts of brown adipocytes were interscapular and subscapular in the anterior subcutaneous depot, inguinal in the posterior subcutaneous depot, and mediastinal, perirenal, and peri-gonadal in the visceral depots. Deep cervical areas (surrounding the carotid and subclavian arteries) and axillary areas are usually thought to belong to the category of subcutaneous fat, but anatomical considerations do not support this idea. As a matter of fact, as shown in Plates 1.2–1.5, these areas are located at the root of the neck where a continuous transition between the visceral thoracic fat (mediastinal) and these areas is present. On the other end, it is evident that the deep cervical and axillary fat is in tight connection with "visceral" structures such as carotid and axillary arteries and other viscera such as those of the visceral unit (composed of the larynx, pharynx, and thyroid and parathyroid glands) in the neck and deep lymph nodes in the axilla. Thus the BAT of these areas should be considered as visceral BAT.

Suggested Reading

Giordano A, et al. Nat Rev Drug Discov. 15:405–24, 2016.

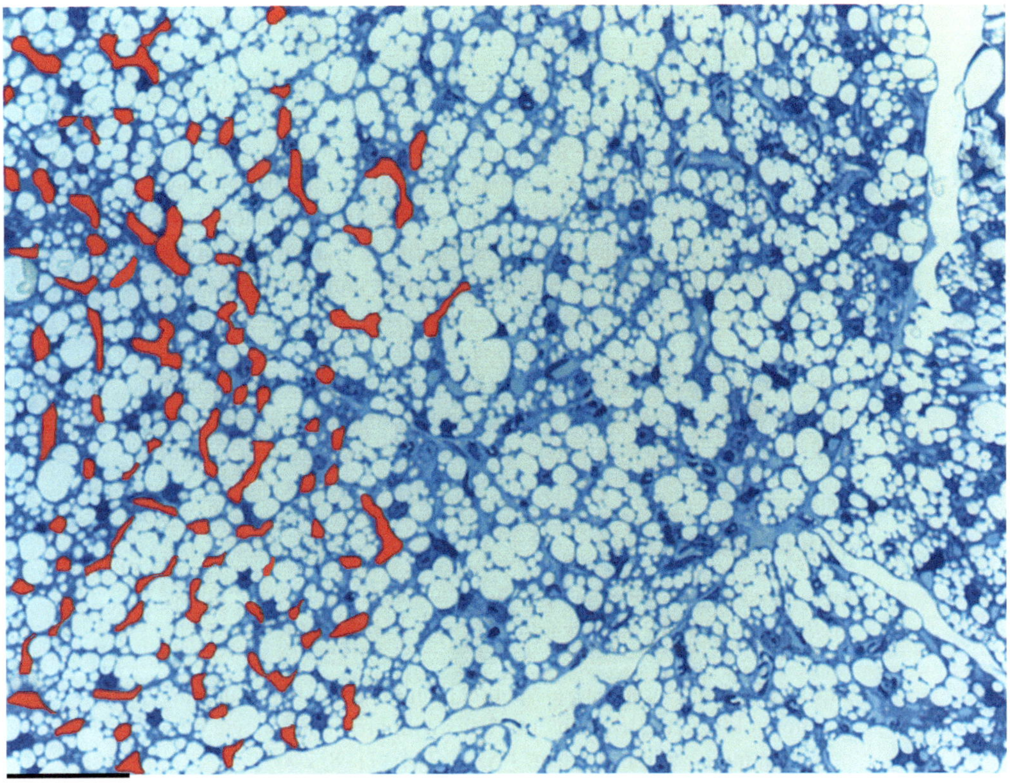

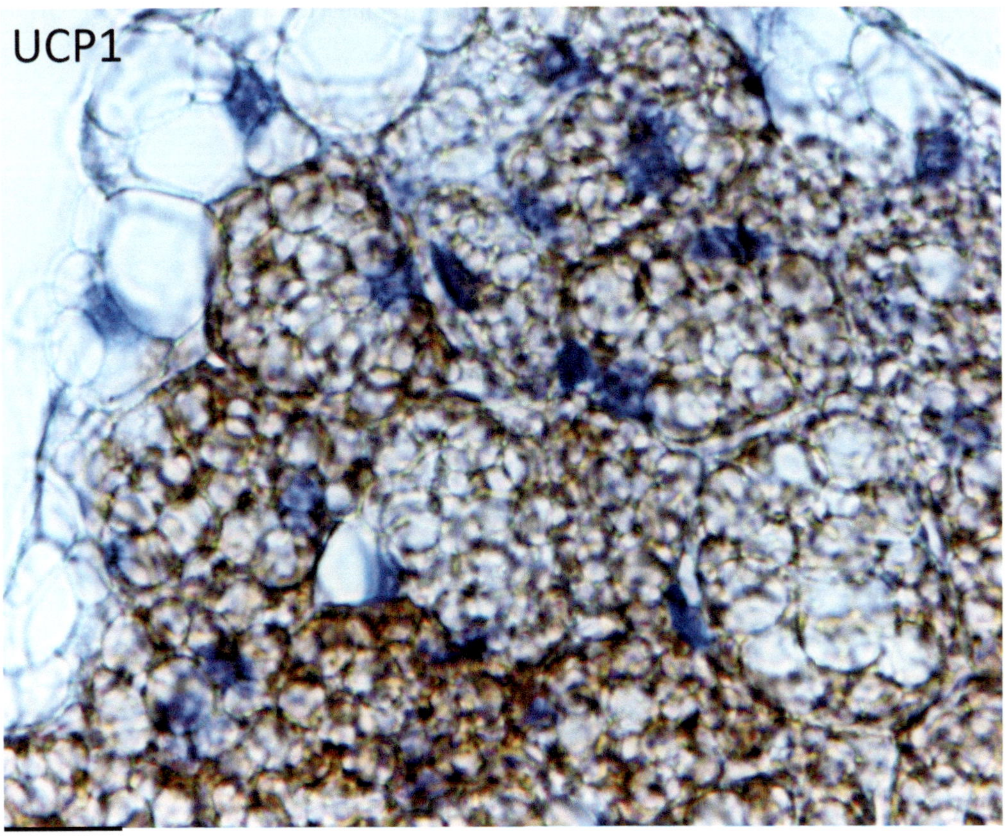

Plate 2.32 Mediastinal BAT of young rat (*upper*) and adult mouse (*lower*). *Upper*: Toluidine blue-stained resin-embedded tissue. *Lower*: ICH, UCP1 ab (1:1,000). LM

PLATE 2.33

Visceral BAT TEM

Electron microscopy of visceral brown adipocytes is comparable to that observed in classic IBAT.
We studied mainly brown adipocytes in mediastinal-periaortic and perirenal fat of rats and mice.
In this plate an example of visceral brown adipocytes from the mediastinal area of the adipose organ of a young mouse maintained at room temperature (22–24 °C) is shown. Note the morphology of mitochondria (lower panel, enlargement of the framed area in the upper panel) and abundance of parenchymal unmyelinated nerve fibers in tight contact with brown adipocytes (arrows). At room temperature BAT is not maximally activated and mitochondria tend to be smaller and elongated. In the lower panel a mitochondrion in the division process is visible (arrows), compared with dividing mitochondria in warm-acclimated animals (Plate 8.4).

Suggested Reading

Giordano A, et al. Presence and distribution of cholinergic nerves in rat mediastinal brown adipose tissue J Histochem Cytochem. 52:923–30, 2004.

Murano I, et al. Noradrenergic parenchymal nerve fiber branching after cold acclimatization correlates with brown adipocyte density in mouse adipose organ. J Anat. 214:171–8, 2009.

Vitali A, et al. The adipose organ of obesity-prone C57BL/6J mice is composed of mixed white and brown adipocytes. J Lipid Res 53:619–29, 2012.

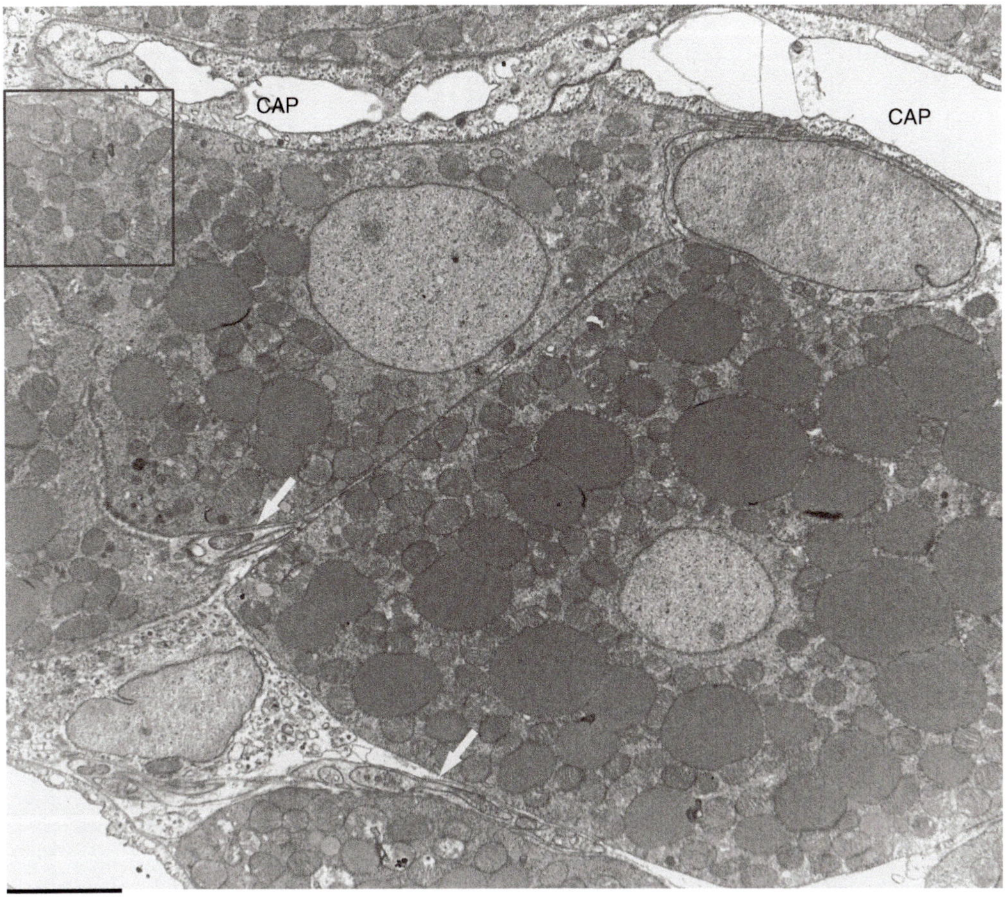

4.0 µm

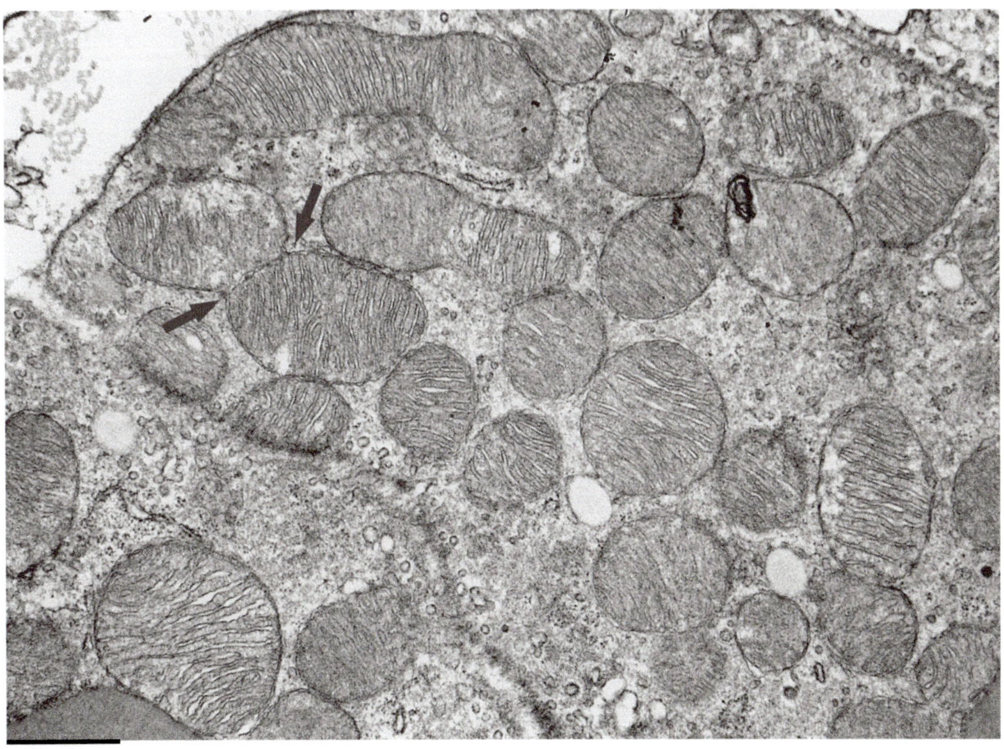

1.0 µm

Plate 2.33 Mediastinal BAT of young mouse. TEM

Human Brown Adipose Tissue

3

S. Cinti, *Obesity, Type 2 Diabetes and the Adipose Organ*, https://doi.org/10.1007/978-3-319-40522-3_3

3.1 Human Brown Adipose Tissue

PLATE 3.1

BAT in Adult Humans

The adipose organ of adult humans contains brown adipocytes. This data was known since many years, but received a worldwide interest when it was demonstrated by a radiologic technique (positron emission tomography, PET). This technique allowed detecting a metabolically active tissue, able to incorporate marked glucose in different amounts under different physiologic environmental conditions. This tissue have been proven to have the histology, electron microscopy, and UCP1 immunoreactivity similar to that of murine brown adipose tissue (BAT). The major site location for BAT in adult humans was described in the area of the adipose organ coincident with what we described in Plate 2.32 as the transition area between subcutaneous and visceral fat at the root of the neck. In our published and unpublished case series of about 50 adults, we were able to detect UCP1-immunoreactive brown adipocytes at the root of the neck (peri-subclavian artery or supraclavicular area) in all patients under 30, in about 25% of patients under 50, and rarely in patients over 60 years old. BAT-positive patients were mostly lean even though we detected BAT in two overweight patients, but never in obese patients. PET studies are in line with our immunohistochemistry data.

Perirenal fat is another major site for BAT in humans, and we found that about 50% of patients under 50 years old were positive for BAT at histology. Recently we found UCP1-immunoreactive BAT in older patients. In this plate UCP1-immunoreactive BAT from 79-year-old lean patients is shown (low magnification in the upper panel and high magnification in the lower panel). See also Plate 6.10 where UCP1-immunoreactive brown adipocytes are dispersed among white adipocytes of perirenal fat in an 83-year-old male, overweight, and diabetic (type 2) patient. In the middle right panel, a fresh pre-embedded tissue is visible. Multilocular cells are easily distinguishable from unilocular cells (some indicated: UL) (see also Plates 4.1 and 5.1 for details on pre-embedded morphology of fat).

Suggested Reading

Cinti S. The role of brown adipose tissue in human obesity. Nutr Metab Cardiovasc Dis. 16:569–74, 2006.

Nedergaard J, et al. Unexpected evidence for active brown adipose tissue in adult humans. Am J Physiol Endocrinol Met. 293:444–452, 2007.

Saito M, et al. High incidence of metabolically active brown adipose tissue in healthy adult humans: effects of cold exposure and adiposity. Diabetes. 58:1526–31, 2009.

Virtanen KA, et al. Functional brown adipose tissue in healthy adults. N Engl J Med. 360:1518–25, 2009.

Cypess AM, et al. Identification and importance of brown adipose tissue in adult humans. N Engl J Med. 360:1509–17, 2009.

van Marken Lichtenbelt WD, et al. Cold-activated brown adipose tissue in healthy men. N Engl J Med. 360:1500–8, 2009.

Vijgen GH, et al. Brown adipose tissue in morbidly obese subjects. PLoS One. 6:e17247, 2011.

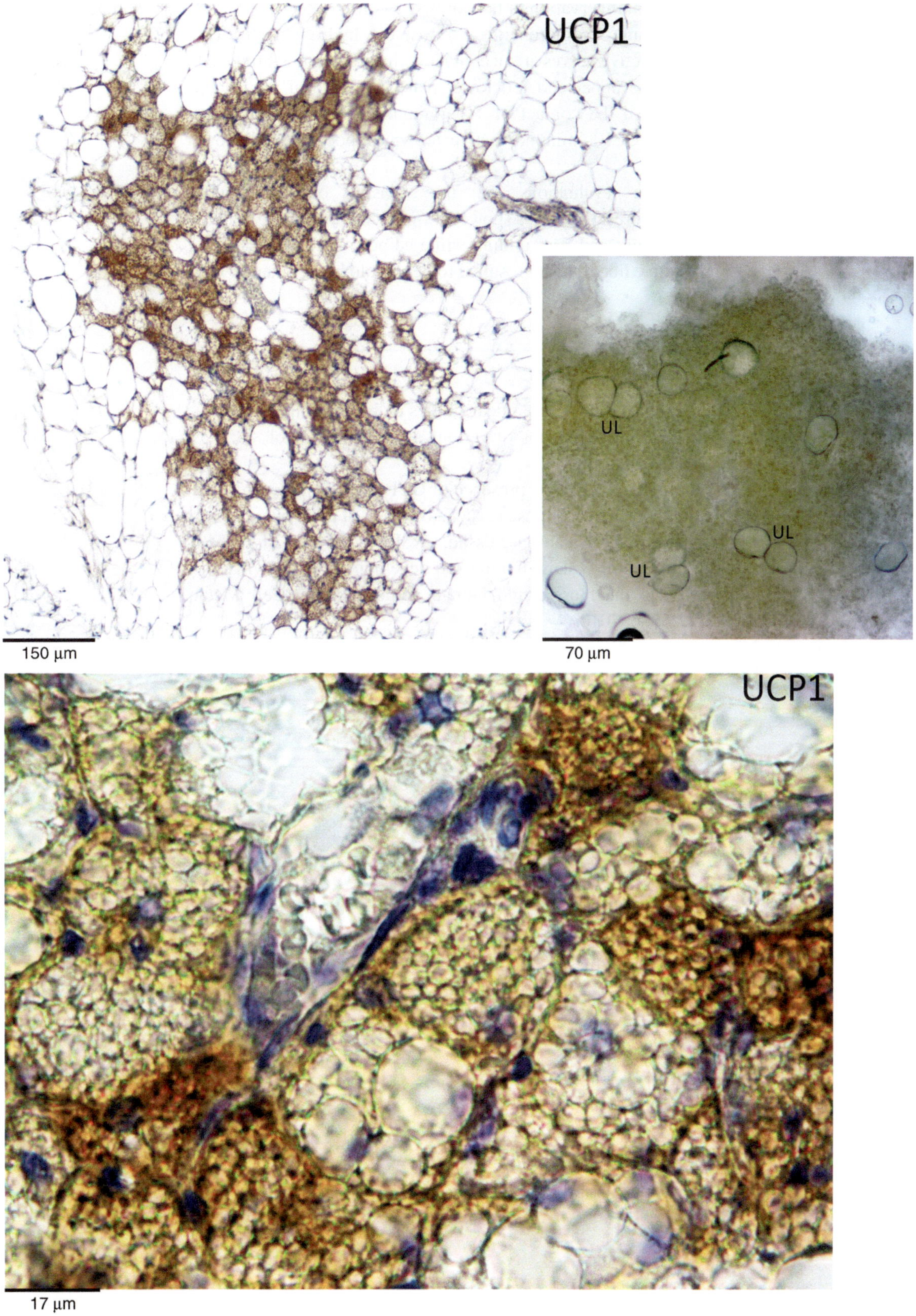

Plate 3.1 Human perirenal BAT from a 79-year-old female. IHC, UCP1 ab (1:500). LM. *Middle*: human BAT fresh tissue from the deep cervical peri-carotid area of an 18-year-old female. LM

PLATE 3.2

Parenchymal Nerves

Parenchymal innervation of human BAT is similar to that of murine BAT. Many noradrenergic tyrosine hydroxylase (TH)-immunoreactive nerves are in contact with parenchymal brown adipocytes (see upper and left lower panels). Confocal microscopy demonstrated the contact of TH-immunoreactive synaptic structures with UCP1-immunoreactive brown adipocytes (right lower panel).

Quantitative evaluations on the density of parenchymal TH-immunoreactive fibers showed a significant difference between the BAT areas and surrounding white adipose tissue (WAT). BAT TH-positive fiber density resulted to be tenfold higher than in WAT areas.

Suggested Reading

Ito T, et al. Arch Morphological studies on brown adipose tissue in the bat and in humans of various ages. Histol Cytol. 54:1–39, 1991.

Zingaretti MC, et al. The presence of UCP1 demonstrates that metabolically active adipose tissue in the neck of adult humans truly represents brown adipose tissue. FASEB J. 9:3113–20, 2009.

Frontini A, Cinti S. Distribution and development of brown adipocytes in the murine and human adipose organ. Cell Metab. 11:253–6, 2010.

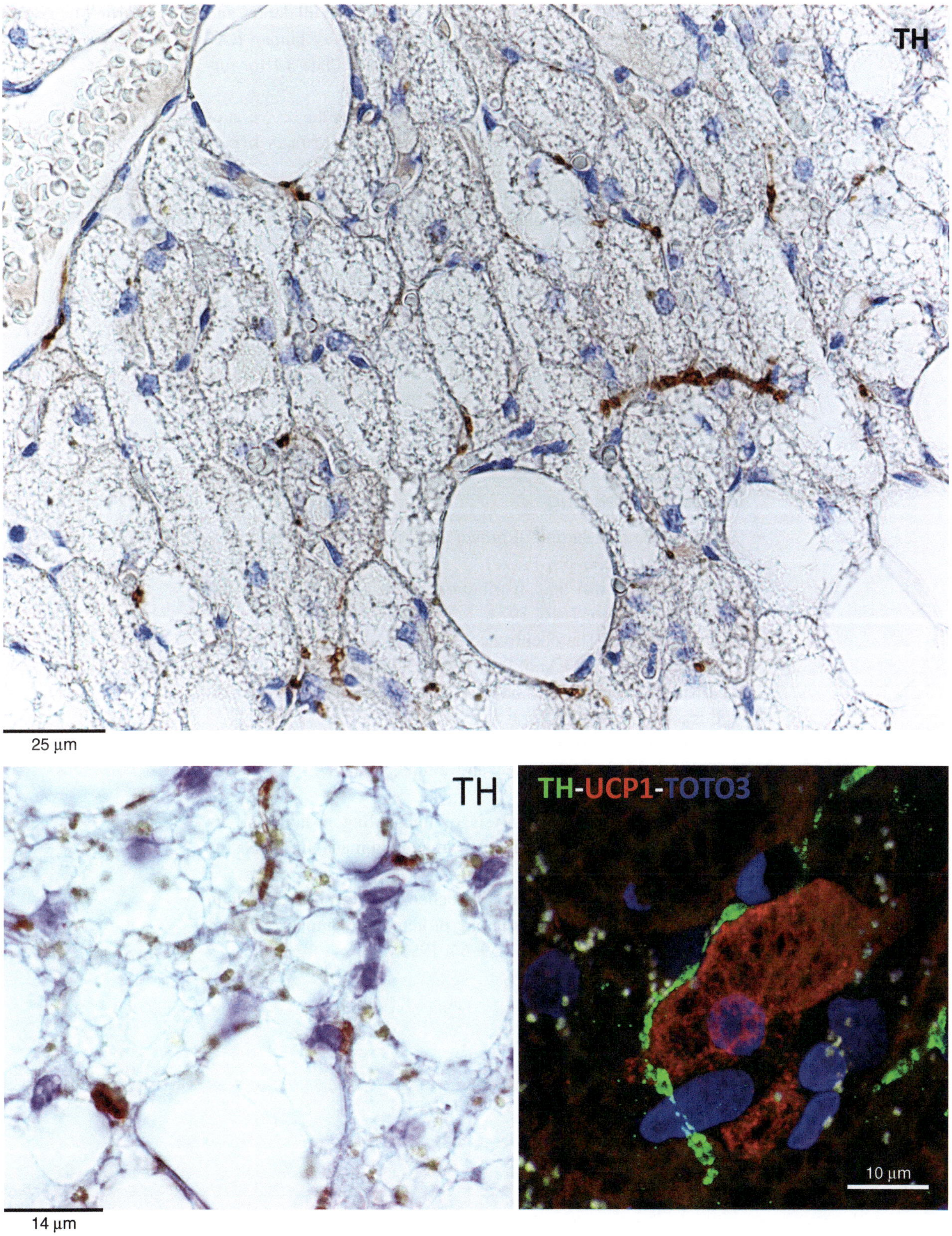

Plate 3.2 Human deep cervical perithyroid BAT of an 18-year-old female. *Lower left*: enlargement of the same tissue in the upper panel in a very densely innervated area. IHC, TH ab (1:600) LM. *Lower right*: double immunolabeling. Red, UCP1; green, TH; blue, TOTO3 (nuclei). Confocal light microscopy. Lower right panel from Smorlesi et al. The adipose organ: white-brown adipocyte plasticity and metabolic inflammation. Obesity Rev. Suppl 2 83–92, 2012, with permission

PLATE 3.3

Electron Microscopy

The ultrastructure of brown adipocytes is the same in all depots and is very similar across species. Low magnifications of human BAT from the deep cervical area (root of the neck; see Plate 3.1 for further details) are shown in this plate.
In the upper panel the BAT sample was collected on the occasion of a parathyroid biopsy performed during surgery for primary hyperparathyroidism on a 16-year-old girl.
In the lower panel a bioptic specimen was taken in occasion of a surgical intervention for goiter in an 18-year-old patient. Note the parenchymal nerve with unmyelinated fibers containing empty vesicles (V, inset: enlargement of the squared area) similar to those in murine BAT parenchymal fibers (compare with Plate 2.22).
In comparison with the electron microscopy of murine BAT presented in Chap. 2, the main difference consists in the abundance of lipofuscins in human brown adipocytes. Lipofuscins (Ly, some indicated) are visible in both patients of this plate (see Plate 5.7 for further discussion of this detail).

Suggested Reading

Heaton J. The distribution of brown adipose tissue in the human. J Anatomy. 112:35–39, 1972.

Merklin RJ. Growth and distribution of human fetal brown fat. Anat Rec. 178:637–46, 1973.

Huttunen P. et al. The occurrence of brown adipose tissue in outdoor workers. Eur J Appl Physiol. 46:339–45, 1981.

Bukowiecki LJ. In “Brown adipose tissue”, Trayhurn and Nichills Eds., Arnold, 1986.

Lean MEJ, et al. Brown adipose tissue uncoupling protein content in human infants, children and adults. Clin Sci. 71:291–97, 1986.

Garruti G, Ricquier D. Analysis of uncoupling protein and its mRNA in adipose tissue deposits of adult humans. Int J Obesity. 16:383–90, 1992.

Kortelainen ML, et al. Immunohistochemical detection of human brown adipose tissue uncoupling protein in an autopsy series. J Histochem Cytochem. 41:759–64, 1993.

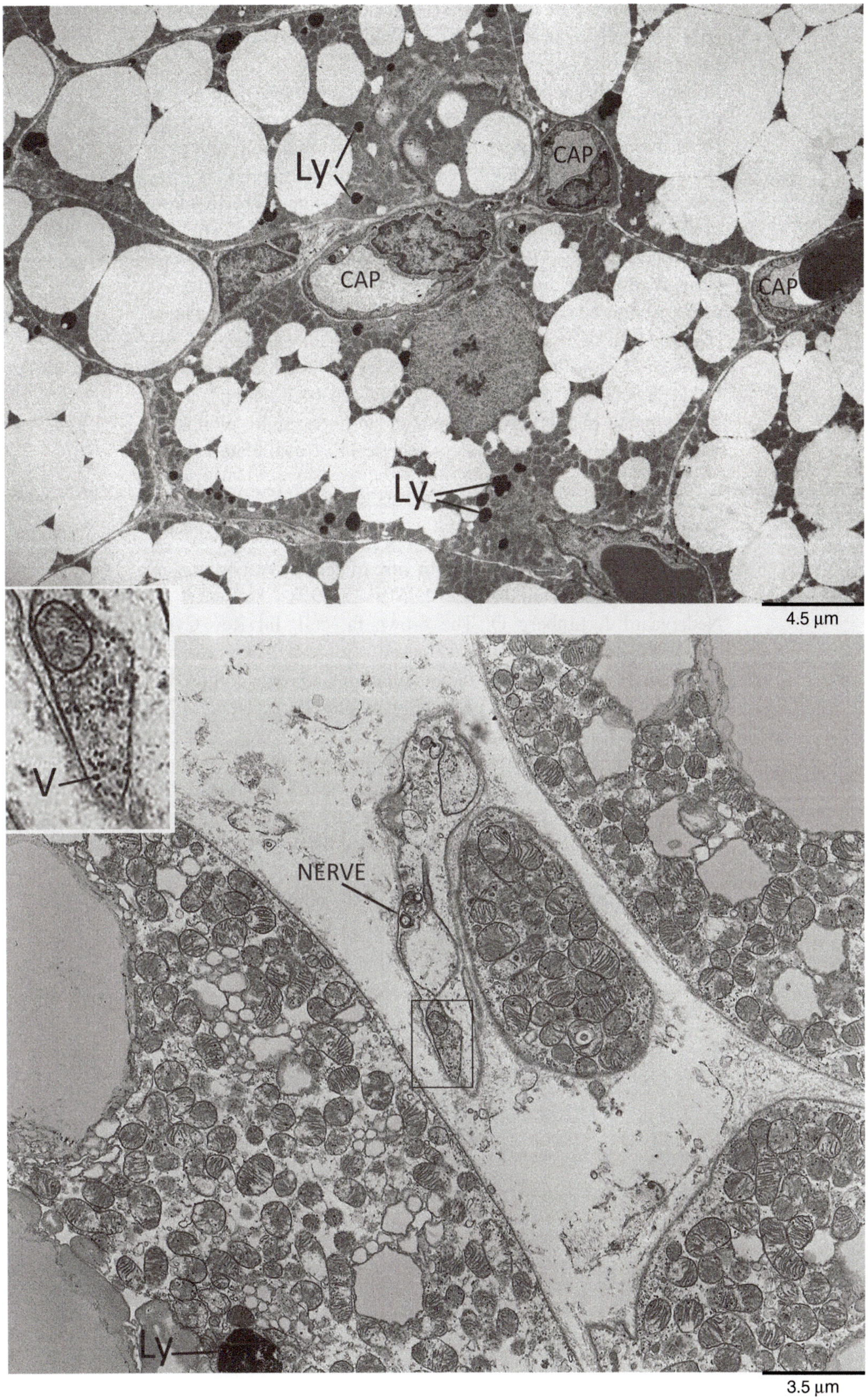

Plate 3.3 Human deep cervical perithyroid BAT of 16 (*upper*)- and 18 (*lower*)-year-old female subjects. CAP, capillary. TEM

PLATE 3.4

Mitochondria

The morphology of human BAT mitochondria is variable and is closely related to the stage of differentiation and the functional status of the brown adipocyte.

In mature brown adipocytes, the number and volume of mitochondria and the number of cristae per mitochondrion increase with the cell's thermogenic activity. Typical mitochondrial morphology is usually associated with UCP1 expression and thermogenesis.

An example of mitochondrial morphology of human brown adipocytes is shown in the upper figure (human sample described in Plate 3.3 upper panel). The mitochondrial morphology in this case strongly resembles that found in a brown adipocyte after 5 days of primary culture of a stromal-vascular fraction (SVF) from the interscapular BAT of a young mouse (shown in the lower panel). Thus, although close to the classic morphology of brown mitochondria found in murine BAT, this morphology can be described as not fully typical, mainly because mitochondria are quite elongated, with indentations, and not always spherical (see also Plate 3.3).

Suggested Reading

Dyer HM, Pirie BJS. The growth in vitro of newborn rat brown and white adipose tissue. J Anat. 125:519–25, 1978.

Nedergaard J, Linberg O. The brown fat cell. Int Rev Cytol. 74:187–286, 1982.

Bouillaud F, et al. Mitochondria of adult human brown adipose tissue contain a 32,000-Mr uncoupling protein. Biosci Rep. 3:775–80, 1983.

Cinti S, et al. Ultrastructure of brown adipocytes mitochondria in cell culture from explants. J Submicrosc Cytol. 18:625–27, 1986.

Ricquier D, Bouillaud F. In "Brown adipose tissue", Trayhurn and Nicholls Eds., Arnold, 86–104, 1986.

Cannon B, Nedergaard J. In "Biology of the adipocytes: research approach", Van Nostrand Reinhold Ed., J. Libbey, 21–51, 1987.

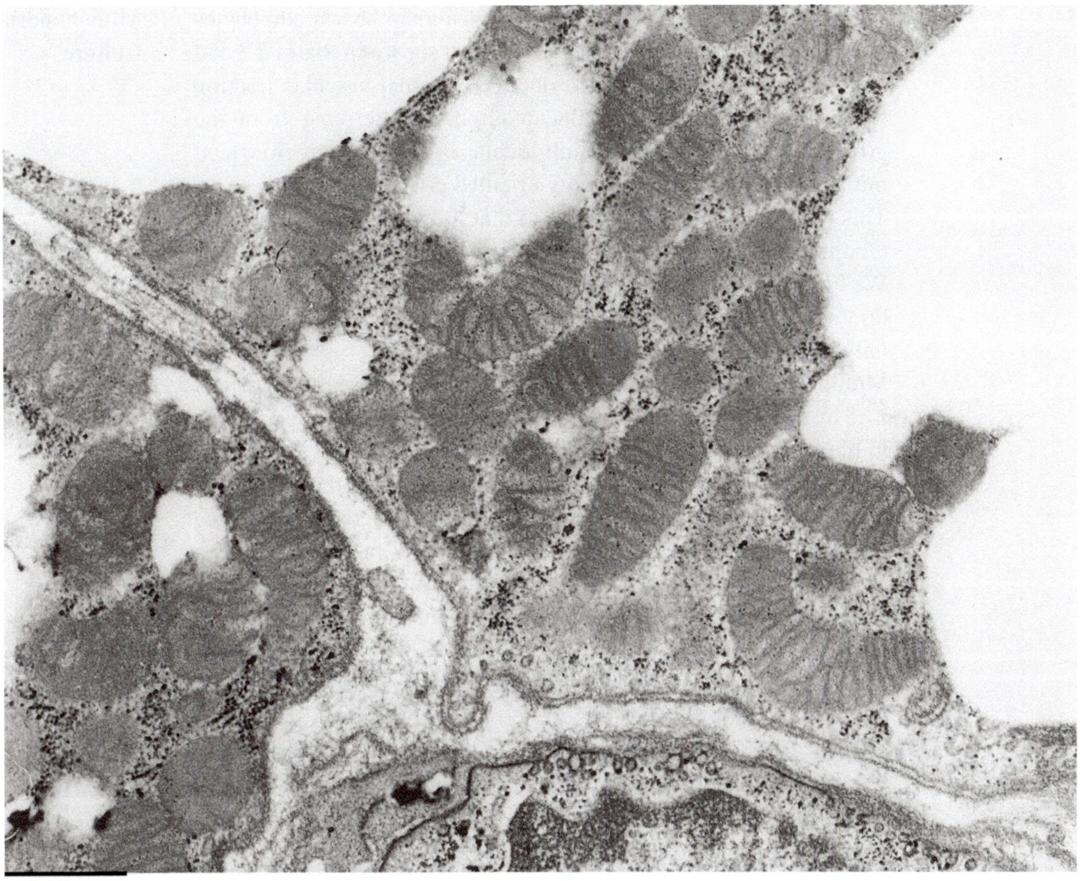

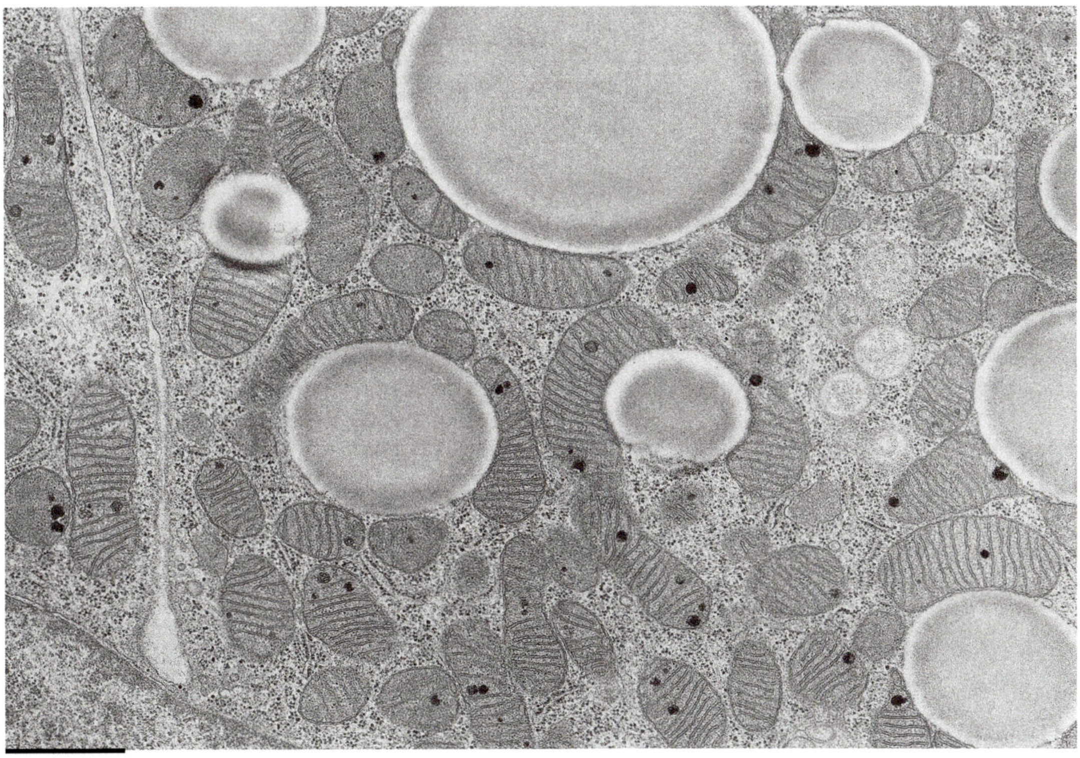

Plate 3.4 Human BAT mitochondria. *Upper*: human tissue. *Lower*: mouse brown adipocyte developing (day 5) in primary culture. TEM

PLATE 3.5

Mitochondria in Culture

The morphology of the mitochondria of human brown adipocytes in culture can differ considerably from that shown in Plates 2.3 and 2.4. When rat BAT is used to obtain a stromal-vascular fraction (SVF), the mature post-confluent adipocytes deriving from the growth of SVF cells have a multilocular lipid depot but elongated mitochondria with few randomly oriented cristae.

This morphology is quite similar to that found in white adipocytes ("nontypical" mitochondria).

We found typical (fully differentiated) and "nontypical" mitochondria in the same cell (post-confluent lipid-laden mature adipocyte) only in human brown adipocytes in vitro.

Multiple symmetric lipomatosis (MSL) is a rare disease characterized by the presence of fat masses symmetrically distributed mainly in the upper part of the body in areas corresponding to anatomical sites for BAT in newborns. Several data suggest that the symmetric fat masses are derived from the proliferation of altered BAT. In cultured adipocytes developed from the SVF of fat biopsied from MSL patients, we observed typical and nontypical brown mitochondria similar to those shown in this plate. Interestingly, some mitochondria with transition aspects (i.e., with a mixed morphology, in part typical and in part nontypical) were found in vitro both in normal human brown adipocytes (upper right panel) and in adipocytes from MSL patients. Similar mixed mitochondria were found in brown adipocytes in the omentum of patients suffering from pheochromocytoma (see Plates 7.20–7.21).

Suggested Reading

Nèchad M, et al. Development of brown fat cells in monolayer culture. I. Morphological and biochemical distinction from white fat cells in culture. Exp Cell Res. 149:105–18, 1983.

Nèchad M. Development of brown fat cells in monolayer culture. II. Ultrastructural characterization of precursors, differentiating adipocytes and their mitochondria. Exp Cell Res. 149:119–27, 1983.

Cinti S, et al. Ultrastructural features of cultured mature adipocyte precursors from adipose tissue in multiple symmetric lipomatosis. Ultrastruct Pathol. 5:145–52, 1983.

Cigolini M, et al. Human brown adipose cells in culture. Exp Cell Res. 159:261–66, 1985.

Cigolini M, et al. Isolation and ultrastructural features of brown adipocytes in culture. J Anat. 145:207–216, 1986.

Cinti S, et al. Effects of noradrenaline exposure on rat brown adipocytes in cultures. An ultrastructural study. Tiss Cell. 19:809–16, 1987.

Kopecky J, et al. Synthesis of mitochondrial uncoupling protein in brown adipocytes differentiated in cell culture. J Biol Chem. 265:22204–09, 1990.

Rehnmark S, Nedergaard J. Alpha- and beta-adrenergic induction of the expression of the uncoupling protein thermogenin in brown adipocytes differentiated in culture. J Biol Chem. 265:16464–71, 1990.

Zancanaro C, et al. Multiple symmetric lipomatosis. Ultrastructural investigation of the tissue and preadipocytes in primary culture. Lab Invest. 63:253–8, 1990.

Klaus S, et al. Development of Phodopus sungorus brown preadipocytes in primary cell culture: effect of an atypical beta-adrenergic agonist, insulin, and triiodothyronine on differentiation, mitochondrial development, and expression of the uncoupling protein UCP. J Cell Biol. 115:1783–90, 1991.

Enzi G, et al. Multiple symmetric lipomatosis: a rare disease and its possible links to brown adipose tissue. Nutr Metab Cardiovasc Dis. 25:347–53, 2015.

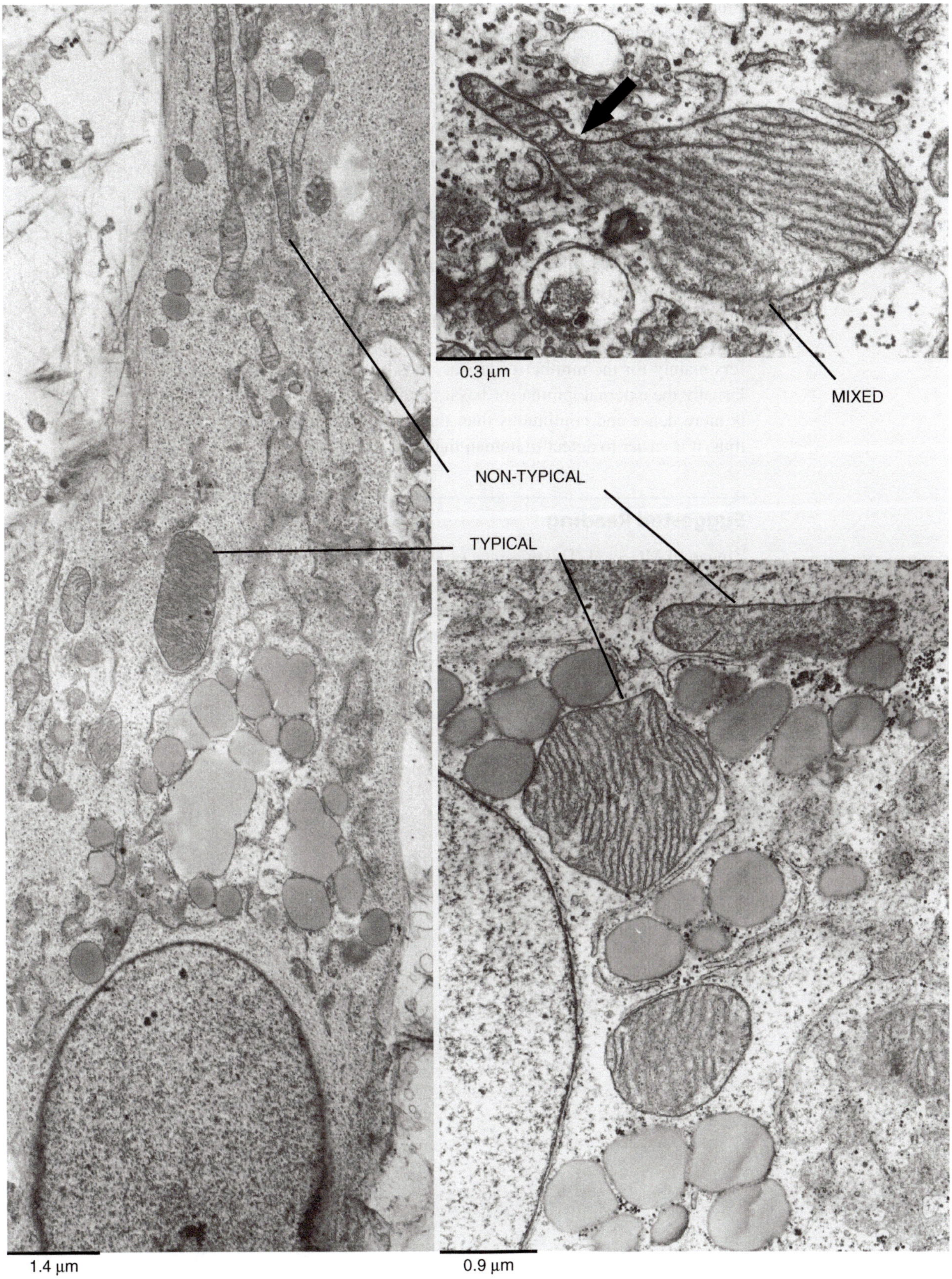

Plate 3.5 Human brown adipocytes in primary culture. Typical and nontypical mitochondria in the same cell. *Upper right*: human brown adipocyte in culture with mixed morphology. The nontypical part is on the left of the arrow, the typical part on the right. Upper right panel from Cigolini M et al. Human brown adipose cells in culture. Exp Cell Res 159:261–6, 1985, with permission. TEM

PLATE 3.6

Preadipocytes

Preadipocytes, with all the ultrastructural characteristics described for BAT murine preadipocytes that allow an easy detection of this cell type by TEM, are present also in human BAT. Their frequency is quite high, and our quantitative analyses revealed that they could be found in every 5–10 capillaries (typical site where preadipocytes are present; see Plates 2.26–2.28).

In this plate a preadipocyte from human BAT is shown in its typical pericapillary site (squared area in the upper panel). In the lower panel an enlargement of the squared area is visible. Note the numerous large "pre-typical" mitochondria (for details, see the above-mentioned murine plates), glycogen granules, and a distinct external lamina (EL). Note that the morphology of "pre-typical" mitochondria in preadipocyte (m) and typical mitochondria in mature brown adipocytes (lower left corner of the lower panel) differs mainly for the number of cristae, but the size is very similar. Usually the external lamina (or basal membrane) of preadipocytes is more dense and continuous than that of murine preadipocytes; thus, it is easier to detect in human than in murine BAT.

Suggested Reading

Zingaretti MC, et al. The presence of UCP1 demonstrates that metabolically active adipose tissue in the neck of adult humans truly represents brown adipose tissue. FASEB J. 9:3113–20.

Xue R, et al. Clonal analyses and gene profiling identify genetic biomarkers of the thermogenic potential of human brown and white preadipocytes. Nat Med. 21:760–8, 2015.

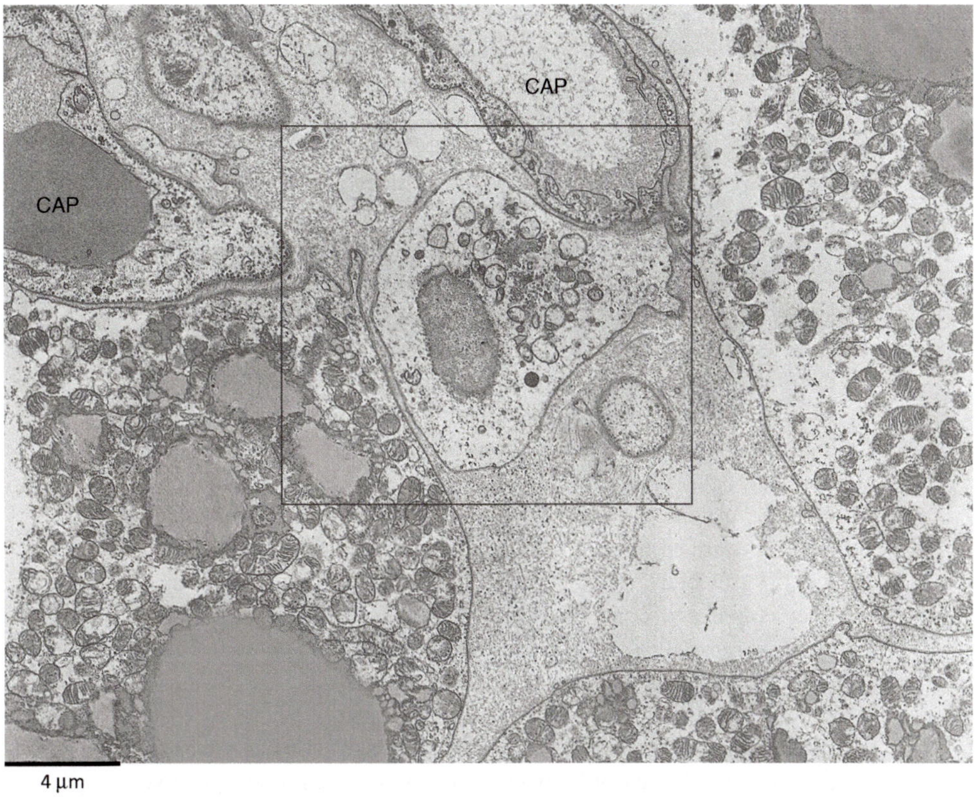

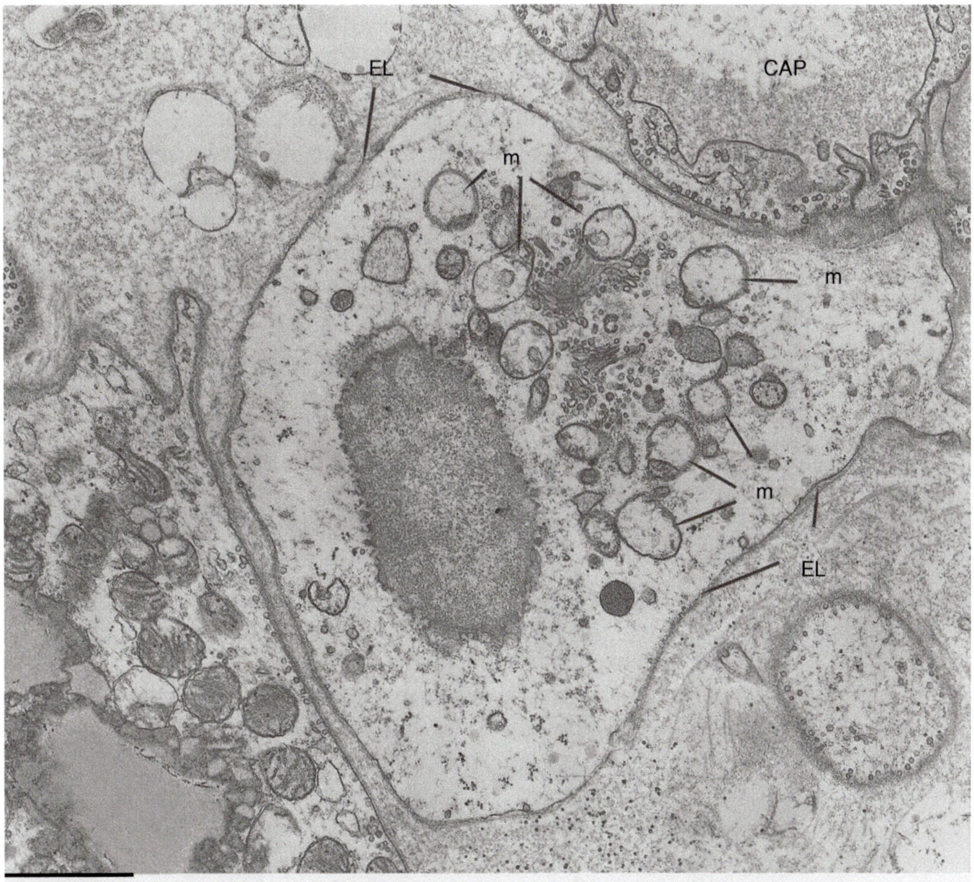

Plate 3.6 Human adult (18-year-old female) BAT preadipocyte. CAP, capillary; m, "pre-typical" mitochondria. TEM

PLATE 3.7

Hibernoma Histology and IHC: UCP1

Hibernomas are benign neoplasms of BAT that reproduce the steps of normal development, enhanced by the neoplastic nature of the tissue. This offers an opportunity to explore some developmental aspects of human adult BAT. In this plate the typical light microscopic appearance of a hibernoma that we recently studied is shown. Most cells of the tumor were multilocular, but the fine morphology and immunostaining (UCP1) were not homogeneous. The smaller cells were intensely UCP1 immunoreactive and showed smaller lipid droplets. Larger cells presented larger lipid droplets and resulted less UCP1 immunoreactive. The largest multilocular cells and unilocular cells (asterisks) were UCP1 negative. These data are in line with the different phenotype of brown adipocytes found in different experimental conditions (see chapters of mixed-, cold-, and warm-acclimated adipose organ) and suggest a possible developmental evolution of the neoplastic cells in hibernoma. One of the most intense UCP1-immunoreactive adipocytes (squared area) is enlarged in the lower left panel. Interestingly this patient lost 5 kg of body weight in the 2 months preceding the surgical intervention and coincident with the clinical appearance of the tumor in line with a possible energy dispersion due to brown adipocyte hyperactivity.

In murine and human adipose organ, the density of noradrenergic parenchymal fibers (TH-immunoreactive fibers) is usually associated with the density of brown adipocytes, and we found a positive correlation between the density of TH-immunoreactive fibers and proportion of UCP1-positive brown adipocytes in different areas of the adipose organ of mice under different experimental conditions (see also chapter on cold-acclimated adipose organ).

In this hibernoma we found only a few TH-immunoreactive fibers (arrow in bottom right panel) in spite of the massive proportion of brown adipocytes versus white adipocytes. The scarce innervation can tentatively be explained by the non-physiologic nature of the tissue. Its neoplastic developmental properties are probably almost totally unlinked to the development of noradrenergic nerve fibers.

Suggested Reading

Allegra SR, et al. Endocrine activity in a large hibernoma. Hum Pathol. 14:1044–52, 1983.

Manieri M, et al. Morphological and immunohistochemical features of brown adipocytes and preadipocytes in a case of human hibernoma. Nutr Metab Cardiovasc Dis. 20:567–74, 2010.

Zancanaro C, et al. Immunohistochemical identification of the uncoupling protein in human hibernoma. Biol Cell. 80:75–8.

Murano I, et al. Noradrenergic parenchymal nerve fiber branching after cold acclimatization correlates with brown adipocyte density in mouse adipose organ. J Anat. 214:171–8, 2009.

Vitali A, et al. The adipose organ of obesity-prone C57BL/6J mice is composed of mixed white and brown adipocytes. J Lipid Res. 53:619–29, 2012.

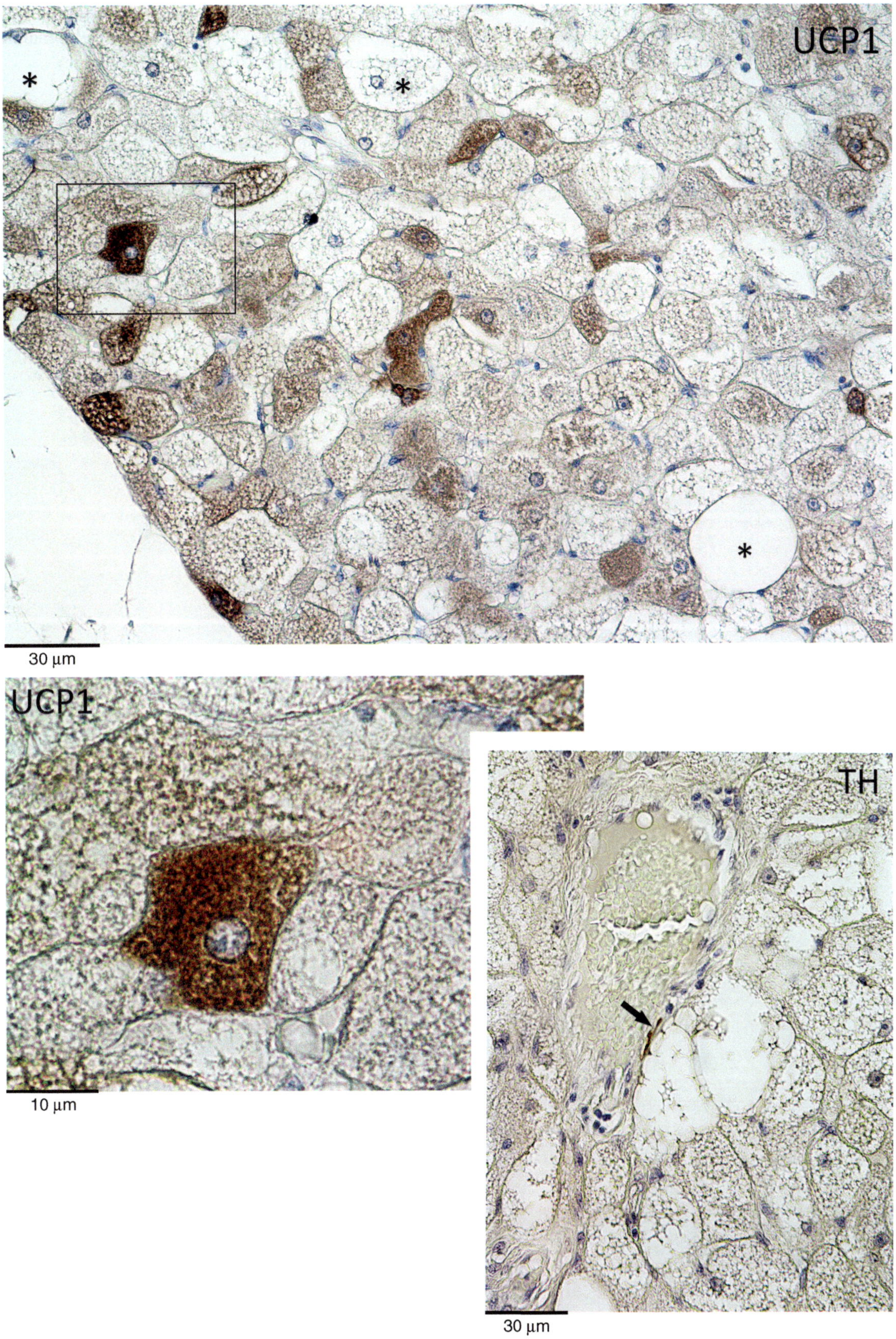

Plate 3.7 Hibernoma excised from rib cage of a 17-year-old male. IHC UCP1 ab (1:4,000) and TH ab (1:300). LM

PLATE 3.8

Hibernoma EM I (Developmental Aspects)

The ultrastructure of brown adipocytes (same hibernoma of previous plate) at low magnification level is shown in this plate. The four adipocytes (beige in the scheme) in close contact with a capillary (red in the scheme) exhibit smaller lipid droplets in comparison with surrounding brown adipocytes (brown in the scheme). Because the usual source for new adipocytes is the niche of vascular walls, it is probable that the cells in contact with the capillary wall represent early-differentiated stages of the neoplastic cells.

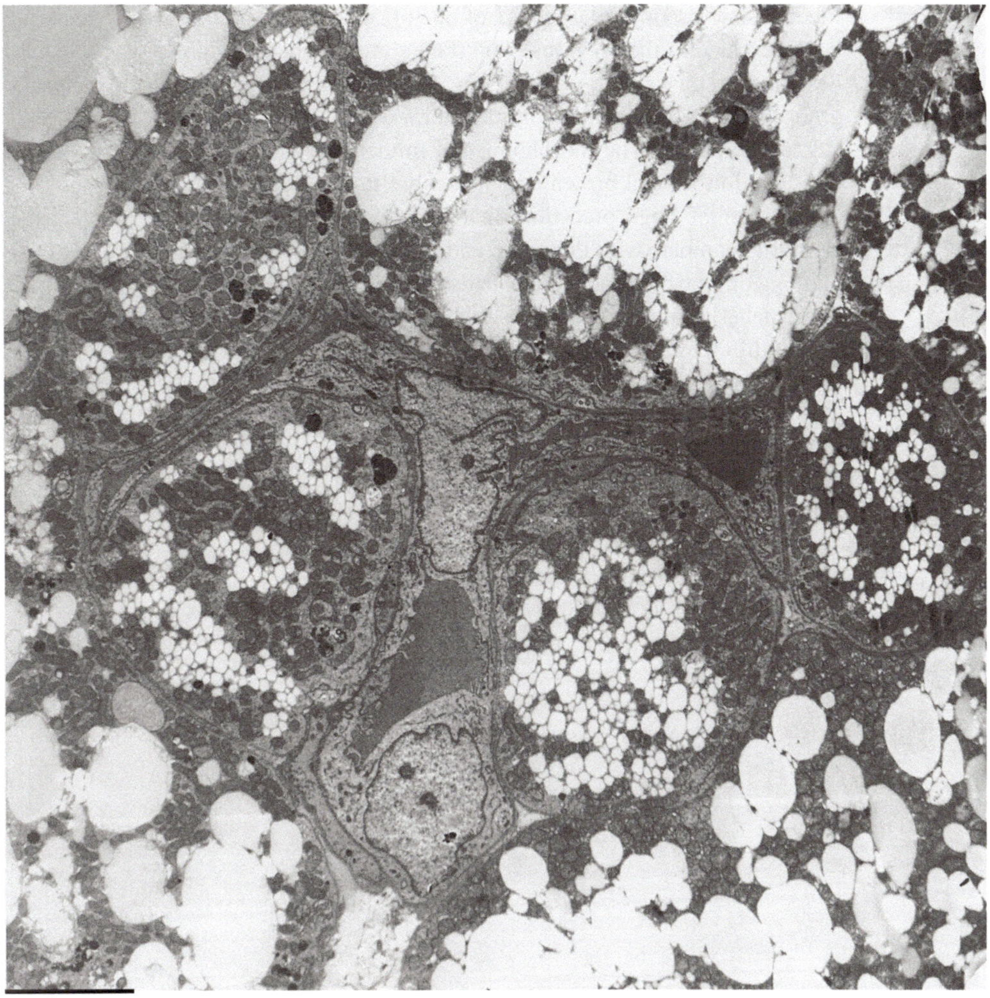

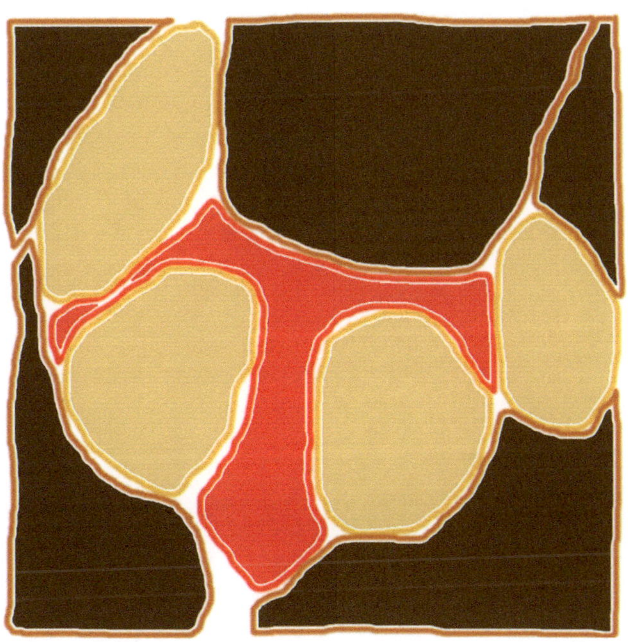

Plate 3.8 Ultrastructure of brown adipocytes in hibernoma (same of Plate 3.7). TEM

PLATE 3.9

Hibernoma EM II (Developmental Aspects)

Electron microscopy enlargement of one of cells close to the capillary presented in the previous plate (beige in the scheme of previous plate) is shown in the present plate. Note the small lipid droplets grouped among the abundant mitochondria and lipofuscin granules (Ly, upper panel). The morphology of mitochondria is similar to that found in normal brown adipocytes but in this cell seems in a developmental stage preceding that of fully differentiated mitochondria (compare with Plates 3.5 and 3.10). Interestingly the morphology of mitochondria in these cells (squared area enlarged in the lower panel) resembles those described in Plates 2.28 and 2.29 for poorly differentiated mitochondria of brown adipocyte precursors. In particular indentations (green arrows) of mitochondria producing "pseudo-holes" (red arrows) are well visible here.

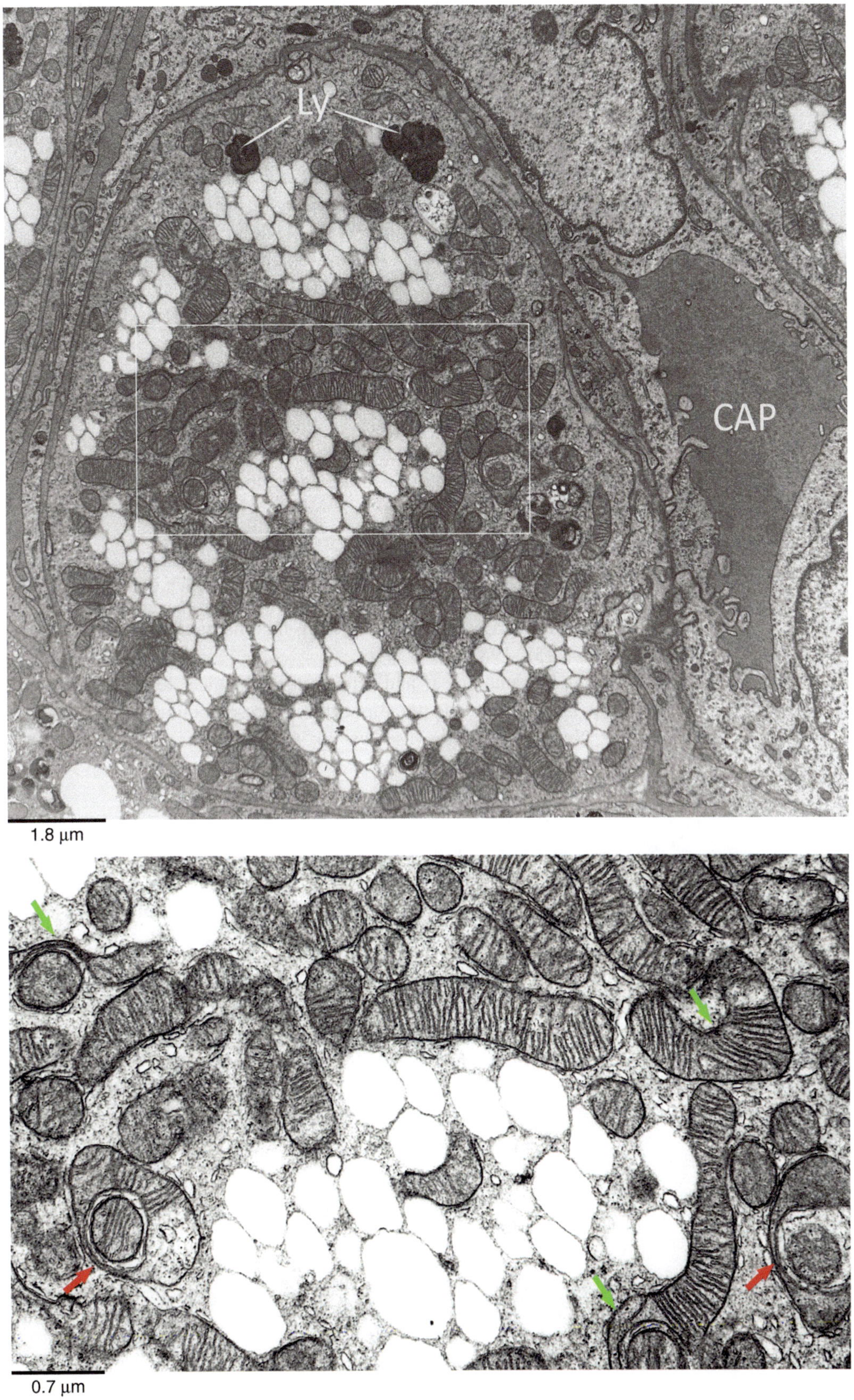

Plate 3.9 Enlargement of a pericapillary cell represented in beige in the scheme of Plate 3.8. *Lower*: enlargement of the squared area in the upper panel. CAP, capillary. TEM

PLATE 3.10

Hibernoma EM III (Endocrine Aspects)

Some brown adipocytes showed a more differentiated morphology than that of the cell presented in the previous plates. The more differentiated developmental stage is supported by the different morphology of mitochondria. Here they are more regularly spherical and packed with laminar cristae (compare with fully differentiated mitochondria in human brown adipocytes developed in culture, Plate 3.5, and with murine BAT mitochondria, Plate 2.3).

The squared area in the upper panel is enlarged in the lower panel. In this area a hypertrophic Golgi complex is visible. It is rare to find such a well-developed Golgi complex in a brown adipocyte, even in adrenergically stimulated brown adipocytes. Furthermore, this Golgi complex area is very rich in medium-dense granules resembling those described in the murine brown adipocytes as endocrine secretory granules for their morphology and size (see Plate 2.7). These data suggest that the cell presented in this plate is a fully differentiated brown adipocyte with intense endocrine activity and that presented in the previous plate is a poorly differentiated brown adipocyte. Other authors have described the endocrine activity of hibernoma also.

Suggested Reading

Allegra SR, et al. Endocrine activity in a large hibernoma. Hum Pathol. 14:1044–52, 1983.

Manieri M, et al. Morphological and immunohistochemical features of brown adipocytes and preadipocytes in a case of human hibernoma. Nutr Metab Cardiovasc Dis. 20:567–74, 2010.

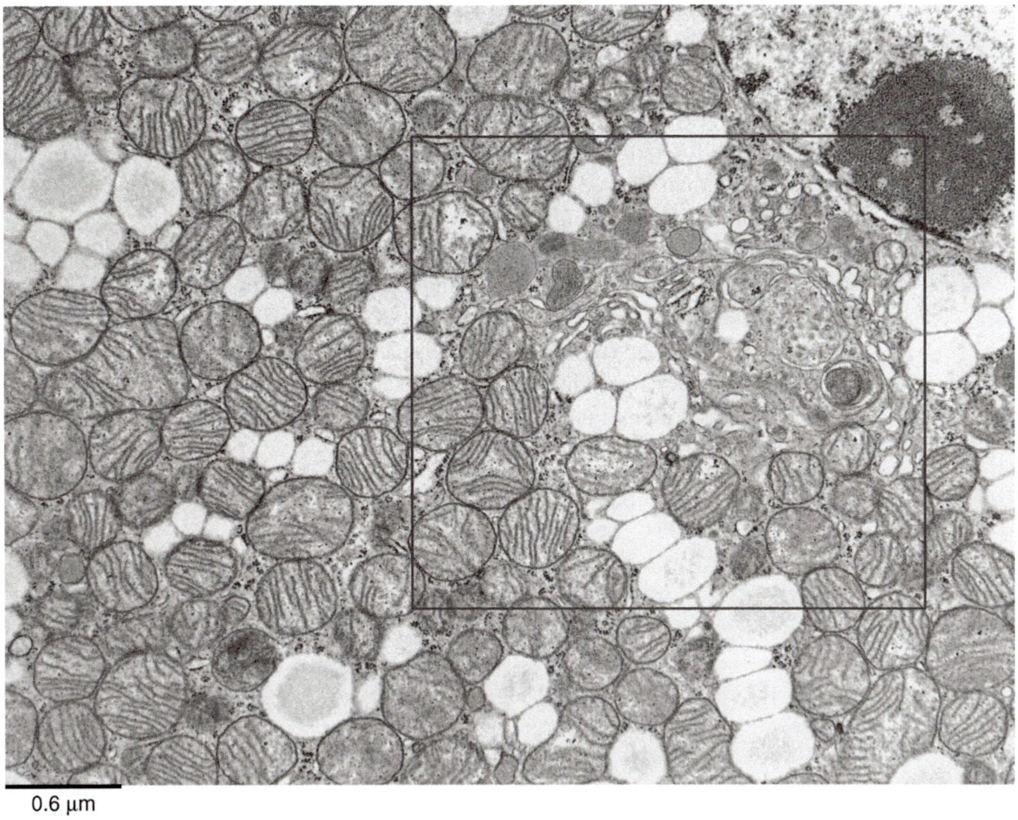

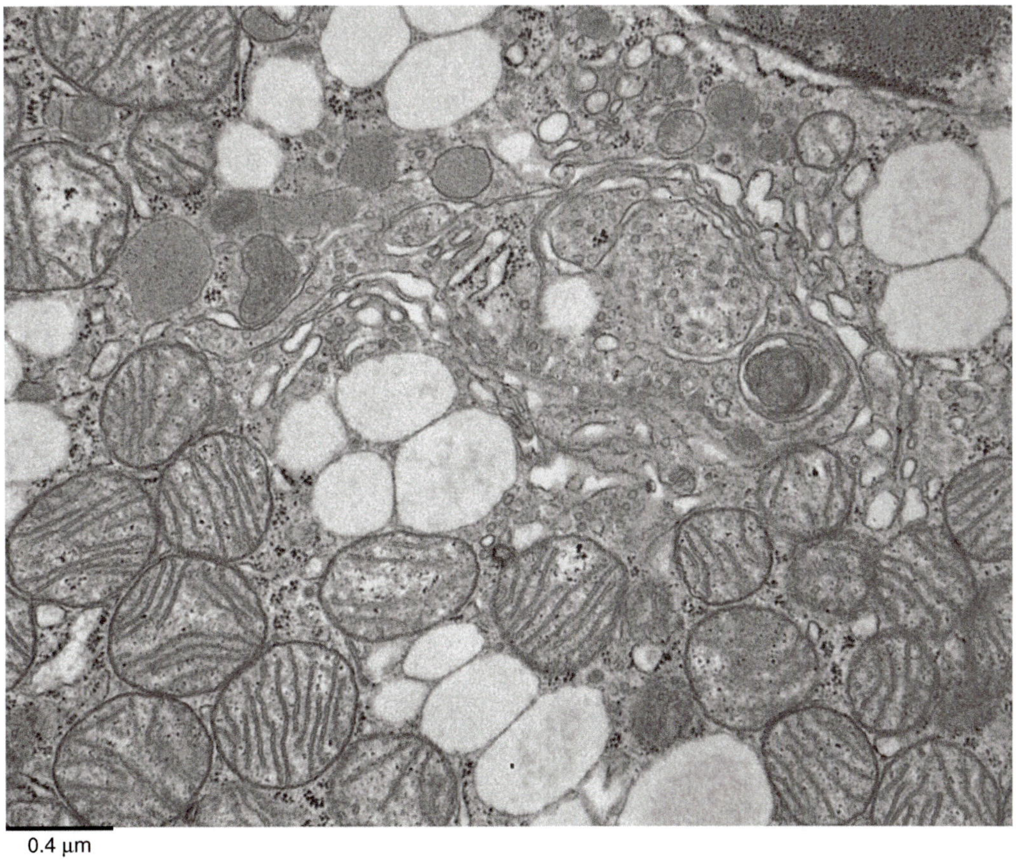

Plate 3.10 Differentiated brown adipocyte in hibernoma with endocrine aspects (same of Plate 3.7). TEM

PLATE 3.11

Hibernoma
Preadipocytes I

Preadipocytes were frequently found in this hibernoma. Our calculations showed a frequency of about sixfold higher than that in normal human BAT, in line with an accelerated developmental biology in neoplastic tissues. The morphology of adipoblast-preadipocyte (see Chap. 2 for details) was similar to that found in normal BAT. Most of them formed cytoplasmic projections included in the doubling of the basal membrane of capillaries (top left panel). Some appeared in a "detaching position," i.e., located with a pole still in contact with the capillary wall and with the other pole projecting to the interstitial space (top right and lower panels). The squared area in the top right panel is enlarged in the bottom panel. The main characteristic features are their location inside doubling of capillary basal membrane, "pre-typical" abundant mitochondria (m), and glycogen particles (G).

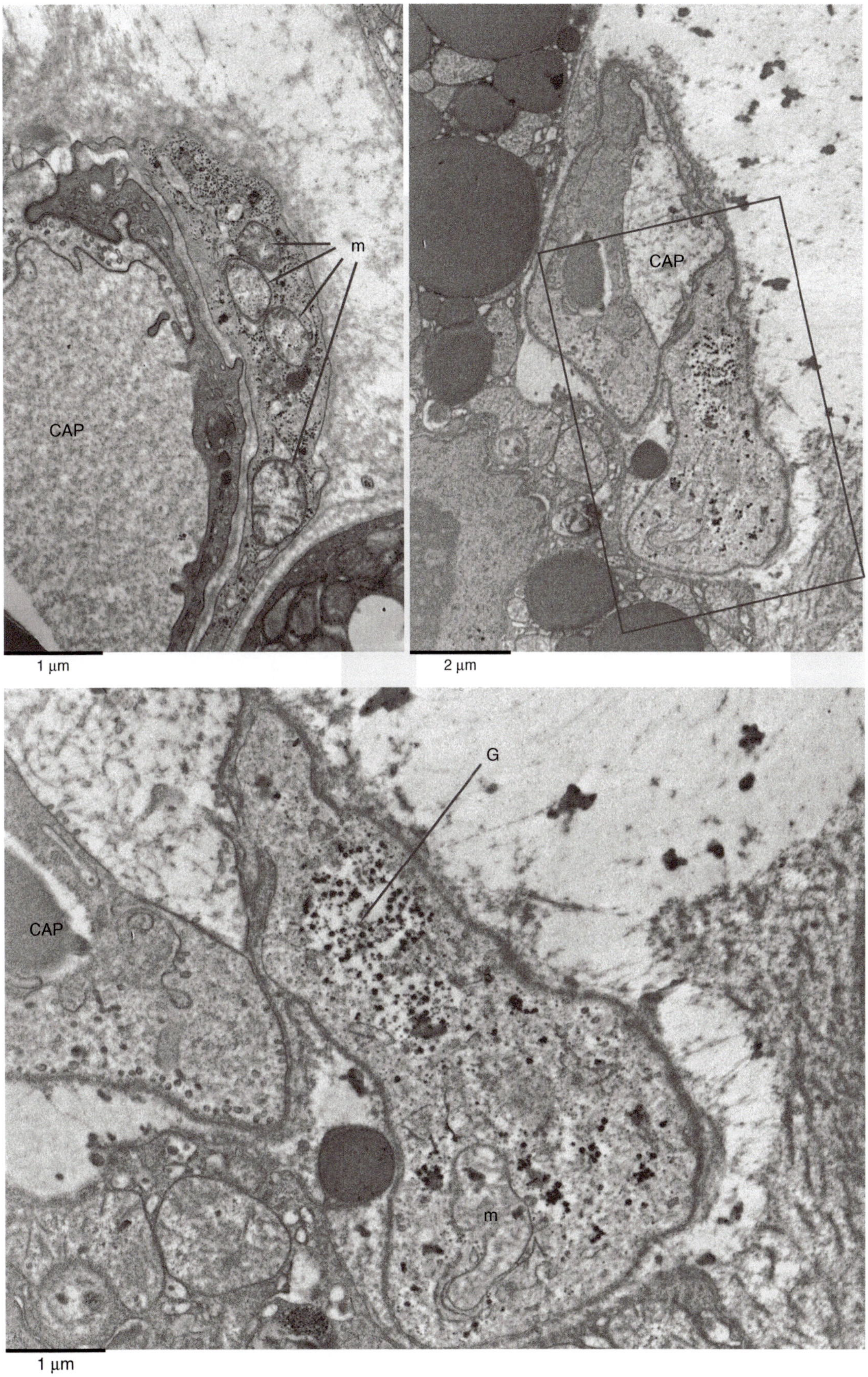

Plate 3.11 Preadipocytes in hibernoma (same of Plate 3.7). CAP, capillary. TEM

PLATE 3.12

Hibernoma
Preadipocytes II

In this plate a preadipocyte (a cell with the ultrastructure suggesting its possible brown preadipocyte nature) in pericyte position in the wall of a capillary (CAP) is visible (squared area, enlarged in the lower panel). Note the nucleus (N) that is not frequently observed in these cells, probably because of their stellate morphology as suggested by some authors.
Note the presence of distinctive features such as external lamina (EL), glycogen particles in the cytoplasm (G), and a "pre-typical" mitochondrion (m).

Suggested Reading

Manieri M, et al. Morphological and immunohistochemical features of brown adipocytes and preadipocytes in a case of human hibernoma. Nutr Metab Cardiovasc Dis. 20:567–74, 2010.
Maumus M, et al. Native human adipose stromal cells: localization, morphology and phenotype. Int J Obes. 35:1141–53, 2011.
Lee YH, et al. Identification of an adipogenic niche for adipose tissue remodeling and restoration. Cell Metab. 18:355–67, 2013.

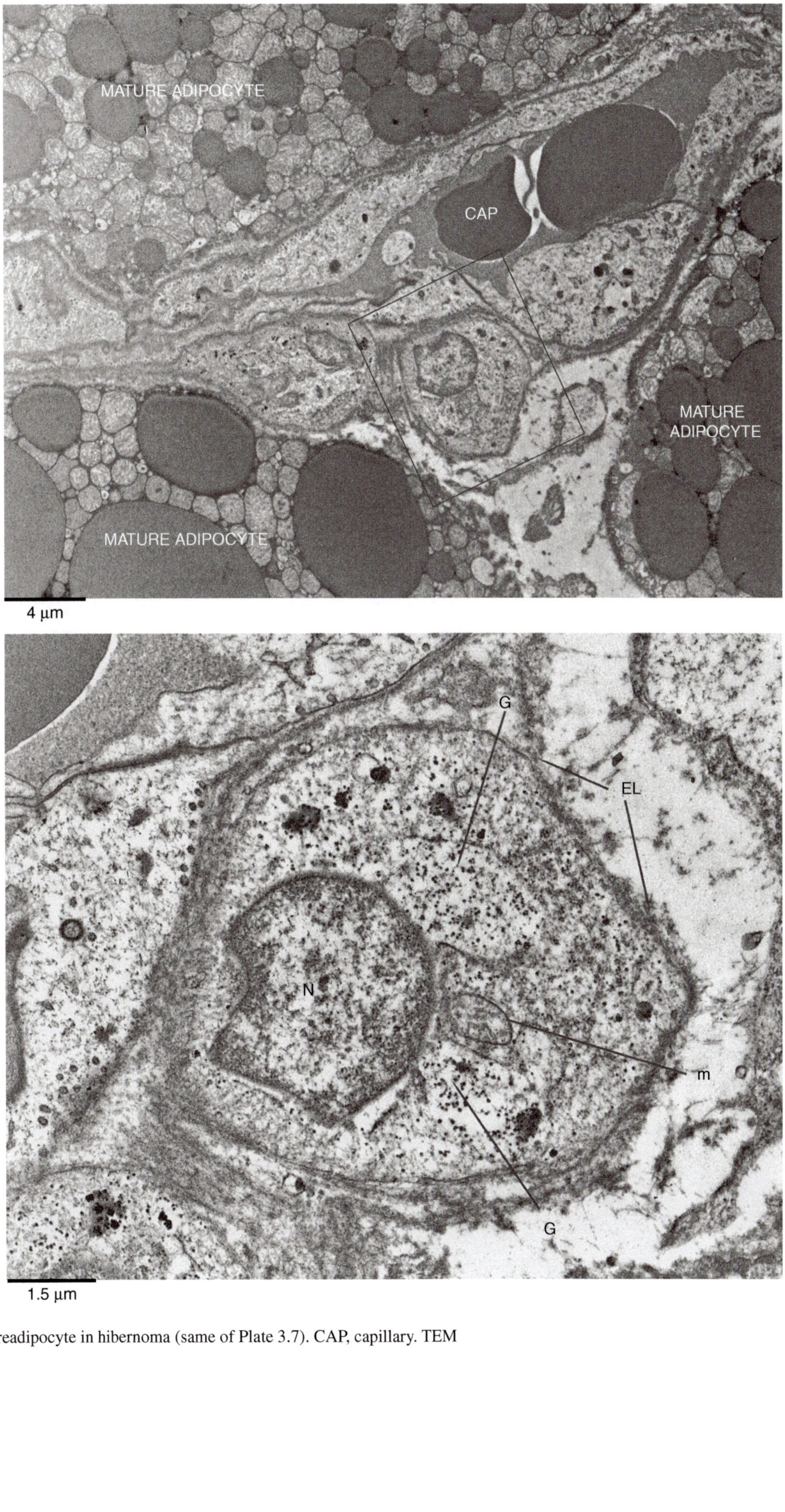

Plate 3.12 Preadipocyte in hibernoma (same of Plate 3.7). CAP, capillary. TEM

4 WAT Murine

S. Cinti, *Obesity, Type 2 Diabetes and the Adipose Organ*, https://doi.org/10.1007/978-3-319-40522-3_4

4.1 WAT Murine

PLATE 4.1

Pre-embedded WAT

Thin parts of adipose organ, fresh or fixed, can be observed at light microscopy before further processing (embedding). In this plate two examples are shown. In the upper plate the external area of a fat lobule from the epididymal fat of a young mouse is shown. Note the extremely regular size of the cells without any artifact due to the embedding procedure. The size of adipocytes in fresh samples is about 20–30% larger than that measured in sections of tissue routinely processed for light microscopy.
In the bottom panel a lobule of omental fat sampled from a young mouse is shown. Interestingly the vasculature tree is well visible and marked in red by the red blood cells. Peripheral branches of vessels are smaller and tightly connected to small adipocytes in line with the well-known correlative relationships between these structures during adipogenesis.

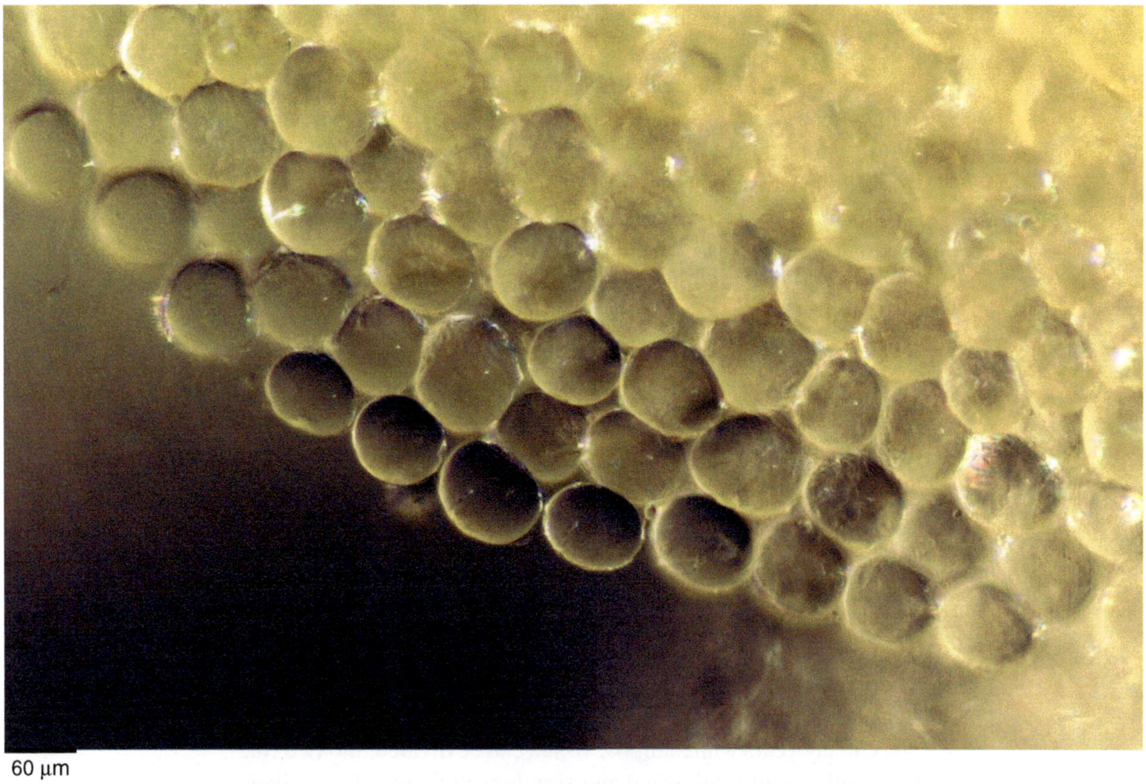

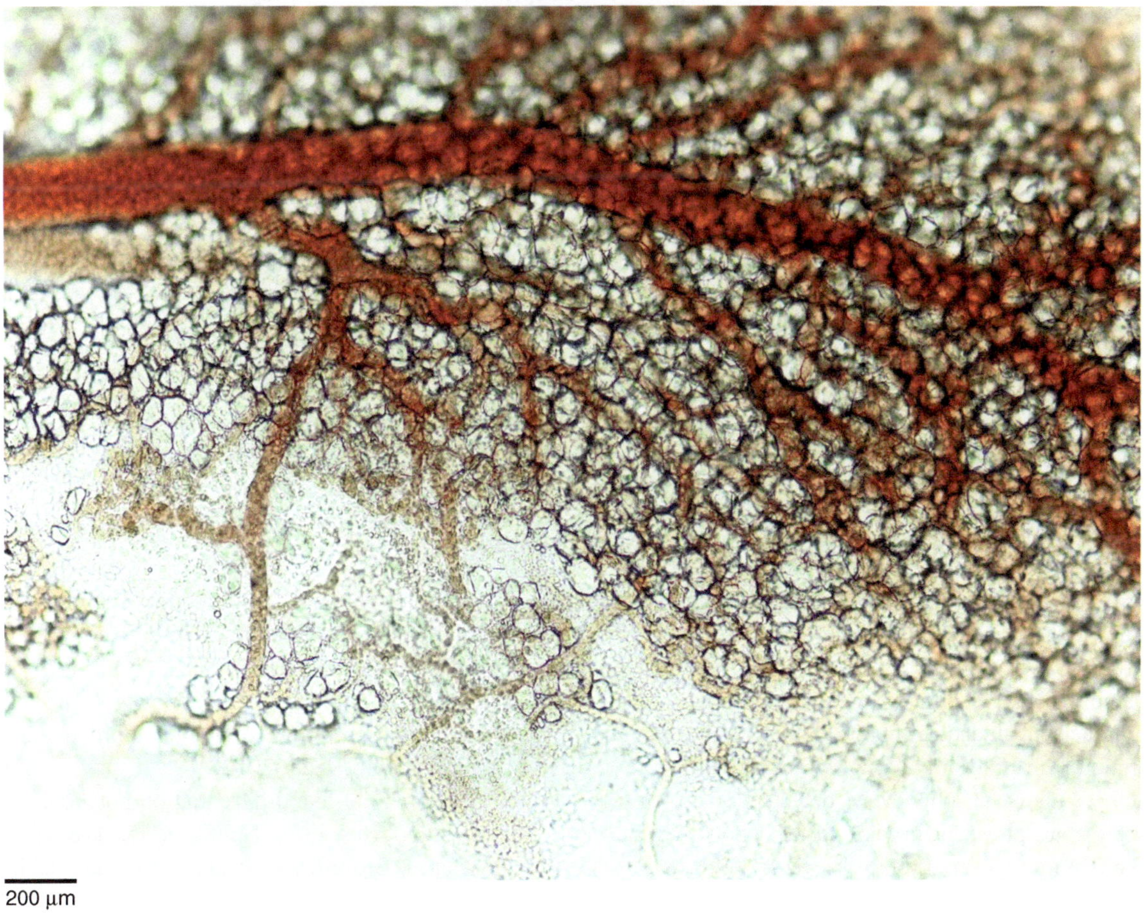

Plate 4.1 Fresh unstained epididymal (*upper*) and omental (*lower*) WAT from young mice. LM

PLATE 4.2

Histology and Cytology of Mature White Adipocytes

The white areas of the adipose organ are constituted of white adipose tissue (WAT). The histology of this tissue is similar in several species (compare with plates in Chap. 5) and shown in the upper panel. White adipocytes are spherical because this shape allows the maximum volume in the minimum space. This is therefore the ideal shape for a cell storing the most important source of energy for the organism. A single lipid droplet surrounded by a thin rim of cytoplasm occupies most of the cell volume. The nucleus is pushed to the periphery. At the light microscopy level, capillaries can be seen running among adipocytes. The size of white adipocytes varies with species, type of depot, nutritional state, and environmental conditions. The adipocytes of subcutaneous depots in B6 mice maintained in standard conditions, chow diet and 22–24 °C (peripheral inguinal area, about 2000–3000 microns square), are usually larger than those of visceral depots (mesenteric, 1000–2300 microns square). Of note, the size of white adipocytes is usually very different also in a specific depot; thus, for example, the size in inguinal subcutaneous depot is smaller in the peri-lymph node area than in the peripheral area. In visceral depots it is smaller in mesenteric than in epididymal depot, and in epididymal fat, it is smaller in the central part (near the epididymis about 2000–2500 microns square) than at the periphery (far from the epididymis about 3000–3500 microns square).

Since many years white adipose tissue can be divided into two fractions with a well-established and simple method based on collagenase separation of the cells and centrifugation. Because of the lipid content in mature adipocytes, these cells are located in the floating fraction after collagenase and centrifugation steps. The rest of the tissue forms the so-called stromal vascular fraction (SVF) mainly enriched with poorly differentiated cells including preadipocytes, cells from vessels (mainly endothelial cells), cells from nerves (mainly Schwann cells), and interstitial cells (including fibroblasts, macrophages, and other blood cells). In case of fat surrounded by serous membrane, serosa epithelium can also be present in the SVF.

In the lower panel mature isolated adipocytes from inguinal fat of an adult mouse are shown. Note the presence of a single well-visible nucleus of each cell.

We recently showed that mouse and human isolated mature adipocytes have stem cell properties and could be used for regenerative medicine.

Suggested Reading

Björntorp P, et al. Isolation and characterization of cells from rat adipose tissue developing into adipocytes. J Lipid Res. 19:316–24, 1978.

DiGirolamo M, et al. Qualitative regional differences in adipose tissue growth and cellularity in male Wistar rats fed ad libitum, Am J Physiol. 274:R1460–67, 1998.

Murano I, et al. Dead adipocytes, detected as crown-like structures, are prevalent in visceral fat depots of genetically obese mice. J Lipid Res. 49:1562–8, 2008.

De Matteis R. et al. In vivo physiological transdifferentiation of adult adipose cells. Stem Cells 27:2761–8, 2009.

Poloni A, et al. Human dedifferentiated adipocytes show similar properties to bone marrow-derived mesenchymal stem cells. Stem Cells. 2012.

Vitali A, et al. The adipose organ of obesity-prone C57BL/6J mice is composed of mixed white and brown adipocytes. J Lipid Res. 53:619–29, 2012.

Poloni A, et al. Glial-like differentiation potential of human mature adipocytes. J Mol Neurosci. 55:91–8, 2015.

Poloni A, et al. Biosafety evidence for human dedifferentiated adipocytes. J Cell Physiol. 230:1525–33, 2015.

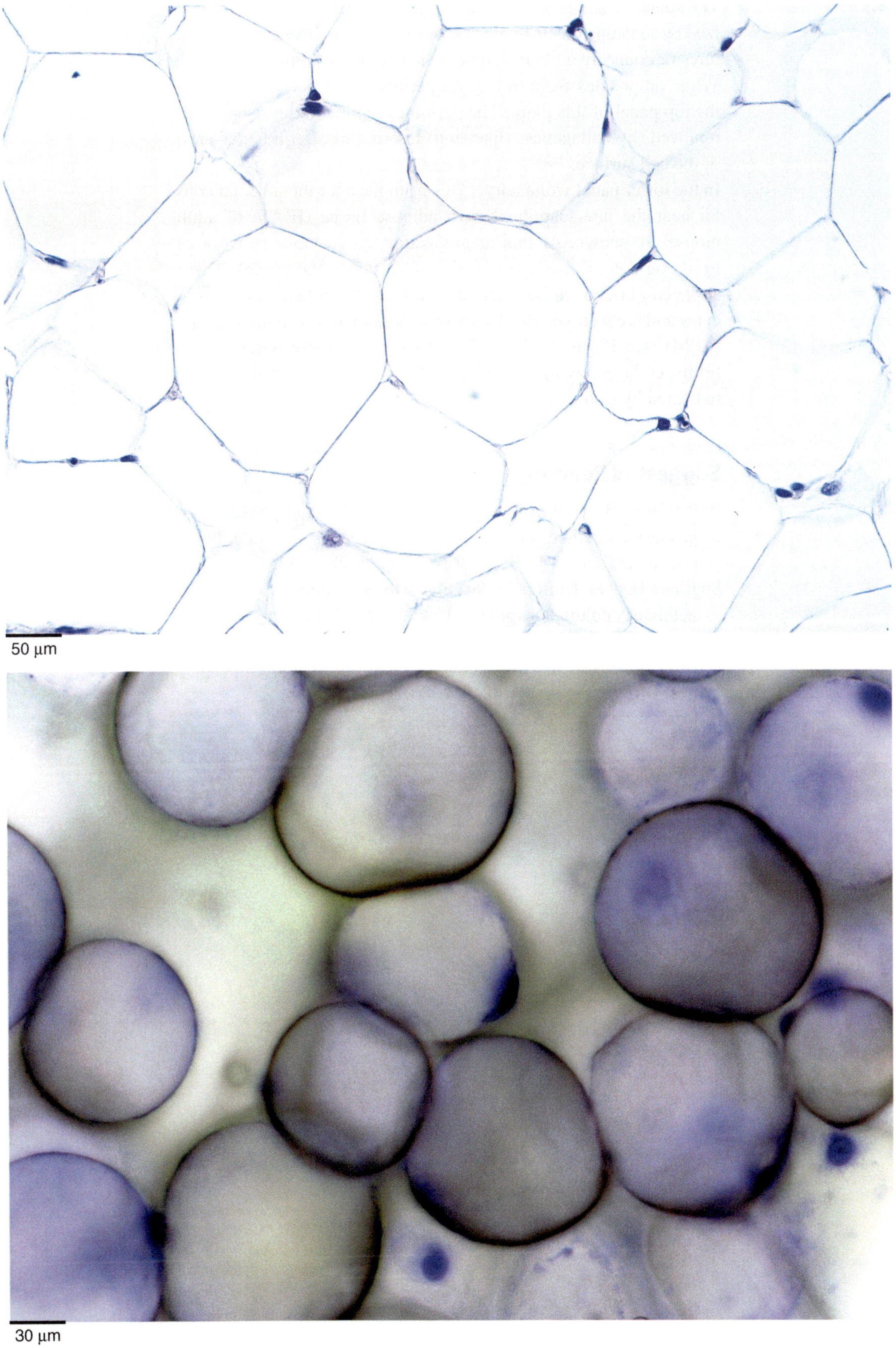

Plate 4.2 Adult rat retroperitoneal WAT (RWAT, *upper*) and isolated mature adipocytes from inguinal WAT of adult mouse (*lower*). H&E. LM

PLATE 4.3

Scanning Electron Microscopy (SEM)

The spherical shape of white adipocytes is particularly well visualized by scanning electron microscopy (SEM). Some vascular structures or connective fibers can be seen among the adipocytes.
White adipocytes from young rat periovarian depot are shown in the top panel of this plate. The peritoneal epithelial layer has been removed (by collagenase digestion) in order to offer a better view of the cell surface.
In the lower panel white adipocytes from the anterior subcutaneous fat near the interscapular brown adipose tissue (IBAT) of adult mouse are shown. At this magnification a fine loose network of fibrils on the cell surface is visible (see inside the circle). These collagen fibrils own the external part of the basal lamina of adipocytes and are well visible also by transmission electron microscopy (TEM) (see Plates 4.10 and 5.5). External to these basal lamina fibrils, collagen owing to the interstitial space is also visible (some indicated by arrows).

Suggested Reading

Richardson RL, et al. Adhesion, proliferation, and adipogenesis in primary rat cell cultures: effects of collagenous substrata, fibronectin, and serum. Cell Tiss Res. 251:123–28, 1988.

Sugihara H, et al. Unilocular fat cells in three-dimensional collagen gel matrix culture J Lipid Res. 29:691–98, 1988.

Sugihara H, et al. Primary culture of unilocular fat cells: characteristics of growth in vitro and changes in differentiation properties. Differentiation. 31:42–9, 1986.

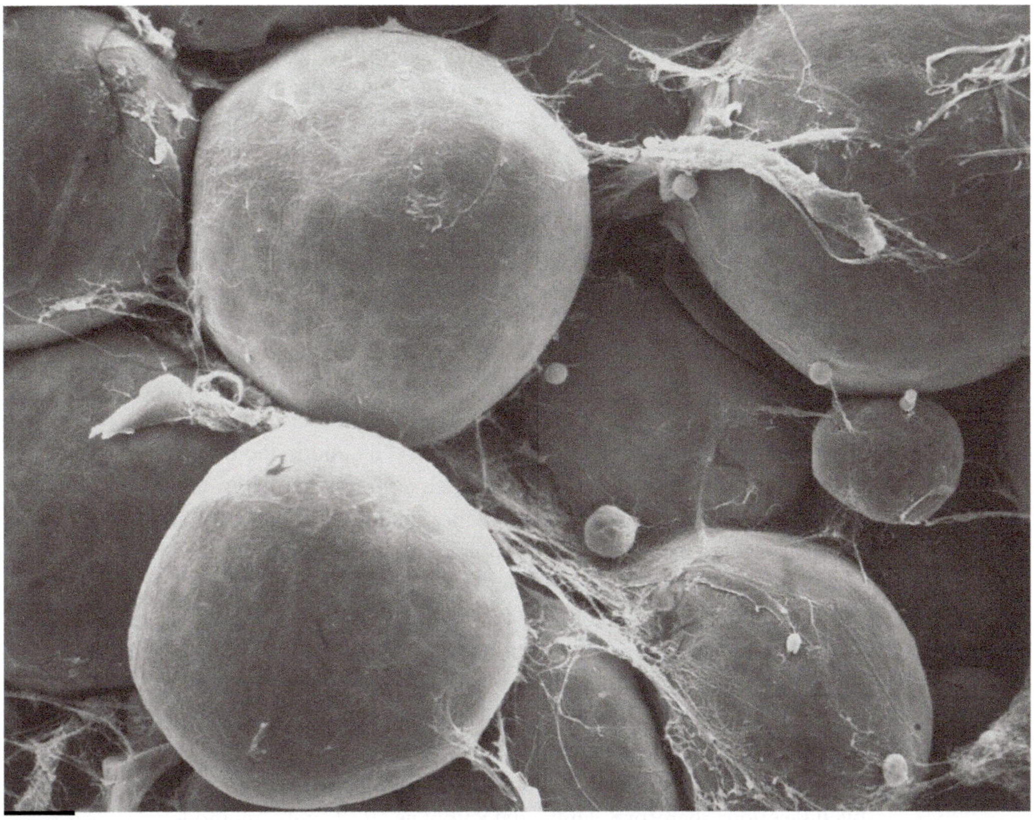

25 µm

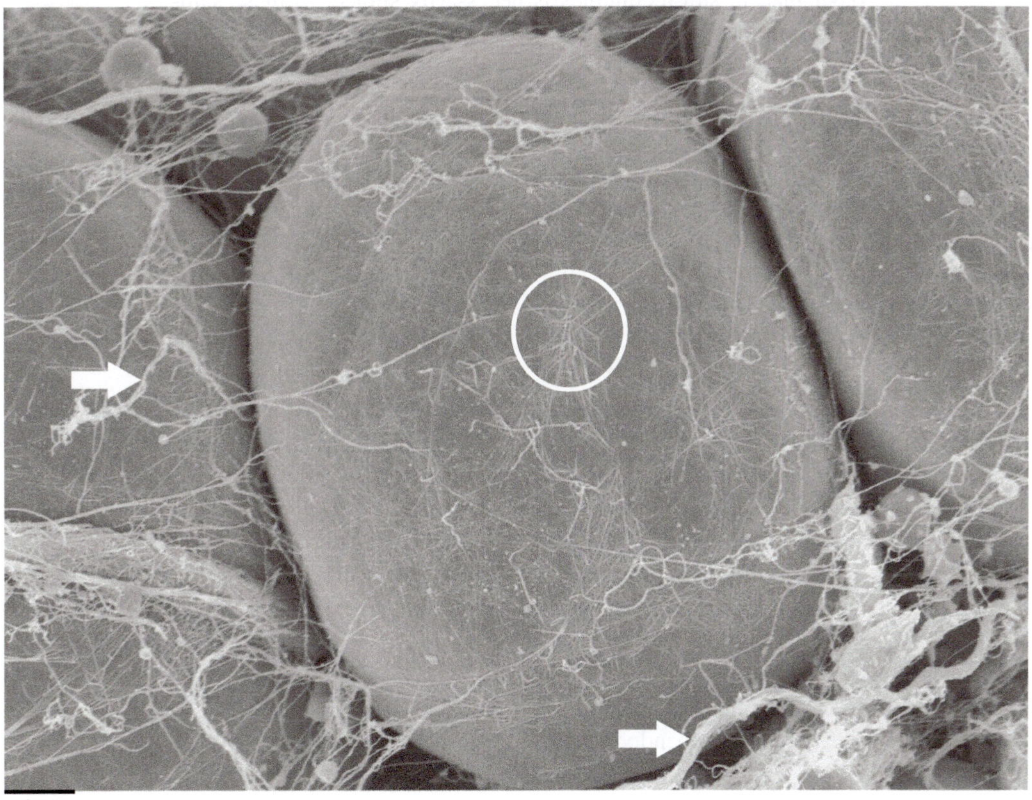

10 µm

Plate 4.3 Adult rat periovarian WAT (*upper*) and adult mouse subcutaneous WAT (*lower*). Basal membrane collagen encircled. *Arrows*: interstitial collagen. SEM

PLATE 4.4

Immunohistochemistry: Leptin

A very important adipocyte secretory product is leptin, which was originally considered the satiety hormone but may in fact have a wider role. Leptin expression is shown in white adipocytes from lean adult rat and obese adult mouse retroperitoneal depot (upper panels). This mouse strain (db/db) lacks the functional form of leptin receptor, so protein expression in situ is very high, and therefore immunostaining is quite intense (brown stain by peroxidase). In animals living in standard conditions or subjected to cold exposure, brown adipocytes do not express sufficient amounts of leptin for immunohistochemistry detection. Interestingly, leptin and UCP1 genes are reciprocally regulated in brown adipocytes. Many other secretory products of white adipocytes have been shown (see also Plate 4.6). Thus, both WAT and BAT have endocrine properties, and the adipose organ can be considered an endocrine organ. This organ is necessary for normal glucose metabolism, and lipoatrophic or lipodystrophic animals and humans are insulin resistant and diabetic. Interestingly one of the first discovered secretory products of WAT, adipsin, has recently been recognized to have an important role for the normal activity of pancreatic beta-cells. BAT also produces several hormone-like molecules.

The lower panel shows leptin-negative brown adipocytes closely apposed to leptin-positive white adipocytes from the interscapular BAT (IBAT) of a mouse maintained at 19 °C. These white unilocular cells are very difficult to separate from multilocular IBAT cells by dissection; therefore, leptin detection in IBAT with methods other than in situ techniques is necessarily subject to these sampling limitations.

Suggested Reading

Zhang Y, et al. Positional cloning of the mouse obese gene and its human homologue. Nature. 372:425–32, 1994.

Tartaglia LA, et al. Identification and expression cloning of a leptin receptor, OB-R. Cell. 83:1263–71, 1995.

Collins S, et al. Role of leptin in fat regulation. Nature. 380:677, 1996.

Cinti S, et al. Immunohistochemical localization of leptin and uncoupling protein in white and brown adipose tissue. Endocrinology. 138:797–804, 1997.

Deng C, et al. Effects of beta-adrenoceptor subtype stimulation on obese gene messenger ribonucleic acid and on leptin secretion in mouse brown adipocytes differentiated in culture. Endocrinology. 138:548–52, 1997.

De Matteis R, et al. Localization of leptin receptor splice variants in mouse peripheral tissues by immunohistochemistry. Proc Nutr Soc. 57:441–8, 1998.

De Matteis R, Cinti S Ultrastructural immunolocalization of leptin receptor in mouse brain. Neuroendocrinoloy. 68:412–19, 1998.

Friedman JM, Halaas JL. Leptin and the regulation of body weight in mammals. Nature. 395:763–70, 1998.

Flier JS, Maratos-Flier E. Obesity and the hypothalamus: novel peptides for new pathways. Cell. 92:437–40, 1998.

Cancello R, et al. Leptin and UCP1 genes are reciprocally regulated in brown adipose tissue. Endocrinology. 139:4747–50, 1998.

Trayhurn P, Beattie JH. Physiologic role of adipose tissue: white adipose tissue as an endocrine and secretory organ. Proc Nutr Soc. 60:329–39, 2001.

Galic S, et al. Adipose tissue as an endocrine organ. Mol Cell Endocrinol. 316:129–39, 2010.

Lo JC, et al. Adipsin is an adipokine that improves cell function in diabetes. Cell. 158:41–53, 2014.

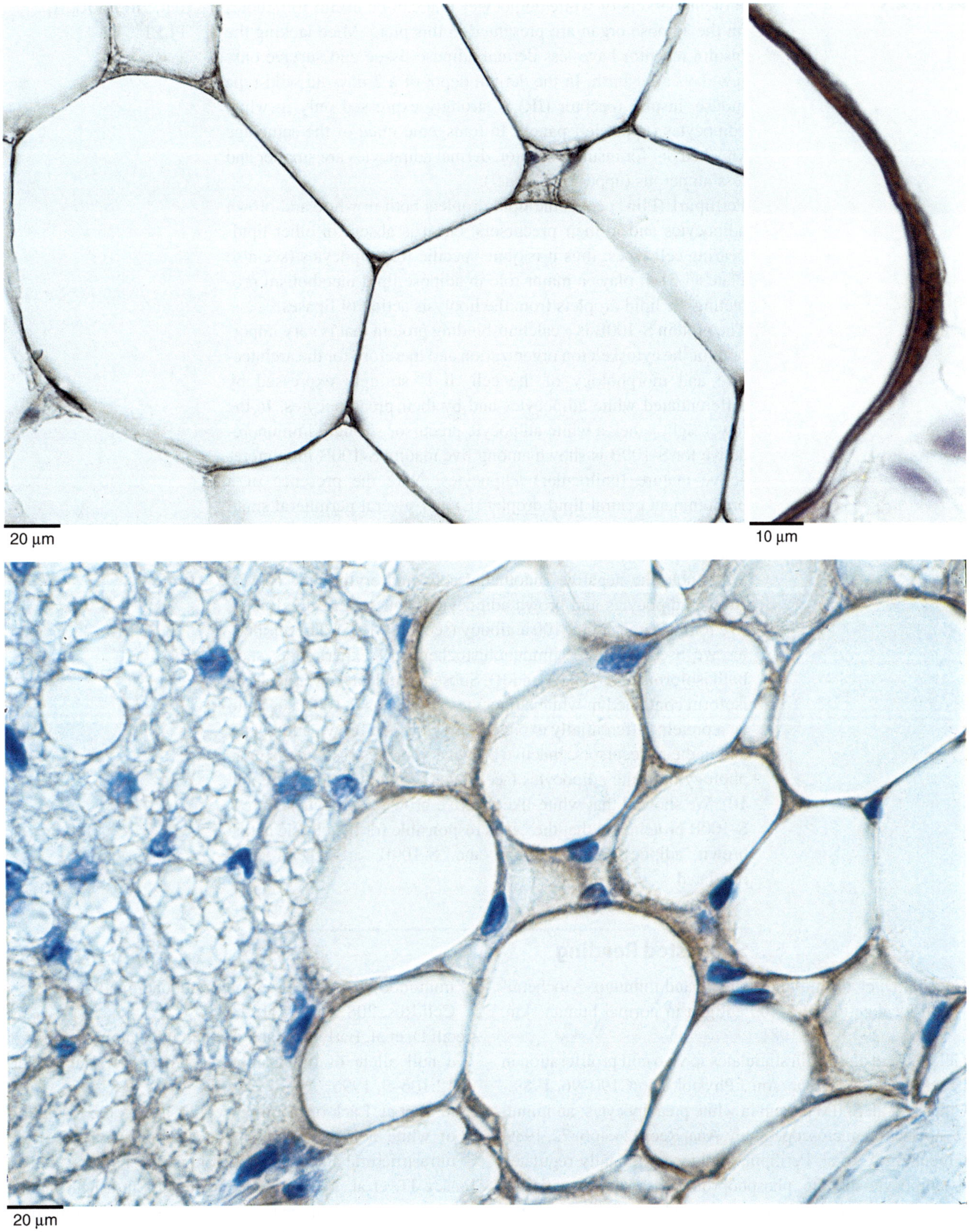

Plate 4.4 Adipocytes immunoreactive for leptin. *Upper left*: retroperitoneal WAT (RWAT) of adult rat. *Upper right*: cytoplasm of an intensely leptin-positive adipocyte in RWAT of adult obese (db/db*)* mouse. *Lower*: IBAT of adult mouse acclimated at 19 °C. Multilocular adipocytes (*left*) are leptin negative; unilocular adipocytes (*right*) are leptin positive. LM. IHC: leptin ab (1:3,000)

PLATE 4.5

IHC: IR, S-100B, PLP1

Protein markers of white adipocytes that can be useful for studies on the adipose organ are presented in this plate. Mice lacking the insulin receptor have less dermal adipose tissue and survive only few days after birth. In the dermal depot of a 2-day-old wild-type mouse, insulin receptor (IR) is strongly expressed only in white adipocytes (upper left panel). In transgenic mice of the same age knocked out for insulin receptor, dermal adipocytes are smaller and less numerous (upper right panel).

Perilipin1 (Plin1) coats the lipid droplets both in white and brown adipocytes and in their precursors, but it is absent in other lipid-bearing cell types; thus it is quite specific for adipocytes (see also Plate 11.3). It plays a major role in adipose lipid metabolism protecting the lipid droplets from the lipolysis action of lipases.

The protein S-100B is a calcium-binding protein that is very important for the cytoskeleton organization and therefore for the architecture and morphology of the cell. It is strongly expressed by differentiated white adipocytes and by their preadipocytes. In the lower right panel, a white adipocyte precursor strongly immunoreactive for S-100B is shown among five mature S-100B immunoreactive mature (unilocular) adipocytes. Note the presence of a predominant central lipid droplet (L) and several peripheral small lipid droplets in the adipocyte precursor. Only adipocytes, adipocyte precursors, and Schwann cells resulted immunoreactive in WAT; note the negative endothelial cells and erythrocyte (CAP). Brown adipocytes and brown adipocyte precursors resulted negative for the same anti-S-100 antibody (see Plate 12.5). The antibodies we used for these immunohistochemistry experiments stain both isoforms of S-100 (A and B). Subsequent data showed that the isoform contained in white adipocytes is B. Thus S-100B seems to be a protein differentially expressed in white and brown adipocytes and in their precursors. Inactive brown adipocytes assume the morphology of white adipocytes (see Plate 2.25 and Chaps. 8, 9, and 10). We showed that white-like inactive brown adipocytes express S-100B protein and that the genes responsible for the classic active brown adipocyte architecture and S-100B are reciprocally regulated.

Suggested Reading

Cocchia D, et al. Immunochemical and immuno-cytochemical localization of S-100 antigen in normal human skin. Nature. 294:85–7, 1981.

Géloën A, et al. Insulin stimulates in vivo cell proliferation in white adipose tissue. Am J Physiol. 256:C190–96, 1989.

Cinti S, et al. S-100 protein in white preadipocytes: an immunoelectron microscopic study. Anat Rec. 224:466–72, 1989.

Greenberg A, et al. Perilipin, a major hormonally regulated adipocyte-specific phosphoprotein associated with the periphery of lipid storage droplets. J Biol Chem. 266:11341–46, 1991.

Barbatelli G, et al. S-100 protein in rat brown adipose tissue under different functional conditions: a morphological, immunocytochemical, and immunochemical study. Exp Cell Res. 208:226–31, 1993.

Accili D, et al. Early neonatal death in mice homozygous for a null allele of the insulin receptor gene. Nat Genet. 12:106–9, 1996.

Cinti S, et al. Lack of insulin receptors affects the formation of white adipose tissue in mice. A morphometric and ultrastructural analysis. Diabetologia. 41:171–7, 1998.

Tansey JT, et al. Perilipin ablation results in a lean mouse with aberrant adipocyte lipolysis, enhanced leptin production, and resistance to diet-induced obesity. PNAS. 98:6494–9, 2001.

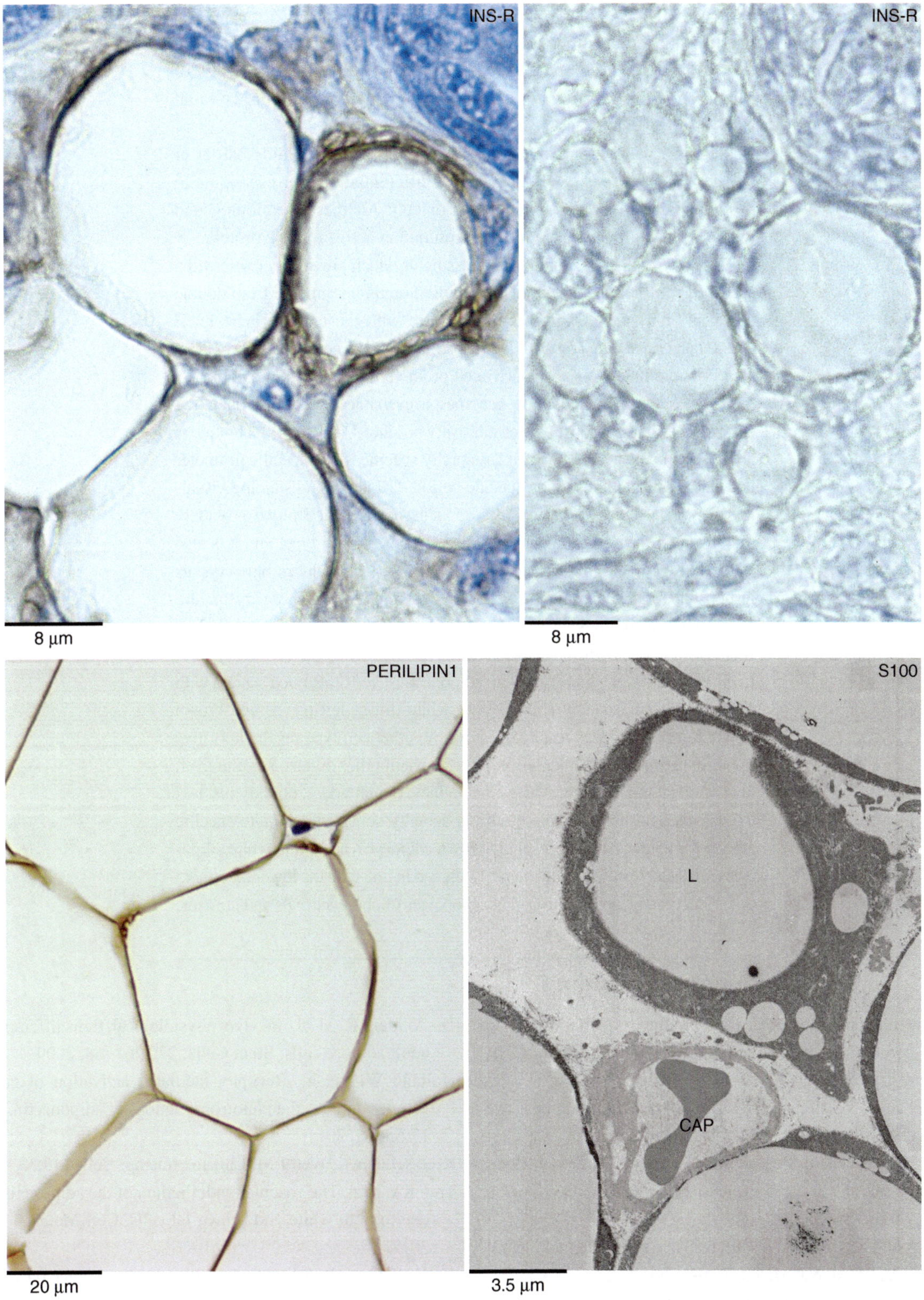

Plate 4.5 *Upper left*: dermal white adipose tissue of newborn mouse. White adipocytes immunoreactive for insulin receptor. *Upper right*: dermal white adipose tissue of newborn mouse lacking the insulin receptor. White adipocytes are negative for insulin receptor. LM. IHC: insulin receptor ab (1:1000). *Lower left*, epididymal WAT of adult mouse: adipocytes are perilipin1 immunoreactive. LM. IHC: perilipin1 ab (1:300). *Lower right*: epididymal WAT of young (3 weeks old) rat. Mature adipocytes and poorly differentiated adipocyte (preadipocyte) resulted intensely immunostained. Endothelial cell of capillary (CAP) is negative. Pre-embedding TEM immunocytochemistry: S-100 ab (1:100) (stain both A and B isoforms but only B is present in adipocytes) (From Cinti S et al. S-100 protein in white preadipocytes: an immunoelectronmicroscopic study Anat Rec 224:466–72, 1989, with permission)

PLATE 4.6

IHC: aP2, ADIPOQ

aP2 or FABP4 (fatty acid-binding protein 4) is a fatty acid carrier protein that is expressed in adipocytes and macrophages. We found this protein in situ with antibodies kindly provided by Dr. Bernlohr (University of Minnesota, Minneapolis) only in adipocytes (both white and brown in all sites of subcutaneous and visceral fat).

In the upper panel immunoreactive white adipocytes of epididymal fat of newborn mouse are in different stages of differentiation (corresponding to different sizes of cytoplasmic lipid droplets). All these developing and mature white adipocytes are intensely immunoreactive for aP2 protein.

In order to visualize in situ a cell expressing or which previously expressed a specific gene, the X-Gal staining can be used on tissue sampled from double transgenic mice derived from crossing mice with the reporter gene LacZ (R26R) and mice carrying a transgene formed by Cre recombinase driven by a specific promoter. When the activated promoter releases Cre recombinase, the process of LacZ activation becomes irreversible, and its product (the enzyme beta-galactosidase) is constitutively produced. Thus, this technique is not only cellular specific but also temporally specific if that specific promoter in a cell is activated only for a specific period of time. X-Gal staining visualizes beta-galactosidase activity in blue. This powerful technique is widely used to study the developmental destiny of a specific cell type, and it is also called lineage tracing technique. The X-Gal reaction produces blue crystals responsible for the blue staining visible by light microscopy. These crystals are electron dense and thus visible by transmission electron microscopy. This is very useful to distinguish the specific cell type expressing the X-Gal crystals.

In the bottom panel adipocytes from adiponectin-Cre/R26R mice stained with X-Gal histochemistry are shown. Both white (lower left panel) and brown (lower right) adipocytes resulted positive; no other cell type resulted positive in our experiments in which we explored several other organs, i.e., the liver, lung, skeletal muscles, heart, intestine, kidney, lymph nodes, epididymis, testis, vessels, and nerves. Adiponectin is actually considered a quite specific marker for adipocytes. Interestingly brown adipocytes and small white adipocytes (all sites) resulted more intensely stained in line with the lower adiponectin production by large hypertrophic adipocytes of obese animals and humans.

Suggested Reading

Baxa CA, et al. Human adipocyte lipid-binding protein: purification of the protein and cloning of its complementary DNA. Biochemistry. 28:8683–90, 1989.

Maeda K, et al. cDNA cloning and expression of a novel adipose specific collagen-like factor, apM1 (AdiPose Most abundant Gene transcript 1). Biochem Biophys Res Commun. 221:286–9, 1996.

Soriano P, Generalized lacZ expression with the ROSA26 Cre reporter strain. Nat Genet. 21:70–1, 1999.

Maeda N, et al. Diet-induced insulin resistance in mice lacking adiponectin/ACRP30. Nat Med. 8:731–7, 2002.

Tosh D, Slack JM. How cells change their phenotype. Nat Rev Mol Cell Biol. 3:187–94, 2002.

Matsuzawa Y, et al. Adiponectin and metabolic syndrome. Arterioscler Thromb Vasc Biol. 24:29–33, 2004.

Morroni M, et al. Reversible transdifferentiation of secretory epithelial cells into adipocytes in the mammary gland. Proc Natl Acad Sci. 101:16801–6, 2004.

De Matteis R, et al. In vivo physiological transdifferentiation of adult adipose cells. Stem Cells. 27:2761–68, 2009.

Holland WL, et al. Receptor-mediated activation of ceramidase activity initiates the pleiotropic actions of adiponectin. Nat Med. 17:55–63, 2011.

Kretzschmar K, Watt FM. Lineage tracing. Cell. 148:33–45, 2012.

Tran KV, et al. The vascular endothelium of the adipose tissue gives rise to both white and brown fat cells. Cell Metab. 15:222–29, 2012.

Ye R, Scherer P. Adiponectin, driver or passenger on the road to insulin sensitivity? Mol Metab. 2:133–41, 2013.

Funahashi T, Matsuzawa Y. Adiponectin and the cardiometabolic syndrome: an epidemiological perspective. Best Pract Res Clin Endocrinol Metab. 28:93–106, 2014.

Hotamisligil GS, Bernlohr DA. Metabolic functions of FABPs—mechanisms and therapeutic implications. Nat Rev Endocrinol. 11:592–605, 2015.

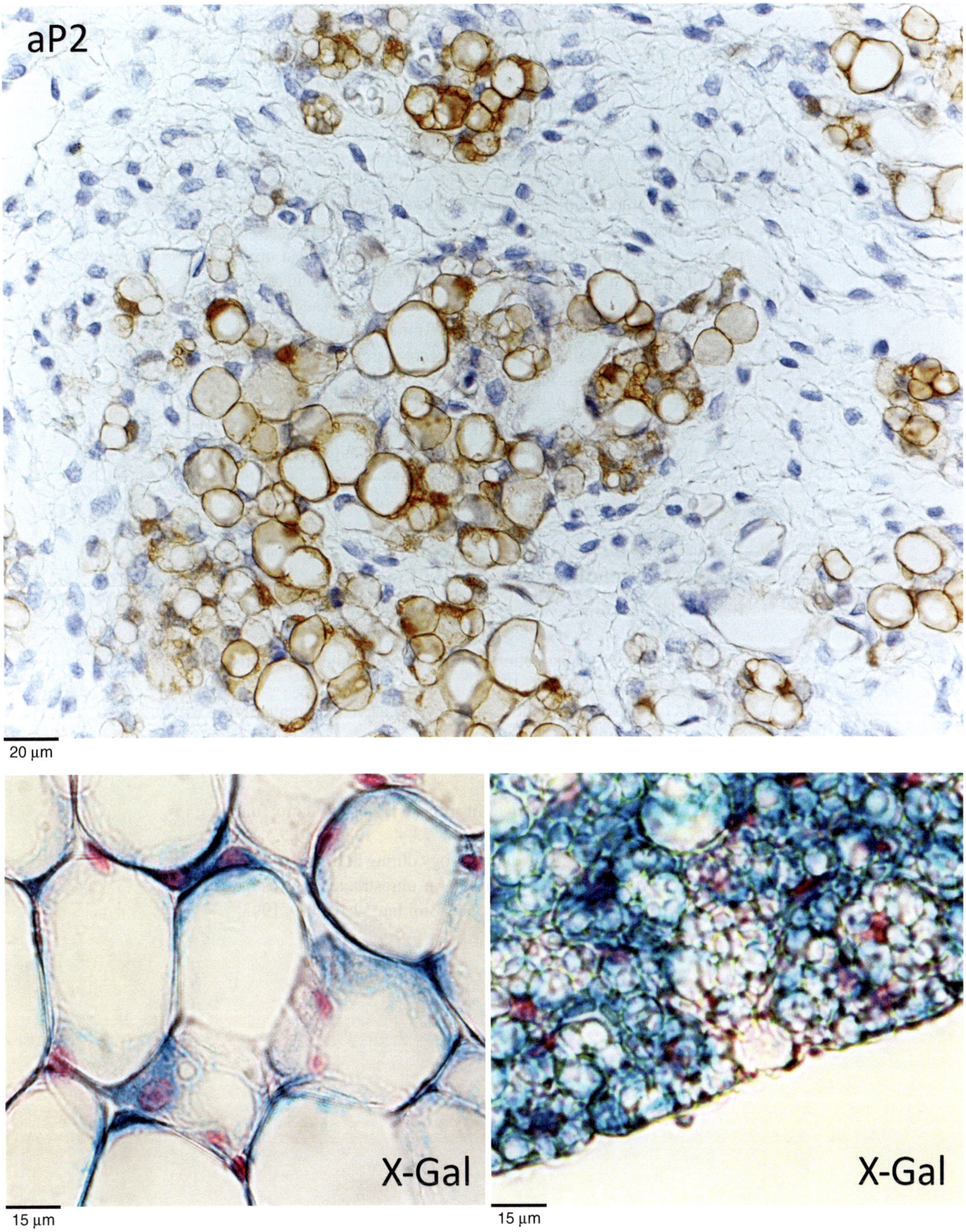

Plate 4.6 *Upper*: epididymal WAT of newborn mouse. LM. IHC: aP2 ab (1.200). *Lower*: subcutaneous WAT (*left panel*) and subcutaneous BAT (*right panel*) of adult adiponectin/Cre-R26R mouse. LM. X-Gal staining

PLATE 4.7

Transmission Electron Microscopy (TEM)

The ultrastructure of young rat epididymal adipose tissue by TEM is shown in this plate. Besides unilocular adipocytes, other cell types are visible: an adipocyte precursor (P) and a fibroblast (F). For details about these two cell types, see Plates 4.15–4.17 and Chap. 12. The unilocular adipocyte in the center of the upper panel is a small adipocyte (compare with the larger adipocyte partially visible on the top). The classic unilocular morphology of white adipocytes is reached at a very early stage of differentiation (see also Plate 4.18); thus small unilocular adipocytes share most of the TEM characteristics of adult mature large white adipocytes, but the peripheral cytoplasmic rim is usually thicker and richer in organelles (including small lipid droplets) in small adipocytes. In the thin peripheral cytoplasmic rim, the squeezed crescent nucleus and some mitochondria are always visible (mitochondria are shown, enlarged, in Plate 4.9). Other organelles are visible in white adipocytes (see the next plate and Chap. 5).

A mature large unilocular adipocyte from the epididymal adipose tissue of a young rat is shown in the lower panel.

Note the flattened crescent nucleus, the mitochondria, and some lipid droplets in the thin cytoplasmic rim. The narrow interstitial space contains a variable amount of collagen fibrils.

Suggested Reading

Barrnett RJ. In "Adipose tissue as an organ", Kinsell Ed., Elsevier, 3–78, 1962.

Hull D, Segall MM. Distinction of brown from white adipose tissue. Nature. 212:469–72, 1966.

Slavin BG. Fine structural studies on white adipocyte differentiation. Anat Rec. 195:63–72, 1979.

Napolitano L. In "Handbook of physiology", Am Physiol Soc., 109–23, 1965.

Slavin B.G. In "New perspectives in adipose tissue: structure, function and development", Butterworth, 23–43, 1985.

Zancanaro C, et al. Adipocyte morphology during hormone-induced lipid deposition and mobilization. An ultrastructural investigation in the perfused cardiac fat. Cell Biol Int. 19:1001–9, 1995.

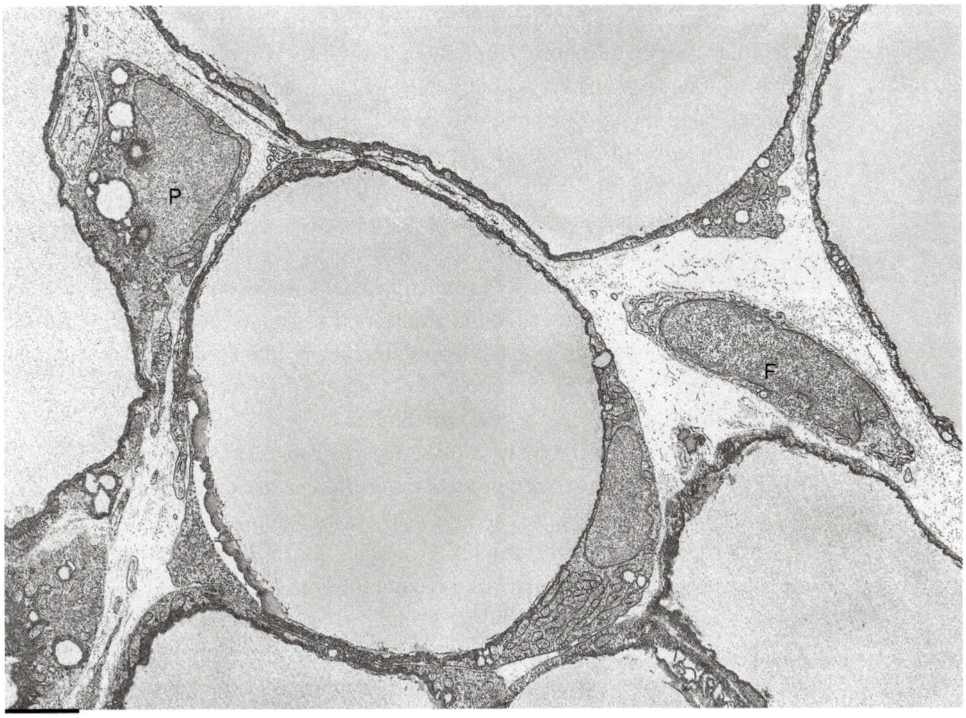

3.6 μm

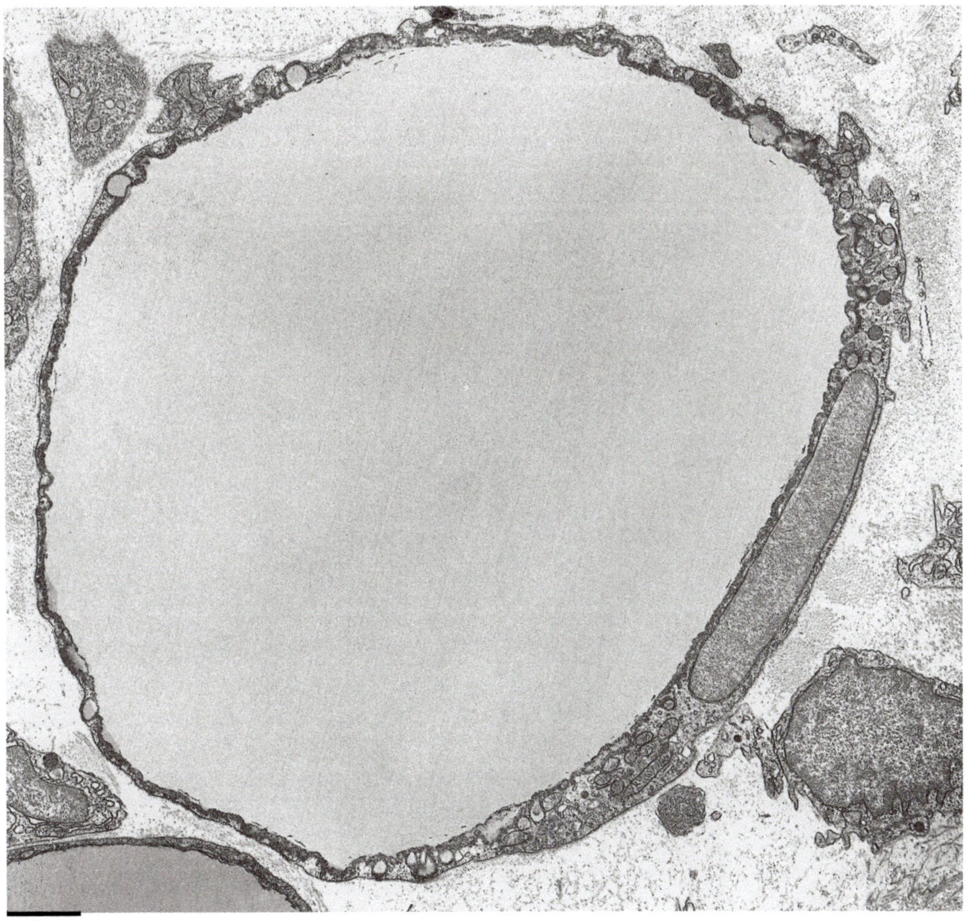
2.6 μm

Plate 4.7 Epididymal WAT of young rat. Mature adipocytes with different amounts of lipid storage. P, adipocyte precursor; F, fibroblast. TEM

PLATE 4.8

Ultrastructure of Organelles in White Adipocytes I

All the organelles usually observed in other cell types are found in the cytoplasmic rim of mature adipocytes. The Golgi complex (Go) is usually more developed in adipocytes that have not differentiated completely, and the cytoplasmic rim is thicker (upper panel) than that found in fully differentiated adipocytes (lower panel). Smooth endoplasmic reticulum (SER) is usually arranged in small vesicular cisternae often located in close apposition to the lipid droplets. Rough endoplasmic reticulum (RER) is usually organized as short strands of cisternae, occasionally grouped in stacks. Ribosomes and polyribosomes are dispersed in the hyaloplasm. Lysosomes are usually rare, but abundant in adipocytes of mammary glands during pregnancy (see Plate 11.4). Secondary lysosomes (lipofuscins) are abundant in omental adipocytes of humans (see Plate 5.7). Mitochondria are shown in the next plate. Microvesicles (MV, some indicated), containing secretory products, of different sizes are visible near the Golgi complex area and near the plasmalemma (see also Plates 5.5–5.6). Pinocytotic vesicles (V) cover the plasma membrane; an external lamina (EL or basal membrane) surrounds the cell. A variable amount of collagen fibrils is always associated with the external membrane (C; see also Plate 4.9). These basal membrane-associated fibrils are more abundant in subcutaneous adipocytes (compare with Plates 4.9 and 5.6) and well visible by scanning electron microscopy (see encircled area in the lower panel of Plate 4.3).

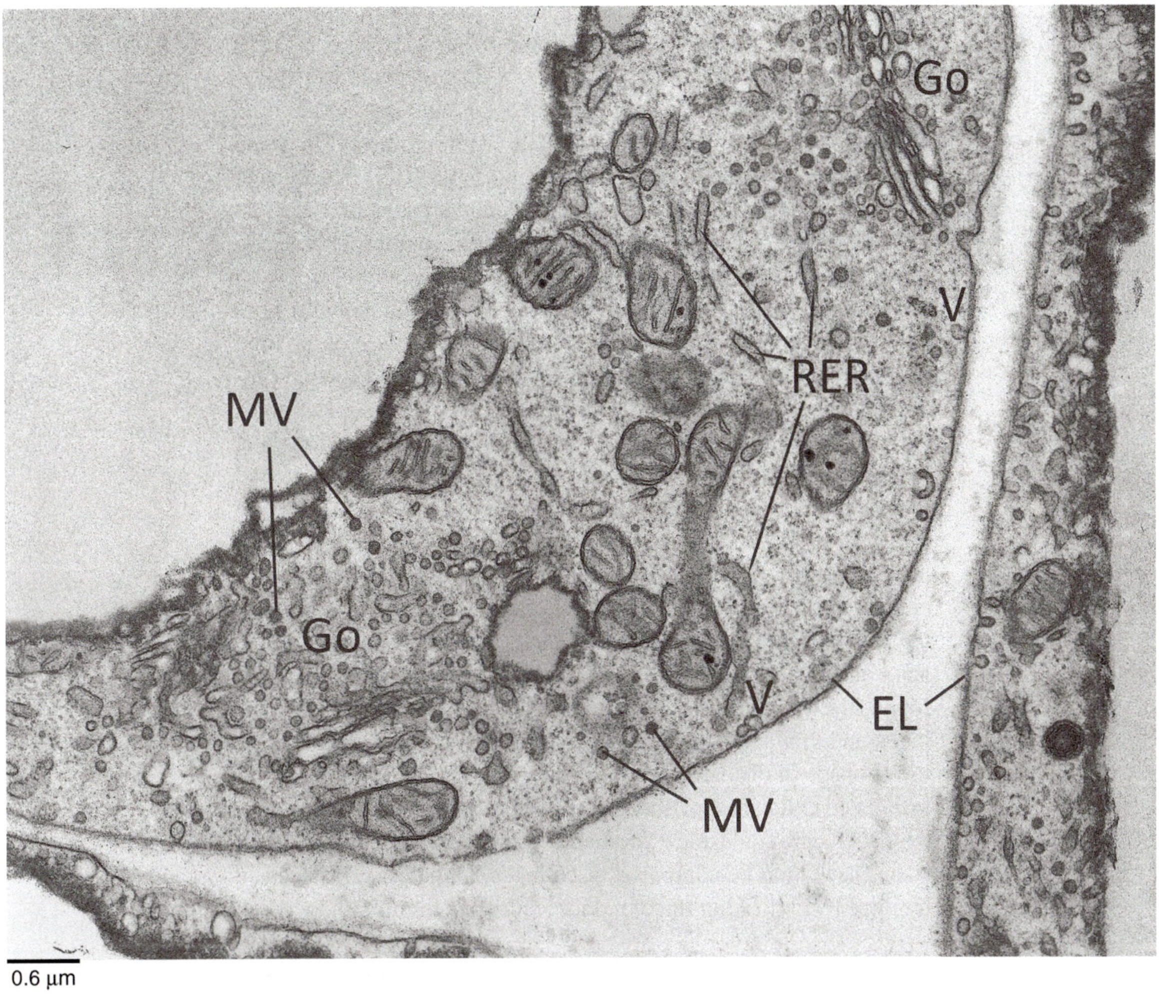

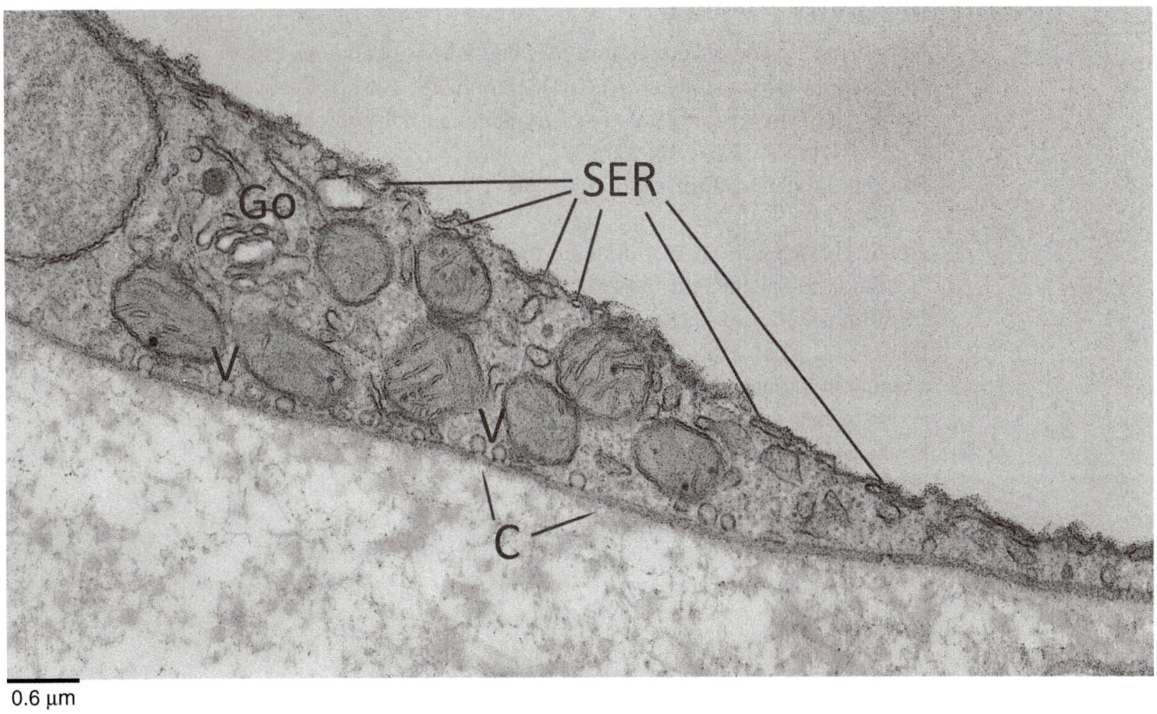

Plate 4.8 Epididymal WAT of young rat. White adipocyte organelles. TEM

PLATE 4.9

Ultrastructure of Organelles in White Adipocytes II

Unilocular white adipocyte classic mitochondria are elongated, and their cristae are randomly oriented both in visceral (upper panel) and subcutaneous (lower panel) WAT. Lipids are stored as triglycerides to form usually a single vacuole (L), but some small lipid droplets (SL, some indicated) are often visible in the cytoplasmic rim, mainly in smaller cells, that are not yet fully differentiated. The maximum cell size is variable in different areas of the organ, in general larger in subcutaneous depots and smaller in visceral depots. Some visceral depots usually contain large adipocytes such as the epididymal depot (comparable size to subcutaneous adipocytes; see also Plate 4.2 for further details). The surface of the lipid droplet is not surrounded by a plasma membrane, and several proteins (among which perilipin1; see Plate 4.5) are associated with its surface. Note the dense "line" (DL) separating the lipid droplet from the cytoplasm containing the organelles. The abovementioned proteins coating the lipid droplets are located at this level and likely responsible for the appearance of this dense line. The hydrophilic portion of the triglycerides contained in lipid droplets (L) is oriented toward the cytoplasm. The adipocyte external plasma membrane is covered with a variable amount of pinocytotic vesicles (V, some indicated). An external lamina (EL) or basal membrane surrounds the adipocyte surface. On the external side of the basal lamina, some thin collagen fibrils are visible (C) (compare with SEM lower image in Plate 4.3; see also Plate 5.5). These external lamina-associated collagen fibrils are usually more abundant in subcutaneous WAT and could have mechanic properties related to the cell size. They could be composed of collagen VI, because its absence (collagen VI knockout mice) induces enlargement of adipocytes.

Suggested Reading

Napolitano L. The differentiation of white adipose cells. An electron microscope study. J Cell Biol. 18:663–79, 1963.

Slavin BG. The cytophysiology of mammalian adipose cells. Int Rev Cytol. 33:297–334, 1972.

Fawcett DW. The Cell. WB Saunders Company. Philadelphia, 1981.

Greenberg AS, et al. Perilipin, a major hormonally regulated adipocyte-specific phosphoprotein associated with the periphery of lipid storage droplets. J Biol Chem. 266: 11341–46, 1991.

Pierleoni C, et al. Fibronectins and basal lamina molecules expression in human subcutaneous white adipose tissue. Europ J Histochem. 42:183–8, 1998.

Souza SC, et al. Overexpression of perilipin A and B blocks the ability of tumor necrosis factor alpha to increase lipolysis in 3T3-L1 adipocytes. J Biol Chem. 273:24665–9, 1998.

Brunk UT, Terman A. Lipofuscin: mechanisms of age-related accumulation and influence on cell function. Free Radical Biol Med. 33:611–19, 2002.

Khan T, et al. Metabolic dysregulation and adipose tissue fibrosis: role of collagen VI. Mol Cell Biol. 29:1575–91, 2009.

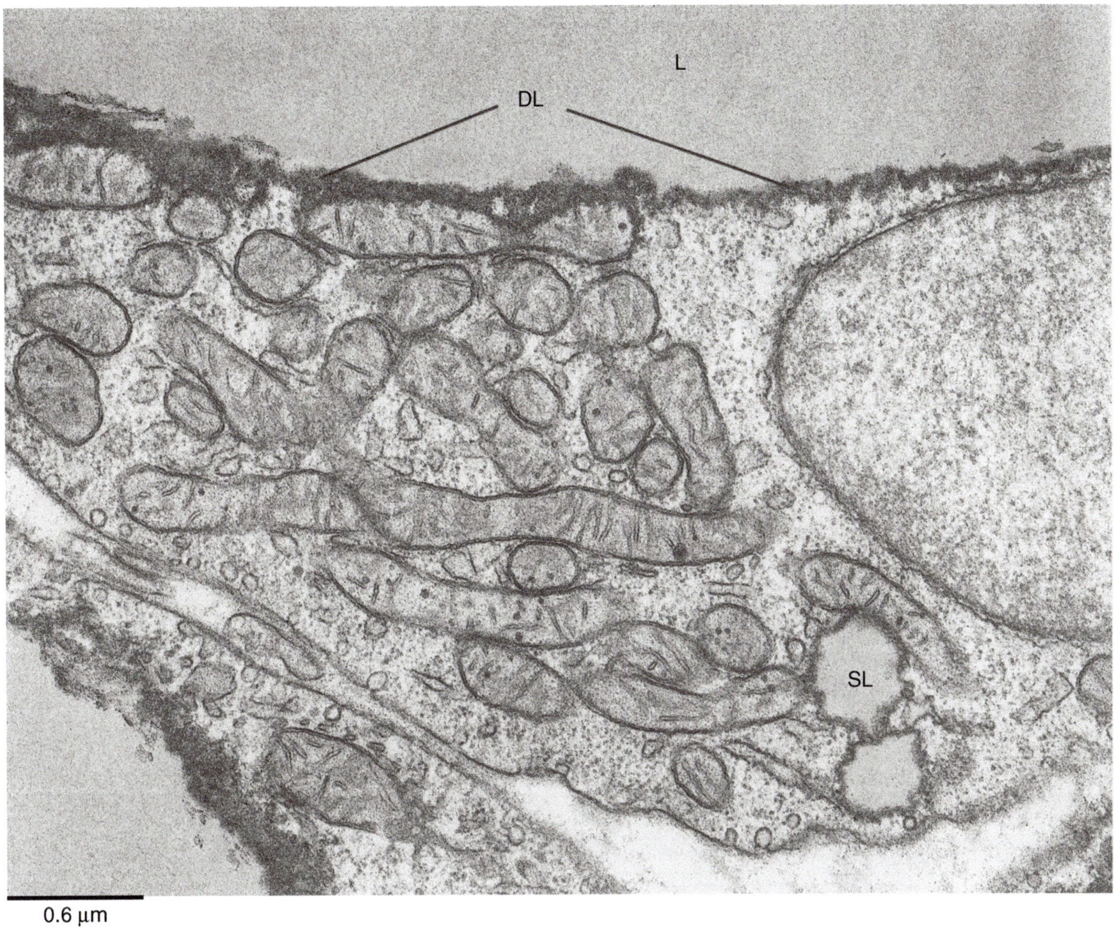

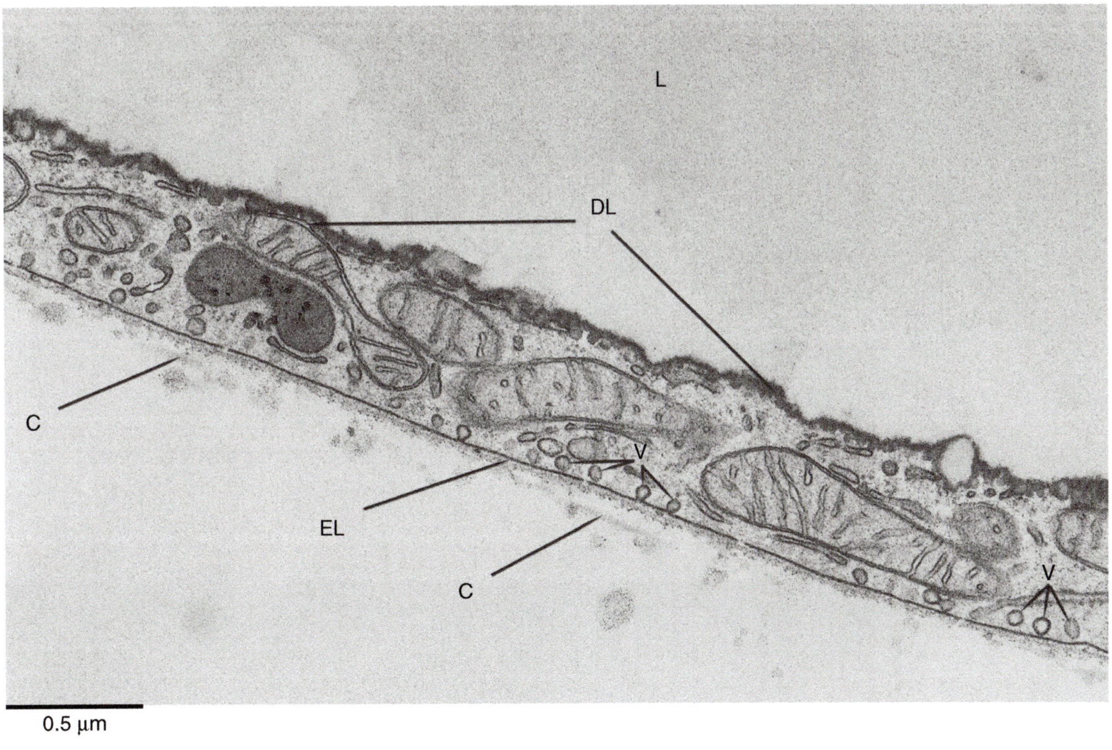

Plate 4.9 Epididymal (*upper*: enlargement of mitochondria shown in the upper panel of Plate 4.7) and inguinal (*lower*) WAT of young rat and adult mouse, respectively. TEM

PLATE 4.10

Subcutaneous Adipocytes with Special Features

In white adipose tissue adjacent to brown adipose areas, some cells have intermediate features between white and brown adipocytes (see also Chap. 6). In these cells, lipids are mainly stored in a single vacuole (L), but several small lipid droplets can also be seen in the thick peripheral cytoplasmic rim. These cells have a large number of mitochondria with an intermediate morphology (lower figure, enlargement of the squared area) between those found in white and brown adipocytes (compare with Plates 2.3 and 4.9). Abundant smooth endoplasmic reticulum (SER, some indicated) is present as a dense network among mitochondria, as frequently observed in brown adipocytes (see Plate 7.7).

Suggested Reading

Daniel H, Derry DM. Criteria for differentiation of brown and white fat in the rat. Can J Physiol Pharmacol. 47:941–45, 1969.

Cameron IL. Age-dependent changes in the morphology of brown adipose tissue in mice. Tex Rep Biol Med. 33:391–96, 1975.

Alexander G, et al. Brown adipose tissue in the new-born calf (Bos taurus). J Physiol. 244:223–34, 1975.

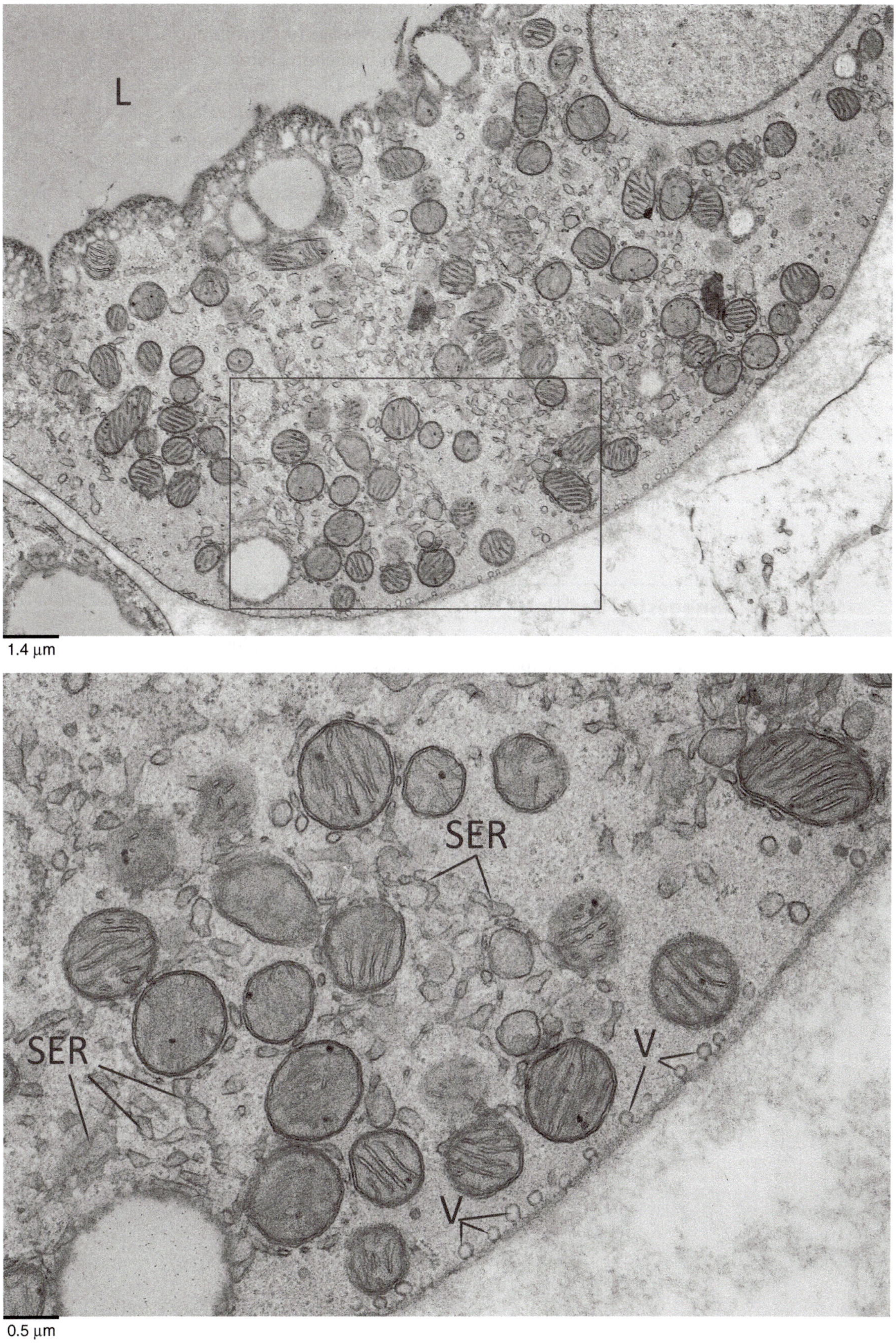

Plate 4.10 Unilocular adipocytes of peri-IBAT WAT of adult rat. TEM

PLATE 4.11

aP2-UCP1
Mitochondria

Transgenic mice overexpressing UCP1 in the adipose organ (driven by aP2 promoter) are obesity resistant. As expected (both white and brown adipocytes express aP2 gene) immunohistochemistry of inguinal fat in these animals revealed intense UCP1 immunoreactivity not only in the multilocular component of this mixed depot (see Chap. 5) but also in unilocular adipocytes (arrows in the top panel).

Electron microscopy revealed unilocular adipocytes with thick cytoplasm (lower right panel) in the same inguinal fat. These adipocytes showed numerous enlarged mitochondria rich in laminar cristae, similar to brown mitochondria of BAT. In unilocular adipocytes of the same depot in control mice, few elongated mitochondria with randomly oriented cristae (classic white mitochondria) were found as expected (lower left panel). Thus, the overexpression of UCP1 induces modifications of mitochondrial morphology in the adipose organ of these transgenic mice. Interestingly, the absence of this protein in UCP1-KO mice also induces drastic changes in the morphology of mitochondria in BAT (see Plate 2.5). These data are in line with the variable morphology of mitochondria in adipocytes under different physiologic environmental conditions (see also Chaps. 6, 7, 8, 9, and 10).

Suggested Reading

Kopecky J, et al. Expression of the mitochondrial uncoupling protein gene from the aP2 gene promoter prevents genetic obesity. J Clin Invest. 96:2914–23, 1995.

Kopecky J, et al. Reduction of dietary obesity in aP2-Ucp transgenic mice: physiology and adipose tissue distribution. Am J Physiol. 270:768–75, 1996.

Rossmeisl M, et al. Expression of the uncoupling protein 1 from the aP2 gene promoter stimulates mitochondrial biogenesis in unilocular adipocytes in vivo. Eur J Biochem. 269:19–28, 2002.

Vitali A, et al. The adipose organ of obesity-prone C57BL/6J mice is composed of mixed white and brown adipocytes. J Lip Res. 53:619–29, 2012.

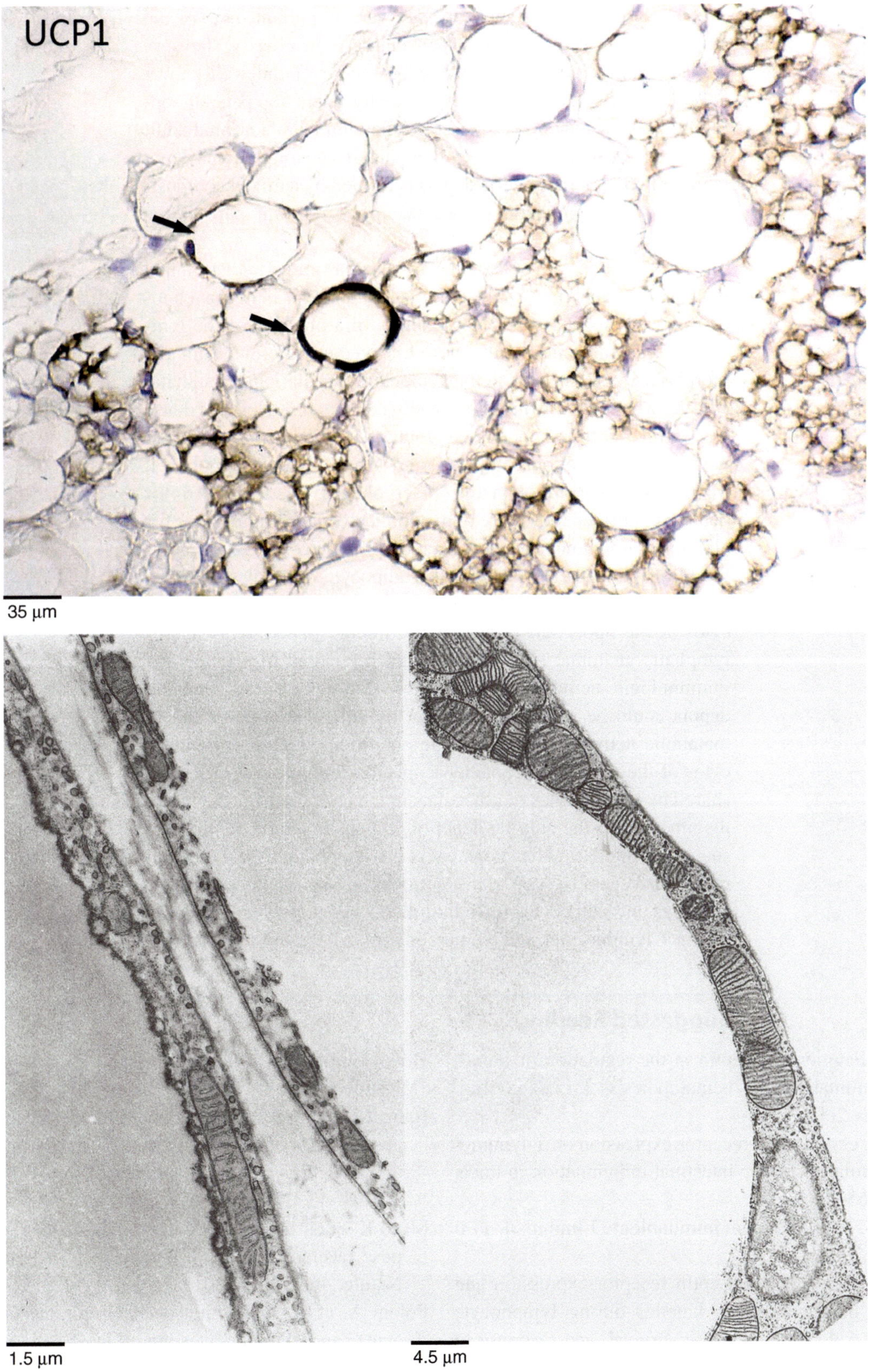

Plate 4.11 *Upper*: inguinal WAT of aP2-UCP1 transgenic mice. IHC. UCP1 ab (1:8000). *Lower left*: representative electron microscope morphology of a unilocular adipocyte from wild-type mouse. *Lower right*: electron microscopy of unilocular adipocyte in aP2-UCP1 transgenic mouse with thick cytoplasm. TEM (lower left from Rossmeisl M et al. Expression of the uncoupling protein 1 from the aP2 gene promoter stimulates mitochondrial biogenesis in unilocular adipocytes in vivo. Eur J Biochem. 269:19–28, 2002, with permission)

PLATE 4.12

Adipo-Lymphatic Tissue

The omentum and mesenteric fat are very important parts of the adipose organ also because, when enlarged in obesity, they are widely believed to be responsible for many of the well-known adverse metabolic consequences of obesity. In the top panel, a representative low magnification of the omentum from a normal adult mouse is shown. It is visually evident that the anatomy of this depot (similar to that of mesenteric depot) is formed by a mixed composition in which lymphatic tissues occupy a relevant part of the parenchyma.

The middle panel is an enlargement of an area similar to that framed in the upper panel. It shows the intima relationships between adipocytes and lymphatic cells. Note that the morphology of the lymphatic cells in contact with the adipocyte is different from the morphology of the rest of the lymphatic population. Lymphatic cells here have a blast-like appearance (i.e., larger nuclei, less dense chromatin, and more abundant cytoplasm). Serial sections stained with perilipin1 (bottom left panel) and MAC2 (bottom right panel, MAC2 is expressed by active macrophages; see Plate 9.6 for details) confirmed the nature of metabolically active adipocytes for all adipocytes shown here and excluded the macrophage nature of the blast-like cells surrounding the adipocyte. Not all adipocytes were surrounded by blast-like lymphocytes (e.g., see the two adipocytes at the upper left corner of the middle panel). This adipo-lymphatic anatomic relationship could be related to a functional immunologic activity of adipocytes. Mesenteric and omental depots could be implicated both in the animal immunity and in metabolic activities in physiologic conditions. Of note, lymphocytes of these two fat depots have specific immune properties not shared by lymphocytes of other sites in the organism. Furthermore, the omentum is the only fat depot of humans in which the first tissue appearing during development is the lymphatic tissue. Old and recent data seem to support a functional interaction between lymphocytes and adipocytes including the expression of leptin receptors in T lymphocytes and the fat body mixed activity in insects.

Suggested Reading

Fantuzzi G, Faggioni R. Leptin in the regulation of immunity, inflammation and hematopoiesis. J Leukoc Biol. 68:437–46, 2000.

Siegmund B, et al. Leptin receptor expression on T lymphocytes modulates chronic intestinal inflammation in mice. Gut. 53:965–72, 2004.

Matarese GS, et al. Leptin in immunology. J Immunol. 174: 3137–42, 2005.

Papathanassoglou E, et al. Leptin receptor expression and signaling in lymphocytes: kinetics during lymphocyte activation, role in lymphocyte survival, and response to high fat diet in mice. J Immunol. 176:7745–52, 2006.

Hotamisligil GS. Inflammation and metabolic disorders. Nature. 444:860–7, 2006.

Rangel-Moreno J, et al. Omental milky spots develop in the absence of lymphoid tissue-inducer cells and support B and T cell responses to peritoneal antigens. Immunity. 30:731–43, 2009.

Moro K, et al. Innate production of T(H)2 cytokines by adipose tissue-associated c-Kit(+)Sca-1(+) lymphoid cells. Nature. 463:540–4, 2010.

Poloni A, et al. Interaction between human mature adipocytes and lymphocytes induces T-cell proliferation. Cytotherapy. 17:1292–301, 2015.

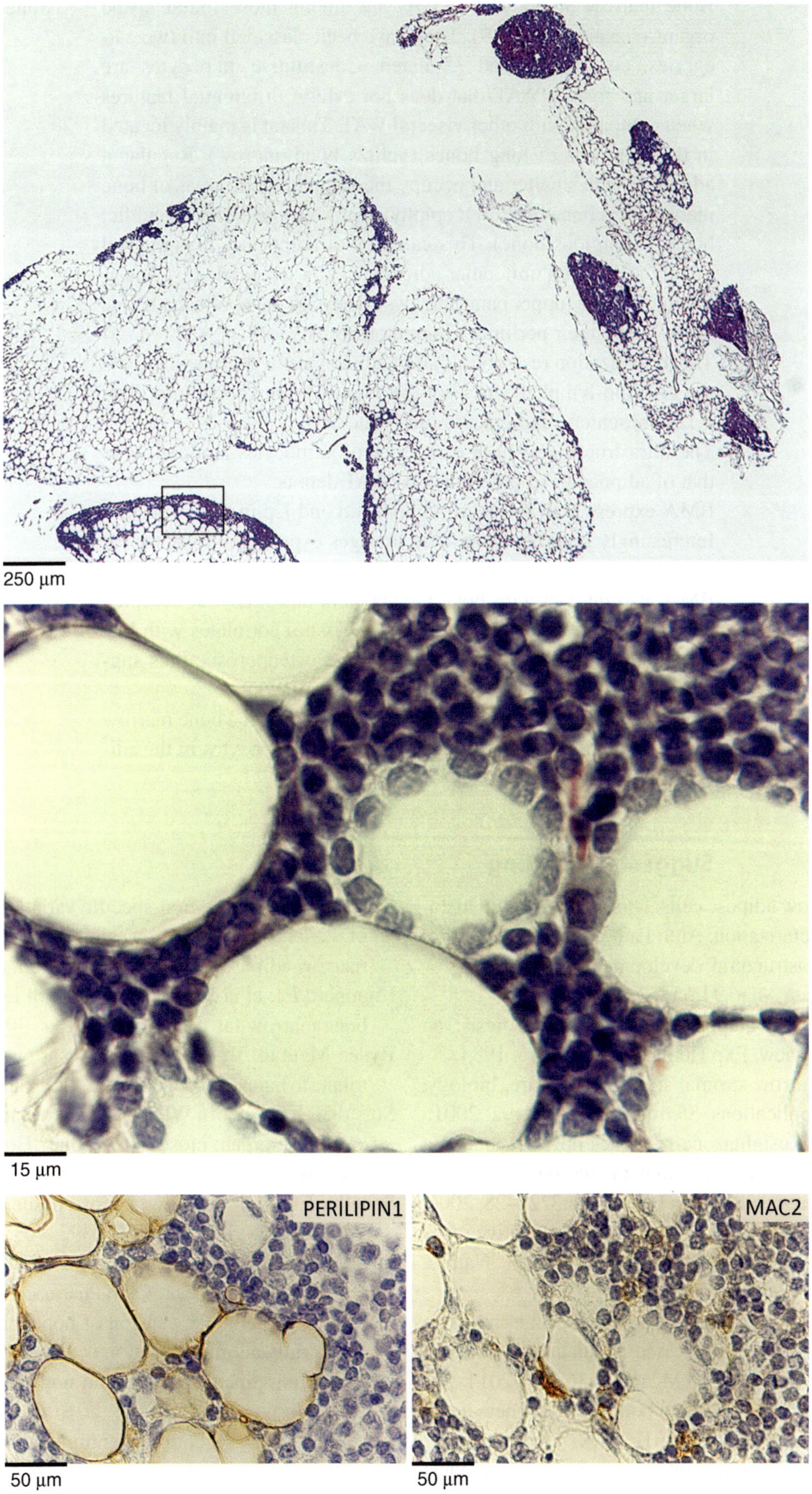

Plate 4.12 *Top*: omentum of adult mouse. LM H&E. *Middle*: enlargement of an area similar to the squared area in the top panel. LM H&E. *Bottom*: IHC. Left perilipin ab (1.300), right MAC2 ab (1.500)

PLATE 4.13

Bone Marrow WAT

Bone marrow adipocytes (BMA) are among those found inside organs (see also Plate 5.9). They have been classified into two categories: constitutive and regulated. Constitutive adipocytes are larger and form a WAT that does not exhibit differential features when compared with other visceral WAT. This fat is mainly located in the diaphysis of long bones (yellow bone marrow). Regulated adipocytes are smaller and occupy the hematopoietic areas of bone marrow (red bone marrow): epiphysis of long and all short and flat bones (spongious bone). This category of adipocytes is organized mainly as isolated unilocular adipocyte cells surrounded by hematopoietic tissue (upper panel, arrows). They are metabolically active as shown by their perilipin1 immunoreactivity.

This organization resembles that of adipocytes in the lymphatic tissue of adipo-lymphatic areas of the adipose organ: omentum (Plate 4.12), mesentery, and epicardium (Plate 5.8).

The ultrastructure of both categories of adipocytes is identical to that of adipocytes of other visceral WAT depots.

BMA express high levels of adiponectin and leptin (lower panel). Interestingly both hematopoietic lineages express the receptor for leptin in line with a role for leptin in normal hematopoiesis.

BMA also interact with bone metabolism, and it is well accepted that increased MAT (Marrow Adipose Tissue) correlates with low bone formation, low mineral density, and osteoporosis, thus suggesting that MAT is a negative regulator of bone mass.

Interestingly, recent data in humans seem to support a bone marrow origin of stem cells able to differentiate into adipocytes in the adipose organ.

Suggested Reading

Tavassoli M. Marrow adipose cells. Ultrastructural and histochemical characterization. Arch Pathol. 98:189–92, 1974.

Tavassoli M. Ultrastructural development of bone marrow adipose cell. Acta Anat. 94:65–77, 1976.

Tavassoli M. Marrow adipose cells and hemopoiesis: an interpretative review. Exp Hematol. 12:139–46, 1984.

Bianco P. Bone marrow stromal stem cells: nature, biology, and potential applications. Stem Cells. 19:180–92, 2001.

Crossno JT, et al. Rosiglitazone promotes development of a novel adipocyte population from bone marrow-derived circulating progenitor cells. J Clin Invest. 116:3220–28, 2006.

Naveiras O, et al. Bone-marrow adipocytes as negative regulators of the haematopoietic microenvironment. Nature. 460:259–63, 2009.

Cawthorn WP, et al. Bone marrow adipose tissue is an endocrine organ that contributes to increased circulating adiponectin during caloric restriction. Cell Metab. 20:368–75, 2014.

Riminucci M, et al. Stem cells and bone diseases: new tools, new perspective. Bone. 70:55–61, 2015.

Hardouin P, et al. New insights into bone marrow adipocytes: report from the First European Meeting on Bone Marrow Adiposity (BMA 2015). Bone. 15:414–7, 2015.

Scheller EL, et al. Region-specific variation in the properties of skeletal adipocytes reveals regulated and constitutive marrow adipose tissues. Nat Commun. 6:7808, 2015.

Limonard EJ, et al. Short-term effect of estrogen on human bone marrow fat. J Bone Miner Res. 30:2058–66, 2015.

Rydén M, et al. Transplanted bone marrow-derived cells contribute to human adipogenesis. Cell Metab. 22:408–17, 2015.

Sulston RJ, Cawthorn WP. Bone marrow adipose tissue as an endocrine organ: close to the bone? Horm Mol Biol Clin Investig. 2016.

Scheller EL, et al. Marrow adipose tissue: trimming the fat. Trends Endocrinol Metab. 27:392–403, 2016.

Suchacki KJ, et al. Bone marrow adipose tissue: formation, function and regulation. Curr Opin Pharmacol. 28:50–6, 2016.

Cawthorn WP, et al. Expansion of bone marrow adipose tissue during caloric restriction is associated with increased circulating glucocorticoids and not with hypoleptinemia. Endocrinology. 157:508–21, 2016.

Chkourko Gusky H, et al. Omentum and bone marrow: how adipocyte-rich organs create tumour microenvironments conducive for metastatic progression. Obes Rev. 2016.

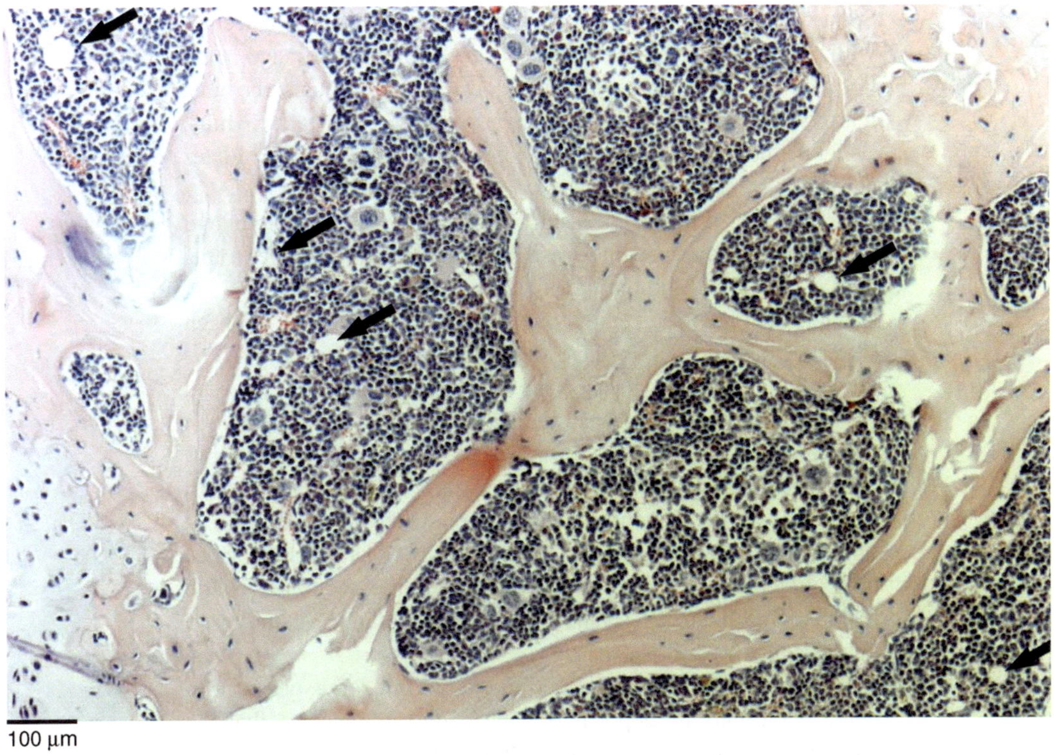

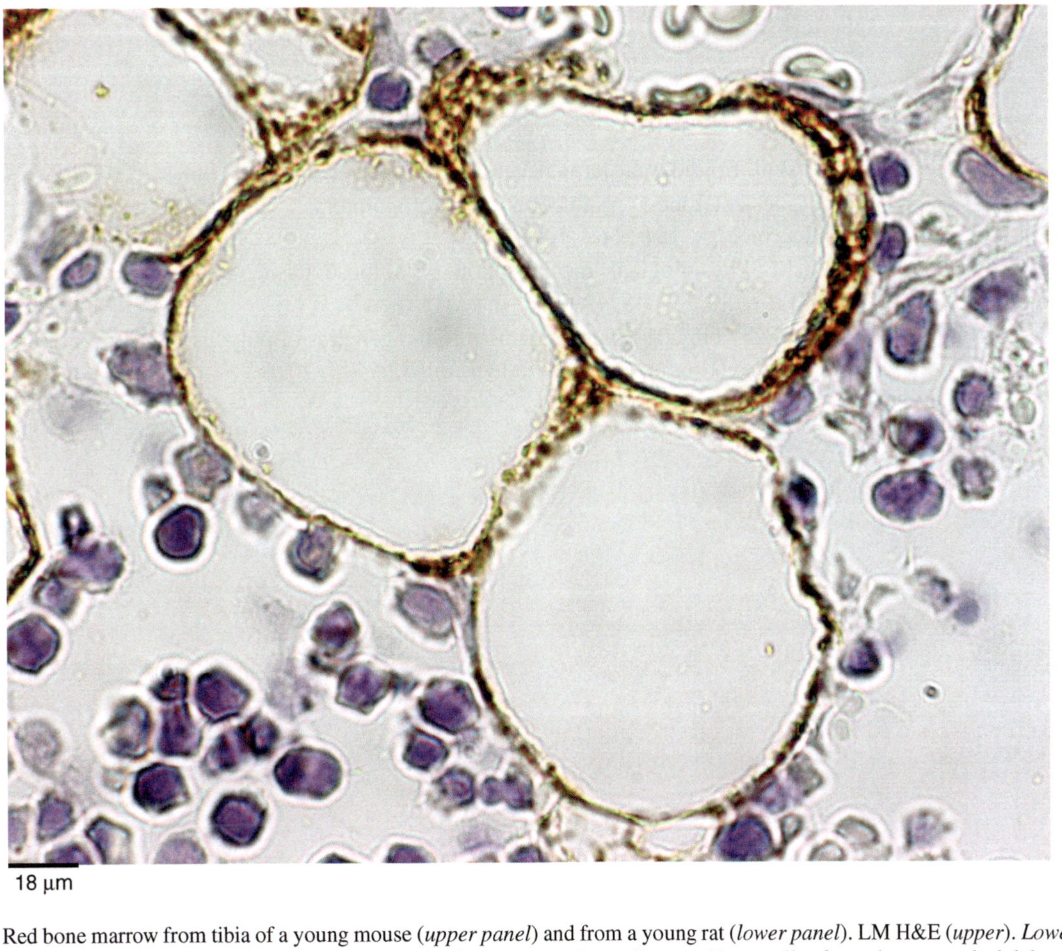

Plate 4.13 Red bone marrow from tibia of a young mouse (*upper panel*) and from a young rat (*lower panel*). LM H&E (*upper*). *Lower*: LM. IHC Leptin ab (1:40) (Lower panel from Morroni M et al. In vivo leptin expression in cartilage and bone cells of growing rats and adult humans. J Anat. 2004 205:291–6, 2004, with permission)

PLATE 4.14

Periovarian WAT

Some visceral adipose depots are in close anatomical connection with some organs, i.e., the gonads, kidney, lymph nodes, and intestine. Furthermore, some white fat is located inside organs: the bone marrow, thymus, parotid gland, parathyroid gland, heart, thymus, skeletal muscles, lymph nodes, and gastrointestinal tract (see Plates 5.4 and 5.9).

Some functional interrelationships between the adipose organ and the other organs are being investigated, but our knowledge in this field is still scarce and requires further studies.

A relationship between epididymal fat and testis function has been shown in rats and mice, where surgical removal of the epididymal fat decreases spermatogenesis, and functional connections between fat and lymph nodes have been shown. Interestingly, 80% of women suffering from polycystic ovary syndrome are obese or overweight.

The anatomical relationships between the ovary and periovarian adipose tissue are shown in the upper panel. This sample was sectioned with a razor blade and observed by SEM (which provides three-dimensional images). The surface of the sectioned ovary, with a corpus luteum (CL) and a secondary follicle (F), can be seen on the right.

The lower panel shows the peripheral portion of a periovarian depot. Note that the depot is organized into lobules and that the adipocytes on their surface are easily recognizable for their regular spherical shape.

Suggested Reading

Chu Y, et al. Epididymal fat is necessary for spermatogenesis, but not testosterone production or copulatory behavior. Endocrinology. 151:5669–79, 2010.

Pond CM. Physiological specialisation of adipose tissue. Prog Lipid Res. 38:225–48, 1999.

Azziz R. PCOS in 2015: new insights into the genetics of polycystic ovary syndrome. Nat Rev Endocrinol. 12:74–5, 2016.

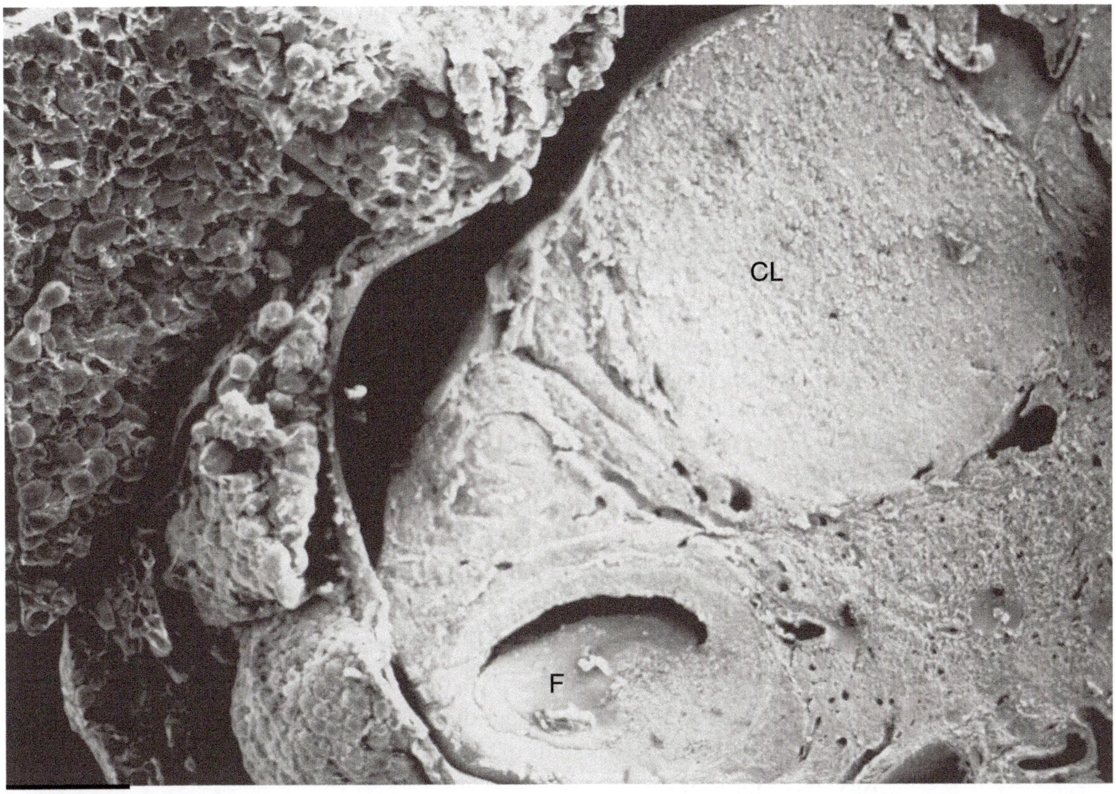

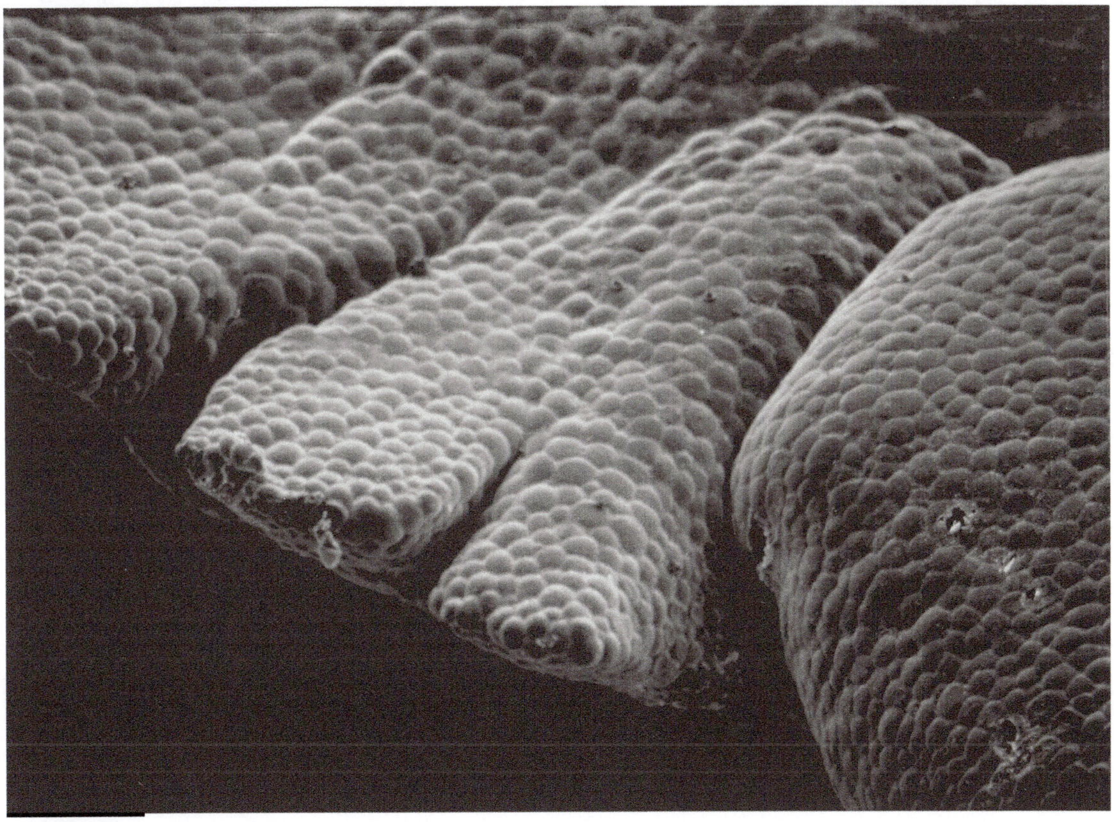

Plate 4.14 *Upper*: adult rat periovarian WAT. *Lower*: adult rat periovarian WAT lobules. SEM

PLATE 4.15

Fibroblasts

Besides the cell types hitherto described, other cytotypes are found in the white areas of the adipose organ: fibroblasts, histiocytes (see Plates 5.5–5.6), mast cells, lymphocytes (see Plates 4.12, 5.4, and 5.8), and granulocytes. The typical aspect of the fibroblasts found in white adipose tissue is shown in this plate. The most distinctive characteristic of this cell type is the abundance of rough endoplasmic reticulum (RER), which occupies almost the entire cytoplasm. Its second most important feature is its close and multiple connections with collagen fibrils (C). The absence of external lamina is also a distinctive ultrastructural feature of these cells. This cell type has been claimed by some authors to be the adipocyte precursor. In our opinion, adipoblasts and adipocyte precursors are derived from cells other than fibroblasts (see Plates 4.15–4.17 for comparison and Chap. 12). Furthermore, the definition of fibroblast-like cell for delipidized adipocytes is widely accepted. This plate strongly outlines the great ultrastructural differences between a delipidized (slimmed) adipocyte and a true fibroblast (compare with the ultrastructure of slimmed adipocytes in Plates 10.6–10.8).

Suggested Reading

Melcher AH, Chan J. Phagocytosis and digestion of collagen by gingival fibroblasts in vivo: a study of serial sections. J Ultrastruct Res. 77:1–36, 1981.

Cho MI, Garant PR. Role of microtubules in the organization of the Golgi complex and the secretion of collagen secretory granules by periodontal ligament fibroblasts. Anat Rec. 199:459–471, 1981.

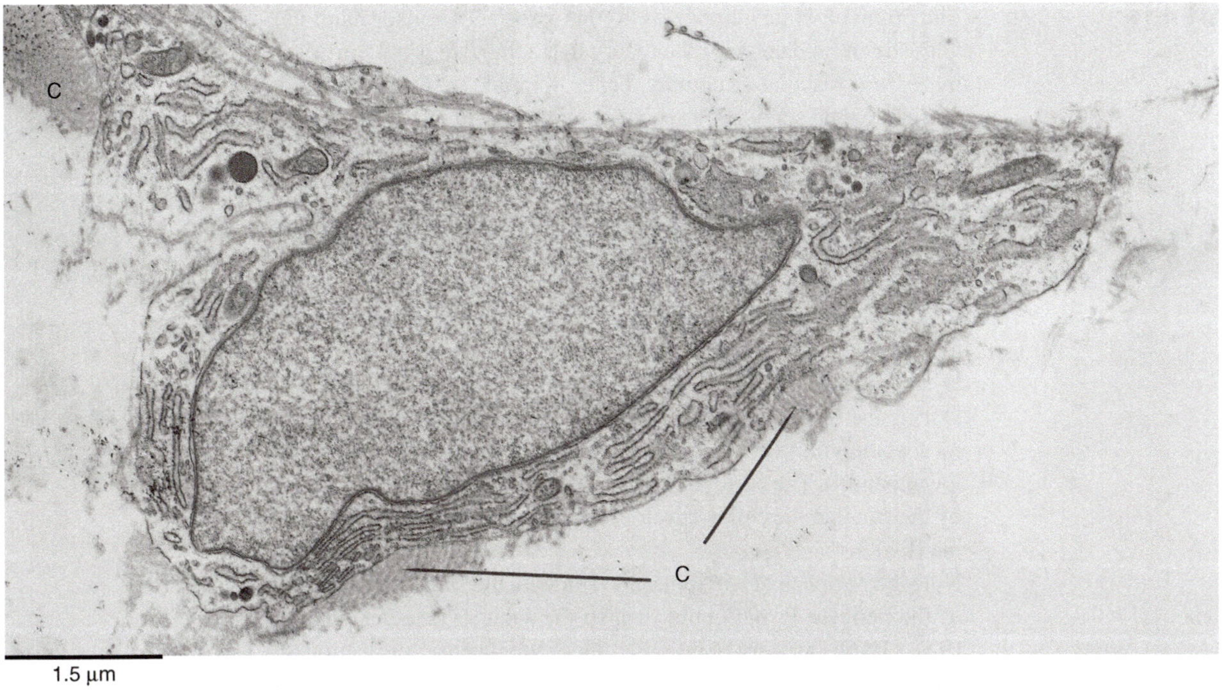

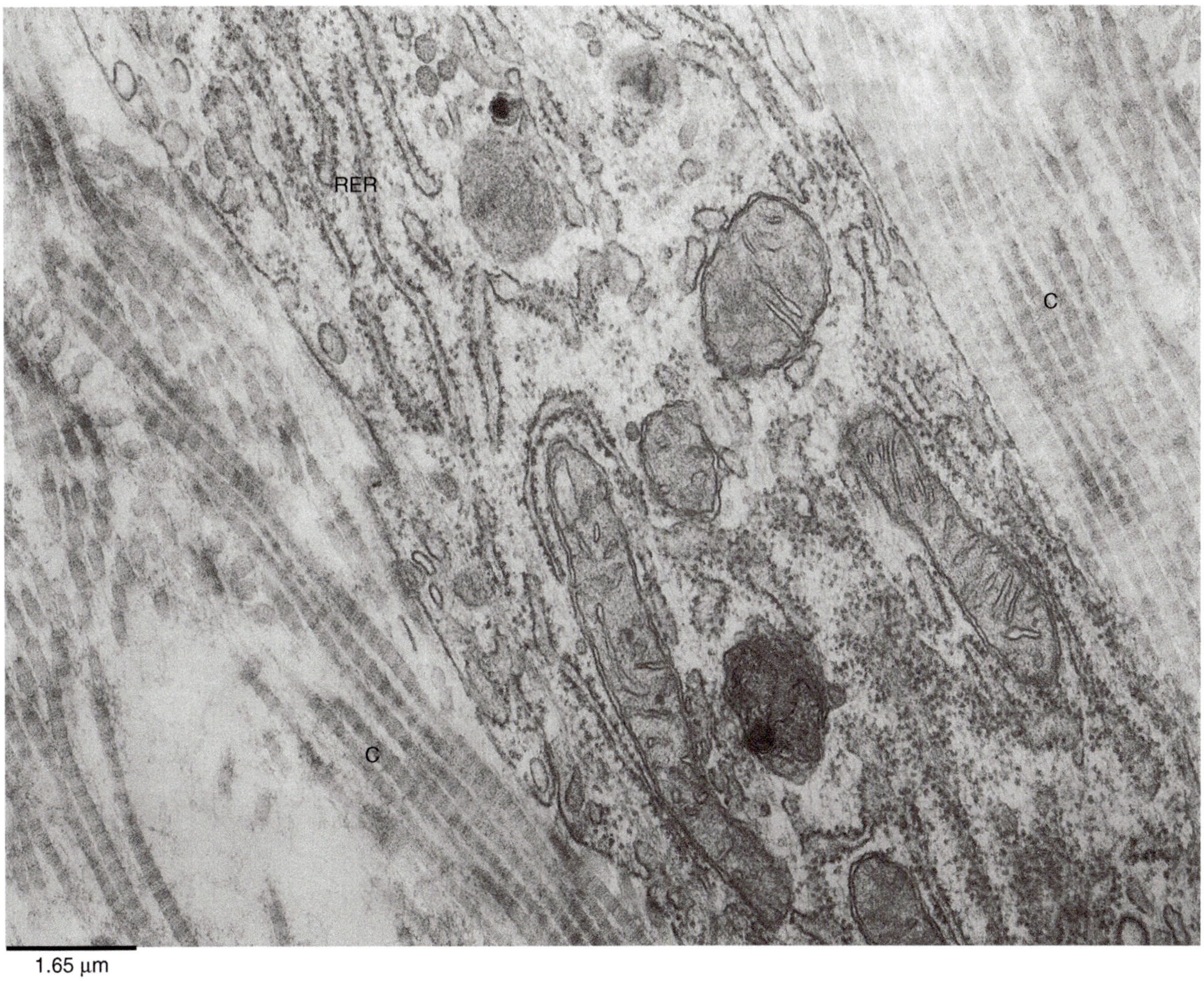

Plate 4.15 Fibroblast in the epididymal fat of young rat. *Lower*: enlargement of the cytoplasm of a fibroblast from the same depot. TEM

PLATE 4.16

Pericytes I

The origin of white adipocytes is controversial (see also Chap. 12). Ultrastructural data favor the theory that adipocyte precursors originate from vascular structures. Plates 4.15 and 4.16 provide some morphological support for the vascular theory. In rats, white adipocytes of epididymal fat appear only after birth, and within few weeks, this depot appears well developed. The in vivo and in vitro analysis of this depot in the neonatal period has allowed the morphological phases of white adipose cell development to be firmly established.

Researchers concur in considering the appearance of lipid droplets and glycogen granules in cells with the general aspect of a blast cell as the first signs of adipocyte differentiation.

During the first weeks of life, the most undifferentiated cell in the rat's epididymal depot is a cell in pericytic position (upper and lower panels). The pericytic position of this cell (P) is demonstrated by the fact that the cell is enveloped by the capillary's external lamina (EL).

Note the presence of a cytoplasmic rim with the same ultrastructure of the pericyte P that could own to the same or another pericyte (P2). These aspects (see also the cytoplasmic projections—arrows—of the pericyte shown in the lower panel) could fit with the stellate morphology of adipocyte precursors described in confocal studies.

The pericyte could be an early form of a blast cell committed to develop into an adipocyte. This hypothesis is based on the following observations: (1) This cell type shows the general aspect of blast cells (high nucleus/cytoplasm ratio, well-developed nucleolus, absence of cytoplasmic differentiation). (2) It is found in great abundance in the tissue only while white depots are developing. (3) Similar cells are frequently detected near capillary walls during depot development. (4) Their size is not proportional with the whole capillary size for a simple pericytic function (in particular this aspect is visually evident in the lower panel).

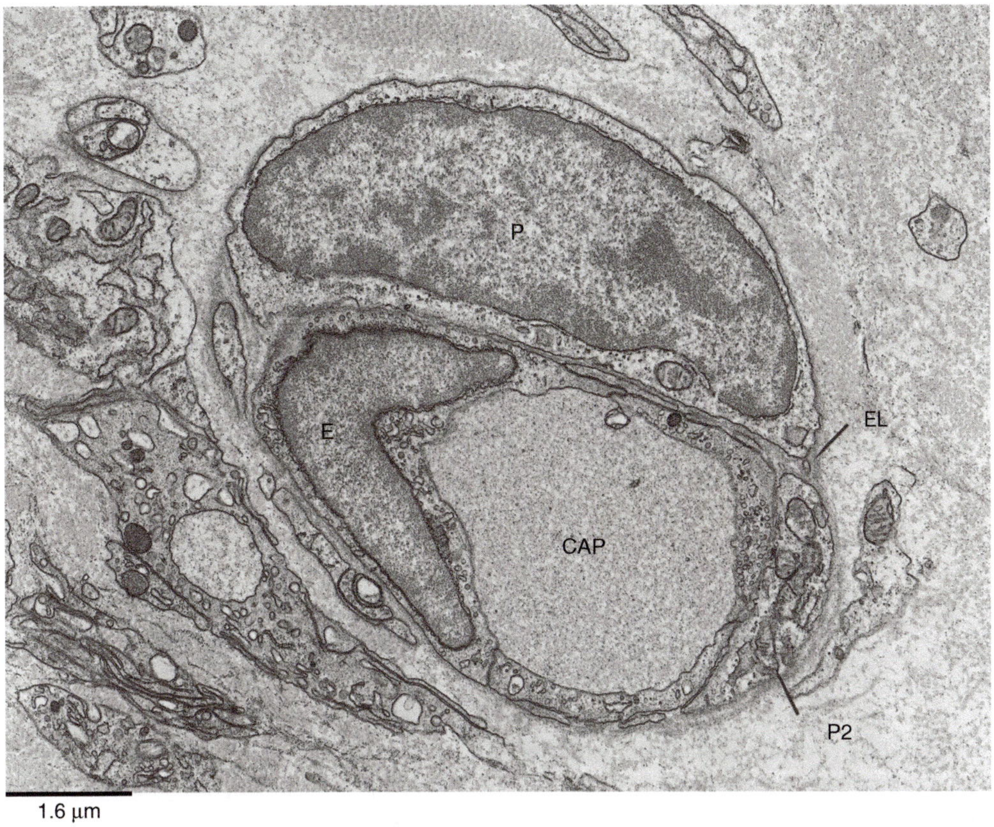

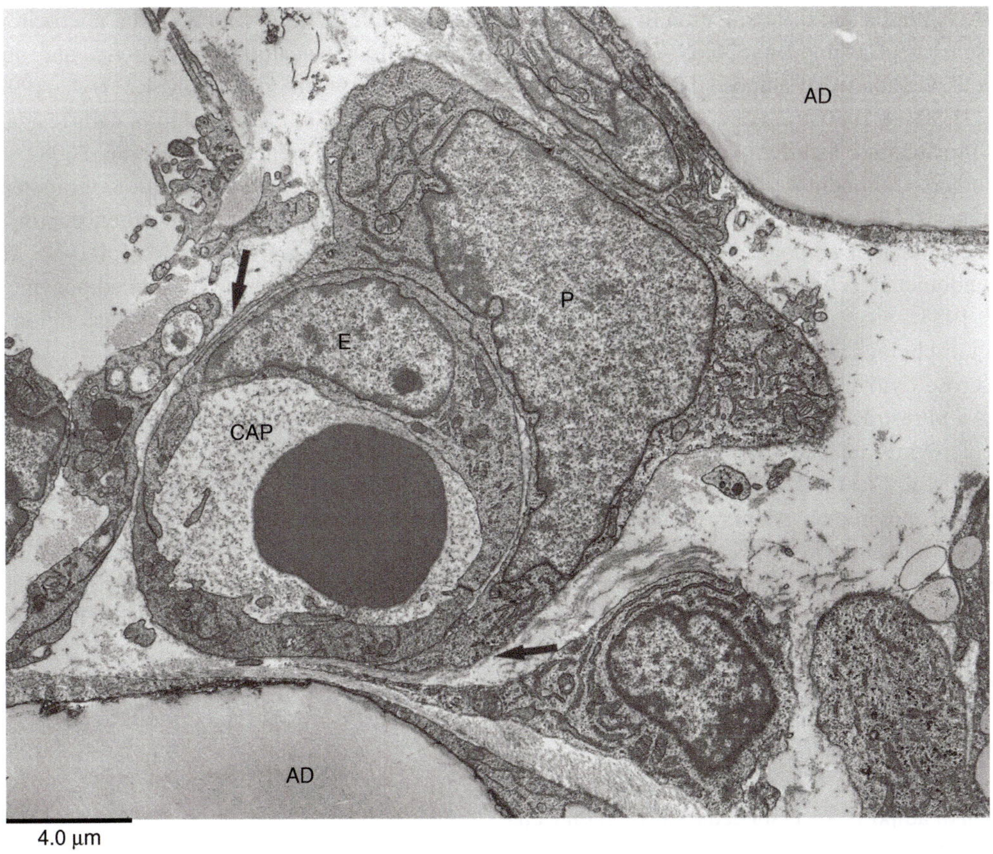

Plate 4.16 *Upper*: cross-sectioned capillaries (CAP) in the epididymal depot of a young rat. E: endothelial cell. *Lower*: same depot. AD: mature white adipocytes. TEM

PLATE 4.17

Pericytes II

(5) Cells sharing these features and exhibiting very early signs of adipocytic differentiation are found during the process of development of white depots (this plate). The cell marked "P" in this plate lies partially in pericytic position (see the external lamina – EL – in the framed areas) and partially in the interstitial space and contains some glycogen granules (G). Other cells in the same position also contain small lipid droplets. It is noteworthy that glycogen granules are rarely seen in pericytes in other organs. Several glycogen granules and lipid droplets are present in the endothelial and pericytic cells of myxoid and round cell liposarcomas. Cells with very early signs of adipocytic differentiation should be considered as specific white adipoblasts-preadipocytes because they exhibit a small number of mitochondria (m) with a different morphology from that of the "pre-typical" mitochondria of brown adipoblasts-preadipocytes (see Plates 2.26–2.30 and Chap. 13).
A series of modern data strongly support the vascular origin of cells committed to develop into white adipocytes (see Chap. 12 for further details).

Suggested Reading

Iyama K, et al. Electron microscopical studies on the genesis of white adipocytes: differentiation of immature pericytes into adipocytes in transplanted preadipose tissue. Virch Arch B 31:143–55, 1979.

Pilgrim C. DNA synthesis and differentiation in developing white adipose tissue. Develop Biol. 26:69–76, 1971.

Desnoyers F, et al. Cellularity of adipose tissue in fetal pig. J Lipid Res. 21:301–8,1980.

Cinti S, et al. Ultrastructural features of cultured mature adipocyte precursors from adipose tissue in multiple symmetric lipomatosis. Ultrastruct Path. 5:145–52, 1983.

Björntorp P. Interactions of adipocytes and their precursor cells with endothelial cells in culture. Exp Cell Res. 149:277–87, 1983.

Cinti S, et al. A morphological study of the adipocyte precursor. J Submicrosc Cytol. 16:243–51, 1984.

Cinti S, et al. An ultrastructural study of adipocyte precursors from epididymal fat pads of adult rats in culture. J Submicrosc Cytol. 17:115–22, 1985.

Rossouw DJ, et al. Liposarcoma. An ultrastructural study of 15 cases. Am J Clin Path. 85:649–67, 1986.

Gregoire F, et al. Ultrastructural analysis of the in vitro differentiation of female rat preadipocytes. Biol Cell. 56:127–36, 1986.

Hauner H. Complete adipose differentiation of 3T3 L1 cells in a chemically defined medium: comparison to serum-containing culture conditions. Endocrinology. 127:865–72, 1990.

Ailhaud G. Extracellular factors, signalling pathways and differentiation of adipose precursor cells. Curr Opion Cell Biol. 2:1043–49, 1990.

Gregoire F, et al. The stroma-vascular fraction of rat inguinal and epididymal adipose tissue and the adipoconversion of fat cell precursors in primary culture. Biol Cell. 69:215–22, 1990.

Crandall DL, et al. A review of the microcirculation of adipose tissue: anatomic, metabolic, and angiogenic perspectives. Microcirculation. 4:211–32, 1997.

Tang W, et al. White fat progenitor cells reside in the adipose vasculature. Science. 322:583–86, 2008.

Lee YH, et al. In vivo identification of bipotential adipocyte progenitors recruited by β3-adrenoceptor activation and high-fat feeding. Cell Metab. 15:480–91, 2012.

Lee YH, et al. Identification of an adipogenic niche for adipose tissue remodeling and restoration. Cell Metab. 18:355–67, 2013.

Tran KV, et al. The vascular endothelium of the adipose tissue gives rise to both white and brown fat cells. Cell Metab. 15:222–29, 2012.

Poulos SP, et al. The increasingly complex regulation of adipocyte differentiation. Exp Biol Med. 241:449–56, 2016.

Hausman GJ, et al. Preadipocyte and adipose tissue differentiation in meat animals: influence of species and anatomical location. Annu Rev Anim Biosci. 2:323–5, 2014.

Berry DC, et al. Emerging roles of adipose progenitor cells in tissue development, homeostasis, expansion and thermogenesis. Trends Endocrinol Metab. 27:574–85, 2016.

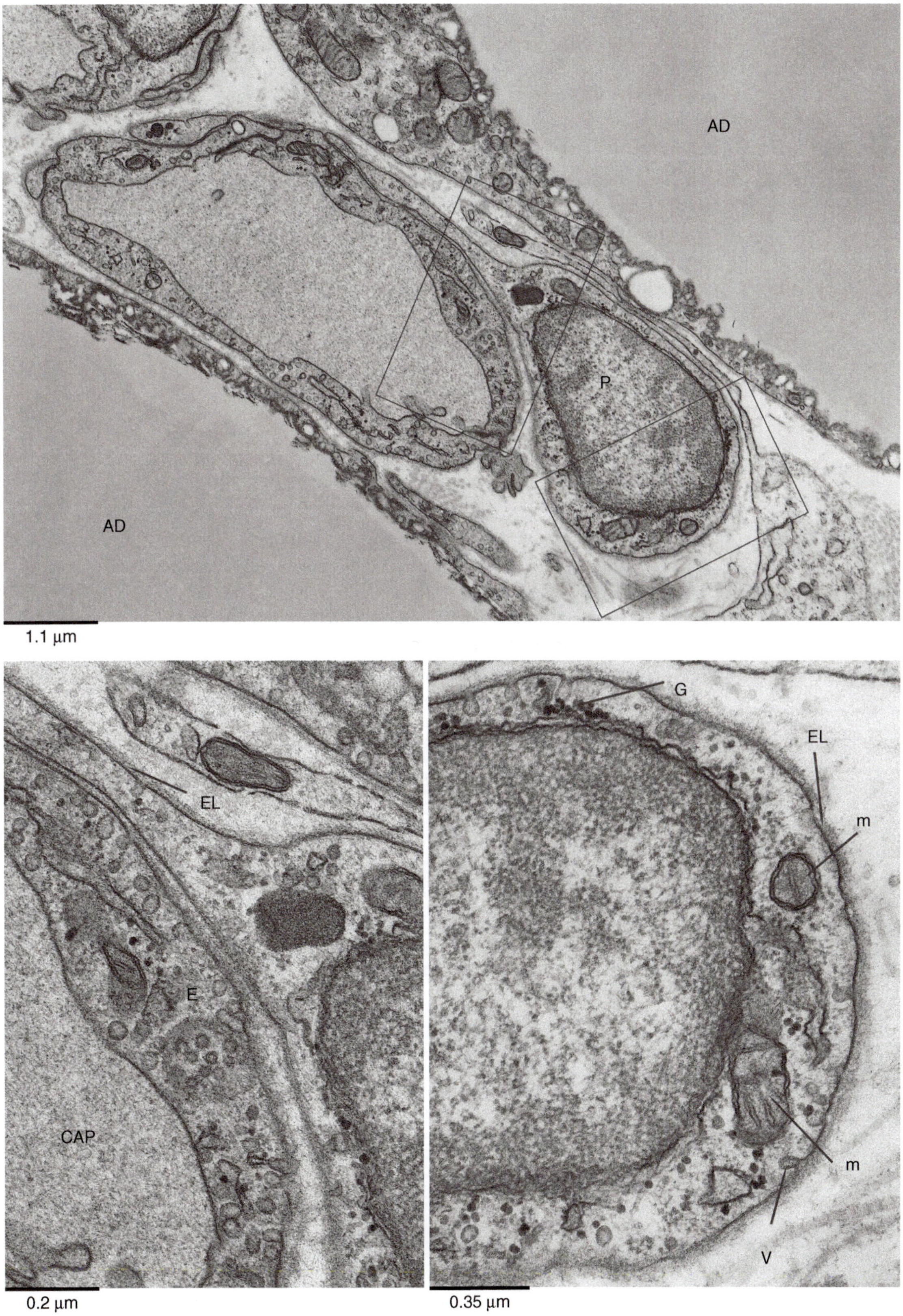

Plate 4.17 *Upper*: depot shown in Plate 4.15. The cell shown in the panel (P) is partly closely apposed to the capillary wall in pericytic position and partly in the interstitium. The framed areas are enlarged in the lower panels. CAP, capillary lumen; AD, mature white adipocytes; V, pinocytotic vesicle; E, endothelial cell; m, mitochondria; G, glycogen; EL, external lamina. TEM

PLATE 4.18

Preadipocytes

Small cells (10–15 μm in diameter) with ultrastructural features similar to those of mature adipocytes are frequently found in developing white depots. The two small adipocytes shown in this plate among mature adipocytes (AD) could be considered as late white preadipocytes (P). The cell near the capillary, which contains three erythrocytes (E), exhibits a paucilocular lipid arrangement (upper panel). This phase of adipocytic differentiation must be very short because in the absence of the activation of the gene(s) responsible for lipid multilocularity, specific of thermogenic brown adipocytes, the aqueous environment of the hyaloplasm causes triglycerides to form quickly a single vacuole (lower figure). Note that the mitochondrial morphology is different from that of brown preadipocytes (compare with Plates 2.28 and 2.29).

Suggested Reading

Dardick I, et al. Ultrastructural observations on differentiating human preadipocytes cultured in vitro. Tiss Cell 8:561–71, 1976.

Van RL, Rocari DA. Complete differentiation of adipocyte precursors. A culture system for studying the cellular nature of adipose tissue. Cell Tiss Res. 317–29, 1978.

Hausman GJ, et al. Adipocyte development in the rat hypodermis. Am J Anat. 165:85–100, 1981.

Roth J, et al. The regenerating fascial sheath in lipectomized Osborne-Mendel rats: morphological and biochemical indices of adipocyte differentiation and proliferation. Int J Obesity 5:131–43, 1981.

Ailhaud G, et al. Cellular and molecular aspects of adipose tissue development. Annu Rev Nutr. 12:207–33, 1992.

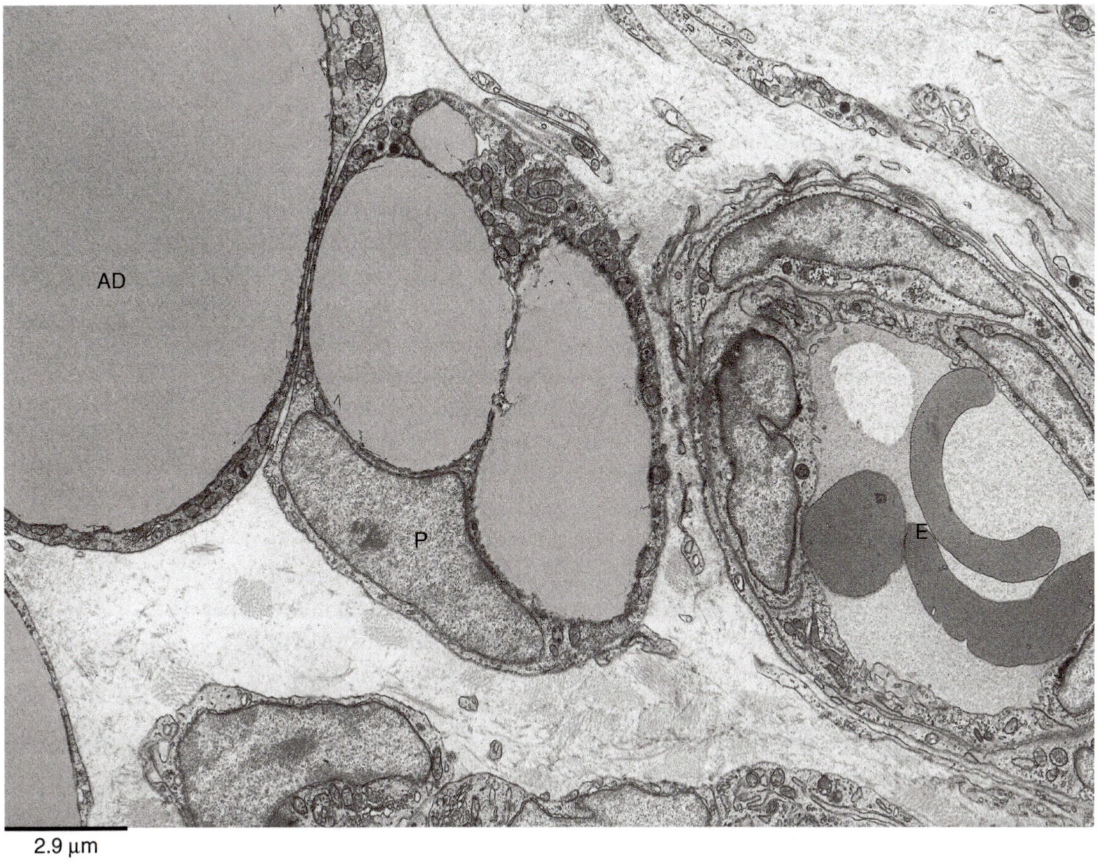

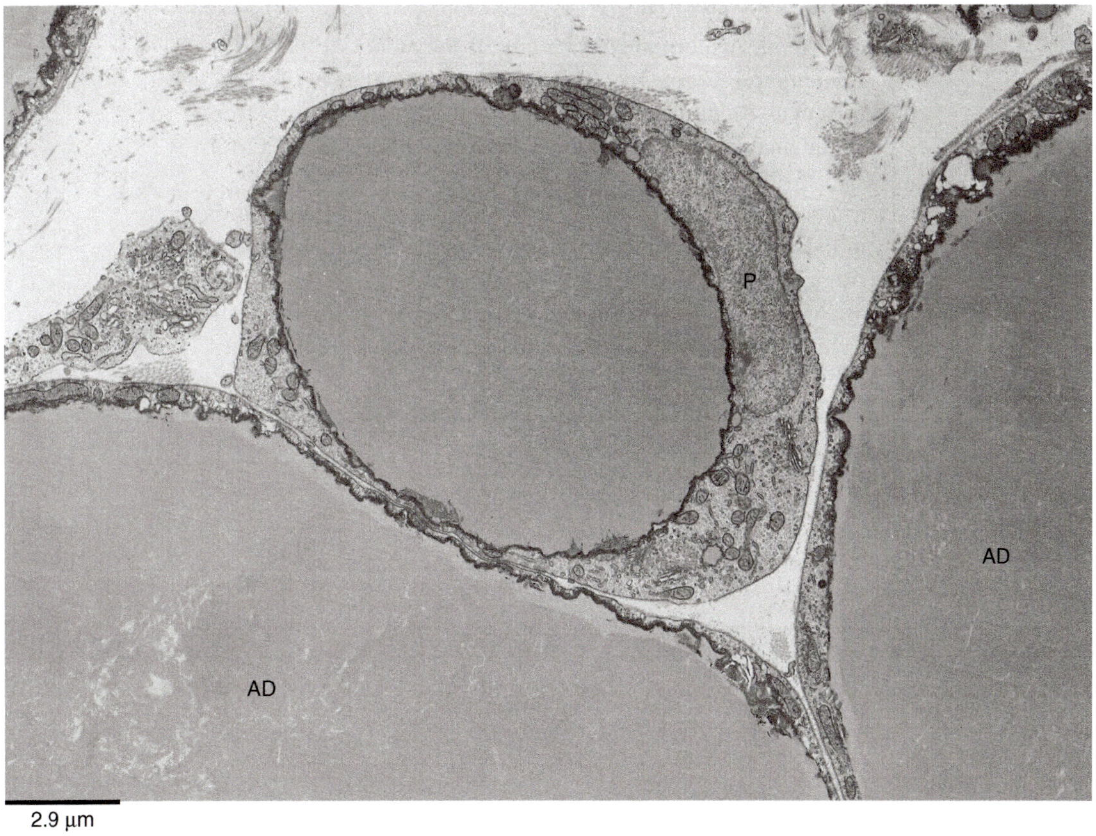

Plate 4.18 Epididymal depot of a young rat. White adipocyte precursors (P). TEM

PLATE 4.19

SVF Electron Microscopy

For many years the technique to isolate mature adipocytes (see Plate 4.2) and the so-called stroma vascular fraction (SVF) (light microscopy: upper panel) has been used in adipose organ research (see also Plate 4.2).

Only a few morphology studies have been performed on the SVF. Here the ultrastructure of isolated preadipocytes is shown together with endothelial cells that are the two most abundant cells found in the SVF (lower panel). Preadipocytes, corresponding to the right squared area in the upper panel, have a diameter of about 7–10 microns; the nucleus is predominantly regular and roundish. In the cytoplasm rough endoplasmic reticulum (RER) and a well-developed Golgi complex (Go) are usually found. Mitochondria are small and numerous. Lipid droplets are small and their frequency is variable. Our quantitative analyses showed that about 50% or 20% of isolated preadipocytes contain lipid droplets if epididymal fat pad from young or adult rats, respectively, is used.

The second frequent cell type (endothelial cells) seen among these pelleted cells is visible in the left side of the lower panel (corresponding to cell aggregates as in the left squared area in the upper panel); nucleus is quite irregular with dense chromatin. The cytoplasm is rich in organelles, but the most distinctive feature is the presence of tight junctions (TJ) joining cells in small groups.

Specific ultrastructural features identify all other cell types present in the SVF.

Suggested Reading

Cinti S, et al. A morphological study of the adipocyte precursor. J Submicrosc Cytol. 16:243–51, 1984.

Cinti S, et al. An ultrastructural study of adipocyte precursors from epididymal fat pads of adult rats in culture. J Submicrosc Cytol. 17:115–22, 1985.

Hausman GJ, et al. Preadipocyte and adipose tissue differentiation in meat animals: influence of species and anatomical location. Annu Rev Anim Biosci. 2:323–51, 2014.

Hausman GJ, Dodson MV. Stromal Vascular Cells and Adipogenesis: Cells within Adipose Depots Regulate Adipogenesis. J Genomics. 1:56–66, 2013.

Hausman DB, et al. The biology of white adipocyte proliferation. Obes Rev. 2:239–54, 2001.

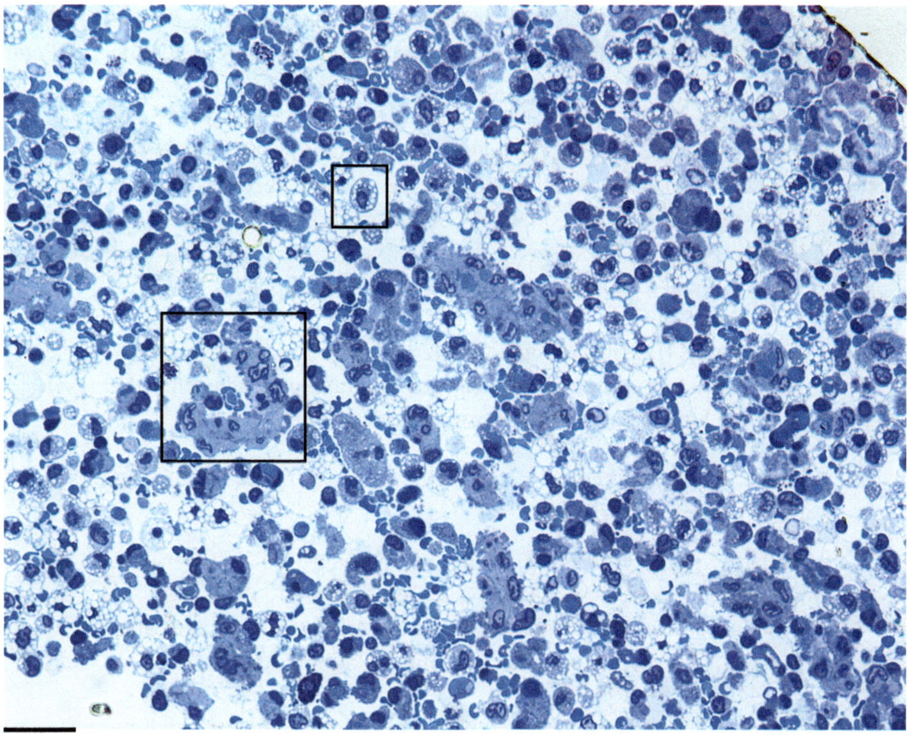
50 µm

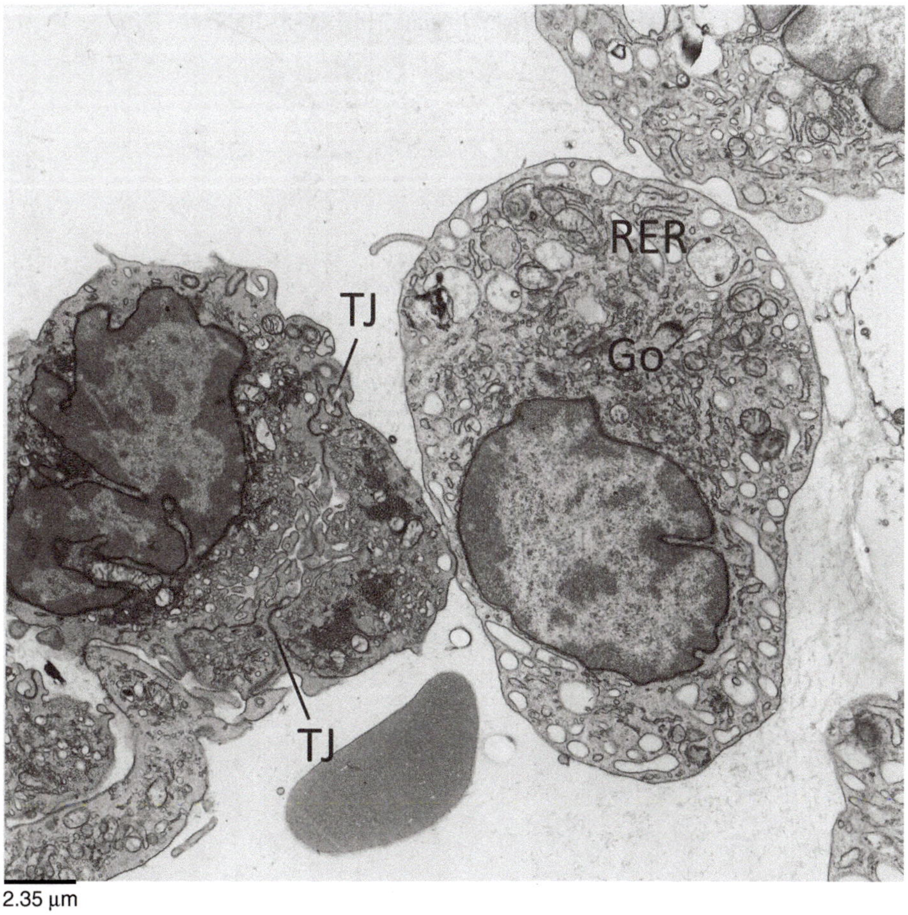

2.35 µm

Plate 4.19 *Upper*: stroma vascular fraction from epididymal WAT of a young rat. Resin-embedded tissue. Toluidine blue staining. LM. *Lower*: SVF from epididymal WAT of a young rat. TEM

PLATE 4.20

Nervous-Vascular Peduncles

In the adipose organ, white areas are also innervated. Nervous-vascular peduncles or exclusively nervous peduncles entering white adipose depots are easy to dissect in adult rats and mice. The left inguinal depot of an adult rat is shown in the upper panel partially dissected to the median third and folded back toward the head of the animal to offer a better view of the depot's nervous-vascular supply (arrows) from collaterals of the femoral nervous-vascular trunk.

In the left epididymal depot of the same rat (lower panel), the depot is displaced outside the surgical window. The urinary bladder (U), vas deferens (D), and seminal vesicles (SV) are marked for orientation. An arrow indicates the nervous-vascular peduncle entering from the lumbar region into the adipose depot.

Suggested Reading

Ballard K, et al. Adrenergic innervation and vascular patterns in canine adipose tissue. Microvasc Res. 8:164–71, 1974.

Crandall DL, et al. Adipocyte blood flow: influence of age, anatomic location, and dietary manipulation. Am J Physiol. 247:R46–51, 1984.

Murano I, et al. Noradrenergic parenchymal nerve fiber branching after cold acclimatization correlates with brown adipocyte density in mouse adipose organ. J Anat. 214:171–8, 2009.

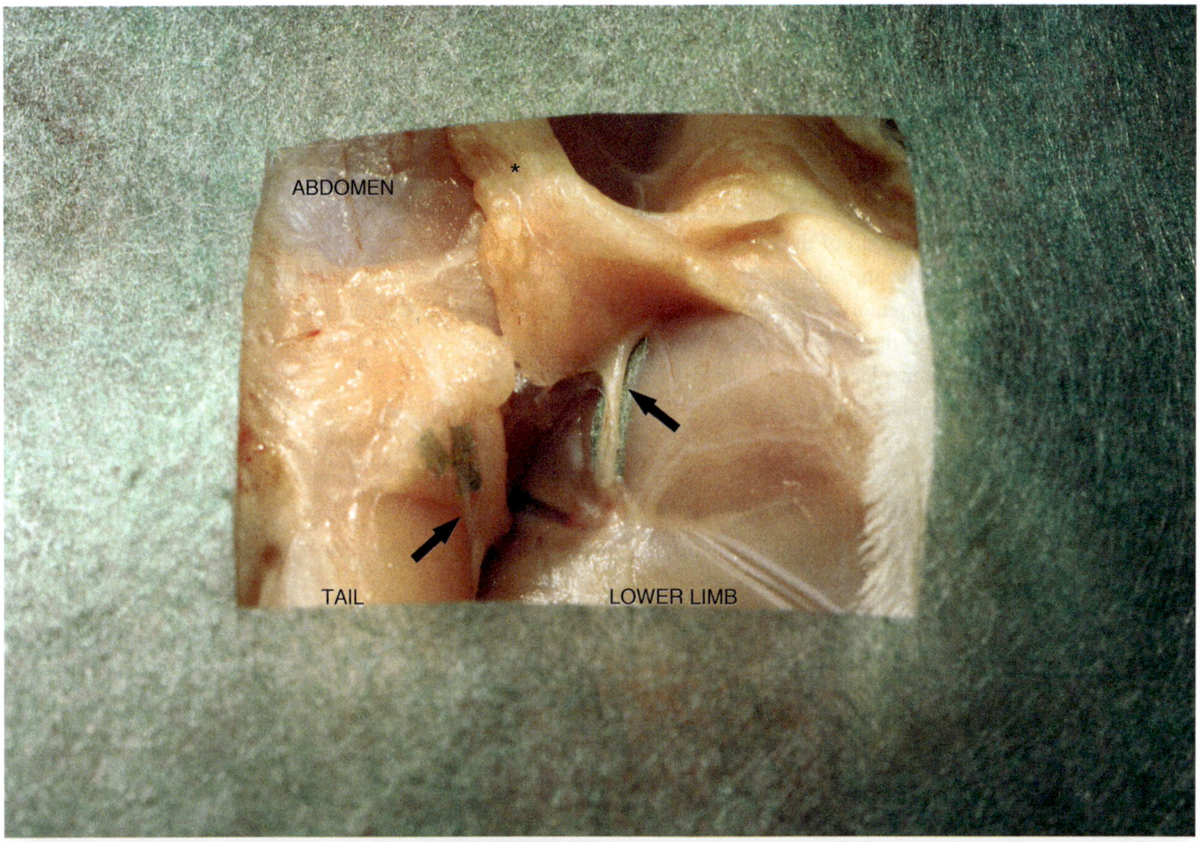

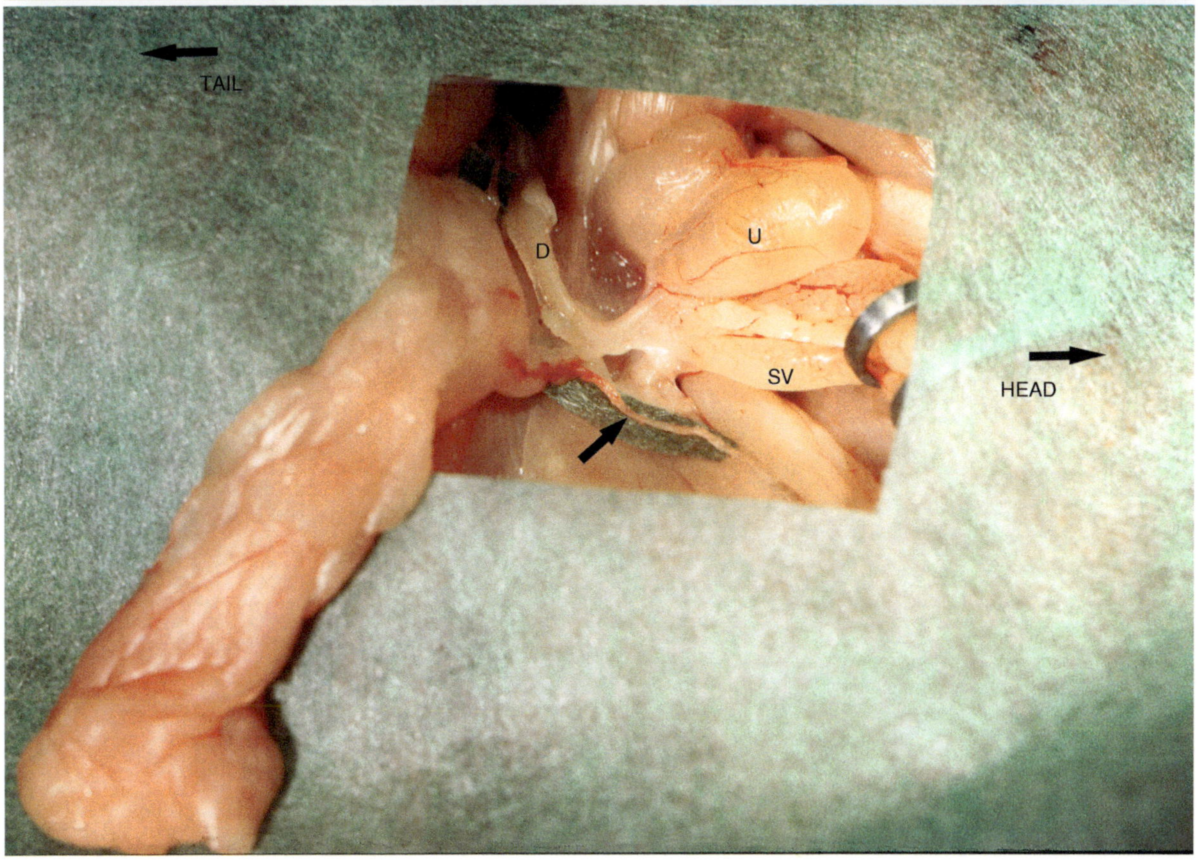

Plate 4.20 *Upper*: adult rat. Nerves to the left inguinal depot (*arrows*). Inguinal depot sectioned and refolded (*asterisk*). *Lower*: nerves to the left epididymal depot (*arrow*)

PLATE 4.21

Nerves

Three nerves (arrows) appear to enter the left retroperitoneal depot of an adult rat (left panel, frontal view). The psoas major muscle (PM) is identified for orientation. Note that the left kidney and the corresponding perirenal depot have not been removed, but displaced to the right of the animal to offer a good view of the posterior surface of the left kidney. The perirenal depot is partially visible on the left (P) of the surgical window. In the right panel, the lower end of the retroperitoneal depot has been displaced to the left of the animal, and the deeper tract of the inferior nerve shown in the left panel is now visible. Only its collaterals enter the retroperitoneal depot (small arrows). Fragments of green surgical sheet have been placed under the dissected nerves better to show their anatomical arrangement.

Suggested Reading

Wirsén C. in "Handbook of Physiology", Am. Physiol. Soc., 197–199, 1965.

Bartness TJ, Bamshad M. Innervation of mammalian white adipose tissue: implications for the regulation of total body fat. Am J Physiol. 275:R1399–411, 1998.

Bamshad M, et al. Central nervous system origins of the sympathetic nervous system outflow to white adipose tissue. Am J Physiol. 275:R291–99, 1998.

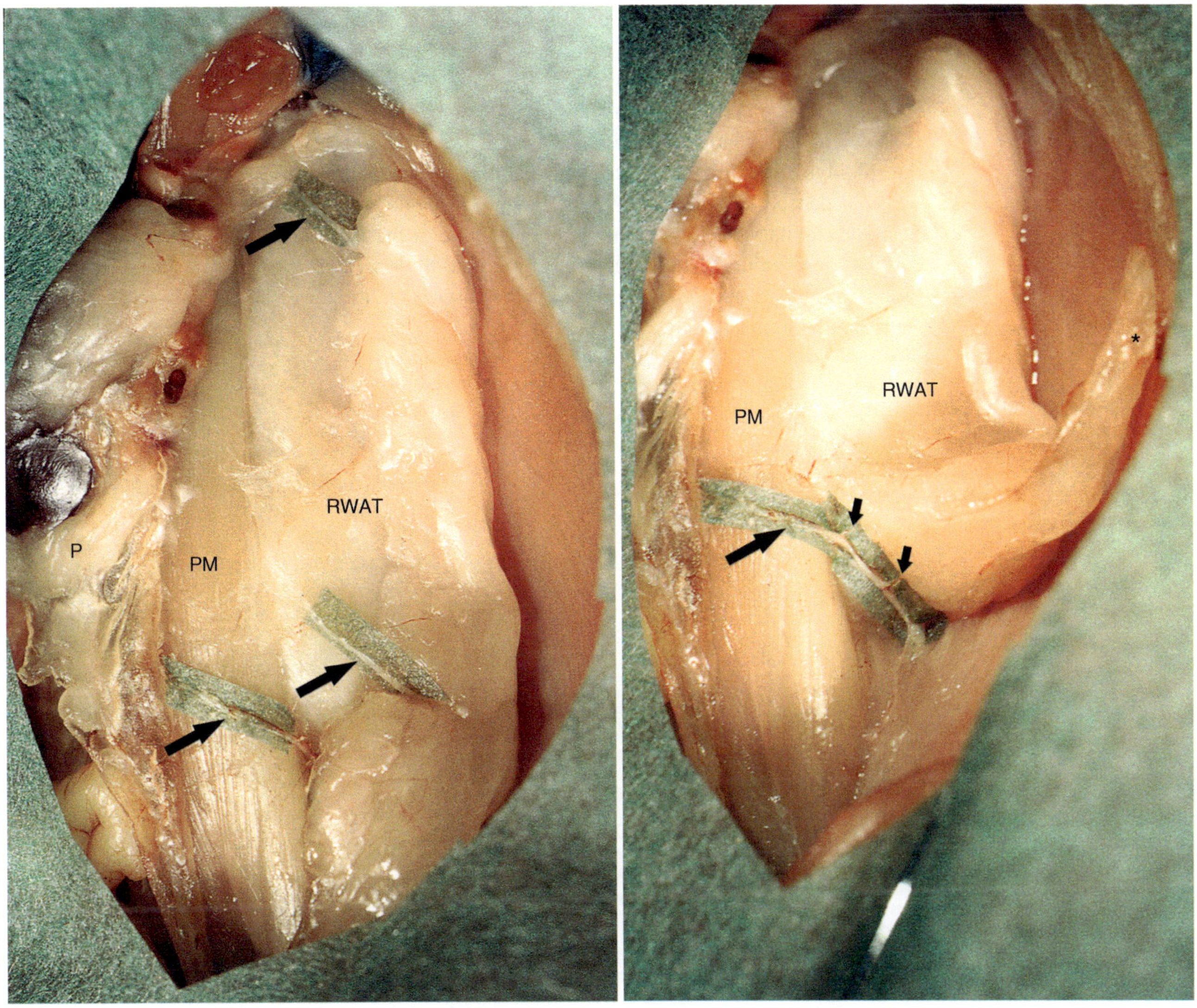

Plate 4.21 Adult rat. Nerves to the left retroperitoneal WAT. *Upper*: three nerves seem to enter the depot (*arrows*). *Lower*: the caudal end of the depot (*asterisk*) is partly displaced to the left. *Small arrows*: collateral nerves

PLATE 4.22

Nerve Ultrastructure I

Parenchymal nerves in WAT are visible by TEM. They are usually in contact with capillaries. All the WAT areas of murine adipose organ contain parenchymal nerves.

A small nerve composed of a small number of unmyelinated axons is shown in close connection with the wall of a capillary (CAP) of the epididymal fat of a young rat. Note that the axons contain vesicles and dense-core granules. About 100 nm separate this nerve from the capillary, but two basal membranes (one of the Schwann cell and one belonging to the capillary) separate these two structures. Cross-sectioned collagen fibrils can be observed in the lower right angle of the enlargement.

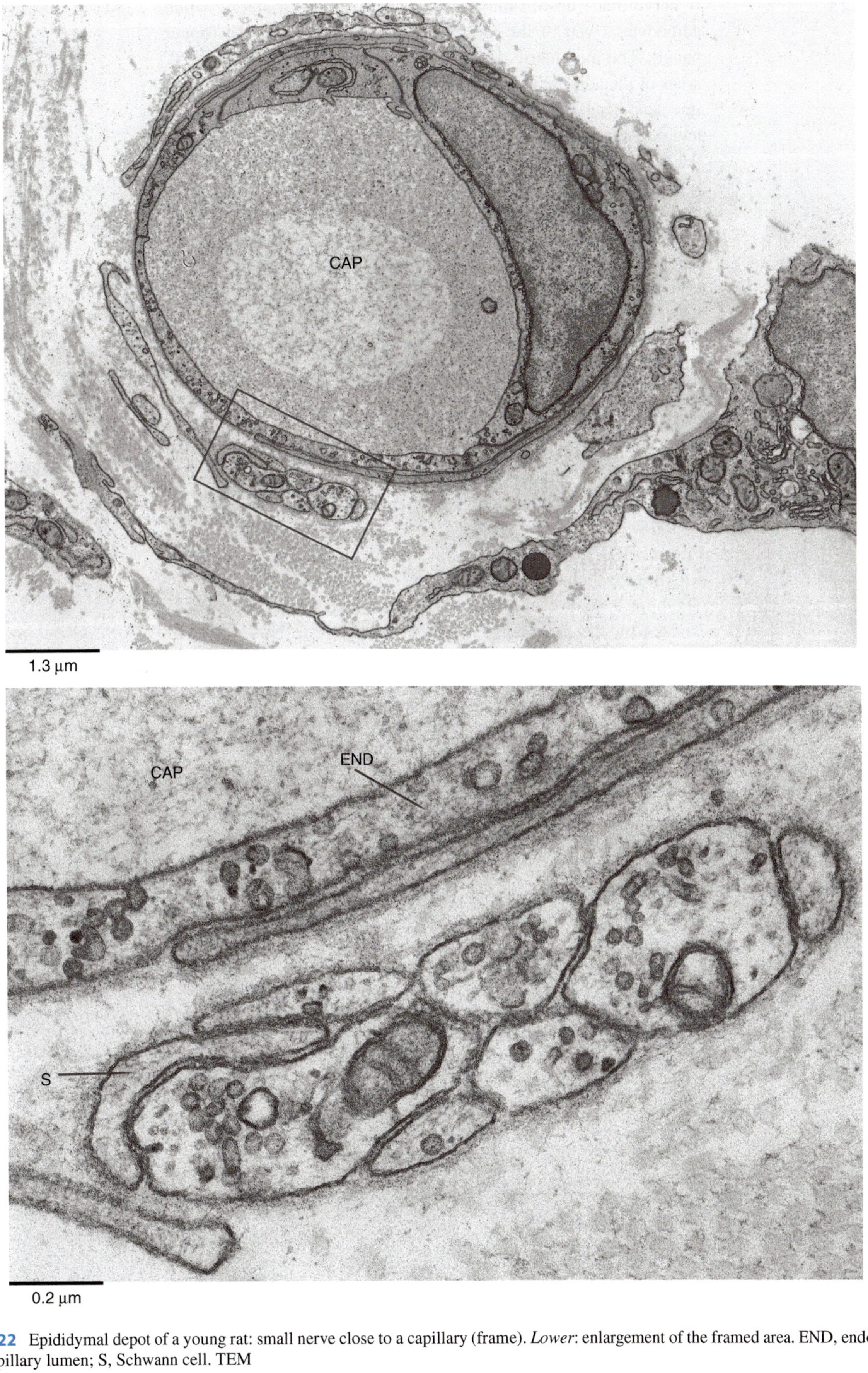

Plate 4.22 Epididymal depot of a young rat: small nerve close to a capillary (frame). *Lower*: enlargement of the framed area. END, endothelium; CAP, capillary lumen; S, Schwann cell. TEM

PLATE 4.23

Nerve Ultrastructure II

A nerve made up of unmyelinated fibers is shown among white adipocytes (AD) of the mesenteric depot of a young rat (upper panel). The mesenteric depot is one of the most innervated WAT areas of the adipose organ. In the white adipose tissue surrounding interscapular BAT, which is also well innervated, small parenchymal nerves run among unilocular adipocytes (AD) (lower panel). In the nerve shown in the lower panel, some unmyelinated fibers (UM, some indicated) and two myelinated (MY, one indicated) ones are present. Note the perineural cells (PE) surrounding the nerve fibers with thin cytoplasmic projections. A collagen fiber made up of collagen fibrils (C) is visible among the adipocytes in close association with a cytoplasmic projection of a fibroblast (F).

Suggested Reading

White JE, Engel FL. A lipolytic action of epinephrine and norepinephrine on rat adipose tissue in vitro. Proc Soc Exp Biol Med. 99:375–78, 1958.

Slavin BG, Ballard K. Morphological studies on the adrenergic innervation of white adipose tissue. Anat Rec. 191:377–90, 1978.

Fishman RB, Dark J. Sensory innervation of white adipose tissue. Am J Physiol. 253:R942–44, 1987.

Trayhurn P, Ashwell M. Control of white and brown adipose tissues by the autonomic nervous system. Proc Nutr Soc. 46: 135–42, 1987.

Rebuffe-Scrive M. Neuroregulation of adipose tissue: molecular and hormonal mechanisms. Int J Obesity. 15:83–6, 1991.

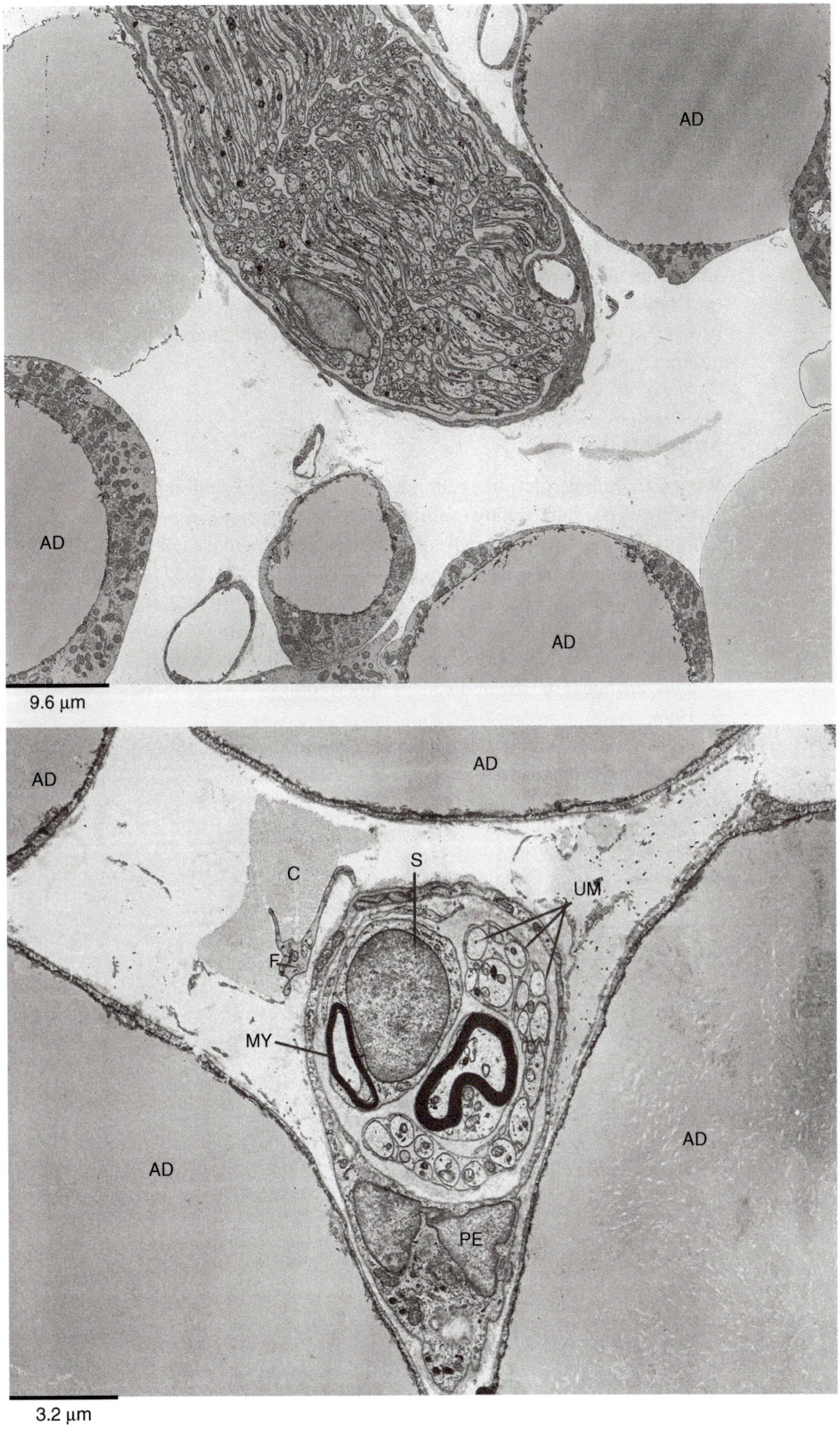

Plate 4.23 *Upper*: mesenteric depot nerve in a young mouse. *Lower*: parenchymal nerves in the white adipose tissue surrounding IBAT in an adult rat. S, Schwann cell. TEM

PLATE 4.24

Nerve IHC, TH-CGRP

Parenchymal nerves and single nerve fibers can also be detected by immunohistochemical methods. Since some proteins are expressed by specific nerve fibers, immunoreactive fibers can be detected and classified using specific antibodies.

The top panel shows noradrenergic fibers immunoreactive for an anti-TH (tyrosine hydroxylase) antibody in close contact with the capillary wall and with adipocytes in the mesenteric depot of a young rat.

Small CGRP-immunoreactive parenchymal nerves running among adipocytes are shown in the middle (retroperitoneal depot) and bottom (epididymal depot) panels. CGRP (calcitonin gene-related peptide) is usually found in sensitive nerve fibers, which also have efferent activity.

Suggested Reading

Wirsen C. Adrenergic innervation of adipose tissue examined by fluorescence microscopy. Nature. 202:913, 1964.

Lafontan M, Berlan M. Fat cell adrenergic receptors and the control of white and brown fat cell function. J Lipid Res. 34:1057–91, 1993.

Cousin B, et al. Local sympathetic denervation of white adipose tissue in rats induces preadipocyte proliferation without noticeable changes in metabolism. Endocrinology. 133:2255–62, 1993.

Giordano A, et al. Adipose organ nerves revealed by immunohistochemistry. Methods Mol Biol. 456:83–95, 2008.

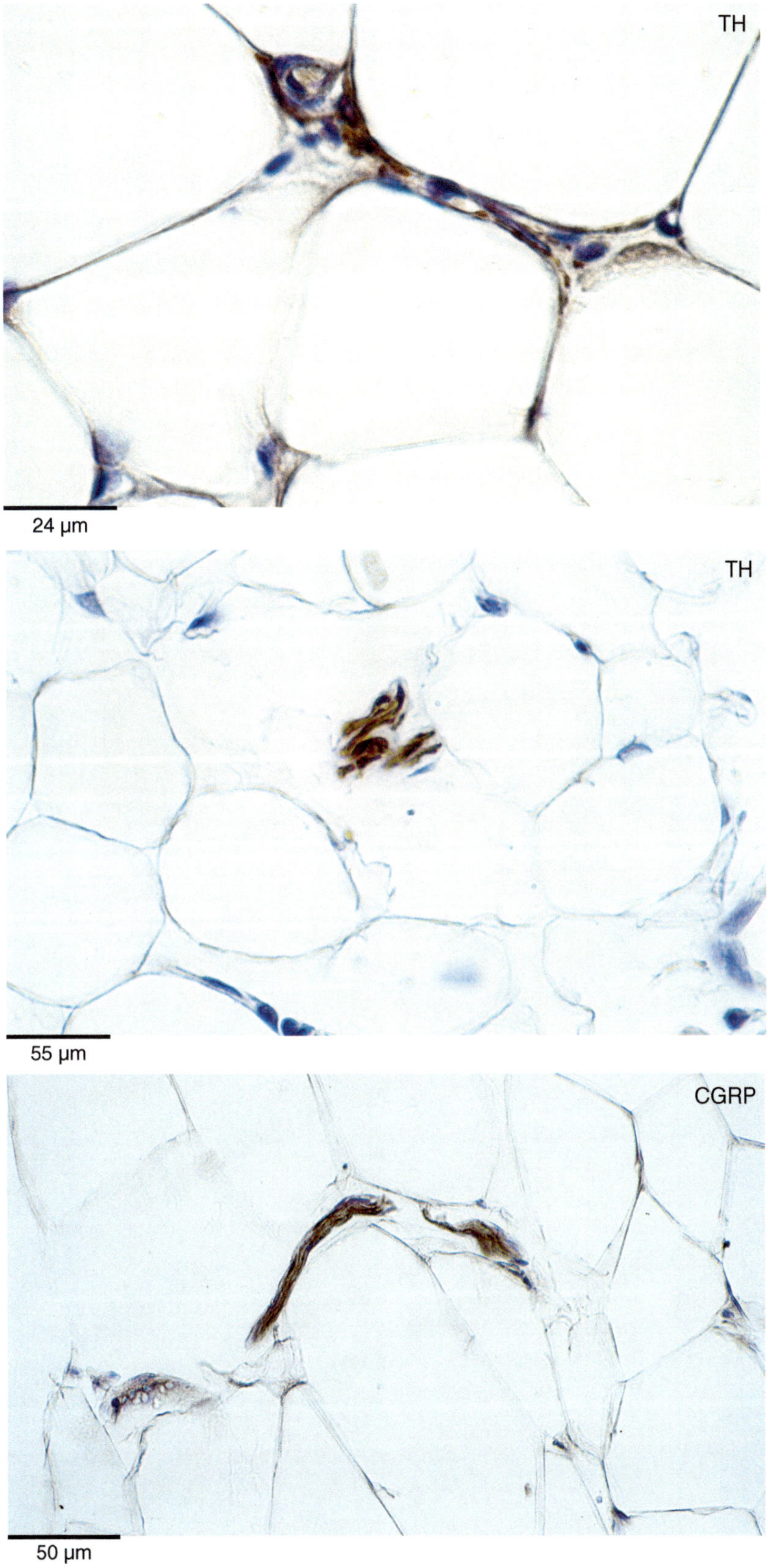

Plate 4.24 *Top*: mesenteric depot of a 30-day-old rat. TH-positive (adrenergic) nerve fibers in close contact with a capillary and adipocytes. LM. IHC: TH ab (1:300). *Middle*: retroperitoneal WAT of adult mouse. TH-immunoreactive (adrenergic) small nerve. LM. IHC: TH ab (1:300). *Bottom*: adult rat epididymal depot. CGRP-positive nerve. LM. IHC: CGRP ab (1.2,000)

5 Human WAT

S. Cinti, *Obesity, Type 2 Diabetes and the Adipose Organ*, https://doi.org/10.1007/978-3-319-40522-3_5

5.1 Human WAT

PLATE 5.1

Pre-embedded WAT

Human adipose tissue (like murine fat; see Plate 4.1), fresh or fixed, can be observed at light microscopy before further processing (embedding). In this plate two examples are shown. In the upper plate visceral fat from the neck (peri-carotid fat) is shown. Note the extremely regular size of the cells without any artifact due to the embedding procedure. The size of adipocytes in fresh samples is about 20–30% larger than that measured in sections of tissue routinely processed for light microscopy also for human fat.
In the bottom panel a lobule of subcutaneous fat sampled from a lean patient is shown. The red areas are due to vascular structures filled with erythrocytes.

Suggested Reading

Englhardt A, et al. Size, lipid and enzyme content of isolated human adipocytes in relation to nutritional state. Diabetologia. 7:51–8, 1971.

Chumlea WC, et al. Size and number of adipocytes and measures of body fat in boys and girls 10 to 18 years of age. Am J Clin Nutr. 34:1791–7, 1981.

Engfeldt P, Arner P. Lipolysis in human adipocytes, effects of cell size, age and of regional differences. Horm Metab Res Suppl. 19:26–9, 1988.

Jernås M, et al. Separation of human adipocytes by size: hypertrophic fat cells display distinct gene expression. FASEB J. 20:1540–2, 2006.

Tchoukalova YD, et al. Subcutaneous adipocyte size and body fat distribution. Am J Clin Nutr. 87:56–63, 2008.

Soula HA, et al. Modelling adipocytes size distribution. J Theor Biol. 332:89–95, 2013.

Parlee SD, et al. Quantifying size and number of adipocytes in adipose tissue. Methods Enzymol. 537:93–122, 2014.

Dankel SN, et al. COL6A3 expression in adipocytes associates with insulin resistance and depends on PPARγ and adipocyte size. Obesity. 22:1807–13, 2014.

Fang L, et al. The cell size and distribution of adipocytes from subcutaneous and visceral fat is associated with type 2 diabetes mellitus in humans. Adipocyte. 4:273–9, 2015.

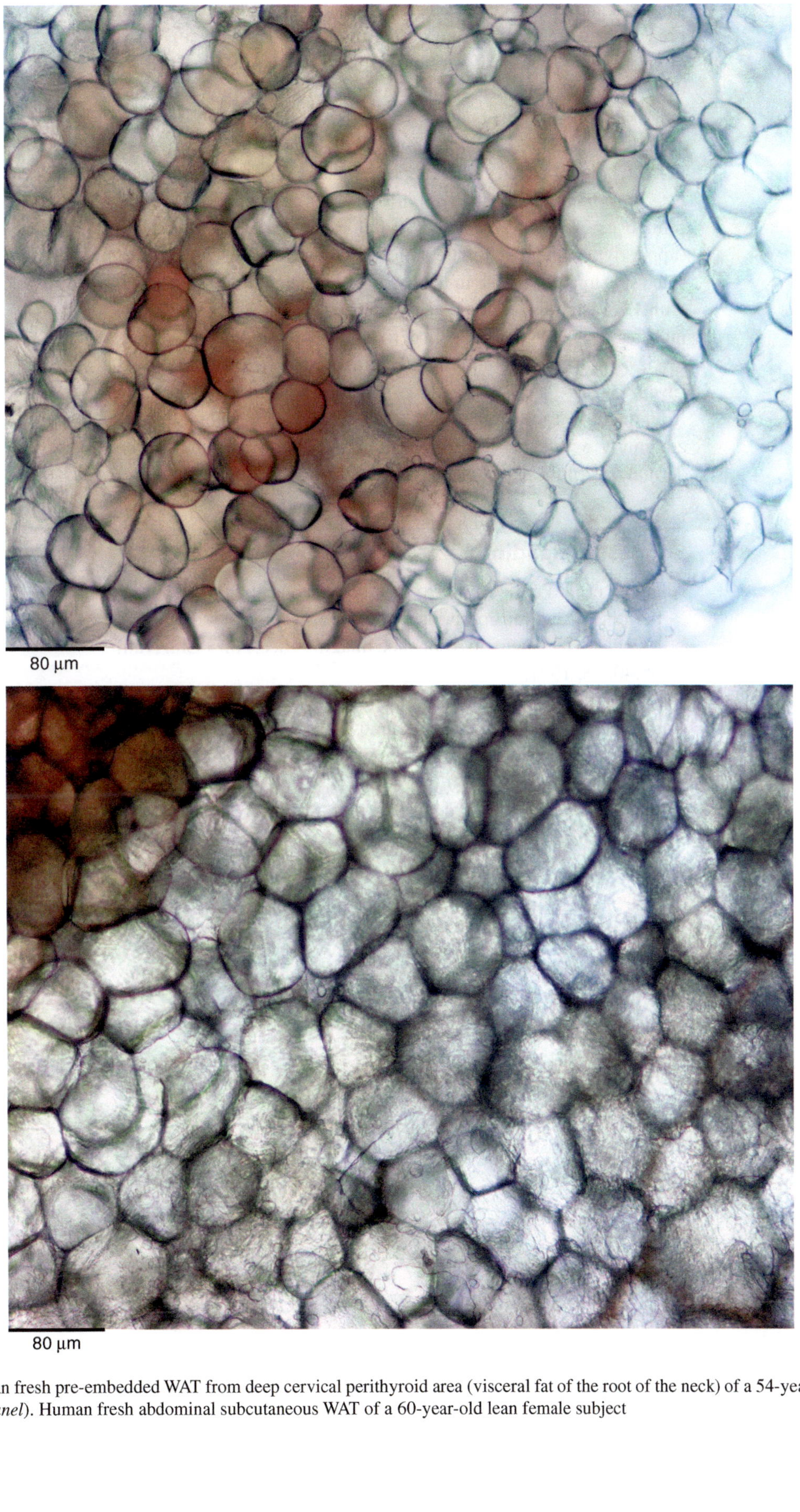

Plate 5.1 Human fresh pre-embedded WAT from deep cervical perithyroid area (visceral fat of the root of the neck) of a 54-year-old lean female subject (*upper panel*). Human fresh abdominal subcutaneous WAT of a 60-year-old lean female subject

PLATE 5.2

Whole Thickness SC Fat

The skin and the subcutaneous fat form a variable thickness membrane that wraps around the human body. Under the skin, fat is organized into lobules of variable size and shape (see Chap. 13 for their fetal development). In this plate an example of human abdominal skin and its subcutaneous fat is shown. Note the connective capsule surrounding each fat lobule. The capsule is visually evident in fresh pre-embedded tissue (upper left panel: one lobule indicated by arrows) and also visualized after xylol clarification during the routine procedure for standard histology by paraffin embedding (upper right panel: one lobule indicated by arrows). A section of the same specimen is visible in the left lower panel at light microscopy with H&E staining. The deeper part is in contact with abdominal muscles fascia. One thick connective layer (denominated Scarpa's fascia—from the Italian anatomist Antonio Scarpa, Motta di Livenza 1747–Pavia 1832) allows separating the deeper part of fat from the rest of the lobules. The most superficial fat lobules are in continuity with skin adnexa, and adipocytes can be found in the dermal part of the skin (lower right panel).

Suggested Reading

Abate N, et al. Prediction of total subcutaneous abdominal, intraperitoneal, and retroperitoneal adipose tissue masses in men by a single axial magnetic resonance imaging slice. Am J Clin Nutr. 65:403–8, 1997.

Clarys JP, et al. Cadaver studies and their impact on the understanding of human adiposity. Ergonomics. 48:1445–61, 2005.

Sbarbati A, et al. Subcutaneous adipose tissue classification. Eur J Histochem. 54:e48, 2010.

Panettiere P, et al. The trochanteric fat pad. Eur J Histochem. 55:e16, 2011.

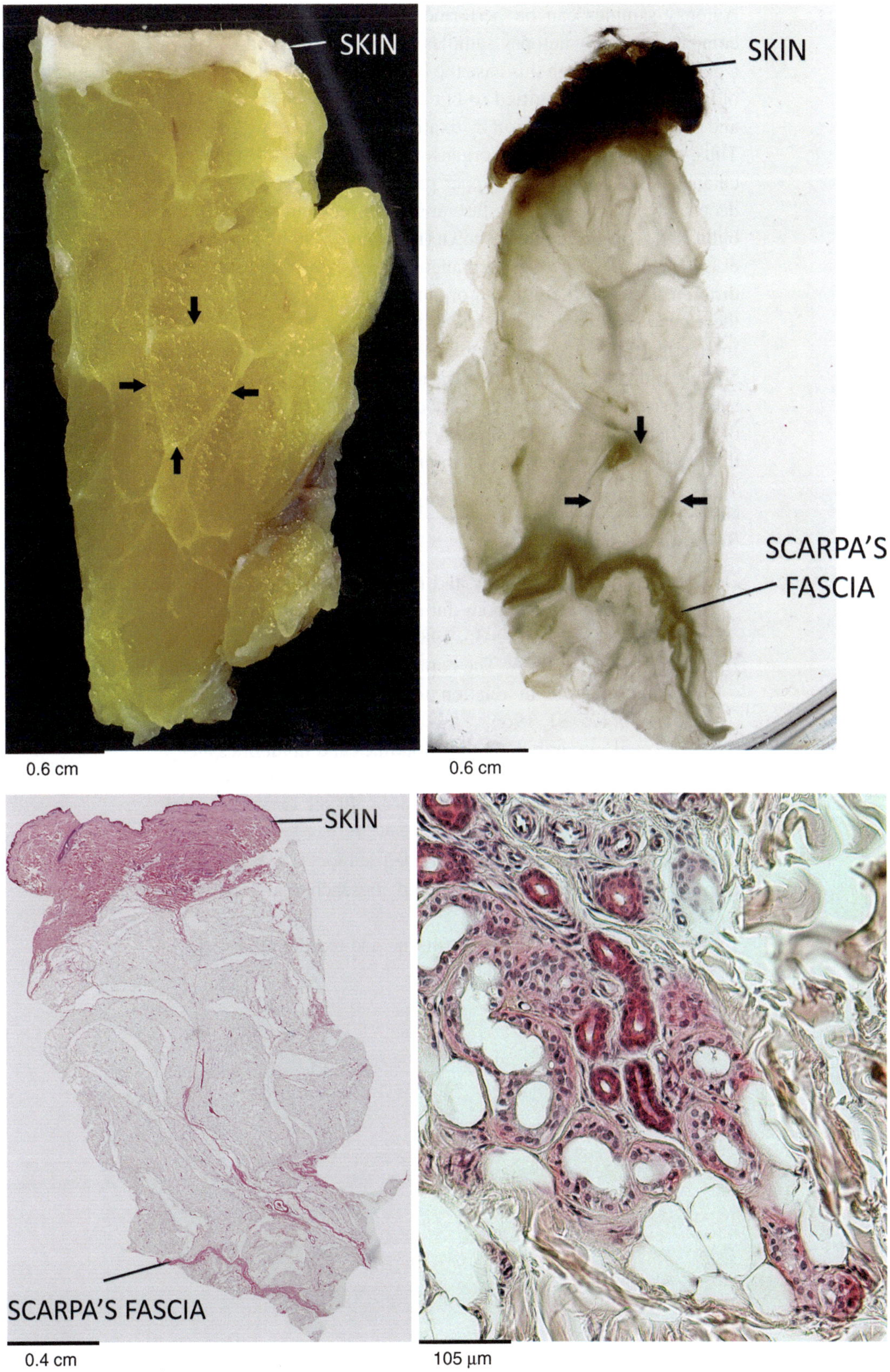

Plate 5.2 Skin and whole thickness subcutaneous fat sampling from a 55-year-old female patient, overweight (BMI, 27), operated for abdominoplasty after 40 kg weight loss achieved by caloric restriction. Gross anatomy of fresh tissue (*upper left*) and after xylol clarification (*upper right*). Histology at very low magnification (*lower left*) of the same sample. LM. H&E. Enlargement of skin from the same sample showing adipocytes in connection with a sweat gland (*lower right*). LM. H&E

PLATE 5.3

WAT from Different Depots of the Same Subject

Autopsy samples can be performed from the same subject and compared. Usually autopsy samples are badly preserved and show a poor morphology. In this case the body of an overweight 83-year-old male subject was gifted to our anatomy lab for scientific use, and a transfemoral perfusion by fixative of the cadaver was allowed. Thus, the preservation of all organs was obtained. In this plate subcutaneous WAT from skin (upper panels: left superficial fat, right deep fat below the Scarpa's fascia; see the previous plate), Bichat bulla, and retro-orbital fat is shown (respectively in the bottom panels). The morphology of subcutaneous adipocytes is similar in the different areas of the adipose organ. Their size is comparable in these depots although quite variable.
Interestingly the size of abdominal subcutaneous adipocytes of a 54-year-old man living in Siberia resulted about one-half of the average size of corresponding adipocytes measured in a case series of lean Italian subjects. The autopsy of this Siberian patient revealed that most of his visceral fat was multilocular (BAT-like).

Suggested Reading

Després JP, et al. Morphology and metabolism of human adipose tissues: relation to sex, body fat and level of training. Arch Int Physiol Biochim. 90:329–35, 1982.

Björntorp P, Martinsson A. The composition of human subcutaneous adipose tissue in relation to its morphology. Acta Med Scand. 179:475–81, 1966.

Caesar R, et al. A combined transcriptomics and lipidomics analysis of subcutaneous, epididymal and mesenteric adipose tissue reveals marked functional differences. PLoS One. 5:e11525, 2010.

Poloni A, et al. Human dedifferentiated adipocytes show similar properties to bone marrow-derived mesenchymal stem cells. Stem Cells. 2012.

Tomskiy M, et al. Brown adipose tissue and extremely severe climate. Yakut Med J. 49:44–5, 2015.

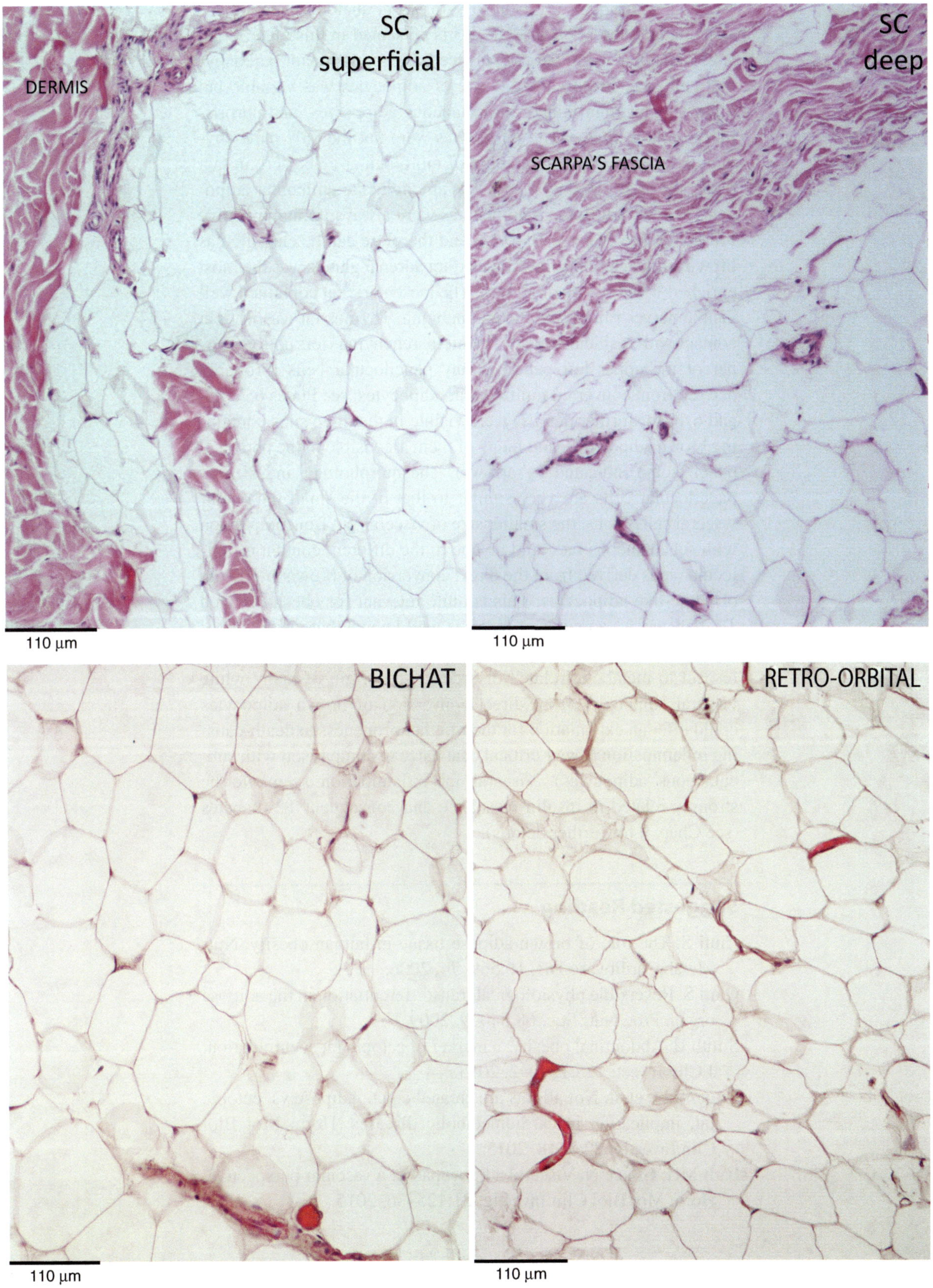

Plate 5.3 WAT samples from different areas of adipose organ of the same subject (cadaver of an overweight 83-year-old male subject). *Upper panels*: abdominal subcutaneous WAT. *Left*, superficial fat; *right*, deep fat. *Lower left panel*: WAT from Bichat bulla. *Lower right panel*: retro-orbital WAT. LM. H&E

PLATE 5.4

Visceral WAT

Visceral fat morphology from five different anatomic sites of the same patient described in Plate 5.3 is presented in this plate. In all sites unilocular white adipocytes were the predominant parenchymal cell type. In all sites the size of adipocytes was variable but often smaller than that of subcutaneous adipocytes, and surprisingly in three sites, white adipocytes were not the only parenchymal cell type. A variable amount of multilocular cells were in fact dispersed or grouped in small islets among white unilocular adipocytes. These multilocular adipocytes were always immunoreactive for UCP1 (see Plates 6.10–6.11) and therefore can be classified as brown adipocytes. The fat surrounding adrenal glands was the most enriched with brown adipocytes. The mesenteric fat contained well visible nerves running in the parenchyma. Thymus fat was in tight contact with residual cells of thymic parenchyma (left bottom corner of the upper left panel). Many paucilocular cells (probably derived from converted multilocular adipocytes; see Plates 6.7, 6.8, and 6.10 for further details) were visible in the three sites containing brown adipocytes, and many of them are visible in the perirenal panel (some indicated by arrows). The morphology and size of paucilocular cells are very similar to that of the small unilocular visceral cells. Thus, the smaller size of visceral WAT in comparison with subcutaneous fat could be due to the different content of unilocular cells derived from the direct conversion of brown into white or white-like adipocytes. This is quite relevant for obesity-related T2 diabetes. As a matter of fact it is well known that visceral obesity is much more dangerous than subcutaneous obesity with respect to metabolic-related disorders. The origin of many white visceral adipocytes from direct conversion of brown adipocytes could offer an explanation for their higher proneness to death-causing inflammation (lower critical death size in comparison with subcutaneous adipocytes). Visceral fat inflammation seems to be strongly related to insulin resistance and consequent T2 diabetes (see Chap. 9 for further details).

Suggested Reading

Cinti S. The role of brown adipose tissue in human obesity. Nutr Metab Cardiovasc Dis. 16:569–74, 2006.

Cinti S. Reversible physiological transdifferentiation in the adipose organ. Proc Nutr Soc. 68:340–9, 2009.

Smith U. Abdominal obesity: a marker of ectopic fat accumulation. J Clin Invest. 125:1790–2. 2015.

Gaggini M, et al. Not all fats are created equal: adipose vs. ectopic fat, implication in cardiometabolic diseases. Horm Mol Biol Clin Investig. 22:7–18, 2015.

Farb MG, Gokce N. Visceral adiposopathy: a vascular perspective. Horm Mol Biol Clin Investig. 21:125–36, 2015.

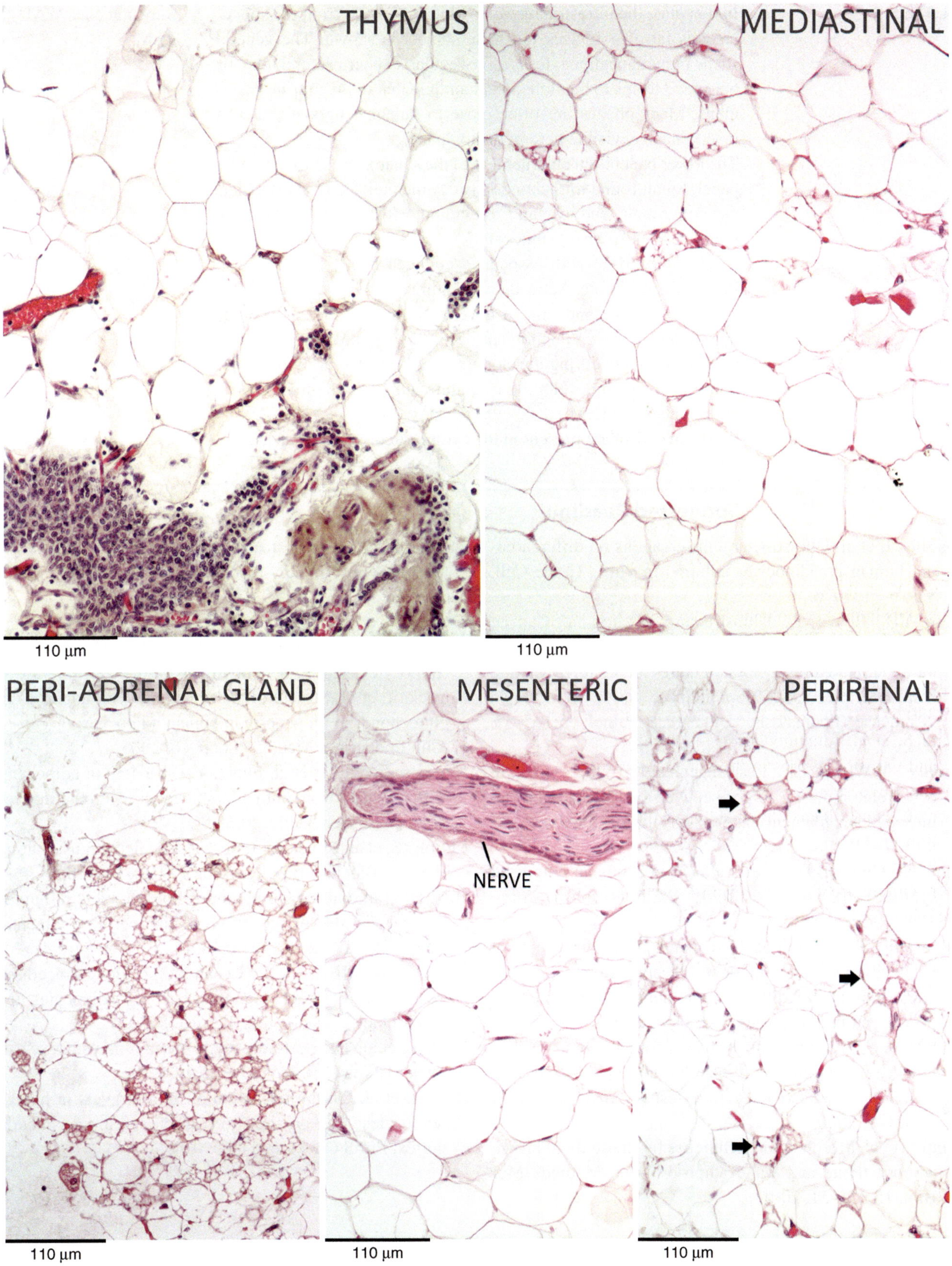

Plate 5.4 Same subject of Plate 5.3. *Upper left*: thymus fat. Upper right: mediastinal fat. *Lower left*: peri-adrenal gland fat. *Lower middle*: mesenteric fat. *Lower right*: perirenal fat. LM. H&E

PLATE 5.5

Subcutaneous WAT: TEM

In this plate the ultrastructure of a white adipocyte from the subcutaneous fat of a 12-year-old male subject is shown. The general shape of human adipocytes is quite regularly spherical, and interstitial space seems to be more abundant than that in the murine specimens. Macrophages are often close to human adipocytes, and a macrophage is visible here in the top panel.

The lower panel is an enlargement of the squared area1 in the upper panel. Small round mitochondria (m, some indicated), short cisternae of rough endoplasmic reticulum (RER, one indicated), microvesicles (ellipse), pinocytotic vesicles (V), and external or basal lamina (EL) with associated collagen fibrils (CF; see also Plate 5.6) are visible. Actin and vimentin microfilaments have been shown in murine and human developing and mature adipocytes in vitro and in vivo. Vimentin has been shown to be associated with the lipid droplets during development in vitro. We rarely observed microfilaments in developing or mature adipose cells treated with our methods for TEM.

Lysosomes (Ly) are present in the cytoplasm of macrophage.

Suggested Reading

Dardick I, et al. Ultrastructural observations on differentiating human preadipocytes cultured in vitro. Tissue Cell. 8:561–71, 1976.

Kim YH, Reiner L. Ultrastructure of lipoma. Cancer. 50:102–6, 1982.

Cinti S, et la. Ultrastructural features of cultured mature adipocyte precursors from adipose tissue in multiple symmetric lipomatosis. Ultrastruct Pathol. 5:145–52, 1983.

Franke WW, et al. Rearrangement of the vimentin cytoskeleton during adipose conversion: formation of an intermediate filament cage around lipid globules. Cell. 49:131–41, 1987.

Kral JG, Crandall DL. Development of a human adipocyte synthetic polymer scaffold. Plast Reconstr Surg. 104:1732–8, 1999.

Bornstein SR, et al. Immunohistochemical and ultrastructural localization of leptin and leptin receptor in human white adipose tissue and differentiating human adipose cells in primary culture. Diabetes. 49:532–8, 2000.

Omata W, et al. Actin filaments play a critical role in insulin-induced exocytotic recruitment but not in endocytosis of GLUT4 in isolated rat adipocytes. Biochem J. 346(Pt 2):321–8, 2000.

Cinti S, et al. Morphologic techniques for the study of brown adipose tissue and white adipose tissue. Methods Mol Biol. 155:21–51, 2001.

Lloreta J, et al. Ultrastructural features of highly active antiretroviral therapy-associated partial lipodystrophy. Virchows Arch. 441:599–604, 2002.

Thorn H, et al. Cell surface orifices of caveolae and localization of caveolin to the necks of caveolae in adipocytes. Mol Biol Cell. 14:3967–76, 2003.

Bogacka I, et al. Structural and functional consequences of mitochondrial biogenesis in human adipocytes in vitro. J Clin Endocrinol Metab. 90:6650–6, 2005.

Karahuseyinoglu S, et al. Functional structure of adipocytes differentiated from human umbilical cord stroma-derived stem cells. Stem Cells. 26:682–91, 2008.

Murphy S, et al. Lipid droplet-organelle interactions; sharing the fats. Biochim Biophys Acta. 1791:441–7, 2009.

Heid H, et al. On the formation of lipid droplets in human adipocytes: the organization of the perilipin-vimentin cortex. PLoS One. 9:e90386, 2014.

Kranendonk ME, et al. Human adipocyte extracellular vesicles in reciprocal signaling between adipocytes and macrophages. Obesity. 22:1296–308, 2014.

Conti G, et al. The post-adipocytic phase of the adipose cell cycle. Tissue Cell. 46:520–6, 2014.

Heid H, et al. On the formation of lipid droplets in human adipocytes: the organization of the perilipin-vimentin cortex. PLoS One. 9:e90386, 2014.

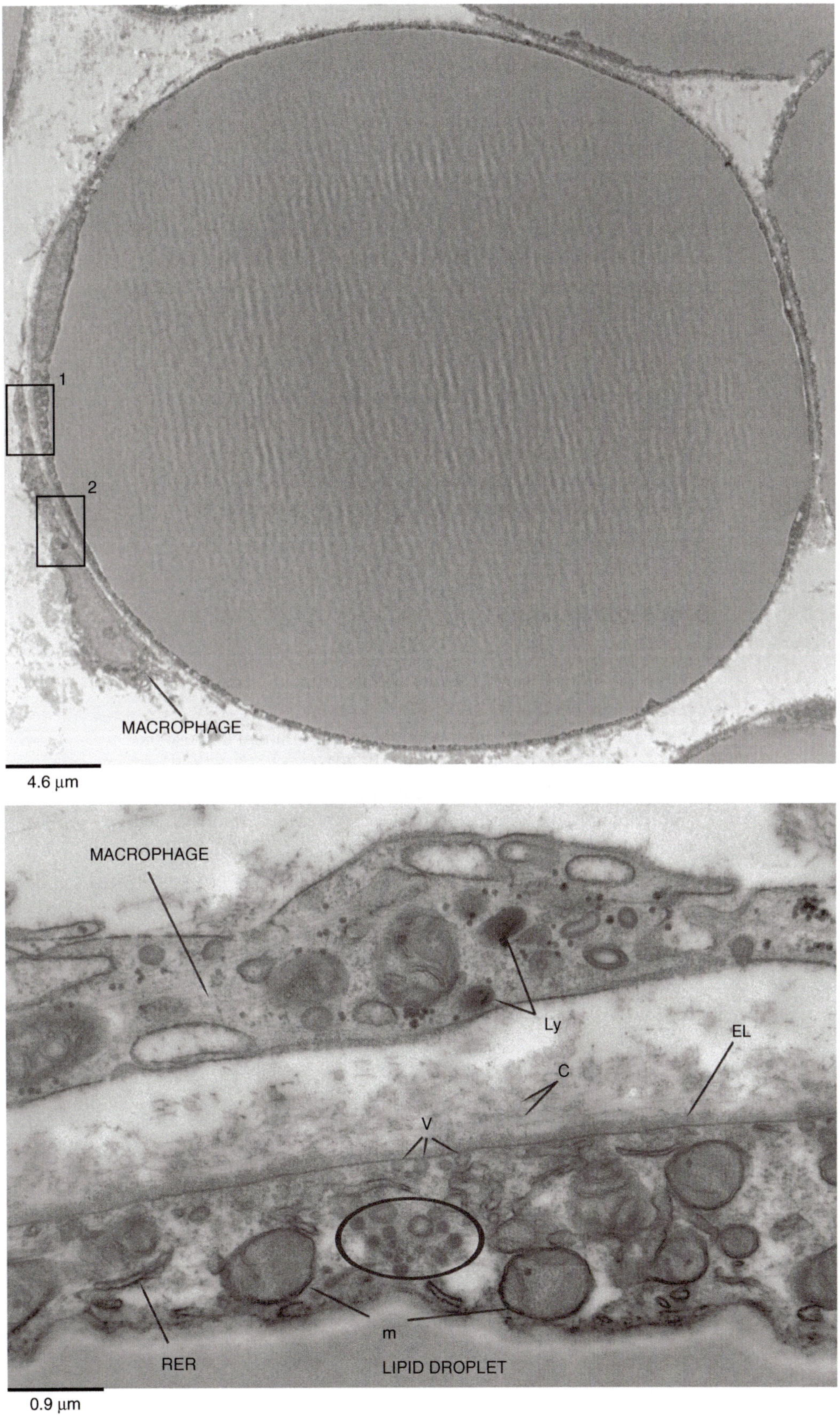

Plate 5.5 Subcutaneous WAT from a 12-year-old male subject. TEM

PLATE 5.6

Subcutaneous Adipocyte Ultrastructure

Enlargements of the squared area 2 of the previous plate are shown here. In the upper panel, part of a macrophage is also visible (N: macrophage nucleus). Three characteristic aspects of macrophage ultrastructure are present in this panel: a big primary lysosome (Ly), dilated cisterna of rough endoplasmic reticulum (RER), and cytoplasmic slender irregular projections (CP).

In the bottom part of the upper panel, the Golgi complex area (Go) in the cytoplasm of this adipocyte is shown.

In the lower panel an enlargement of the Golgi complex area of the adipocyte is visible. Three different-sized vesicles are visible here: the largest (about 120–150 nm) are pinocytotic vesicles (V), and the smallest are very small microvesicles (SMV, about 30–40 nm). Microvesicles with intermediate size (MV, about 30–80 nm) are also visible.

At the external side of the plasma membrane, a thick external lamina (EL) mainly composed of collagen IV is present. Collagen fibrils (C) associated with the external lamina are also visible. The transverse-sectioned collagen fibrils are on the left (T), those longitudinally sectioned are on the right (L), and in these last fibrils, the classic periodicity is evident.

Suggested Reading

Pierleoni C, et al. Fibronectins and basal lamina molecules expression in human subcutaneous white adipose tissue. Eur J Histochem. 42:183–8, 1998.

Arner E, et al. Adipocyte turnover: relevance to human adipose tissue morphology. Diabetes. 59:105–9, 2010.

Michaud A, et al. Abdominal subcutaneous and omental adipocyte morphology and its relation to gene expression, lipolysis and adipocytokine levels in women. Metabolism. 63:372–81, 2014.

Heinonen S, et al. Adipocyte morphology and implications for metabolic derangements in acquired obesity. Int J Obes. 38:1423–31, 2014.

Gao H, et al. Early B cell factor 1 regulates adipocyte morphology and lipolysis in white adipose tissue. Cell Metab. 19:981–92, 2014.

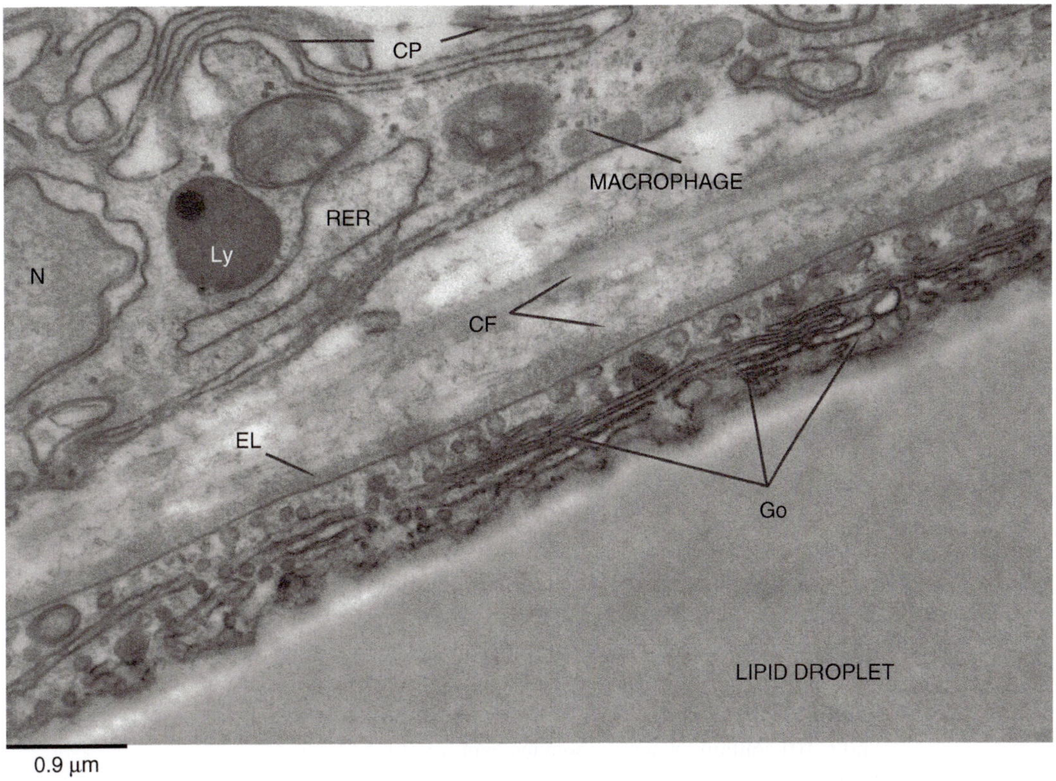

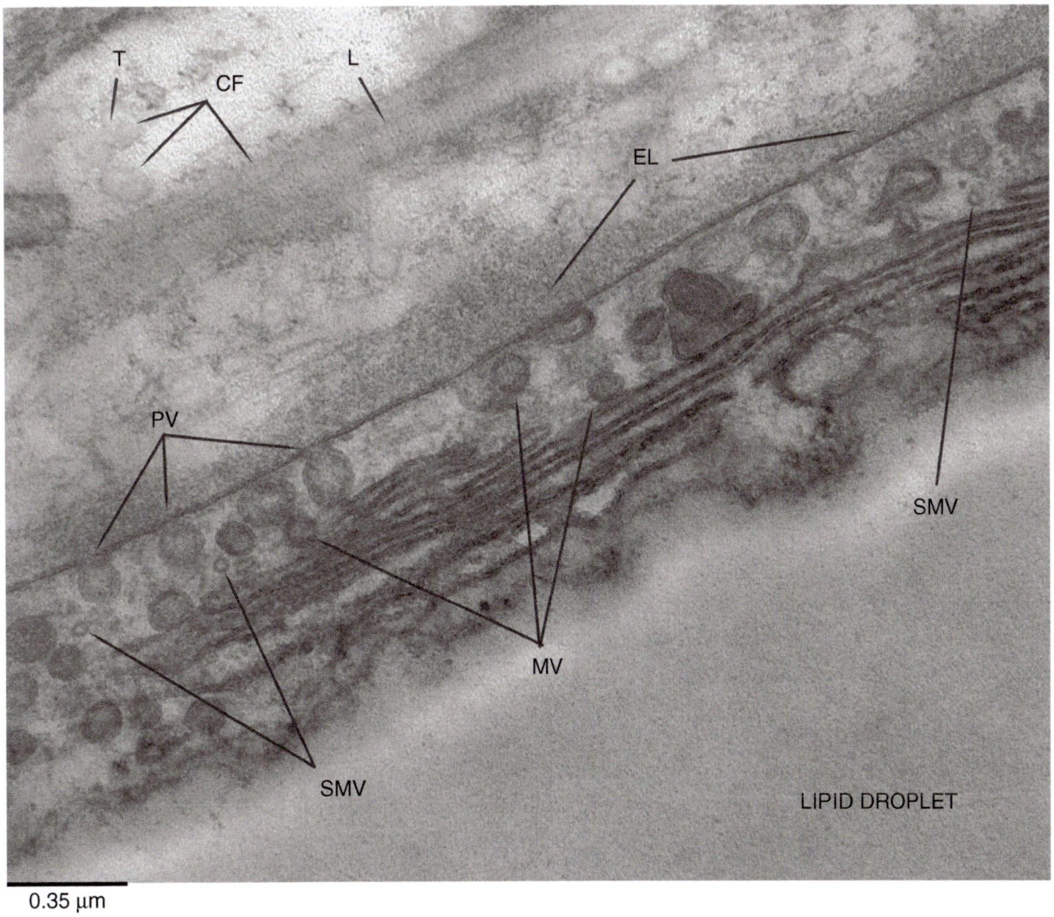

Plate 5.6 Same subject of Plate 5.5. White adipocyte ultrastructure of organelles. TEM

PLATE 5.7

Visceral Adipocyte Ultrastructure

Besides the size difference described in Plates 4.2–4.3 and 5.4, the ultrastructure of visceral adipocytes is similar to that of subcutaneous adipocytes. We observed only a few differences. Collagen fibrils associated with the external lamina are more abundant in subcutaneous adipocytes (compare lower panels in Plates 5.5 and 5.6). This seems to be in line with the tendency to fibrosis of subcutaneous fat in obese subjects. Furthermore visceral white adipocytes show a higher number of lipofuscins. In particular, omental adipocytes of lean subjects with abundant cytoplasmic lipofuscins (LP, some indicated) are shown in this plate.

We found similar lipofuscins also in lipoatrophic adipocytes of subcutaneous fat of diabetic patients treated with recombinant insulin. The lipoatrophic fat corresponded to the site of insulin injection. The presence of lipofuscin granules could be due to increased oxidative activity to eliminate the free fatty acid excess resulting from an accelerated lipolysis due to local insulin resistance.

Interestingly lipofuscins are also a sign of autophagy that is an important mechanism to maintain the white phenotype of adipocytes. Thus, their abundance in visceral fat could be due to the intense activity of the cellular mechanisms converting visceral brown into white adipocytes (see Chap. 7). In this regard it is noteworthy that most visceral fat of the adipose organ (see Plates 3.1 and 6.10) contain brown adipocytes even in old subjects.

Suggested Reading

Brunk UT, Terman A. Lipofuscin: mechanisms of age-related accumulation and influence on cell function. Free Radical Biol & Med. 33:611–19, 2002.

Singh R, et al. Autophagy regulates adipose mass and differentiation in mice. J Clin Invest. 119(11):3329–39, 2009.

Milan G, et al. Lipoatrophy induced by subcutaneous insulin infusion: ultrastructural analysis and gene expression profiling. J Clin Endocrinol Metab. 95:3126–32, 2010.

Kovsan J, et al. Altered autophagy in human adipose tissues in obesity. J Clin Endocrinol Metab. 96:E268–77, 2011.

Sun K, et al. Fibrosis and adipose tissue disfunction. Cell Metab. 18:470–7, 2013.

Martinez-Lopez N, et al. Autophagy in Myf5+ progenitors regulates energy and glucose homeostasis through control of brown fat and skeletal muscle development. EMBO Rep. 14:795–803, 2013.

Tam CS, et al. Weight gain reveals dramatic increases in skeletal muscle extracellular matrix remodeling. J Clin Endocrinol Metab. 99:1749–57, 2014.

Cairó M, et al. Thermogenic activation represses autophagy in brown adipose tissue. Int J Obes. 2016.

Martinez-Lopez N, et al. Autophagy in the CNS and periphery coordinate lipophagy and lipolysis in the brown adipose tissue and liver. Cell Metab. 23:113–27, 2016.

Giordano A, et al. Convertible visceral fat as a therapeutic target to curb obesity. Nat Rev Drug Discov 15:405–24, 2016.

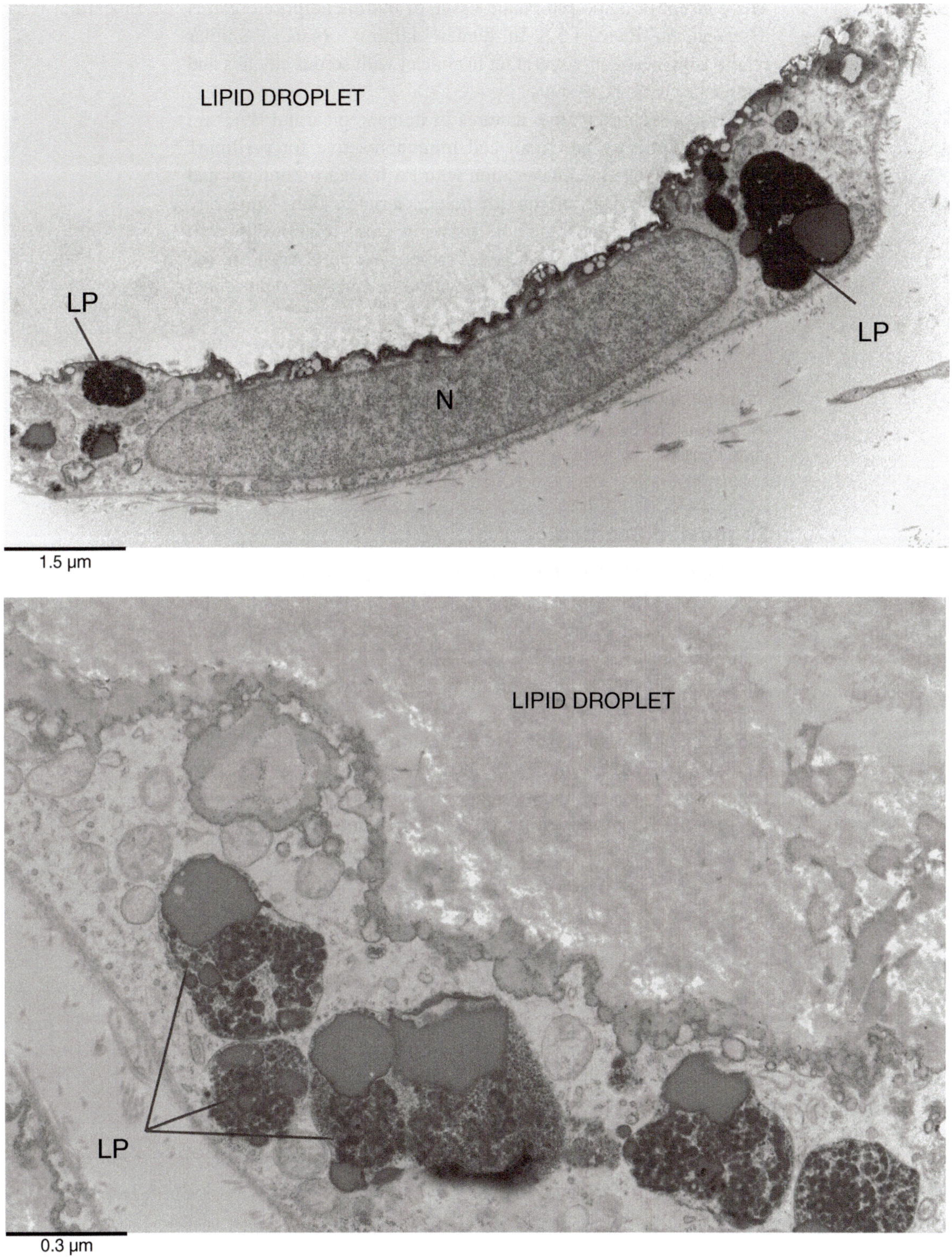

Plate 5.7 Omental adipocytes from a 56-year-old lean patient. TEM

PLATE 5.8

Epicardial WAT

The concept of adipo-lymphatic tissue of murine adipose organ is described in Plate 4.12. In human adipose organ, a similar relationship between visceral fat in contact with serous cavities and lymphatic tissue is present.

In this plate representative features of human epicardial WAT are shown. Adipocytes are small and immunoreactive for perilipin1 (unpublished data in collaboration with Prof. Mauro Zamboni and Dr. Elena Zoico, Dpt Internal Medicine, Geriatric Unit, University of Verona). Note the lymphatic tissue in close relationship with perilipin immunoreactive (viable) adipocytes (enlarged in the bottom panel). Note the similarities with mice omental fat presented in Plate 4.12.

Epicardial fat and omentum are both proximal to serous cavities, and the adipo-lymphatic tissue could be related to some immunological role specific for these anatomic sites.

Several studies suggest that epicardial adipocytes share intermediate characteristics between white and brown adipocytes.

Suggested Reading

Marchington JM, Pond CM. Site-specific properties of pericardial and epicardial adipose tissue: the effects of insulin and high-fat feeding on lipogenesis and the incorporation of fatty acids in vitro. Int J Obes. 14:1013–22, 1990.

Sacks HS, Fain JN. Human epicardial adipose tissue: a review. Am Heart J. 153:907–17, 2007.

Sacks HS, et al. Adult epicardial fat exhibits beige features. J Clin Endocrinol Metab. 98:E1448–55, 2013.

Iacobellis G. Local and systemic effects of the multifaceted epicardial adipose tissue depot. Nat Rev Endocrinol. 11(6):363–71, 2015.

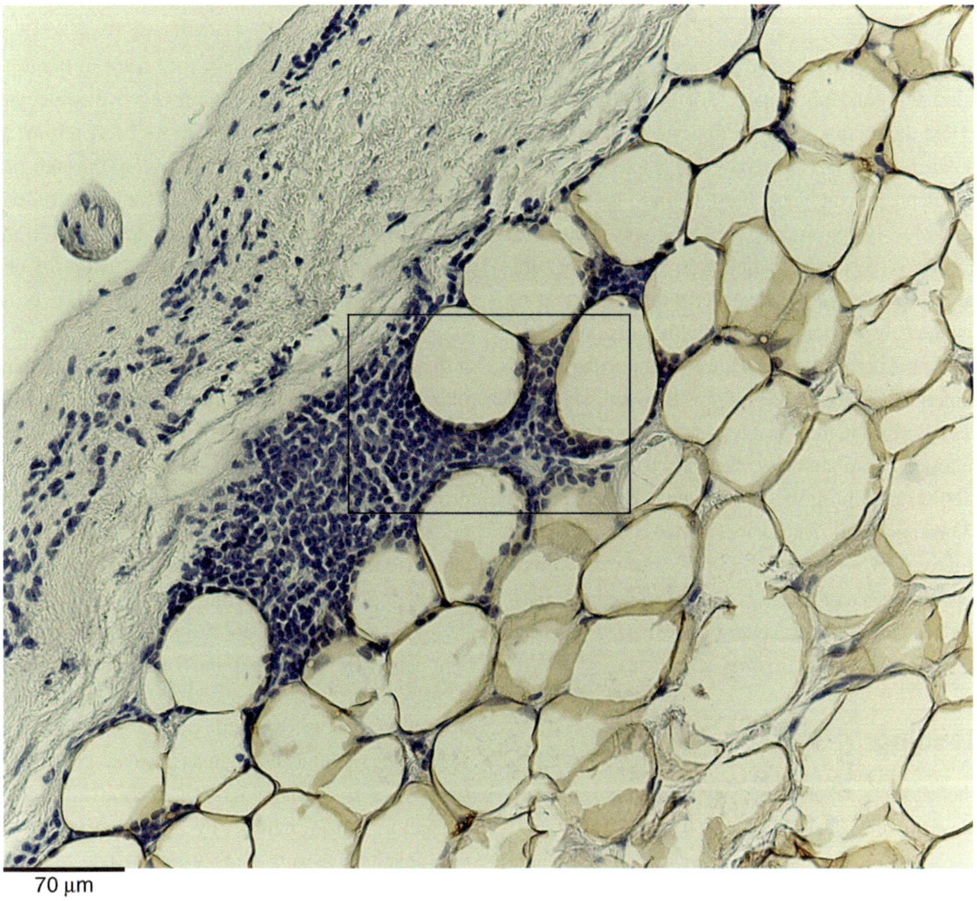

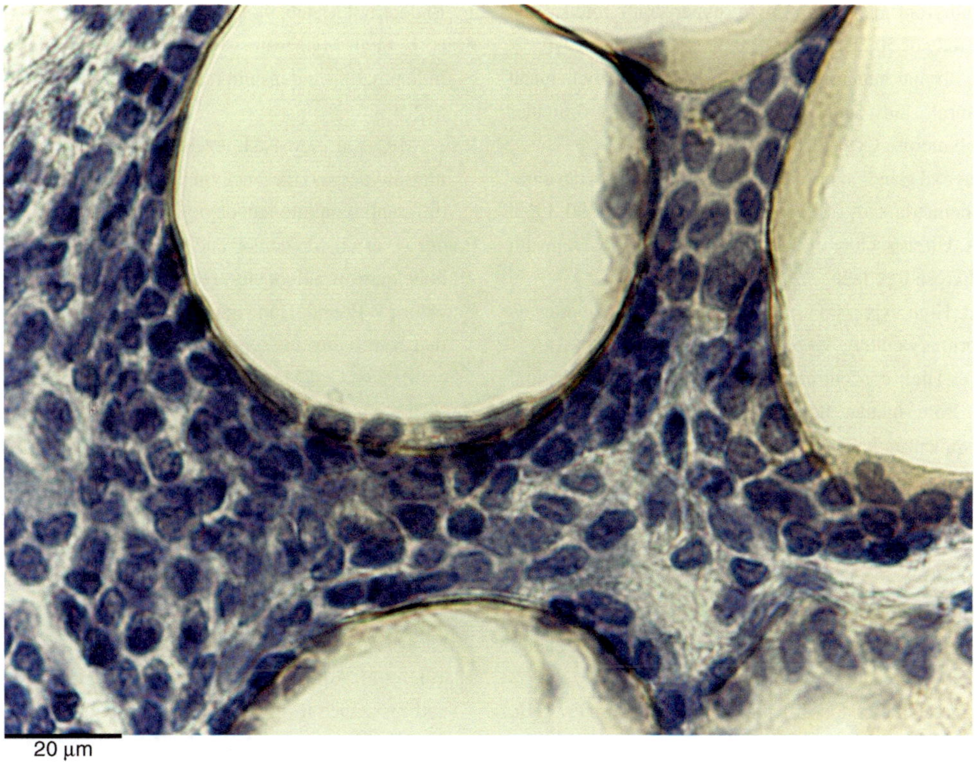

Plate 5.8 Epicardial fat from a lean 80-year-old subject. IHC. Perilipin1 ab (1:300). LM

PLATE 5.9

Many organs, in normal conditions, have adipocytes inside their parenchyma. The fine morphology and functional role of these adipocytes are largely unknown. Here the morphology of adipocytes found in some human organs is shown. In all organ explored by light microscopy (bone marrow, parathyroid gland, parotid gland, heart, thymus, gastrointestinal tract, skeletal muscles, lymph nodes), we found only adipocytes with the unilocular morphology of white adipocytes. Some authors suggested the presence of brown adipocyte characteristics in murine bone marrow fat, but we never observed intra-organ multilocular adipocytes both in murine and human normal tissues. However unilocular adipocytes can express intermediate molecular features between white and brown adipocytes as described in the previous plate. All intraparenchymal adipocytes we tested by immunohistochemistry with the specific perilipin1 antibodies resulted positive (heart, lymph nodes, parotid glands, atrium, and bone marrow). The adipocyte marker and secretory product: adiponectin resulted more expressed in the bone marrow than in all other fat depots. Recently a protective role of adiponectin for mesenchymal stem cells and hematopoietic cells of bone marrow has been suggested (see also Plate 4.13 for bone marrow adipocytes).

In this plate some examples are shown: in the top panel and in the middle panel, perilipin1 immunoreactive adipocytes among parotid glands and myocardial cells in the heart atrium (respectively) are visible. The bottom panels show a normal parathyroid gland, removed during thyroidectomy, composed of parenchymal chief cells mixed with unilocular adipocytes. Electron microscopy of this gland (bottom left) shows the ultrastructure of chief cells in close proximity to a parenchymal adipocyte. The ultrastructure of the parenchymal adipocyte is not different from that found in other sites of the adipose organ. Here, a distinct external lamina (EL) and small mitochondria (m) are visible in the thin cytoplasmic rim; a unilocular lipid droplet forms the rest of the cell. Note the presence of a long slender cytoplasmic projection of an unidentified interstitial cell (arrows), running in the narrow space between endocrine cells and this adipocyte. Secretory granules of chief cells are oriented to the adipocyte (some encircled). Note the presence of lipid droplets (L) in the cytoplasm of chief cells (L). In many chief cells lipid droplets are abundant (visible also at light microscopy level in the bottom right panel) and contained into lipofuscin-like granules.

Suggested Reading

Cinti S, et al. Morphometric evaluation of intracytoplasmic lipid in normal and pathological parathyroid glands. J Pathol. 160:31–4, 1990.

Cinti S, et al. Parathyroid glands in primary hyperparathyroidism: an ultrastructural morphometric study of 25 cases. J Pathol. 167:283–90, 1992.

Cinti S, et al. Parathyroid glands in primary hyperparathyroidism: an ultrastructural study of 50 cases. Hum Pathol. 17:1036–46, 1986.

Cinti S, et al. The normal human parathyroid gland. A histochemical and ultrastructural study with particular reference to follicular structures. J Submicrosc Cytol. 15:661–79, 1983.

Cinti S, et al. Parathyroid glands in primary hyperparathyroidism: an ultrastructural morphometric study of 25 cases. J Pathol. 167:283–90, 1992.

Cinti S, Sbarbati A. Ultrastructure of human parathyroid cells in health and disease. Microsc Res Tech. 32:164–79, 1995.

Laharrague P, et al. High expression of leptin by human bone marrow adipocytes in primary culture. FASEB J. 12:747–52, 1998.

Laharrague P, et al. High concentration of leptin stimulates myeloid differentiation from human bone marrow CD34+ progenitors: potential involvement in leukocytosis of obese subjects. Int J Obes Relat Metab Disord. 24:1212–6, 2000.

Cinti S, et al. Secretory granules of endocrine and chief cells of human stomach mucosa contain leptin. Int J Obes Relat Metab Disord. 24:789–93, 2000.

Cinti S, et al. Leptin in the human stomach. Gut. 49:155, 2001.

De Matteis R, et al. Intralobular ducts of human major salivary glands contain leptin and its receptor. J Anat. 201:363–70, 2002.

Oliver P, et al. Perinatal expression of leptin in rat stomach. Dev Dyn. 223:148–54, 2002.

Corre J, et al. Human bone marrow adipocytes support complete myeloid and lymphoid differentiation from human CD34 cells. Br J Haematol. 127:344–7, 2004.

Morroni M, et al. In vivo leptin expression in cartilage and bone cells of growing rats and adult humans. J Anat. 205:291–6, 2004.

Rossi A, et al. Quantification of intermuscular adipose tissue in the erector spinae muscle by MRI: agreement with histological evaluation. Obesity. 18:2379–84, 2010.

Sacks HS, et al. Adult epicardial fat exhibits beige features. J Clin Endocrinol Metab. 98:E1448–55, 2013.

Zoico E, et al. Myosteatosis and myofibrosis: relationship with aging, inflammation and insulin resistance. Arch Gerontol Geriatr. 57:411–6, 2013.

Rippo MR, et al. Low FasL levels promote proliferation of human bone marrow-derived mesenchymal stem cells, higher levels inhibit their differentiation into adipocytes. Cell Death Dis. 4:e594, 2013.

Poloni A, et al. Molecular and functional characterization of human bone marrow adipocytes. Exp Hematol. 41:558–66, 2013.

Cawthorn WP, et al. Bone marrow adipose tissue is an endocrine organ that contributes to increased circulating adiponectin during caloric restriction. Cell Metab. 20:368–75, 2014.

Heid H, et al. On the formation of lipid droplets in human adipocytes: the organization of the perilipin-vimentin cortex. PLoS One 9:e90386, 2014.

Luche E, et al. Differential hematopoietic activity in white adipose tissue depending on its localization. J Cell Physiol. 230:3076–83, 2015.

Mazzali G, et al. Heart fat infiltration in subjects with and without coronary artery disease. J Clin Endocrinol Metab. 100:3364–71, 2015.

Zhao L, et al. Adiponectin enhances bone marrow mesenchymal stem cell resistance to flow shear stress through AMP-activated protein kinase signaling. Sci Rep. 6:28752, 2016.

Masamoto Y, et al. Adiponectin enhances antibacterial activity of hematopoietic cells by suppressing bone marrow inflammation. Immunity. 44:1422–33, 2016.

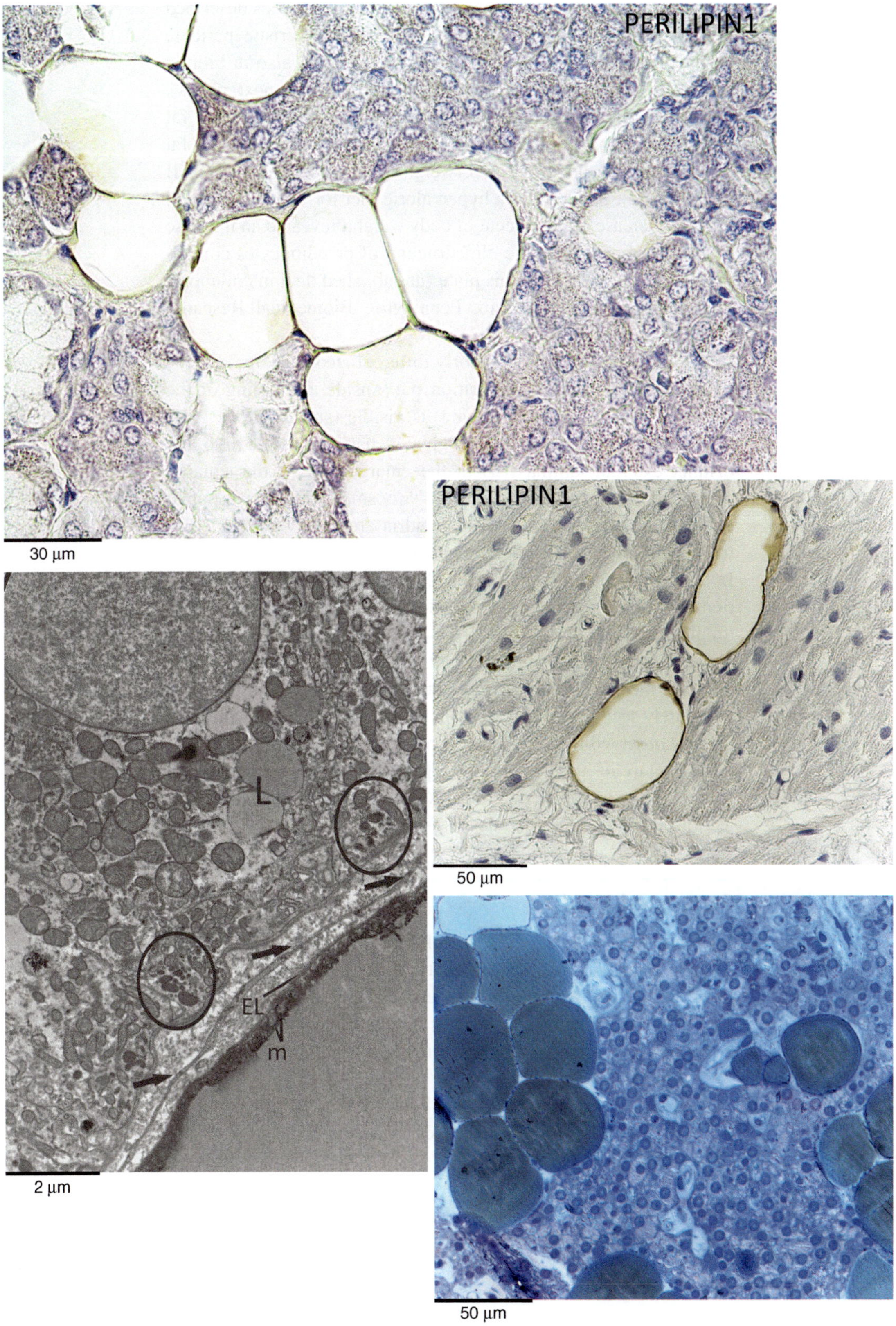

Plate 5.9 Intra-organ human adipocytes. *Top panel*: normal parotid gland of adult lean subject. Perilipin1 immunoreactive unilocular adipocytes among normal salivary glands. LM. IHC Perilipin1 ab (1:300). *Middle panel*: normal atrium of adult lean subject. Two perilipin1 immunoreactive unilocular adipocytes among myocardial cells. LM. IHC Perilipin ab (1:300). *Bottom right*: normal parathyroid gland of adult lean subject. Resin-embedded tissue. LM. Toluidine blue. *Bottom left*: same subject of the bottom right panel. TEM

PLATE 5.10

Adipocyte Precursors

We found cells with all the ultrastructural characteristics described for murine preadipocytes, including their characteristic pericyte and pericapillary positions (see Plates 4.16–4.17), also in bioptic specimen from human adipose organ (present and next plates). Preadipocytes were found both in subcutaneous and in visceral fat at any age and gender. Quantitative analyses in the subcutaneous fat of voluntary adult normal, overweight, and obese patients (BMI range 22–32), undergoing a hypercaloric diet for 8 weeks with an average increase of 10 percent of body weight, revealed an increase in density of cells with the ultrastructure of preadipocytes comparable to that presented in this plate (unpublished data in collaboration with Dr. Eric Ravussin, Pennington Biomedical Research Center, Baton Rouge).

In the upper panel a classic poorly differentiated preadipocyte (P) (or adipoblast) in pericyte position (i.e., inside a doubling of the capillary—CAP—external lamina) is visible (subcutaneous WAT of adult lean subject). Note the high nucleus/cytoplasmic ratio, the distinct external lamina (EL in the enlargement of the squared area), and the glycogen granules (G, very small diffuse or grouped cytoplasmic black points). Mitochondria are poorly developed in these preadipocytes (see the next plate).

In the lower panel a preadipocyte (P) in pericapillary (CAP) position, with some signs of adipose differentiation (glycogen and lipid droplets; see also Plate 4.16–19), is visible. Glycogen (G) is abundant and small lipid droplets (L) are visible in the middle of glycogen (see the enlargement of the squared area). Lipid droplets are very rarely seen in preadipocytes in pericyte position. They are frequently observed in pericapillary preadipocytes. Note the different ultrastructure of an adjacent macrophage (MAC). This last cell is lacking the external lamina and shows irregular cytoplasmic projections (arrow) and lysosomes (Ly).

Suggested Reading

Johannsen DL, et al. Effect of 8 weeks of overfeeding on ectopic fat deposition and insulin sensitivity: testing the "adipose tissue expandability" hypothesis. Diabetes Care. 37:2789–97, 2014.

Tam CS, et al. Weight gain reveals dramatic increases in skeletal muscle extracellular matrix remodeling. J Clin Endocrinol Metab. 99:1749–57, 2014.

Heid H, et al. On the formation of lipid droplets in human adipocytes: the organization of the perilipin-vimentin cortex. PLoS One. 9:e90386, 2014.

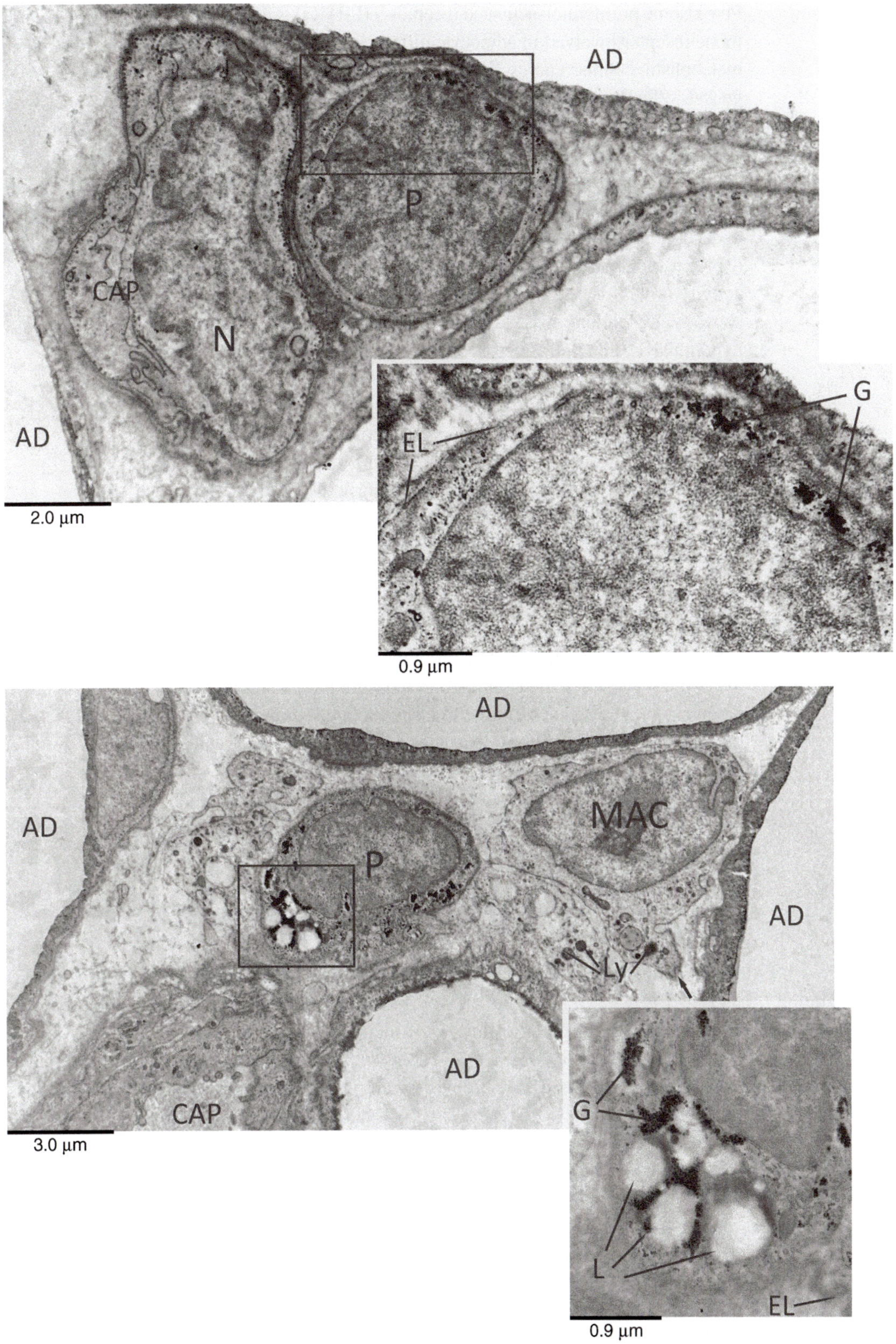

Panel 5.10 Human preadipocytes. Subcutaneous WAT from a 79-year-old lean subject. TEM. AD: mature adipocyte

PLATE 5.11

Ultrastructure of Adipocyte and Preadipocyte from a Subject with PPARγ Dominant-Negative Mutation (P467L)

Peroxisome proliferator-activated receptor-γ (PPARγ) is a nuclear hormone receptor involved in adipocyte differentiation, lipid and glucose metabolism, cellular energy homeostasis, inflammation, and carcinogenesis. PPARγ is required for adipogenesis. In addition to its important role in promoting adipocyte differentiation, PPARγ is also a modulator of insulin sensitivity; in fact synthetic agonists (thiazolidinediones) are used in type 2 diabetic patients as insulin sensitizers.

In this plate the morphology of a representative mature adipocyte and a preadipocyte from the abdominal subcutaneous fat of a patient (32-year-old lean male) with markedly attenuated transcriptional activity of wild-type PPARγ gene in a dominant-negative manner is shown. The patient was severely insulin resistant, diabetic, and hypertensive. The light microscopy of the abdominal subcutaneous adipose tissue of the subject with the P467L PPARG mutation showed classic white adipose tissue morphology with unilocular adipocytes. Adipocyte size showed no significant differences compared with the values of control subjects with similar BMI.

Electron microscopy revealed classic morphology with normal mitochondria (m), isolated strands of rough endoplasmic reticulum, abundant pinocytotic vesicles, and a distinct basal lamina of mutant subject adipocytes (upper panels, framed area enlarged on the right; N: nucleus of adipocyte). Poorly differentiated cells in pericytic position with the electron microscopic features of adipocyte precursors (compare with previous plate) are shown in the lower panels (framed area enlarged in the right panel; N, nucleus of preadipocyte). Elongated mitochondria, isolated strands of endoplasmic reticulum, glycogen particles, many pinocytotic vesicles, and a distinct external lamina (EL) characterized these cells.

These data suggest that this mutation does not interfere with a normal morphology of abdominal subcutaneous adipocytes and preadipocytes.

Suggested Reading

Spiegelman BM, et al. PPAR gamma and the control of adipogenesis. Biochimie. 79:111–2, 1997.

Spiegelman BM. PPAR-gamma: adipogenic regulator and thiazolidinedione receptor. Diabetes. 47:507–14, 1998.

Wu Z, et al. Transcriptional activation of adipogenesis. Curr Opin Cell Biol. 11:689–94, 1999.

Rosen ED, et al. PPAR gamma is required for the differentiation of adipose tissue in vivo and in vitro. Mol Cell. 4:611–17, 1999.

Barroso I, et al. Dominant negative mutations in human PPARgamma associated with severe insulin resistance, diabetes mellitus and hypertension. Nature. 402:880–3, 1999.

Sewter C, Vidal-Puig A. PPARgamma and the thiazolidinediones: molecular basis for the treatment of 'Syndrome X'. Diabetes Obes Metab. 4:239–48, 2002.

Savage DB, et al. Human metabolic syndrome resulting from dominant-negative mutations in the nuclear receptor peroxisome proliferator-activated receptor-gamma. Diabetes. 52:910–17, 2003.

Gray SL, et al. Mouse models of PPAR-gamma deficiency: dissecting PPAR-gamma's role in metabolic homeostasis. Biochem Soc Trans. 33:1053–8, 2005.

Totonoz P, Spiegelman BM. Fat and beyond: the diverse biology of PPARgamma. Annu Rev Biochem. 77:289–312, 2008.

Savage DB, et al. Complement abnormalities in acquired lipodystrophy revisited. J Clin Endocrinol Metab. 94:10–6, 2009.

Christodoulides C, Vidal-Puig A. PPARs and adipocyte function. Mol Cell Endocrinol. 318:61–8, 2010.

Boiani R, et al. Abdominal subcutaneous adipose tissue morphology in a patient with a dominant-negative mutation (P467L) in the nuclear receptor peroxisome proliferator-activated receptor-gamma (PPARG) gene. Nutr Metab Cardiovasc Dis. 20:e11–2, 2010.

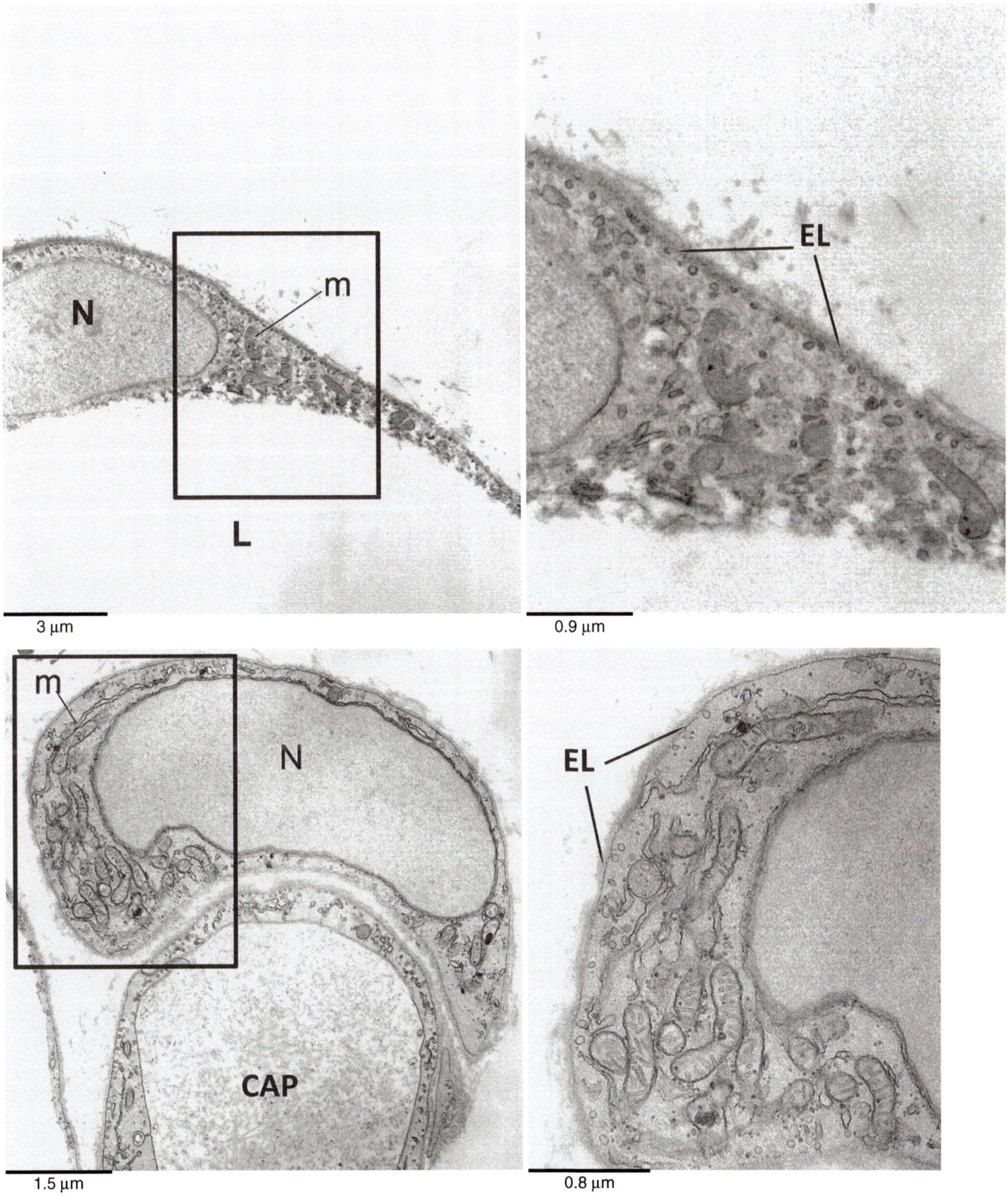

Panel 5.11 Abdominal subcutaneous fat from a subject with a PPARγ dominant-negative mutation (P467L). CAP, capillary. TEM (From: Boiani R et al. Abdominal subcutaneous adipose tissue morphology in a patient with a dominant-negative mutation (P467L) in the nuclear receptor peroxisome proliferator-activated receptor-gamma (PPARG) gene. Nutr Metab Cardiovasc Dis. 20:e11–2, 2010, with permission)

6 Mixed Areas of Adipose Organ

S. Cinti, *Obesity, Type 2 Diabetes and the Adipose Organ*, https://doi.org/10.1007/978-3-319-40522-3_6

6.1 Mixed Areas of Adipose Organ

PLATE 6.1

Gross Anatomy

It is visually evident that even in animals maintained at room temperature or even near thermoneutrality (see Plate 8.1), the brown part of the adipose organ (corresponding to brown adipose tissue (BAT) at histology level) is not restricted to the interscapular area of the adipose organ, but is present also in other areas of the subcutaneous fat, mainly in the anterior depot, such as in the subscapular and axillary areas and in several visceral areas such as the periaortic mediastinal area, interrenal area, and pelvic areas.

It is also visually evident that an anatomic net boundary between white areas (corresponding to WAT at histology level) and brown areas (BAT) does not exist; thus, several "transition areas" between BAT and WAT are present in subcutaneous and visceral areas of adipose organ.

Transition areas formed about 5–10% of the adipose organ volume both in B6 and Sv129 mice maintained at 28 °C and increased (up to about 15–20%) in Sv129 maintained at 6 °C. In B6 mice the increase in cold-acclimated mice was less relevant.

Suggested Reading

Murano I, et al. The adipose organ of Sv129 mice contains a prevalence of brown adipocytes and shows plasticity after cold exposure. Adipocytes. 1:121–30, 2005.

Murano I, et al. Noradrenergic parenchymal nerve fiber branching after cold acclimatisation correlates with brown adipocyte density in mouse adipose organ. J Anat. 214:171–8, 2009.

Cinti S. The adipose organ at a glance. Dis Model Mech. 5:588–94, 2012.

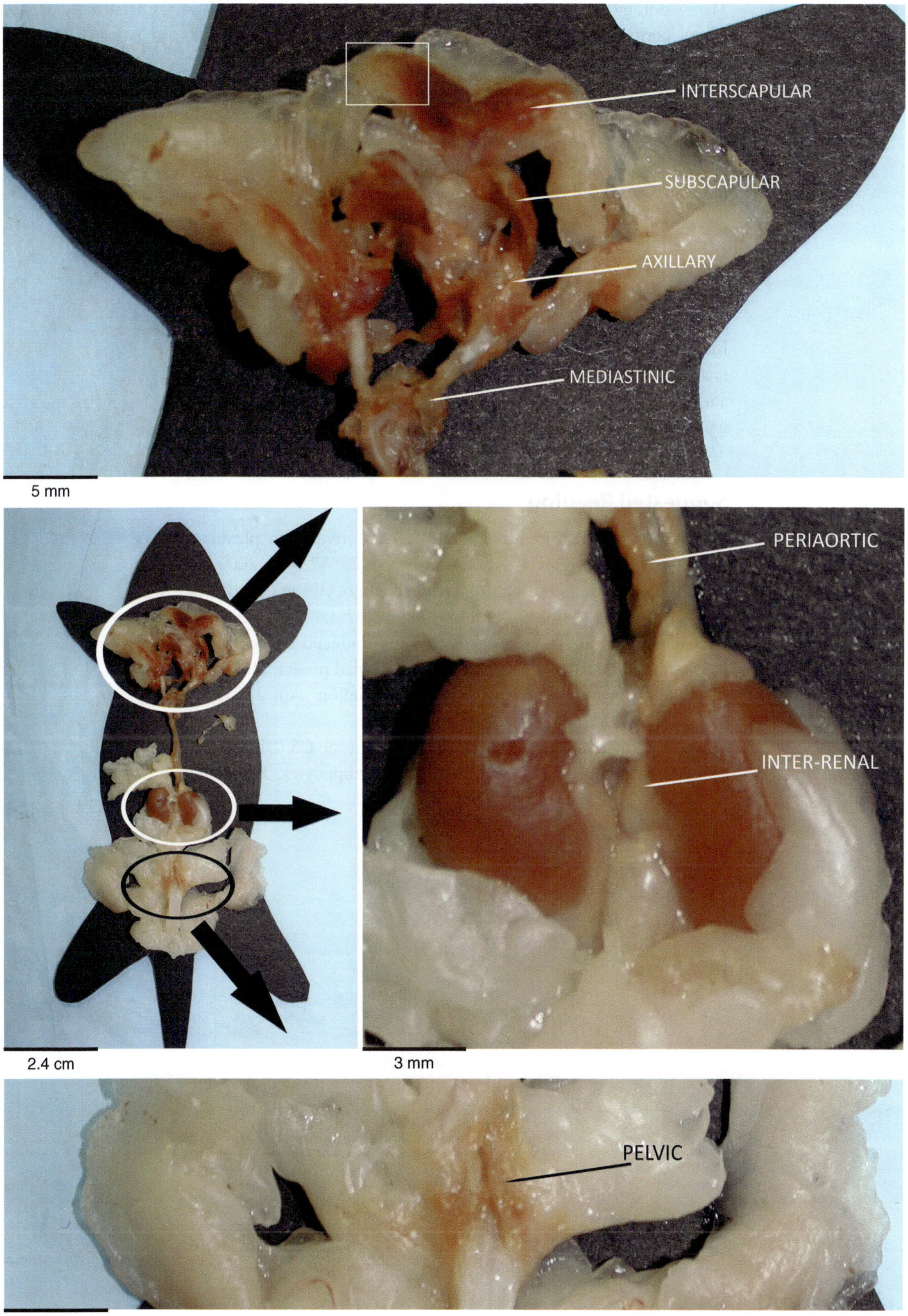

Plate 6.1 Adipose organ of adult Sv129 female mouse maintained at 24 °C

PLATE 6.2

Histology of Transition Areas

The histology of a transition area of the anterior subcutaneous depot, corresponding to the squared area in the top panel of the previous plate, is presented here. Adipocytes in the transition areas have intermediate features between those characteristics of unilocular adipocytes in WAT and those of multilocular adipocytes in BAT. Many of them maintain a certain degree of multilocularity, but lipid vacuoles are less numerous and larger than those found in multilocular adipocytes of frankly BAT areas and can be denominated as paucilocular adipocytes. Among paucilocular adipocytes several morphologic categories can be described: from those with few vacuoles of equivalent size to those with a predominant central vacuole and several small peripheral vacuoles. Of note, these small peripheral vacuoles usually correspond to the size of vacuoles found in adjacent adipocytes of BAT. The size of paucilocular cells is also variable from the smallest, close to the size of multilocular adipocytes of BAT, to the largest that are close to the size of unilocular adipocytes of WAT.

Suggested Reading

Cinti S. Adipocyte differentiation and transdifferentiation: plasticity of the adipose organ. J Endocrinol Invest. 25: 823–35, 2002.

Cinti S. Transdifferentiation properties of adipocytes in the adipose organ. Am J Physiol Endocrinol Metab. 297: E977–86, 2009.

Barbatelli G, et al. The emergence of cold-induced brown adipocytes in mouse white fat depots is determined predominantly by white to brown adipocyte transdifferentiation. Am J Physiol Endocrinol Metab. 298:E1244–53, 2010.

Vitali A, et al. The adipose organ of obesity-prone C57BL/6J mice is composed of mixed white and brown adipocytes. J Lip Res. 53:619–29, 2012.

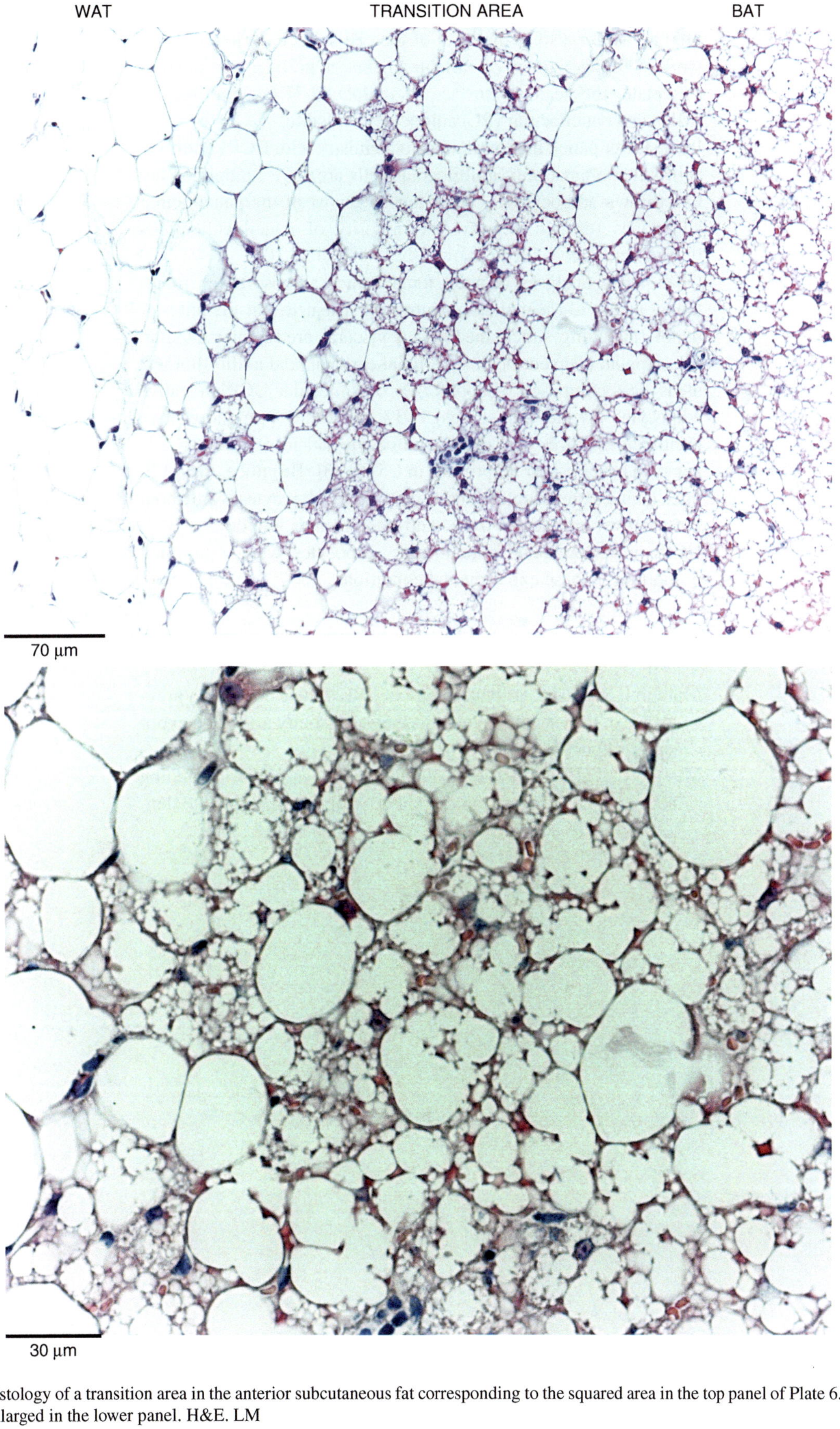

Plate 6.2 Histology of a transition area in the anterior subcutaneous fat corresponding to the squared area in the top panel of Plate 6.1. The transition area is enlarged in the lower panel. H&E. LM

PLATE 6.3

SEM and UCP1-IHC of Transition Areas

The scanning electron microscopy of transition areas reveals its mixture aspect also at the level of the cell surface. Below the network of collagen fibers of variable thickness, in the upper panel of this plate, the scanned surface of unilocular (UL), multilocular (ML), and paucilocular (PL) adipocytes is visible.

In the lower panel, the immunohistochemistry with UCP1 antibody shows that almost only multilocular cells are UCP1 immunoreactive (brown adipocytes). Unilocular and most of the paucilocular adipocytes resulted negative. A minority of paucilocular cells resulted immunostained (arrow) (see also Plate 6.10).

Quantitative analyses in adult female mice adipose organ maintained at 28 °C (near thermoneutrality) revealed that the anterior depot (including subcutaneous and visceral areas: interscapular, subscapular, deep cervical, superficial cervical, and axillo-thoracic areas) was composed of about 73% of unilocular UCP1-negative adipocytes (white adipocytes), 15% of UCP1-immunoreactive multilocular adipocytes (brown adipocytes), and 10% of UCP1-negative paucilocular adipocytes in C57BL/6J (B6) mice. In Sv129 mice (same experimental conditions), white adipocytes were about 20%, brown adipocytes 70%, and paucilocular adipocytes 10%. UCP1-immunoreactive paucilocular adipocytes were a minimal proportion in these experimental conditions.

Suggested Reading

Murano I, et al. The Adipose Organ of Sv129 mice contains a prevalence of brown adipocytes and shows plasticity after cold exposure. Adipocytes. 1:121–30, 2005.

Murano I, et al. Noradrenergic parenchymal nerve fiber branching after cold acclimatization correlates with brown adipocyte density in mouse adipose organ. J Anat. 214(1):171–8, 2009.

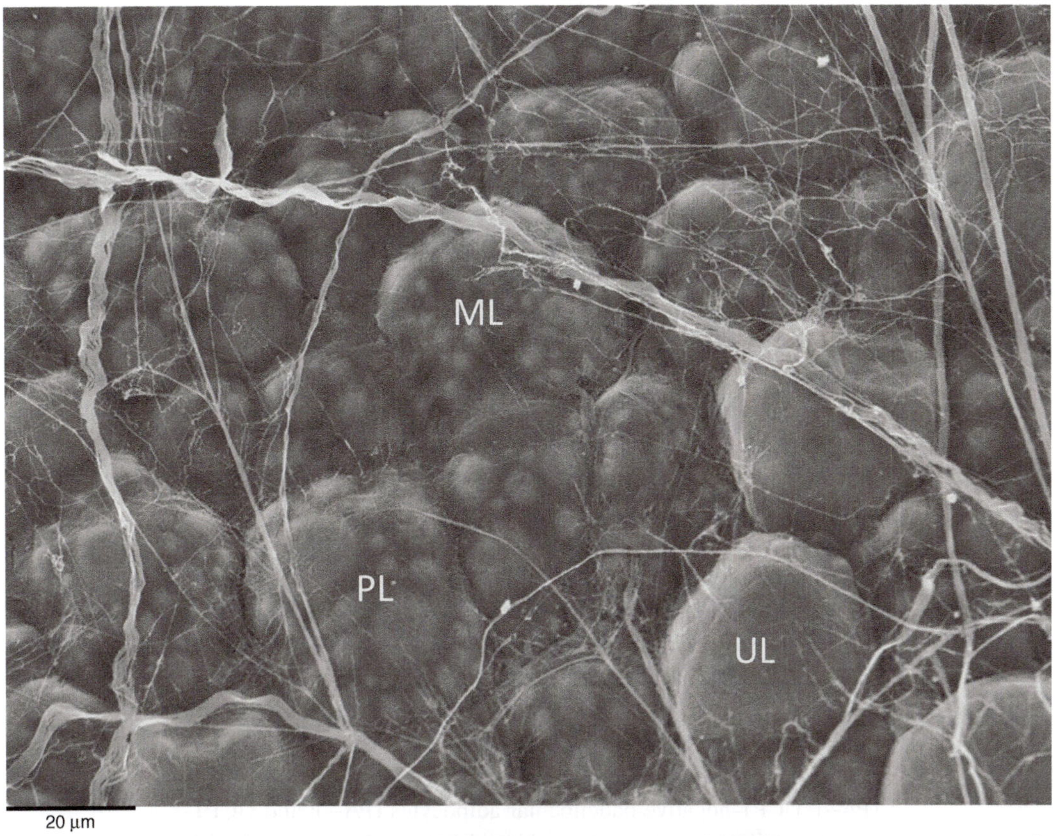

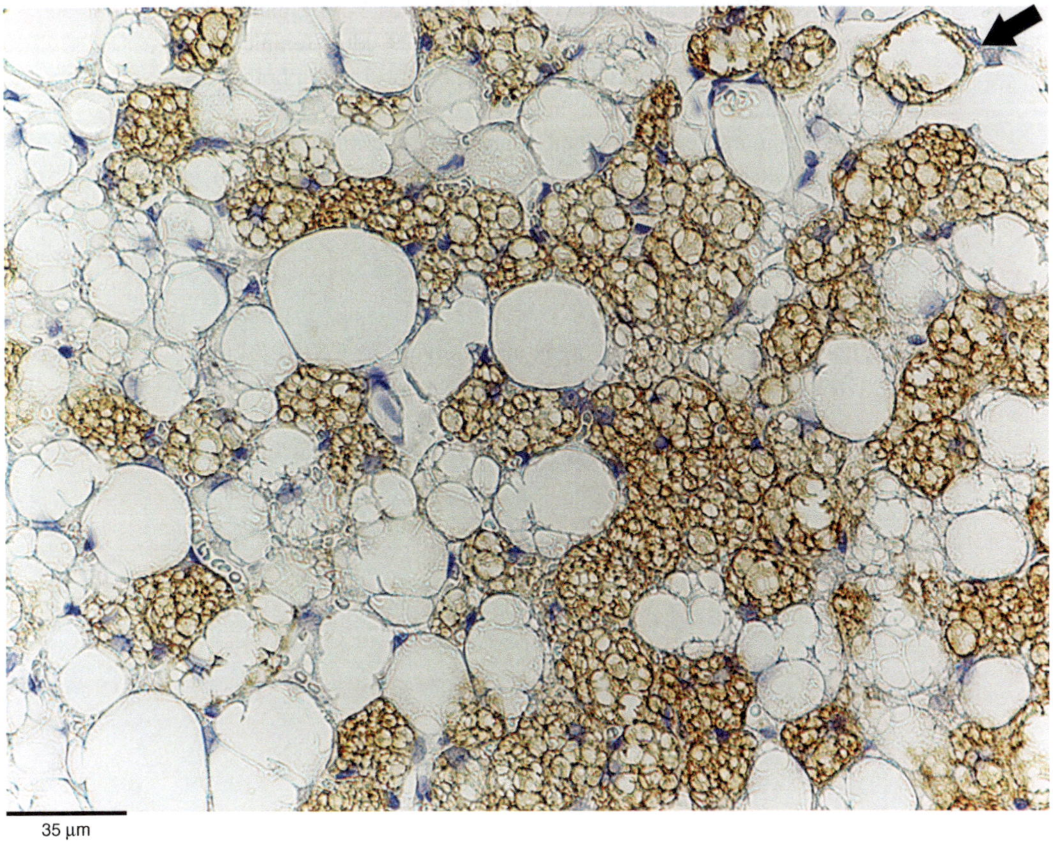

Plate 6.3 Transition areas in the anterior subcutaneous fat (corresponding to the framed area in the top panel of Plate 6.1) of adult mouse. *Upper*: SEM. *Lower*: IHC. UCP1 ab (1:3000). LM

PLATE 6.4

Inguinal WAT

The inguinal area of the subcutaneous posterior depot of normal mice maintained at room temperature (22–24 °C) is a classic example of mixed subcutaneous fat.

The top panel shows the histology of a whole mount preparation of a young (3 weeks old) mouse. This technique allows seeing the whole sampled tissue by transparency. Note the dense central part of the tissue due to BAT lobules. The peripheral part is more transparent due to WAT. The oval dense structure is a lymph node. The nipple with ramified ducts is also visible (arrow). At this age (3 weeks old), the mammary gland ducts are poorly developed, and most of the inguinal area (corresponding to the fourth mammary gland in adult female mice during pregnancy and lactation) is formed almost only by fat.

The middle left panel is a routine section of paraffin-embedded and hematoxylin-eosin-stained inguinal tissue of a young adult mouse. The nerve-vascular supply (NV) occupies the central part of the tissue, and it is surrounded mainly by BAT. Note the dense oval structure corresponding to the lymph node.

The middle right panel is an enlargement of an area corresponding to the squared area shown in the middle left panel in an adult mouse. UCP1 immunohistochemistry shows the presence of a mixture of adipocytes (see enlargement of squared area in the bottom panel): UCP1-immunoreactive multilocular adipocytes (brown adipocytes, BA), rare UCP1-immunoreactive paucilocular adipocytes (PA+), UCP1-negative paucilocular adipocytes (PA−), and UCP1-negative unilocular adipocytes (white adipocytes, WA). Quantitative analyses of warm-acclimated B6 and Sv 129 adult female mice (10 days at 28 °C) showed the following composition in both: 95% of WA and 5% of PA−, with rare PA+.

Age, strain, and environmental temperature are important factors for the determination of the adipocyte cell-type composition in mixed fat.

Suggested Reading

Vitali A, et al. The adipose organ of obesity-prone C57BL/6J mice is composed of mixed white and brown adipocytes. J Lip Res. 53:619–29, 2012.

Cinti S. The adipose organ at a glance. Dis Model Mech. 5:588–94, 2012.

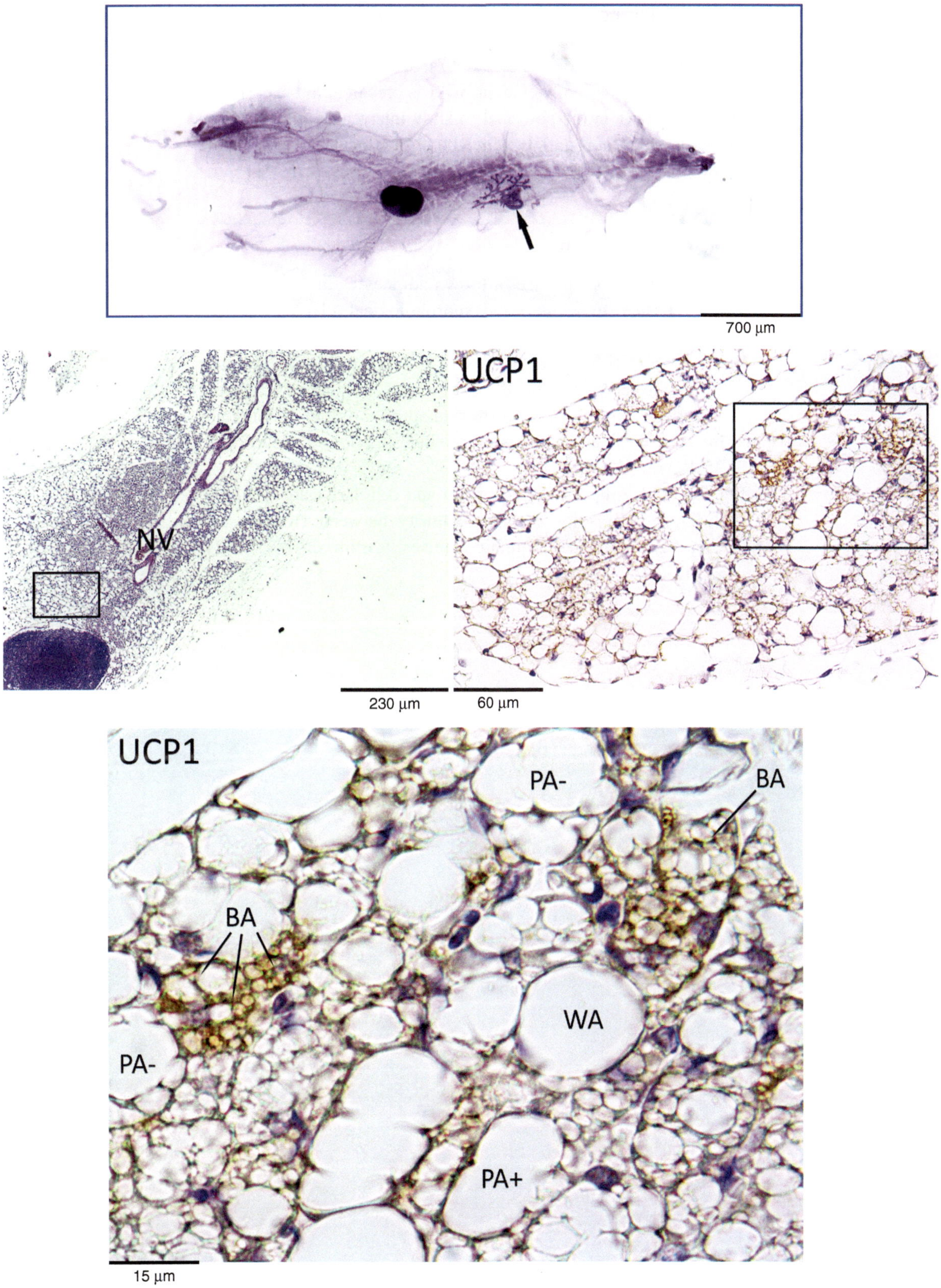

Plate 6.4 Inguinal area of posterior subcutaneous depot of normal mice maintained at room temperature (22–24 °C). *Top*: whole mount of 3-week-old female mouse. Carmine alum solution staining. LM (from: DeMatteis R et al. In Vivo Physiological Transdifferentiation of Adult Adipose Cells. Stem Cells 27:2761–8, 2009, with permission). *Middle left*: 6-week-old male mouse histology. LM. H&E. *Middle right*: 2-month-old male mouse. IHC UCP1 ab (1:400). *Bottom*: enlargement of the squared area in the middle right panel. IHC UCP1 ab (1:400). LM

PLATE 6.5

Mixed Visceral Fat
Gross Anatomy

Most visceral areas of the adipose organ are mixed both in the thorax and abdomen. In this plate several areas of the abdominal part of the adipose organ of an adult rat are visible. The mixture of WAT and BAT is visually evident. WAT is prevalent in the periovarian fat and BAT in the perirenal (mainly interrenal) and periaortic fat. Parametrial fat is mainly white, but brown striae are also visible (arrow).

Suggested Reading

Cousin B, et al. Occurrence of brown adipocytes in rat white adipose tissue: molecular and morphological characterization. J Cell Sci. 103:931–42, 1992.

Giordano A, et al. Tyrosine hydroxylase, neuropeptide Y, substance P, calcitonin gene-related peptide and vasoactive intestinal peptide in nerves of rat periovarian adipose tissue: an immunohistochemical and ultrastructural investigation. J Neurocytol. 25:125–36, 1996.

Taga H, et al. Adipocyte metabolism and cellularity are related to differences in adipose tissue maturity between Holstein and Charolais or Blond d'Aquitaine fetuses. J Anim Sci. 89:711–21, 2011.

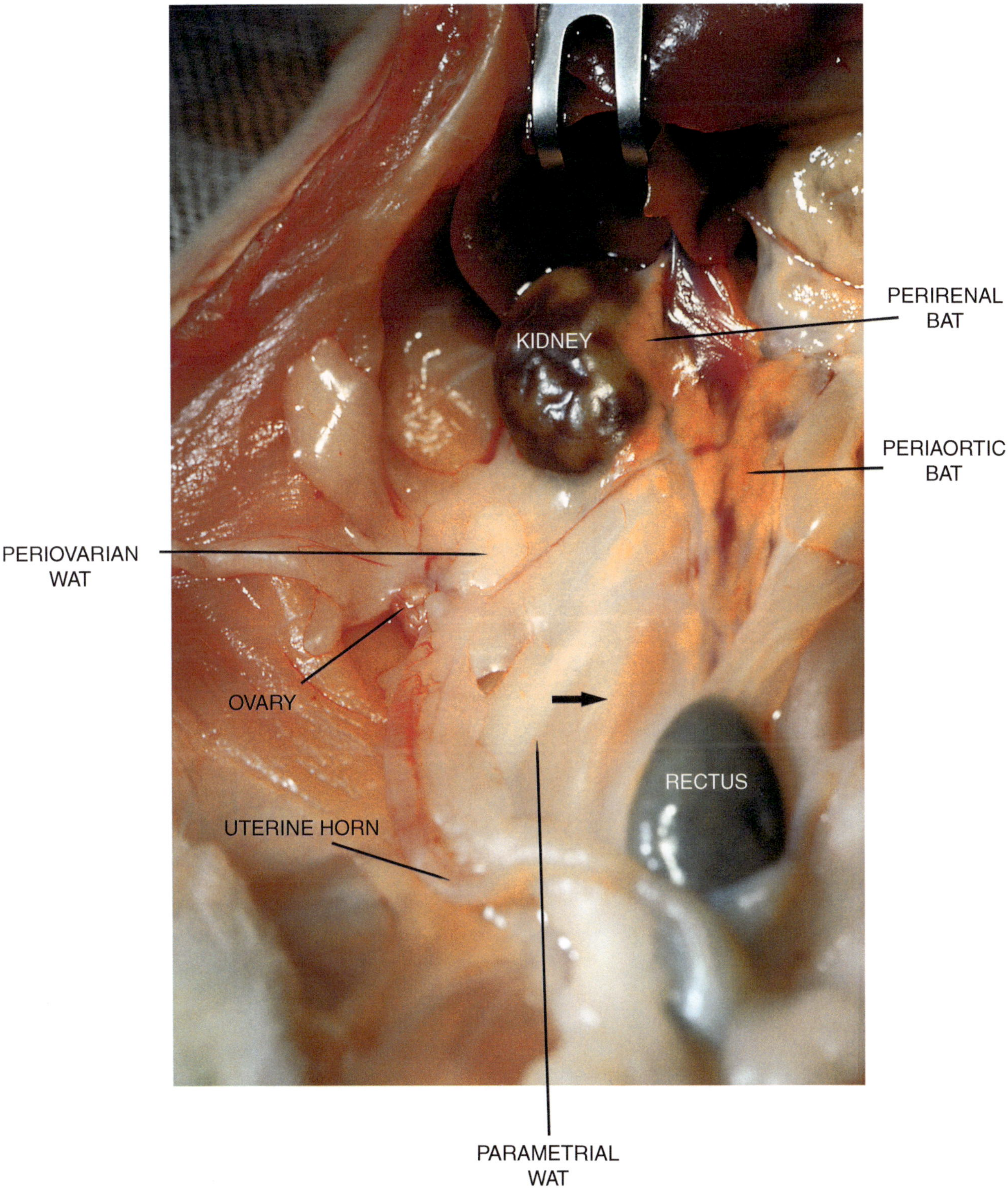

Plate 6.5 Mixed abdominal fat of an adult rat. Gross anatomy

PLATE 6.6

UCP1-immunoreactive multilocular adipocytes are visible among paucilocular and unilocular UCP1-negative adipocytes in two different visceral areas of adipose organ in this plate.
Note the different staining intensity revealed in multilocular cells with different morphology. The more intense staining is present in cells with the smallest vacuoles (in line with the well-known notion that this aspect is indicative of the higher thermogenic activity).

Mixed Visceral Fat
UCP1-IHC

Suggested Reading

Young P, et al. Brown adipose tissue in the parametrial fat pad of the mouse. FEBS Lett. 167:10–14, 1984.

Trayhurn P, et al. Presence of the brown fat-specific mitochondrial uncoupling protein and iodothyronine 5′-deiodinase activity in subcutaneous adipose tissue of neonatal lambs. FEBS Lett. 322:76–8, 1993.

Rossell M, et al. Brown and white adipose tissues: intrinsic differences in gene expression and response to cold exposure in mice. Am J Physiol Endocrinol Metab. 306:E945–64, 2014.

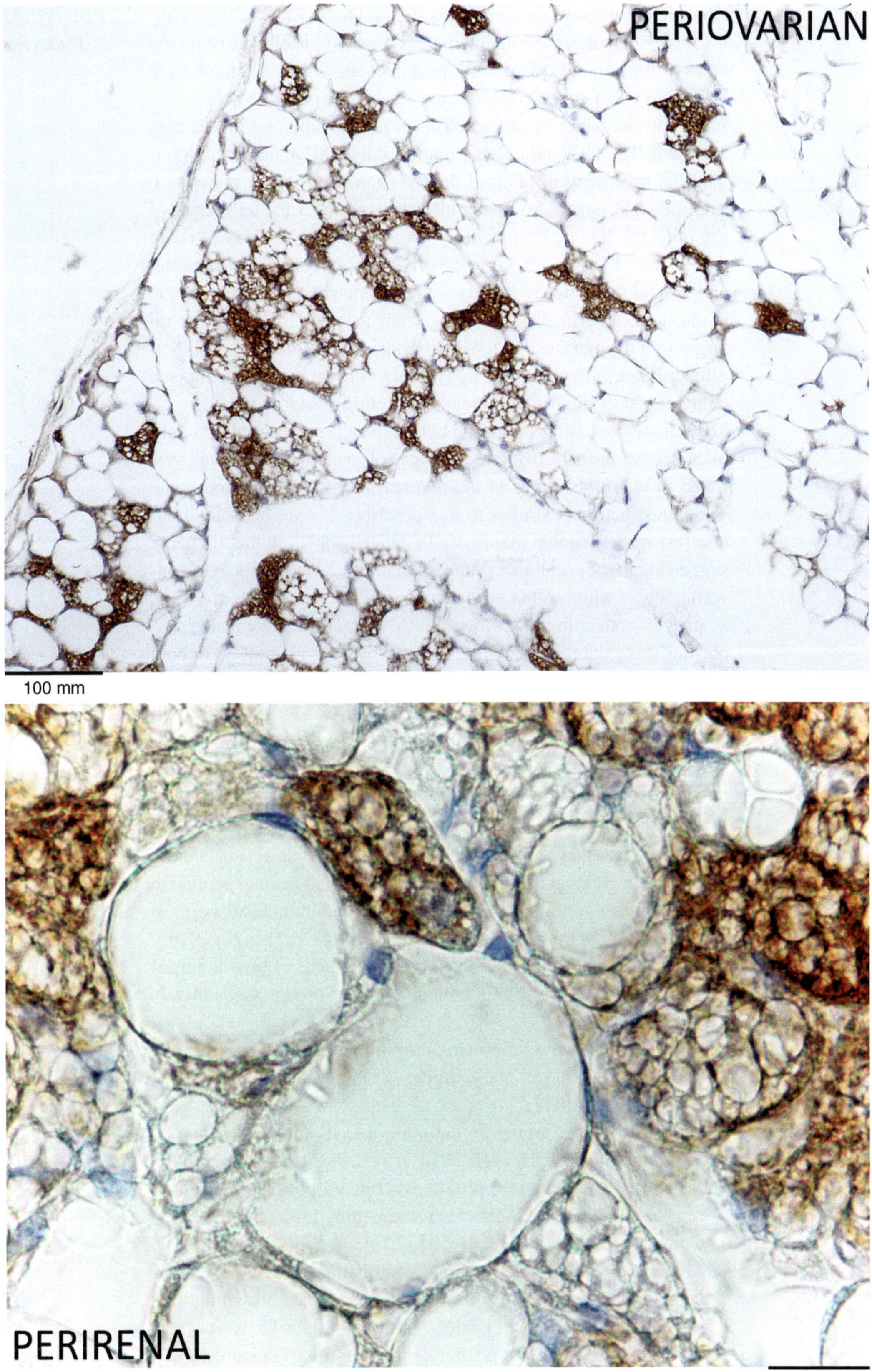

Plate 6.6 *Upper*: periovarian fat of adult rat. IHC. UCP1 ab (1:10,000). *Lower*: perirenal fat of adult mouse. IHC. UCP1 ab (1.3,000). LM

PLATE 6.7

Paucilocular Adipocytes

Considering what was described in the previous plates of this chapter, it is evident that the characteristic parenchymal cell type of mixed areas of the adipose organ is the paucilocular cell. In this plate light microscopy and electron microscopy details are presented.

In the top left panel, scanning electron microscopy of a mixed area is shown. The unilocular (UL), multilocular (ML), and paucilocular (PL) organization of lipid droplets into adipocytes is evident. The top right panel shows the ultrastructure of a PL adipocyte of the inguinal depot of a normal young mouse maintained at room temperature (22–24 °C). Note the predominant central lipid droplet and several small lipid droplets at the cytoplasmic periphery. Some of these peripheral lipid droplets seem to stem from the central large lipid droplet (arrows). Mitochondria are numerous, and their ultrastructure is similar to those typical of brown mitochondria (see enlargement of the squared area in the left top-middle panel).

The left middle (color) panel and bottom panels are examples at light microscopy and electron microscopy of paucilocular adipocytes found in the mixed areas in the inguinal fat of cold-exposed mice. The ultrastructure is similar to that described above, but mitochondria (m) are less brown than those in the cell shown in the top panel suggesting that the cell in the upper panel is a brown adipocyte converting into a white adipocyte and those in the lower panels are white adipocytes converting into brown adipocytes. Thus, paucilocular adipocytes show the morphology of an intermediate phenotype in both converting directions between white and brown adipocytes. The ultrastructure of their mitochondria seems to remain closer to their starting morphology in this intermediate step of conversion.

Suggested Reading

Giordano A, et al. Tyrosine hydroxylase, neuropeptide Y, substance P, calcitonin gene-related peptide and vasoactive intestinal peptide in nerves of rat periovarian adipose tissue: an immunohistochemical and ultrastructural investigation. J Neurocytol. 25:125–36, 1996.

Frontini A, Cinti S. Distribution and development of brown adipocytes in the murine and human adipose organ. Cell Metab. 11:253–6, 2010.

Giordano A, et al. White, brown and pink adipocytes: the extraordinary plasticity of the adipose organ. Eur J Endocrinol. 170:R159–71, 2014.

Rajan S. Adipocyte transdifferentiation and its molecular targets. Differentiation. 87:183–92, 2014.

Shen W, et al. Acupuncture promotes white adipose tissue browning by inducing UCP1 expression on DIO mice. BMC Complement Altern Med. 14:501, 2014.

Jankovic A, et al. Two key temporally distinguishable molecular and cellular components of white adipose tissue browning during cold acclimation. J Physiol. 593:3267–80, 2015.

Wang J, et al. Influence of phenotype conversion of epicardial adipocytes on the coronary atherosclerosis and its potential molecular mechanism. Am J Transl Res. 7:1712–23, 2015.

Lombardi A, et al. 3,5-Diiodo-L-thyronine activates brown adipose tissue thermogenesis in hypothyroid rats. PLoS One. 10:e0116498, 2015.

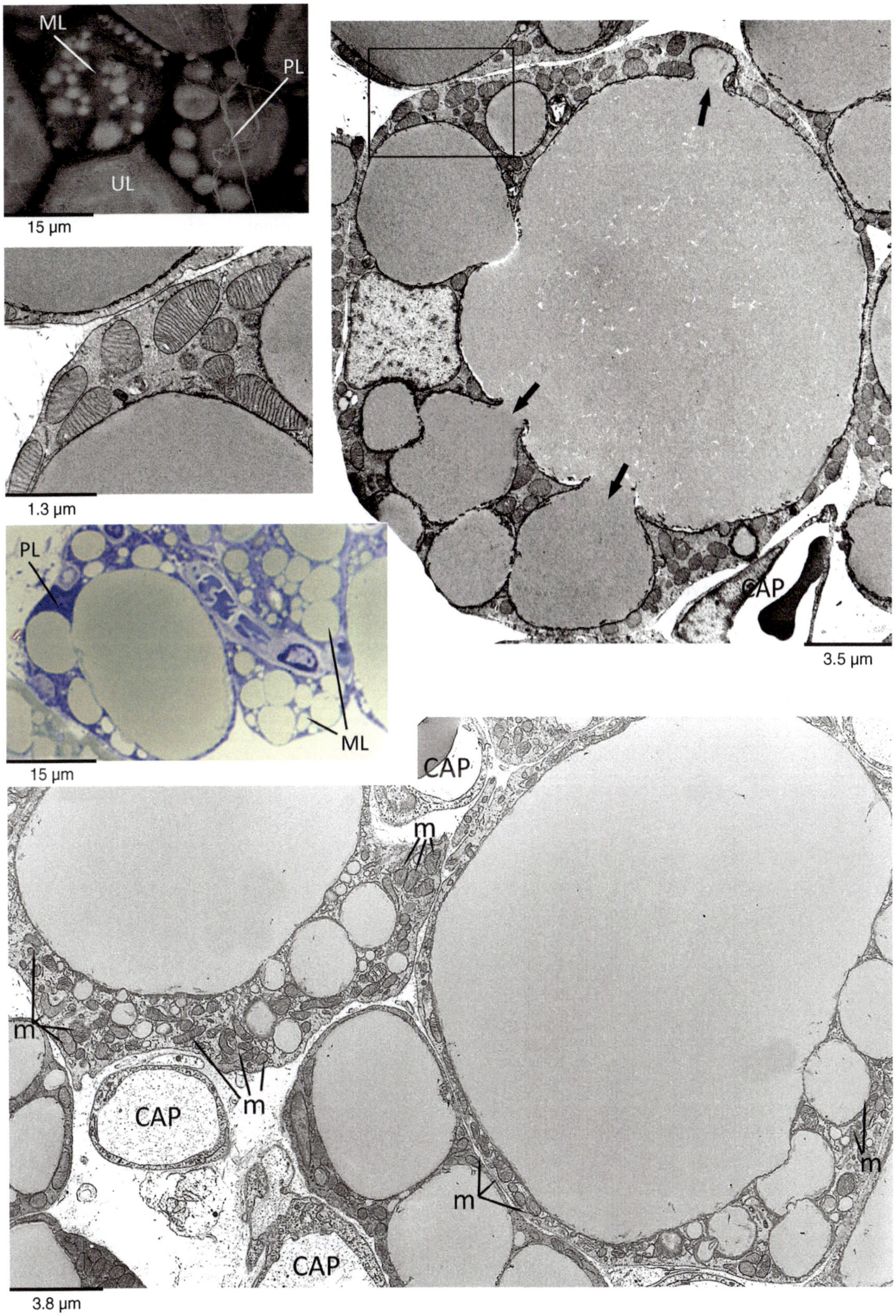

Plate 6.7 *Top left*: anterior subcutaneous fat of adult mouse. SEM. *Top right*: inguinal fat of young adult (6 weeks old) mouse maintained at room temperature (22–24 °C). TEM. *Middle-top*: enlargement of squared area in the top right. TEM. *Middle color*: inguinal fat of cold-exposed adult mouse (6 °C for 5 days) in the resin-embedded tissue. Toluidine blue (from: Istologia Medica, Maraldi and Tacchetti, Chapter 16, The Adipose Organ. Edi Ermes Milan, 2016, with permission). LM. *Bottom*: inguinal fat of cold-exposed adult mouse (6 °C for 5 days). *CAP* capillary, *m* mitochondria (some indicated). TEM

PLATE 6.8

Mitochondria of Paucilocular Adipocytes

In this plate the morphology of mitochondria in paucilocular adipocytes (bottom and middle panel) found in the inguinal area of the posterior subcutaneous depot of a 6-week-old mouse maintained at room temperature (22–24 °C) is compared with that in unilocular adipocytes (top panel) from the same fat depot. In the top panel, two adjacent unilocular adipocytes are visible. Lipids form a single vacuole (L). Note the absence of small lipid droplets in the peripheral rim of the cytoplasm in both adipocytes. The mitochondria (m) are very small, elongated, and with few randomly oriented cristae (white mitochondria).
The paucilocular adipocyte in the bottom panel is slightly more multilocular than the one shown in the middle panel. Note the abundance of small lipid droplets (SL, some indicated) in the cytoplasmic rim and the predominant central lipid droplet (L). In parallel with the degree of multilocularity of the cell, the morphology of mitochondria approaches that typical of brown adipocyte mitochondria (m, some indicated).

Suggested Reading

Barbatelli G, et al. The emergence of cold-induced brown adipocytes in mouse white fat depots is determined predominantly by white to brown adipocyte transdifferentiation. Am J Physiol Endocrinol Metab. 298:E1244–53, 2010.

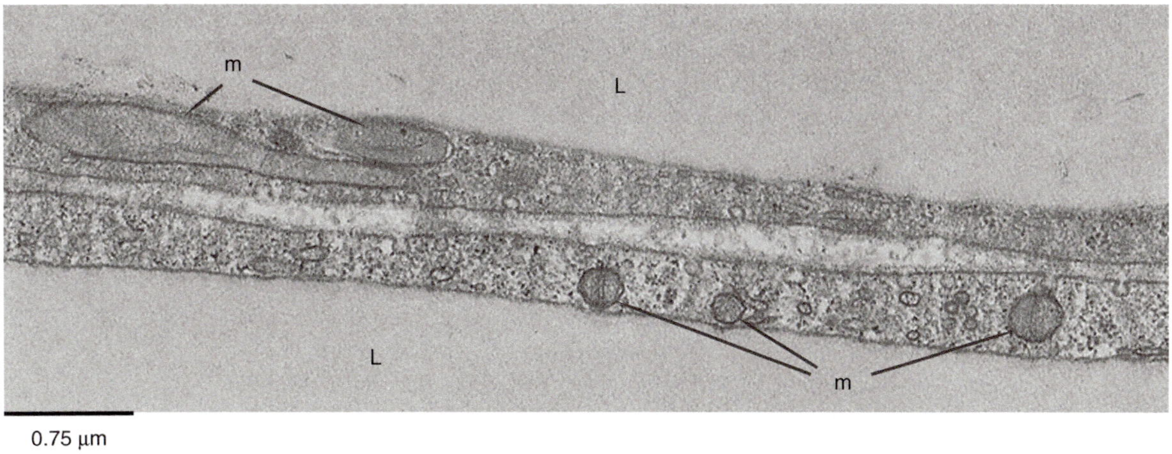

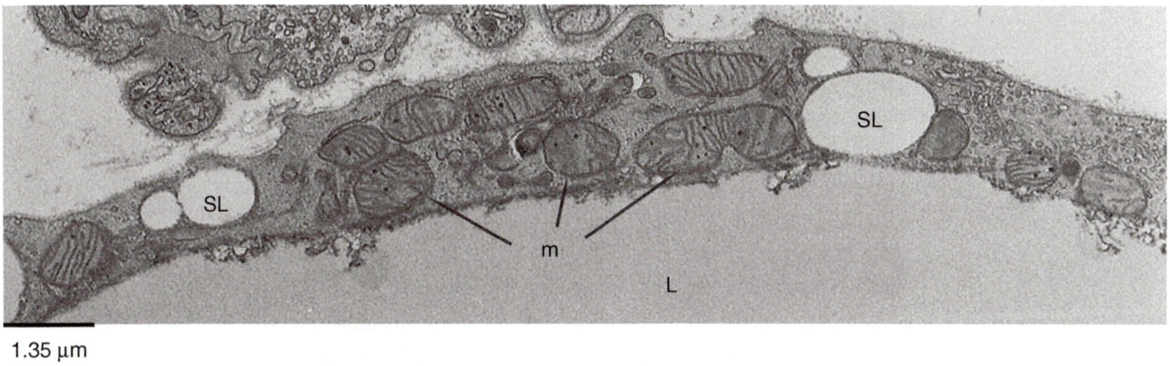

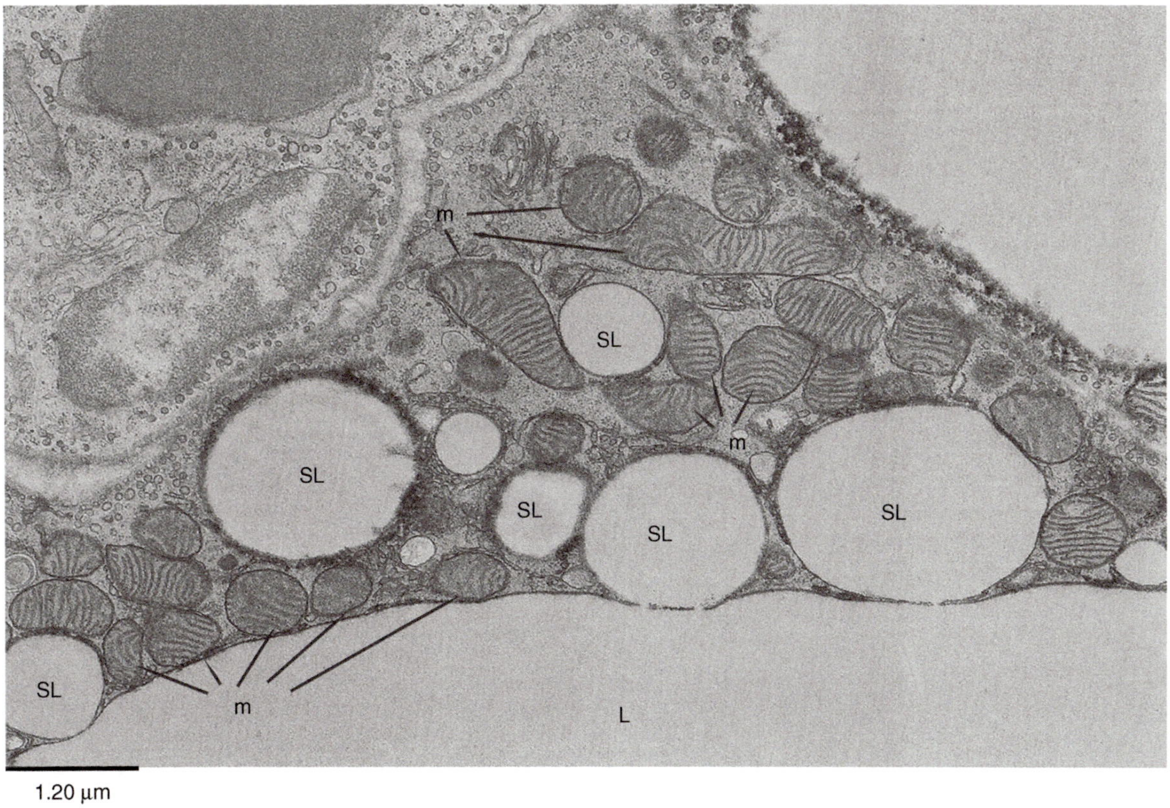

Plate 6.8 Inguinal fat of a 6-week-old mouse maintained at room temperature (22–24 °C). *Top*: cytoplasmic rim of two adjacent unilocular adipocytes. *Middle*: paucilocular adipocyte with few peripheral small lipid droplets. *Bottom*: paucilocular adipocyte with several peripheral lipid droplets. TEM

PLATE 6.9

Adipocyte Precursors in Mixed Fat

In addition to the brown and white precursors shown and described in Plates 2.26–2.29 and 4.15–4.18, respectively, we observed in visceral depots of young (15 days old) rat's adipocyte precursors with features differing from those of the two types (white and brown) of precursor cells. In this plate, the cells labeled "A" are poorly differentiated; they are in close connection with capillary walls and show "attenuated" brown precursor features. The most distinctive characteristic of these cells is the presence of a significant number of mitochondria (m) with intermediate ultrastructure between typical (brown) and "nontypical" (white) mitochondria.

The other characteristic feature of this poorly developed cell type is the presence of small lipid droplets in the cytoplasm. A variable number of mature brown adipocytes (B) are always found in close connection with these precursors. These mature brown cells have large lipid droplets (a sign of weak thermogenesis). Precursors and mature brown cells form small foci surrounded by paucilocular adipocytes. These paucilocular adipocytes closest to brown cell foci (C) have mitochondria with intermediate features.

Some researchers have described white adipose tissue exhibiting intermediate features as "convertible adipose tissue."

Suggested Reading

Loncar D, Afzelius B. Ontogenetical changes in adipose tissue of the cat: convertible adipose tissue. J Ultrastruct Mol Struct Res. 102:9–23, 1989.

Cousin B, et al. Adipose tissues from various anatomical sites are characterized by different patterns of gene expression and regulation. Biochem J. 292:873–76, 1993.

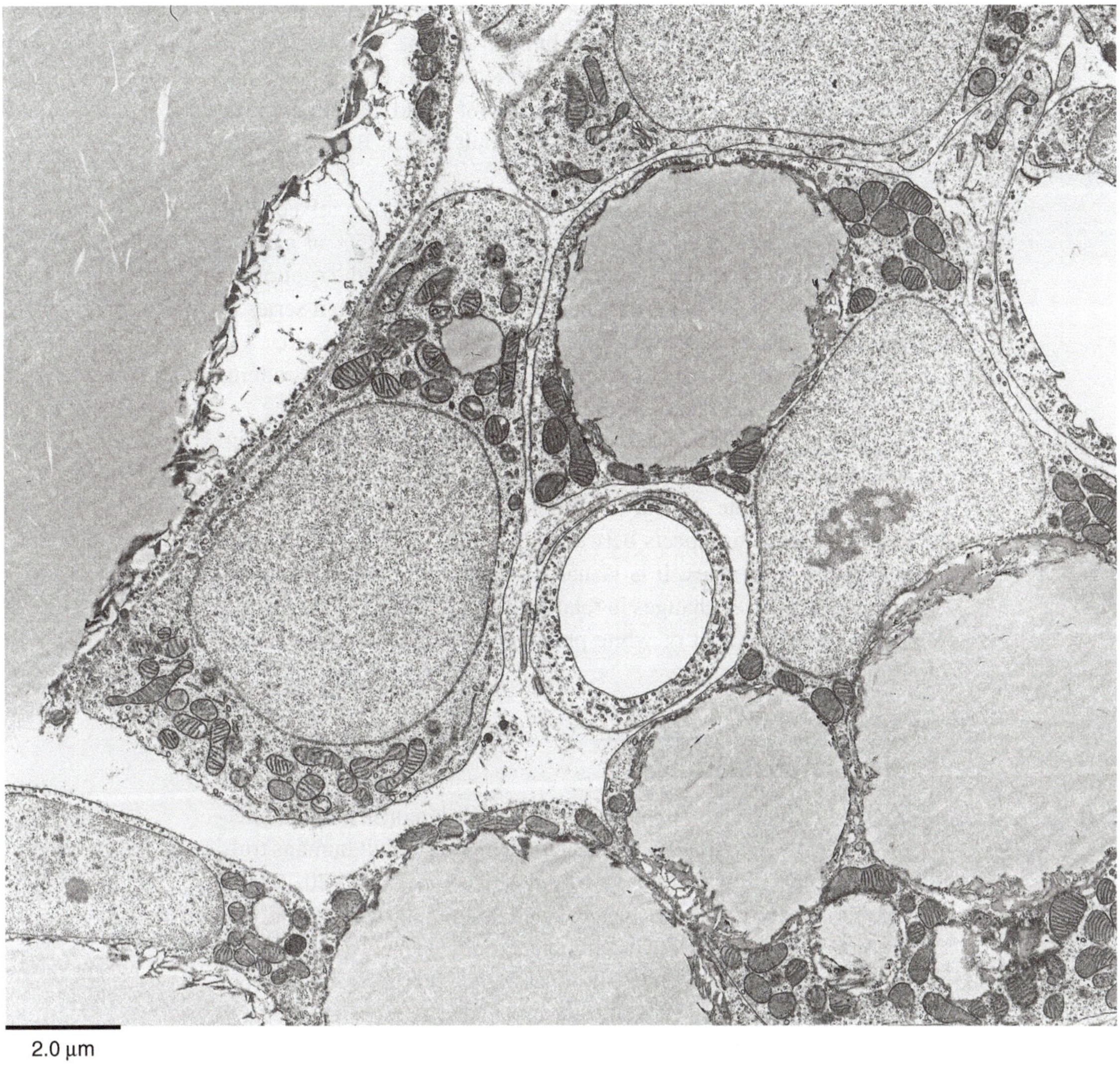

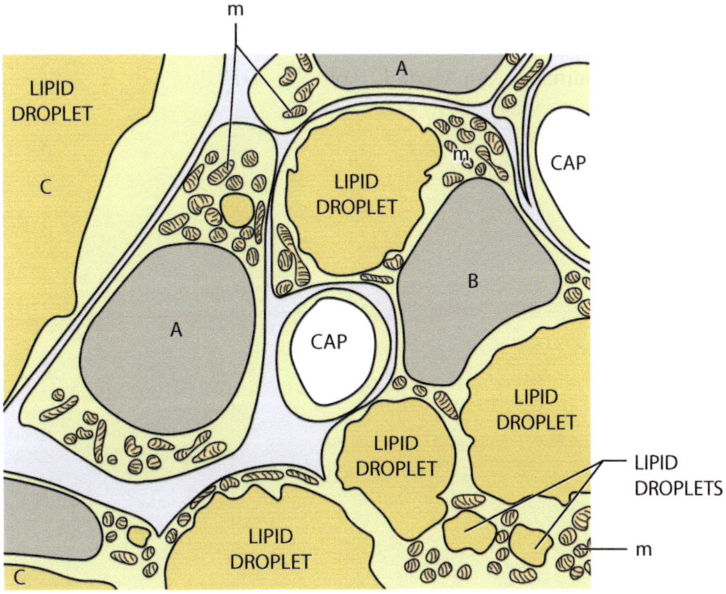

Plate 6.9 Retroperitoneal WAT of a 15-day-old rat. The cross-sectioned capillary (CAP) is surrounded by cells at different stages of differentiation. TEM. A ⇨ B ⇨ C: Possible differentiation steps of the same cell type

PLATE 6.10

Human-Mixed Fat

Adult humans have reduced thermal dispersion due to the high surface/volume ratio. Thus, the human adipose organ is mainly composed of WAT. Compact BAT areas, such as those shown and described in Chaps. 1 and 2 in mice, are not found in adult humans, but only in newborns (see Chap. 12). Adult human BAT should be described as a mixed fat.

We found UCP1-immunoreactive brown adipocytes mixed with white adipocytes in all patients under 30, in about 25% of patients under 50, and rarely in patients over 60 years old at the root of the neck (peri-subclavian artery or supraclavicular area) in a series of about 50 subjects (see also Plate 3.1). In the perirenal fat, UCP1-immunoreactive brown adipocytes were found also in old patients (present plate and Plate 3.1).

Together with UCP1-immunoreactive multilocular adipocytes, several UCP1-immunoreactive paucilocular adipocytes (PL+) were also present. Note the variable morphology of paucilocular cells with intermediate aspects between classic multilocular and classic unilocular adipocytes. It is visually evident that the size of paucilocular adipocytes changes in relationship with their phenotype: the largest approach that of white phenotype, and the smallest that of brown phenotype.

Suggested Reading

Zingaretti MC, et al. The presence of UCP1 demonstrates that metabolically active adipose tissue in the neck of adult humans truly represents brown adipose tissue. FASEB J. 23:3113–20, 2009.

Manieri M, et al. Morphological and immunohistochemical features of brown adipocytes and preadipocytes in a case of human hibernoma. Nutr Metab Cardiovasc Dis. 20:567–74, 2010.

Townsend KL, Tseng YH. Of mice and men: novel insights regarding constitutive and recruitable brown adipocytes. Int J Obes Suppl. 5:S15–20, 2015.

Cereijo R, et al. Thermogenic brown and beige/brite adipogenesis in humans. Ann Med. 47:169–77, 2015.

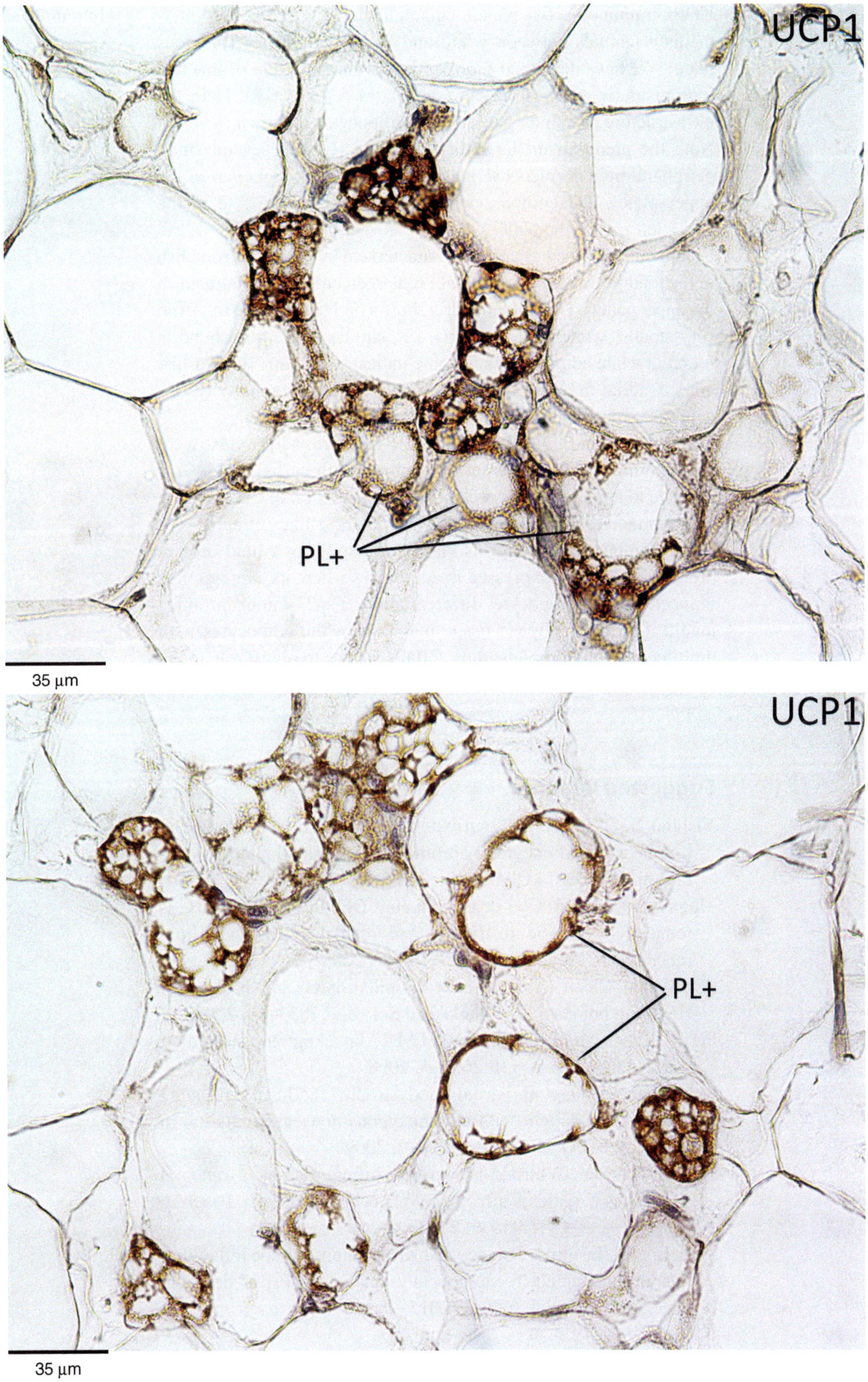

Plate 6.10 Perirenal fat of an 83-year-old overweight male patient. IHC. UCP1 ab (1:3,000). LM

PLATE 6.11

Human Paucilocular Adipocyte's Ultrastructure

UCP1-immunoreactive paucilocular adipocytes are cells with intermediate features between white and brown adipocytes (previous plate). We have described thoroughly the ultrastructure of this cell type in murine adipose organ (see Plates 6.7 and 6.8). Here the ultrastructure of human paucilocular adipocytes is shown.

Note the predominant large lipid vacuole (L) and several small peripheral lipid droplets (SL) in paucilocular cells (right part of the upper plate), and compare with the unilocular adipocyte in the upper left part of the plate.

Paucilocular adipocytes are also characterized by numerous roundish mitochondria; see the lower panel (enlargement of squared area in the upper panel). The mitochondria show a highly variable size, from very small ("white" mitochondria, i.e., similar to the mitochondria found in white adipocytes; sm, some indicated) to large (brown-like mitochondria; m, some indicated). Note the dense capillary (CAP) network (typical of BAT) associated with paucilocular cells.

Paucilocular and multilocular UCP1-negative adipocytes were found in the subcutaneous fat of a subject with partial lipodystrophy due to a homozygous premature stop mutation in CIDEC (cell death-inducing DNA fragmentation factor-α-like effector C). CIDEC (mouse orthologue is known as Fsp27) is a lipid droplet protein most highly expressed in adipocytes where its expression is induced during adipocyte differentiation. Fsp27-knockout mice manifest reduced adipose tissue mass and white adipocytes with multilocular lipid droplets; thus, CIDEC seems to play a role in the unilocular organization of the cytoplasmic lipid droplets in human adipocytes.

Suggested Reading

Nishino N, et al. FSP27 contributes to efficient energy storage in murine white adipocytes by promoting the formation of unilocular lipid droplets. J Clin Invest. 118:2808–21, 2008.

Magnusson B, et al. Cell death-inducing DFF45-like effector C is reduced by caloric restriction and regulates adipocyte lipid metabolism. Metabolism. 57:1307–13, 2008.

Puri V, et al. Cidea is associated with lipid droplets and insulin sensitivity in humans. Proc Natl Acad Sci. 105: 7833–38, 2008.

Puri V, Czech MP. Lipid droplets: FSP27 knockout enhances their sizzle. J Clin Invest. 118:2693–6, 2008.

Rubio-Cabezas O, et al. Partial lipodystrophy and insulin resistant diabetes in a patient with a homozygous nonsense mutation in CIDEC. EMBO Mol Med. 1:280–7, 2009.

Frontini A, et al. White-to-brown transdifferentiation of omental adipocytes in patients affected by pheochromocytoma. Biochim Biophys Acta. 1831:950–9, 2013.

Zhou L, et al. Insulin resistance and white adipose tissue inflammation are uncoupled in energetically challenged Fsp27-deficient mice. Nat Commun. 6:5949, 2015.

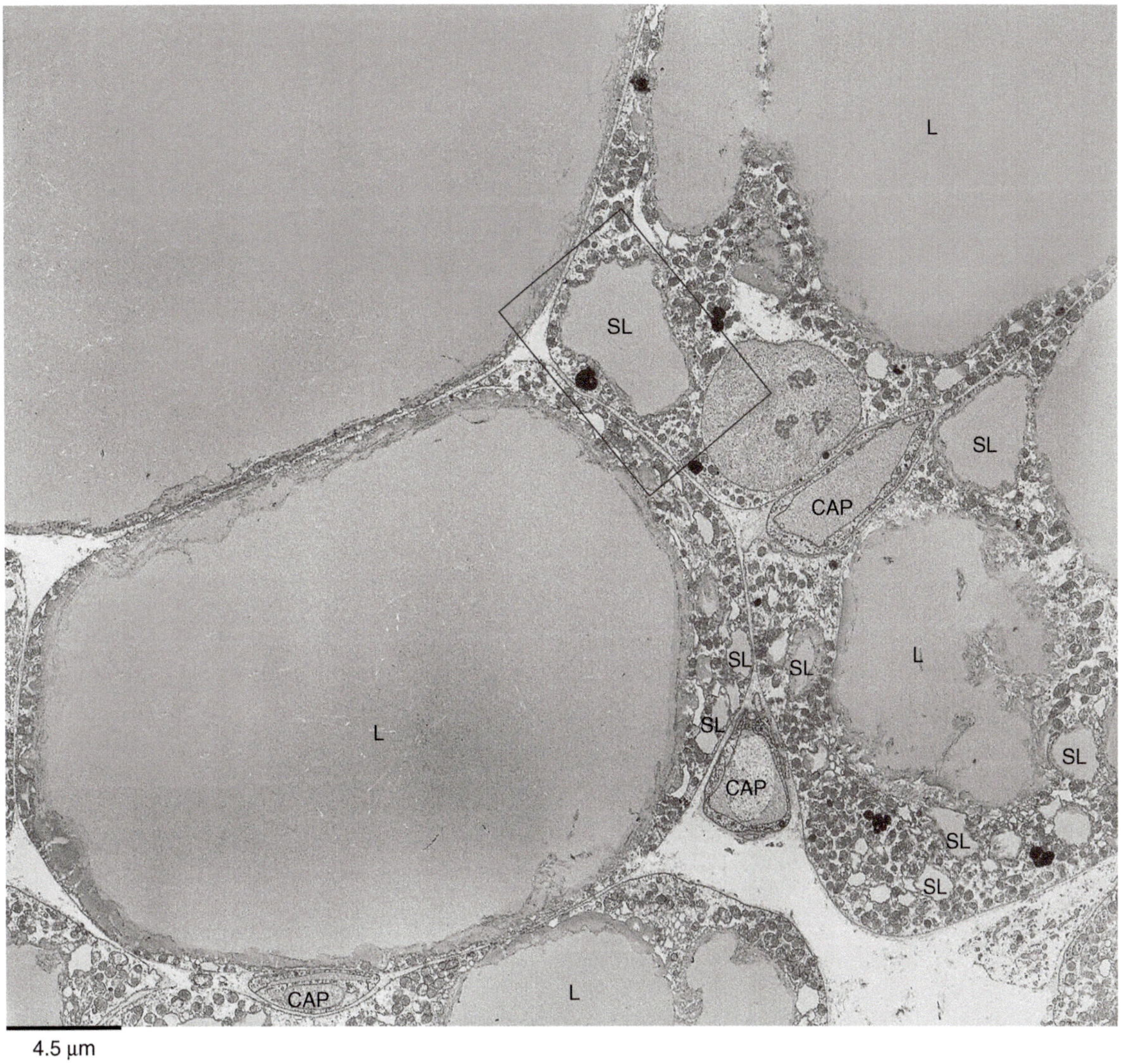

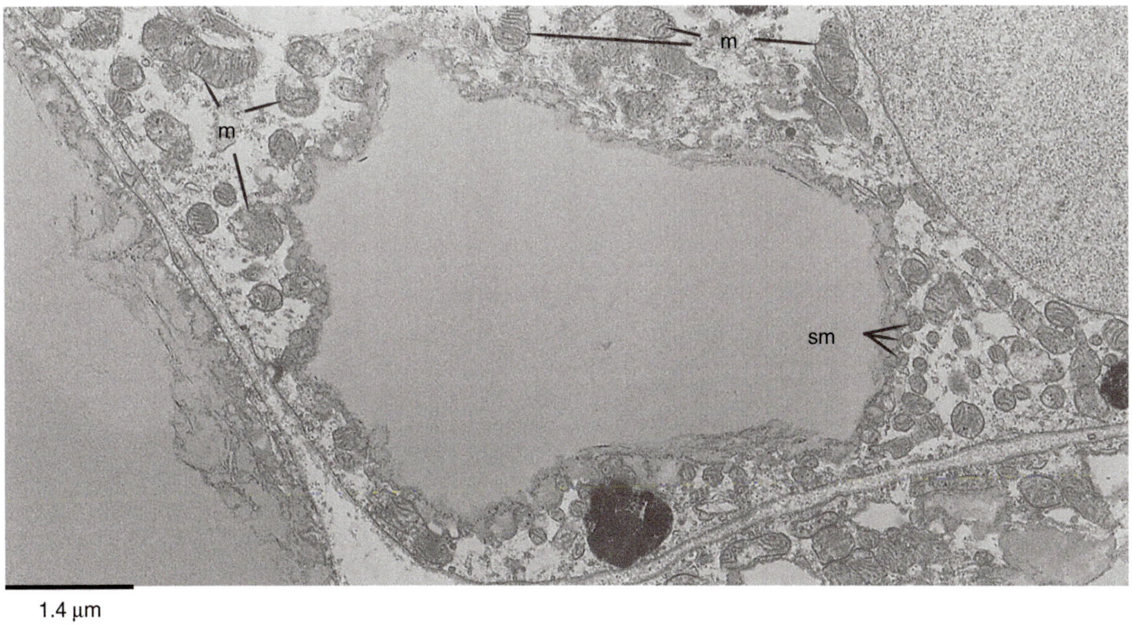

Plate 6.11 Deep cervical perithyroid fat of lean adult female. Human paucilocular adipocytes. TEM

7 The Adipose Organ: Cold Acclimation

S. Cinti, *Obesity, Type 2 Diabetes and the Adipose Organ*, https://doi.org/10.1007/978-3-319-40522-3_7

7.1. The Adipose Organ Cold Acclimation

PLATE 7.1

Cold-Exposed Adipose Organ

In cold-exposed and adapted mice (10 days or more), the color of the adipose organ changes dramatically. In this plate adult female mice Sv129 maintained at 28 °C (left) or 6 °C (right) for 10 days are shown. It is visually evident that the browning of white areas of the organ is diffused to the whole organ with only some areas in both visceral and subcutaneous fat remaining paler. Areas most resistant to browning included gluteal (in the posterior subcutaneous depot), mesenteric, and superficial cervical of the anterior subcutaneous depot. Our calculations on mice of this strain and on mice B6, tested in the same experimental conditions, showed that the cold-adapted adipose organ does not change the total number of adipocytes. In both strains the number of brown adipocytes increased, and the number of white adipocytes decreased to an amount equivalent to the increased number of brown adipocytes. The paucilocular cell (intermediate forms between white and brown adipocytes, described in the previous chapter) number did not change significantly although the UCP1-immunoreactive paucilocular cells seemed to be more frequently found, even if not calculated. We did not observe morphologic signs of apoptosis carefully searched in all depots, and neither did we find signs of proliferation or mitosis (with the exception of the interscapular area). Of note, cold exposure with its increase in noradrenaline content of tissue protects against apoptosis. Data from single depots showed an increase of the total cell number only in the interscapular area of the anterior subcutaneous depot.

These data, together with many other molecular data (e.g., absence of DNA increase, increased expression of the antimitotic gene C/EBP, no change in Ccna1), strongly suggest that browning is due predominantly to a direct transdifferentiation of white to brown adipocytes in agreement with old experiments from our and others' laboratories (see also Plates 7.12–7.14).

Recent lineage tracing experiments support the idea that white adipocytes can convert into brown adipocytes under adrenergic stimuli.

Suggested Reading

Loncar D. Convertible adipose tissue in mice. Cell Tissue Res. 266:149–61, 1991.

Himms-Hagen J, et al. Multilocular fat cells in WAT of CL-316243-treated rats derive directly from white adipocytes. Am J Physiol Cell Physiol. 279:C670–81, 2000.

Cinti S. Anatomy of the adipose organ. Eat Weight Disord. 5:132–42, 2000.

Nisoli E, et al. Protective effects of noradrenaline against tumor necrosis factor- alpha-induced apoptosis in cultured rat brown adipocytes: role of nitric oxide-induced heat shock protein 70 expression. Int J Obes Relat Metab Disord. 25:1421–30, 2001.

Cinti S. The adipose organ: endocrine aspects and insights from transgenic models. Eat Weight Disord. 6:4–8, 2001.

Cinti S. Adipocyte differentiation and transdifferentiation: plasticity of the adipose organ. J Endocrinol Invest. 25:823–35, 2002.

Cannon B, Nedergaard J. Brown adipose tissue: function and physio-logical significance. Physiol Rev. 84: 277–359, 2004.

Cinti S. The adipose organ. Prostaglandins Leukot Essent Fatty Acids. 73:9–15, 2005.

Wang QA, et al. Tracking adipogenesis during white adipose tissue development, expansion and regeneration. Nat Med. 19:1338–44, 2013.

Rosenwald M, et al. Bi-directional interconversion of brite and white adipocytes. Nat Cell Biol. 15:659–67, 2013.

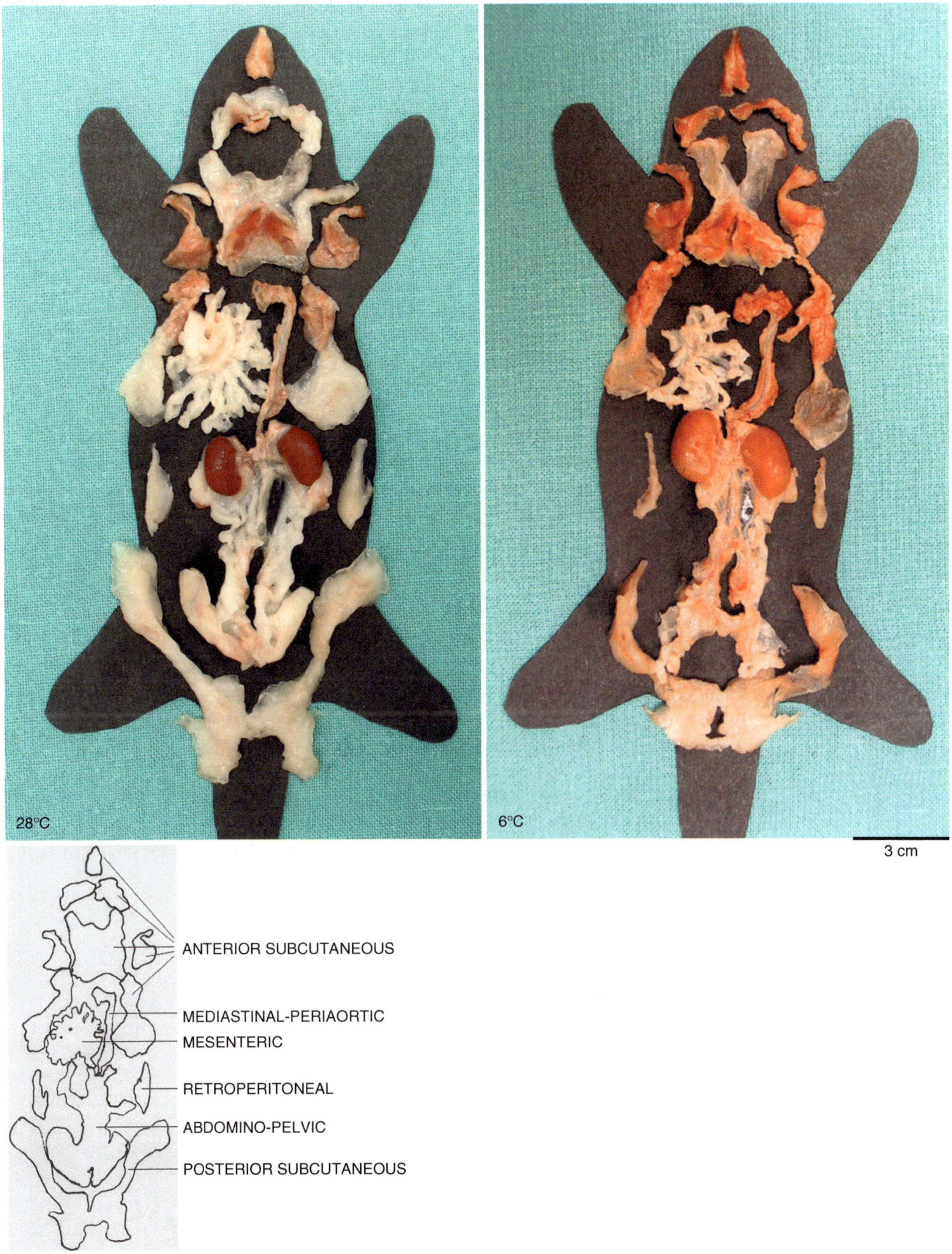

Plate 7.1 Adipose organs of adult female Sv129 mice maintained at 28 °C (*left*) or 6 °C (*right*) for 10 days. Gross anatomy (from Murano I et al. The Adipose Organ of Sv129 mice contains a prevalence of brown adipocytes and shows plasticity after cold exposure. Adipocytes 1:121–30, 2005 with permission)

PLATE 7.2

Brown adipose tissue (BAT) in cold-exposed and acclimated mice has a classic morphology and UCP1 immunostaining. In the upper panel the interscapular area (left) of the anterior subcutaneous depot appear intensely and homogeneously immunostained. The white adipose tissue (WAT) area of the same depot appears unstained (right). Between these two areas, there is a transition area that is mainly formed by UCP1-immunoreactive multilocular cells on the left (near interscapular BAT (IBAT)) and mainly formed by UCP1-negative paucilocular and multilocular adipocytes on the right (near WAT).

In the bottom panel a higher magnification from the transition area (near IBAT) of the upper panel shows that immunostaining of brown adipocytes is not homogeneous. In this panel UCP1-immunoreactive multilocular adipocytes are present. Among them it is evident that the intensity of immunostaining is variable from intense to weak, and some multilocular adipocytes are clearly negative. Furthermore some paucilocular UCP1-negative adipocytes are also present. This nonhomogeneous UCP1 immunostaining could be due to the Harlequin phenomenon described in Plate 7.4 and to the presence in this area of transdifferentiation stages from white to brown adipocytes.

IBAT Histology-IHC-UCP1

Suggested Reading

Guerra C, et al. Emergence of brown adipocytes in white fat in mice is under genetic control. Effects on body weight and adiposity. J Clin Invest. 102:412–20, 1998.

Cinti S. Adipocyte differentiation and transdifferentiation: plasticity of the adipose organ. J Endocrinol Invest. 25:823–35, 2002.

Jimenez M, et al. Beta 3-adrenoceptor knockout in C57BL/6J mice depresses the occurrence of brown adipocytes in white fat. Eur J Biochem. 270:699–705, 2003.

Granneman JG, et al. Metabolic and cellular plasticity in white adipose tissue I: effects of β3-adrenergic receptor activation. Am J Physiol Endocrinol Metab. 289:E608–16, 2005.

Cinti S. Transdifferentiation properties of adipocytes in the adipose organ. Am J Physiol Endocrinol Metab. 297:E977–86, 2009.

Barbatelli G, et al. The emergence of cold-induced brown adipocytes in mouse white fat depots is determined predominantly by white to brown adipocyte transdifferentiation. Am J Physiol Endocrinol Metab. 298:E1244–53, 2010.

Lee YH, et al. Adipose tissue plasticity from WAT to BAT and in between. Biochim Biophys Acta. 1842:358–69, 2014.

Rosenwald M, Wolfrum C. The origin and definition of brite versus white and classical brown adipocytes. Adipocyte. 3:4–9, 2014.

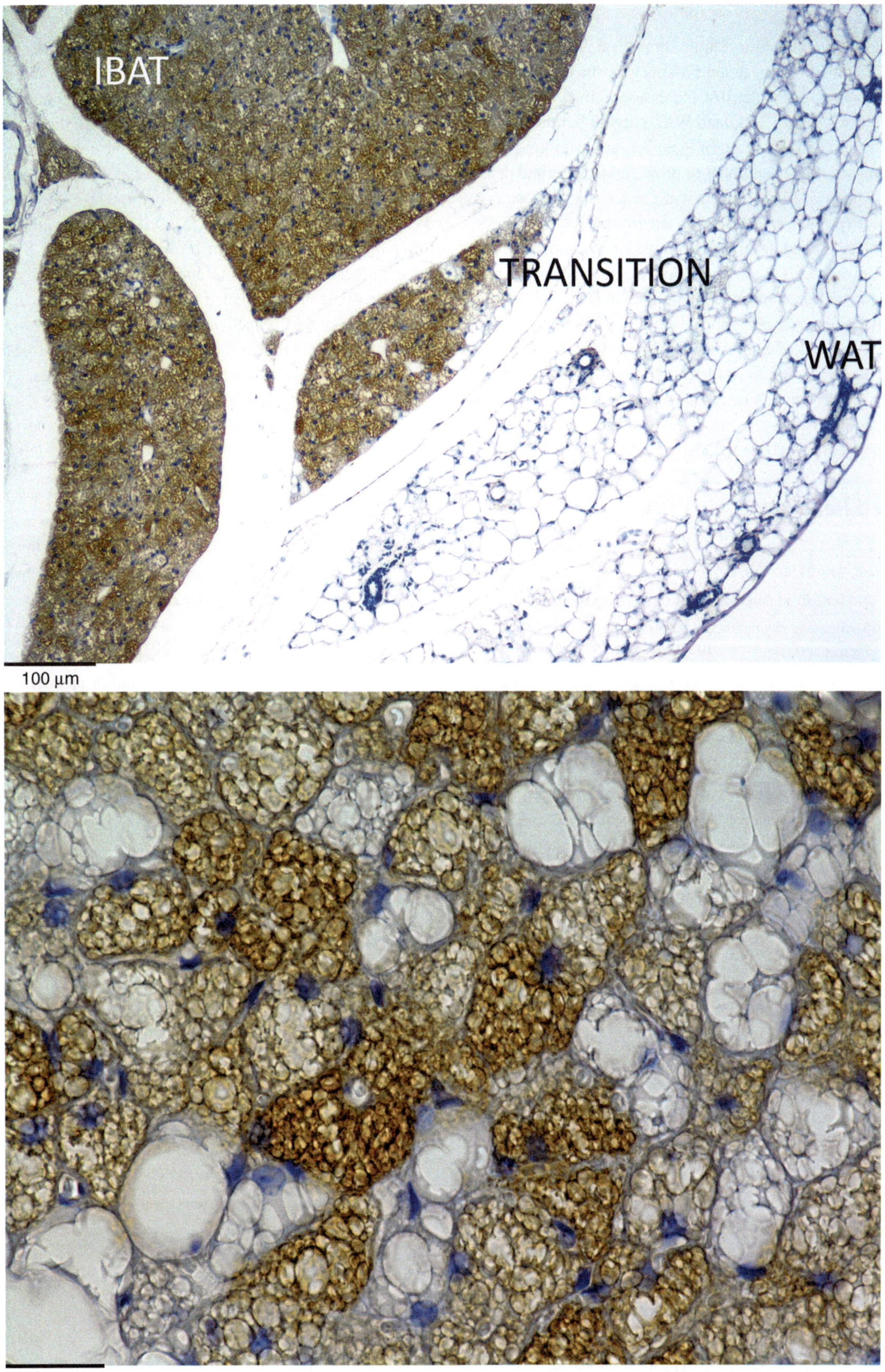

Plate 7.2 *Upper*: anterior subcutaneous depot of adult female Sv129 cold-acclimated (10 days) mouse. Transition area between interscapular BAT (IBAT) and surrounding WAT. IHC. UCP1 ab (1:3,000). LM

PLATE 7.3

Parenchymal innervation of the adipose organ (i.e., nerve fibers running in the interstitial space among adipocytes) increases in cold-acclimated animals. Their density increases both in BAT (upper panel, compare with Plate 2.21) and WAT areas in parallel with the browning phenomenon described in Plate 7.1, and we found a positive correlation between the number of brown adipocytes and density of tyrosine hydroxylase-immunoreactive fibers in the adipose organ of animals exposed to different environmental conditions. Morphometric data in adult female B6 mice cold acclimated (6 °C) for 10 days showed that TH-immunoreactive parenchymal fiber density increased in all mixed areas (containing both BAT and WAT; see Chap. 6) of the adipose organ: about sixfold in the anterior subcutaneous depot, 1.5-fold in the mediastinal fat, twofold in the abdominopelvic depot, and threefold in the posterior subcutaneous depots. Adult female Sv129 mice under the same experimental conditions induced a 3.5-fold increase in the anterior subcutaneous depot, no increase in the mediastinal depot, 2.3-fold increase in the abdominopelvic depot, and 12-fold increase in the posterior subcutaneous depot. The absence of increase in mediastinal fat of these mice could be explained with the fact that this depot in this strain showed the highest density of TH-immunoreactive fibers in the adipose organ of warm (28 °C for 10 days) adapted mice, and all adipocytes were already brown adipocytes in this depot at 28 °C. In general, noradrenergic parenchymal fiber density in the whole organ was higher in Sv129 than in B6 in warm-acclimated animals in line with the five times higher total number of brown adipocytes in Sv129 than B6 mice in these environmental conditions. Interestingly Sv129 mice are more obese and T2 diabetes resistant than B6 mice.

Parenchymal nerve fiber activity is necessary for the browning phenomenon, and activated brown adipocytes produce nerve growth factors.

Furthermore, cold exposure and acclimation increases the intensity of TH- and NPY-positive vascular nerve fibers.

At the ultrastructural level, axons and even small nerves are easier to observe among the cells (lower panel) in cold-adapted mice.

Suggested Reading

Steiner G, et al. Effect of denervation on brown adipose tissue metabolism. Am J Physiol. 218(2):566–70, 1970.

Seydoux J, et al. Short-lived denervation of brown adipose tissue of the rat induced by chemical sympathetic denervation. J Physiol (Paris). 77:1017–22, 1981.

Dulloo AG, Miller DS. Energy balance following sympathetic denervation of brown adipose tissue. Can J Physiol Pharmacol. 62:235–40, 1984.

Granneman JG, et al. Effects of sucrose feeding and denervation on lipogenesis in brown adipose tissue. Metabolism. 33:257–61, 1984.

Minokoshi Y, et al. Metabolic and morphological alterations of brown adipose tissue after sympathetic denervation in rats. J Auton Nerv Syst. 15:197–204, 1986.

Minokoshi Y, et al. Sympathetic denervation impairs responses of brown adipose tissue to VMH stimulation. Am J Physiol. 251:R1005–8, 1986.

Benzi RH, et al. Prepontine knife cut-induced hyperthermia in the rat. Effect of chemical sympathectomy and surgical denervation of brown adipose tissue. Pflugers Arch. 411:593–9, 1988.

Hamilton JM, et al. Effects of norepinephrine and denervation on brown adipose tissue in Syrian hamsters. Am J Physiol. 257:R396–404, 1989.

Gong TW, et al. The effects of 2-deoxy-D-glucose and sympathetic denervation of brown fat GDP binding in Sprague-Dawley rats. Life Sci. 46:1037–44, 1990.

Himms-Hagen J, et al. Sympathetic and sensory nerves in control of growth of brown adipose tissue: effects of denervation and of capsaicin. Neurochem Int. 17:271–9, 1990.

Néchad M, et al. Production of nerve growth factor by brown fat in culture: relation with the in vivo developmental stage of the tissue. Comp Biochem Physiol. 107A:381–88, 1994.

Klingenspor M, et al. Effect of unilateral surgical denervation of brown adipose tissue on uncoupling protein mRNA level and cytochrom-c-oxidase activity in the Djungarian hamster. J Comp Physiol B. 163:664–70, 1994.

Nisoli E, et al. Expression of nerve growth factor in brown adipose tissue: implications for thermogenesis and obesity. Endocrinology. 137:495–503, 1996.

Giordano A, et al. Tyrosine hydroxylase, neuropeptide Y, substance P, calcitonin gene-related peptide and vasoactive intestinal peptide in nerves of rat periovarian adipose tissue: an immunohistochemical and ultrastructural investigation. J Neurocytol. 25:125–36, 1996.

De Matteis R, et al. TH-, NPY-, SP-, and CGRP-immunoreactive nerves in interscapular brown adipose tissue of adult rats acclimated at different temperatures: an immunohistochemical study. J Neurocytol. 27:877–86, 1998.

Giordano A, et al. Sema3a is produced by brown adipocytes and its secretion is reduced following cold acclimation. J Neurocytol. 30:5–10, 2001.

Giordano A, et al. Sibutramine-dependent brown fat activation in rats: an immunohistochemical study. Int J Obes Relat Metab Disord. 26:354–60, 2002.

Giordano A, et al. Sema3A and neuropilin-1 expression and distribution in rat white adipose tissue. J Neurocytol. 32:345–52, 2003.

Cereijo R, et al. Non-sympathetic control of brown adipose tissue. Int J Obes. 5:S40–4, 2015.

Almind K, et al. Ectopic brown adipose tissue in muscle provides a mechanism for differences in risk of metabolic syndrome in mice. Proc Natl Acad Sci 104:2366–71, 2007.

Severi I, et al. Constitutive expression of ciliary neurotrophic factor in mouse hypothalamus. J Anat. 220:622–31, 2012.

Jung KM, et al. 2-arachidonoylglycerol signaling in forebrain regulates systemic energy metabolism. Cell Metab. 15:299–310, 2012.

Harris RB. Sympathetic denervation of one white fat depot changes norepinephrine content and turnover in intact white and brown fat depots. Obesity. 20:1355–64, 2012.

Vaughan CH, Bartness TJ. Anterograde transneuronal viral tract tracing reveals central sensory circuits from brown fat and sensory denervation alters its thermogenic responses. Am J Physiol Regul Integr Comp Physiol. 302:R1049–58, 2012.

Severi I, et al. Opposite effects of a high-fat diet and calorie restriction on ciliary neurotrophic factor signaling in the mouse hypothalamus. Front Neurosci. 7:263, 2013.

Severi I, et al. Activation of transcription factors STAT1 and STAT5 in the mouse median eminence after systemic ciliary neurotrophic factor administration. Brain Res. 1622:217–29, 2015.

Senzacqua M, et al. Action of administered ciliary neurotrophic factor on the mouse dorsal vagal complex. Front Neurosci. 10:289, 2016.

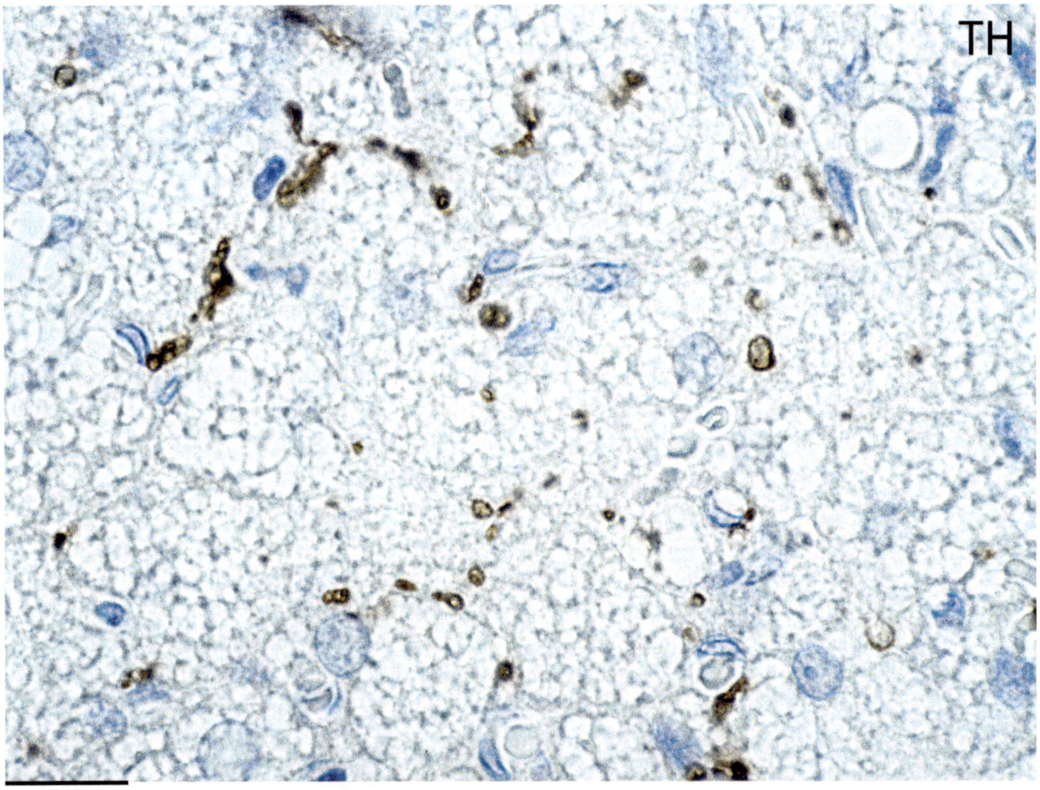

11 μm

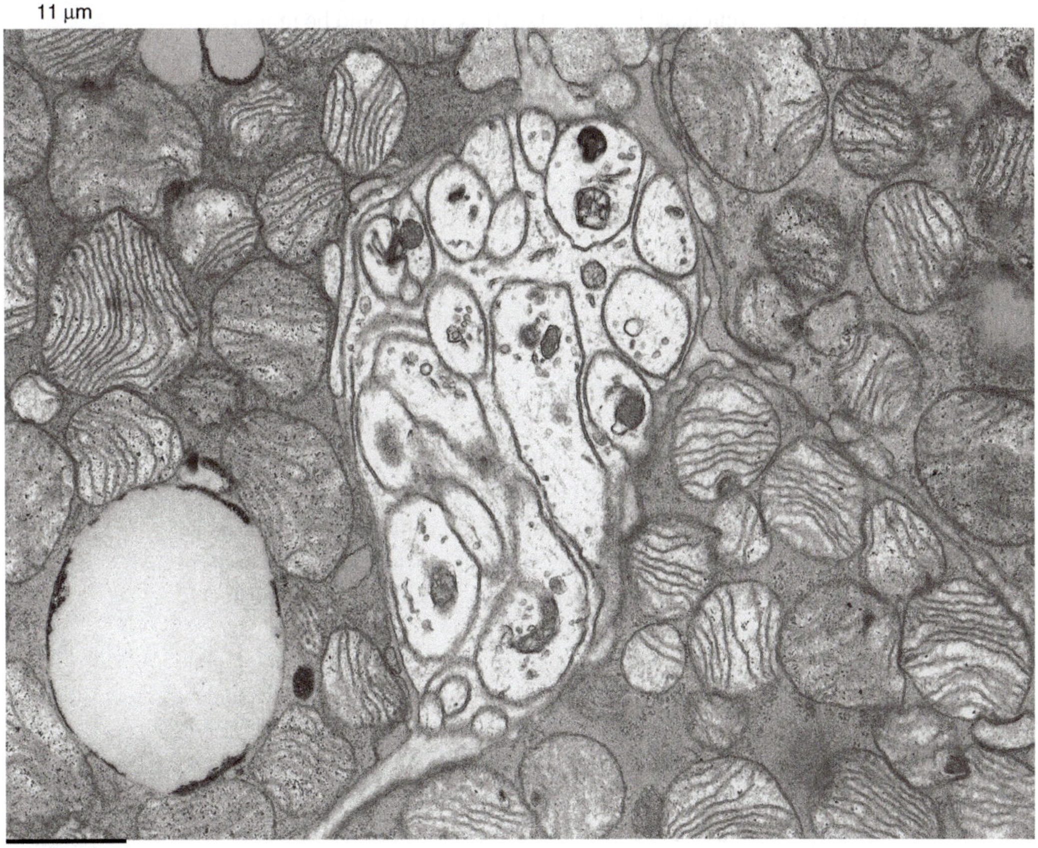

0.65 μm

Plate 7.3 Interscapular BAT of adult rat acclimated at 4 °C for 14 days. TH-immunoreactive (noradrenergic) fibers are visible among the adipocytes (*brown dots*). IHC: TH ab (1:300). LM. *Lower*: a small parenchymal nerve with several unmyelinated fibers is visible among three brown adipocytes. TEM

PLATE 7.4

The Harlequin Secret

Immunohistochemical BAT staining with anti-UCP1 antibodies results in a motley staining pattern that we denominated "the Harlequin secret."

This phenomenon is more evident in BAT of cold-acclimated animals, where intensely stained adipocytes are found among weakly stained or negative ones (upper left panel; see also Plate 7.2).

The same staining pattern is observed in BAT of ß3 agonist-treated animals (lower left panel).

We showed by in situ hybridization with a nonradioactive probe (digoxigenin) on tissue processed for immunohistochemistry that UCP1 mRNA exhibits a similar expression pattern (lower right).

The Harlequin phenomenon is more pronounced after acute cold exposure. We noticed that the UCP1 immunoreactivity of brown adipocytes is more intense after acute cold exposure (such as 3–6 h) than after prolonged (days) cold exposure. In this chronic exposure, the Harlequin phenomenon strongly attenuates in parallel with a generalized reduction of UCP1 immunoreactivity; thus we thought that it could be in relationship to its thermogenic activity. In acute cold exposure, the intense stimulus for thermogenesis is concentrated to the few multilocular brown adipocytes ready for thermogenesis. In fact the browning phenomenon described in Plate 7.1 strongly expands the number of thermogenic cells. Thus the few acute responders could be maximally requested in their thermogenic activity with the risk of heat damages at single cell level. In order to prevent heat damages, UCP1 activity could be inhibited by heat shock proteins induced by heat. We tested the presence of heat shock proteins and found an intense expression and a striking correspondence between the nuclei strongly expressing heat shock proteins and the intensely stained brown adipocytes by immunohistochemistry. Of note, heat shock proteins inhibit UCP1 gene expression, and adrenergically stimulated brown adipocytes in vitro reduce UCP1 gene expression after a heat shock (unpublished data in collaboration with Prof Enzo Nisoli, Dpt Medical Biotechnology and Translational Medicine, University of Milan).

Suggested Reading

Strosberg AD. Structure, function, and regulation of adrenergic receptors. Protein Sci. 2:1198–202, 1993.

Lafontan M. Differential recruitment and differential regulation by physiological amines of fat cell beta-1, beta-2 and beta-3 adrenergic receptors expressed in native fat cells and in transfected cell lines. Cell Signal. 6:363–92, 1994.

Bengtsson T, et al. Down-regulation of beta3 adrenoreceptor gene expression in brown fat cells is transient and recovery is dependent upon a short-lived protein factor. J Biol Chem. 271:33366–75, 1996.

Giordano A, et al. Expression and distribution of heme oxygenase-1 and -2 in rat brown adipose tissue: the modulatory role of the noradrenergic system. FEBS Lett. 487:171–5, 2000.

Cinti S, et al. CL316,243 and cold stress induce heterogeneous expression of UCP1 mRNA and protein in rodent brown adipocytes. J Histochem Cytochem. 50:21–31, 2002.

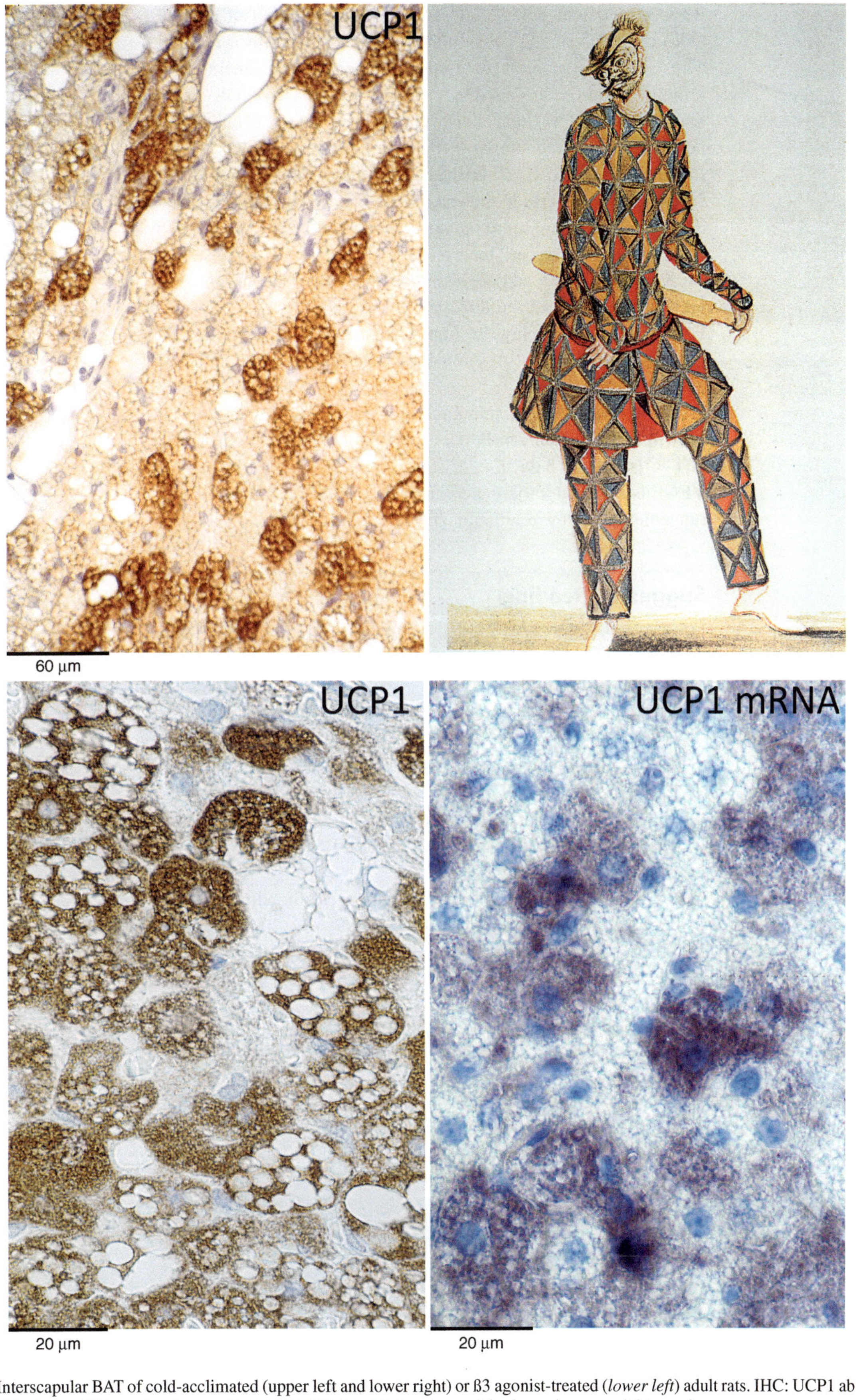

Plate 7.4 Interscapular BAT of cold-acclimated (upper left and lower right) or ß3 agonist-treated (*lower left*) adult rats. IHC: UCP1 ab (1:10,000). In situ hybridization: mRNA probe (*lower right*). ISH. LM. The Harlequin mask is shown in upper right panel

PLATE 7.5

IHC: iNOS-VEGF

Besides increased innervation and UCP1 expression, other molecules can be localized by immunohistochemistry in brown adipocytes of cold-acclimated animals. The upper panel shows immunodetection of inducible nitric oxide synthase (iNOS) in rats maintained at 20 °C (left) or at 4 °C (right) for 3 days. eNOS immunostaining was quite similar to that of iNOS shown here.

Interestingly, serial BAT sections from animals acclimated to cold for two different periods showed that both cytoplasmic and nuclear eNOS and iNOS are more intensely expressed, in the same brown adipocytes that are more intensely positive, for UCP1. Thus, NOS expression in brown adipocytes is positively correlated with cellular activation and heat production.

Furthermore eNOS plays an important role also in mediating the adrenergic induction of mitochondrial biogenesis in brown adipocytes.

The lower panels show immunoreactivity of vascular endothelial growth factor (VEGF) in BAT of rats maintained at 20 °C (left) or at 4 °C (right) for 3 days.

VEGF is believed to play a crucial role in BAT vascular bed rearrangement and flow regulation during cold acclimation.

Suggested Reading

Nisoli E, et al. Effects of nitric oxide on proliferation and differentiation of rat brown adipocytes in primary cultures. Brit J Pharmacol. 125:888–94, 1998.

Tonello C, et al. Role of sympathetic activity in controlling the expression of vascular endothelial growth factor in brown fat cells of lean and genetically obese rats. FEBS Letters. 442:167–72, 1999.

Giordano A, et al. Evidence for a functional nitric oxide synthase system in brown adipocyte nucleus. FEBS Lett. 514:135–40, 2002.

Xue Y, et al. Hypoxia-independent angiogenesis in adipose tissues during cold acclimation. Cell Metab. 9:99–109, 2009.

Nisoli E, et al. Calorie restriction promotes mitochondrial biogenesis by inducing the expression of eNOS. Science. 310:314–7, 2005.

Nisoli E, et al. Mitochondrial biogenesis in mammals: the role of endogenous nitric oxide. Science. 299:896–9, 2003.

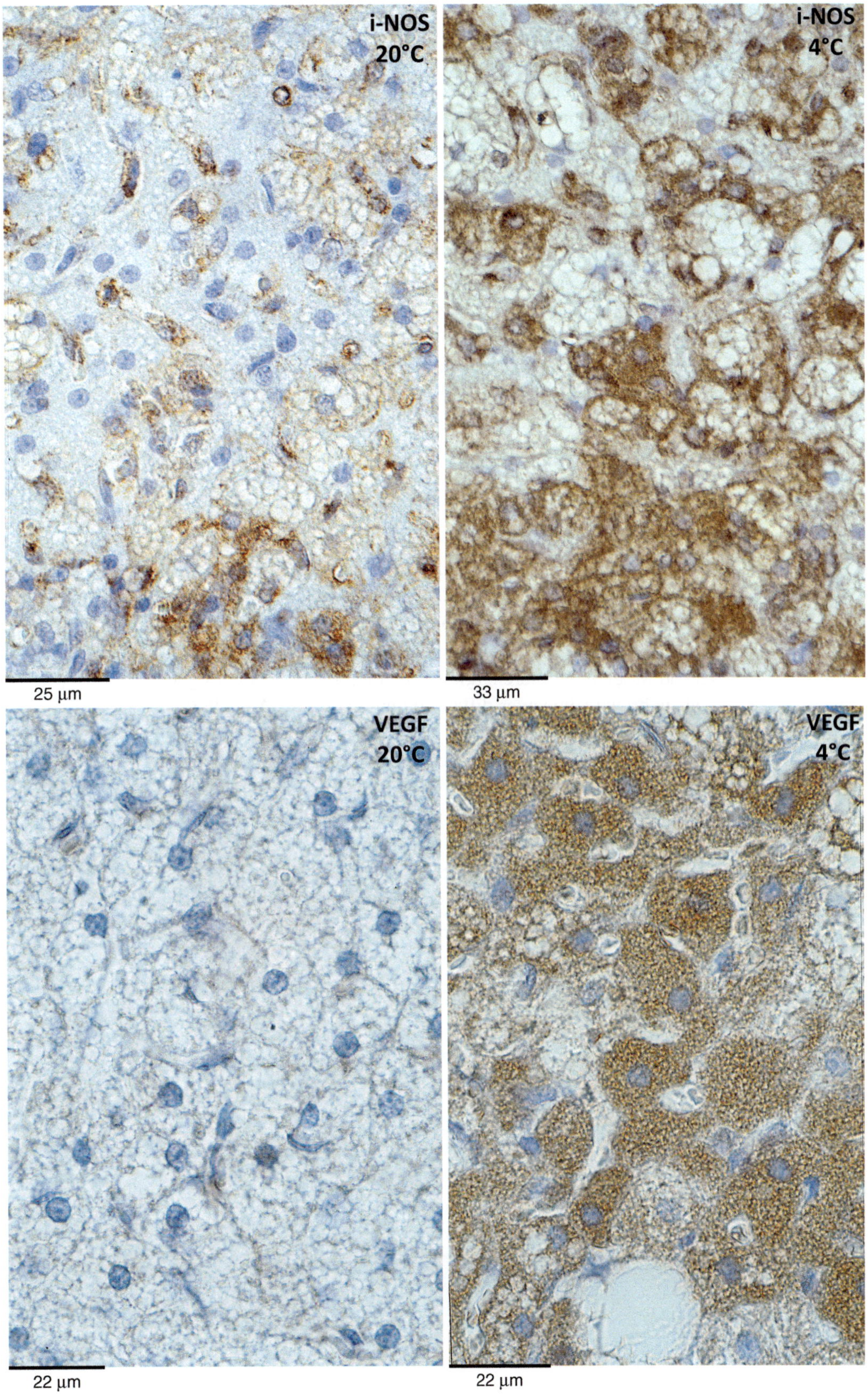

Plate 7.5 Interscapular BAT of adult rats acclimated at 20 °C (*left*) and 4 °C (*right*). Inducible nitric oxide synthase (iNOS) (*upper*) and vascular endothelial growth factor (VEGF) (*lower*). IHC: iNOS ab (1:500), VEGF ab (1:50). LM

PLATE 7.6

Electron Microscopy

In cold-acclimated animals, the brown adipose tissue appears activated: brown adipocytes are rich in mitochondria and lipid droplets are small and numerous in most cells. Capillaries (CAP) are numerous and show flattened endothelial cells (upper panel). The connection between adipocytes and capillaries can be so close that some capillaries can appear completely surrounded by the cytoplasm of a brown adipocyte (CAP1). Peroxisomes, organelles rich in oxidase and catalase enzymes capable of reducing oxygen to hydrogen peroxide and hydrogen peroxide to water, are abundant in brown adipocytes of cold-acclimated and newborn animals (lower panels). Peroxisomes are easy to identify by their morphology: extremely electron dense pleomorphic structures, often grouped near the Golgi complex. In the lower left panel, a brown adipocyte with a consistent amount of peroxisomes on the left part of the cell is shown (enlarged in the lower right panel). In the cervical BAT of a cold-acclimated adult rat, we found some brown adipocytes showing an extraordinary abundance of peroxisomes.

Suggested Reading

Kramar R, et al. Beta-oxidation in peroxisomes of brown adipose tissue. Biochim Biophys Acta. 531:353–6, 1978.

Ahlabo I, Barnard T. Observations on peroxisomes in brown adipose tissue of the rat. J Histochem Cytochem. 19:670–5, 1971.

Nechad M, et al. Noradrenergic stimulation of mitochondriogenesis in brown adipocytes differentiating in culture. Am J Physiol. 253:C889–94, 1987.

Alexson SE, et al. The presence of acyl-CoA hydrolase in rat brown-adipose-tissue peroxisomes. Biochem J. 262:41–6, 1989.

Guardiola-Diaz HM, et al. Rat peroxisome proliferator-activated receptors and brown adipose tissue function during cold acclimatization. J Biol Chem. 274:23368–77, 1999.

Bagattin A, et al. Transcriptional coactivator PGC-1alpha promotes peroxisomal remodeling and biogenesis. Proc Natl Acad Sci USA. 107:20376–81, 2010.

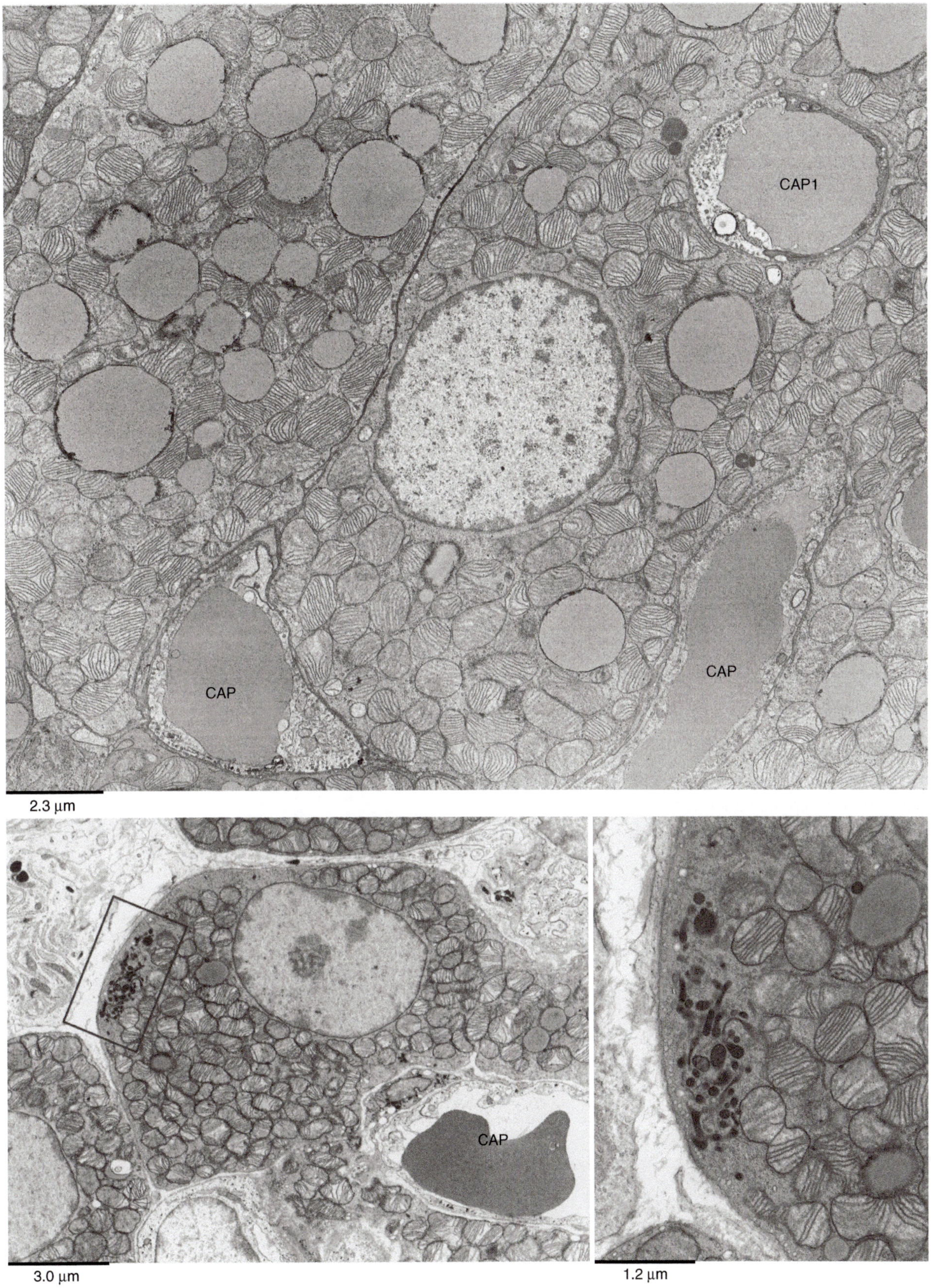

Plate 7.6 *Upper*: brown adipocytes of adult rats acclimated at 4 °C for 14 days from interscapular BAT. *Lower left*: interscapular BAT of newborn rat. *Lower right*: enlargement of squared area in the *lower left panel*. TEM

PLATE 7.7

Mitochondria I

In cold-acclimated and cold-exposed animals, especially in mouse BAT, brown adipocyte mitochondria are numerous and hypertrophic with numerous cristae. This morphological feature usually correlates with abundant expression of UCP1. Peroxisome proliferator-activated receptor gamma coactivator 1-alpha (PGC-1α) plays a pivotal role in mitochondriogenesis.

The smooth endoplasmic reticulum is also always hypertrophic (arrows) in these cells.

The high-resolution scanning microscopy applied to samples processed with the osmium maceration technique allows us to demonstrate that mitochondria of cold-stimulated brown adipocytes acquire mainly spheroidal shape (middle panel).

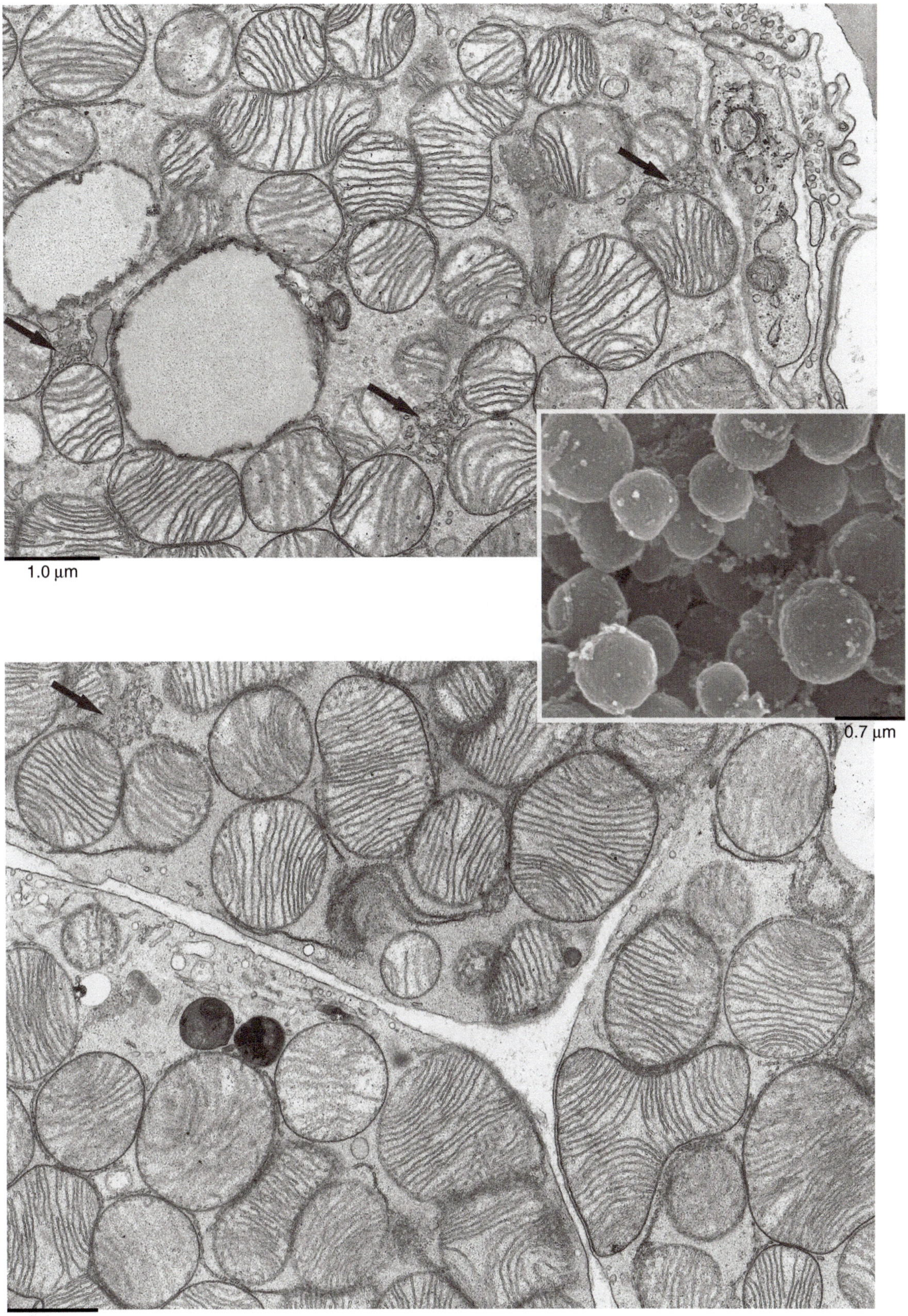

Plate 7.7 Interscapular BAT of cold-acclimated adult rat (*upper*) and mouse (*lower*). TEM. Middle: spherical mitochondria from interscapular BAT of adult mouse exposed to 6 °C for 24 h. High-resolution SEM

PLATE 7.8

Mitochondria II

In cold-acclimated animals, the size of IBAT mitochondria is variable (upper figure). This feature correlates with the possibility of fractioning mitochondria by centrifugation into different subpopulations termed heavy, medium, and light mitochondria. In interscapular BAT brown adipocytes, the smooth endoplasmic reticulum is hypertrophic and is arranged as small networks among mitochondria (arrow in the lower panel of this plate and arrows in Plate 7.7).

Note the dilated area at low density among cristae in the matrix of large mitochondrion in the upper plate (arrow). This dilatation is due to the presence of filamentous structures corresponding to the morphology of mitochondrial DNA.

Suggested Reading

Thomson JF, et al. Ultrastructural and biochemical changes in brown fat in cold-exposed rats. J Cell Biol. 41:312–34, 1969.

Lindgren G, Barnard T. Changes in interscapular brown adipose tissue of rat during perinatal and early postnatal development and after cold acclimation. IV. Morphometric investigation of mitochondrial membrane alterations. Exp Cell Res. 70:81–90, 1972.

Fawcett DW. The Cell. WB Saunders Company, Philadelphia, 1981.

Moreno M, et al. Cold exposure induces different uncoupling-protein thermogenin masking/unmasking processes in brown adipose tissue depending on mitochondrial subtypes. Biochem J. 300:463–68, 1994.

Goglia F, et al. Light mitochondria and cellular thermogenesis BBRC. 151:1241–49, 1988.

Wu Z, et al. Mechanisms controlling mitochondrial biogenesis and respiration through the thermogenic coactivator PGC-1. Cell. 98:115–24, 1999.

Lin J, et al. Defects in adaptive energy metabolism with CNS-linked hyperactivity in PGC-1alpha null mice. Cell. 119:121–35, 2004.

Wikstrom JD, et al. Hormone-induced mitochondrial fission is utilized by brown adipocytes as an amplification pathway for energy expenditure. EMBO J. 33:418–36, 2014.

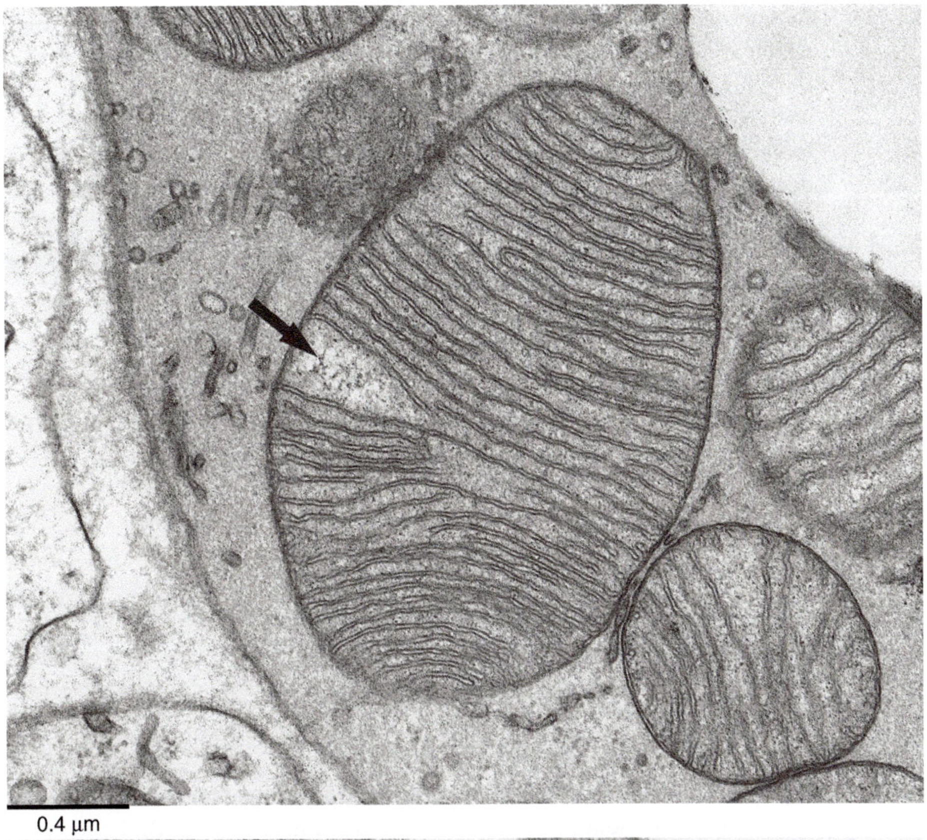

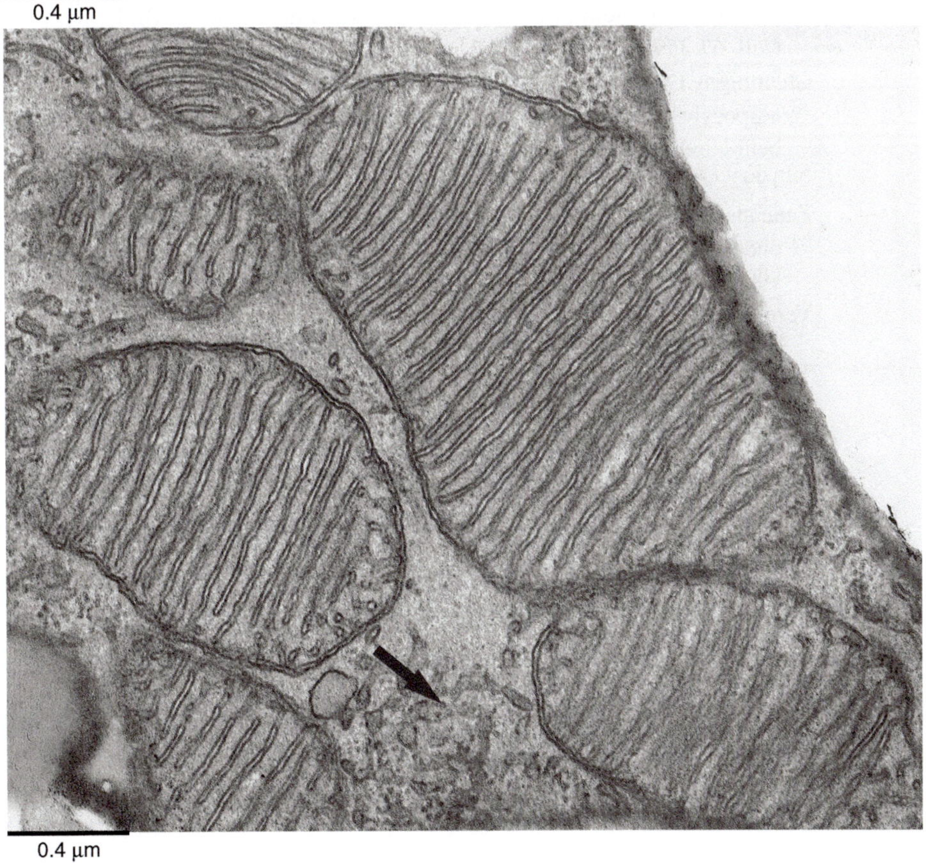

Plate 7.8 Interscapular BAT mitochondria of cold-acclimated adult mouse. TEM

PLATE 7.9

Mitochondria UCP1-IGS

Immuno-gold staining (IGS) is an immunocytochemical technique, which allows antigens to be localized at ultrastructural level. This section was processed with anti-UCP1 antibodies at 1:100 dilution and visualized with an anti-IgG linked to spherical particles of colloidal gold 10 nm in diameter. Colloidal gold particles are electron dense and visible at TEM; thus these dense particles correspond to UCP1 protein. The reaction was performed directly on thin sections of BAT from a cold-acclimated adult mouse. Mitochondrial morphology is still recognizable, although these procedures, which aim at preserving the immunoreactivity of the tissue, are different from those used for standard TEM. Of note, BAT mitochondria in mice lacking UCP1 or the mitochondrial transcription factor A (TFAM) change their morphology (lower panel) (see Plate 2.4 for UCP1-KO mitochondria). Recently we also observed altered morphology of brown mitochondria in adiponectin-Cre-mediated FH (fumarate hydratase, an integral Krebs cycle enzyme that catalyzes the reversible hydration of fumarate to malate) KO mice.

Suggested Reading

Sundin U, et al. Thermogenin amount and activity in hamster brown fat mitochondria: effect of cold acclimation. Am J Physiol. 252:R822–32, 1987.

Cinti S, et al. Immunoelectron microscopical identification of the uncoupling protein in brown adipose tissue mitochondria. Biol Cell. 67:359–62, 1989.

Champigny O, et al. Regulation of UCP gene expression in brown adipocytes differentiated in primary culture. Effects of a new beta-adrenoceptor agonist. Mol Cell Endocrinol. 86:73–82, 1992.

Zancanaro C, et al. Immunohistochemical identification of the uncoupling protein in human hibernoma. Biol Cell. 80:75–8, 1994.

Vernochet C, et al. Adipose-specific deletion of TFAM increases mitochondrial oxidation and protects mice against obesity and insulin resistance. Cell Metab. 16:765–76, 2012.

Hao Y, et al. Adipose-specific deficiency of fumarate hydratase in mice protects against obesity, hepatic steatosis, and insulin resistance. Diabetes. 65:1–14, 2016.

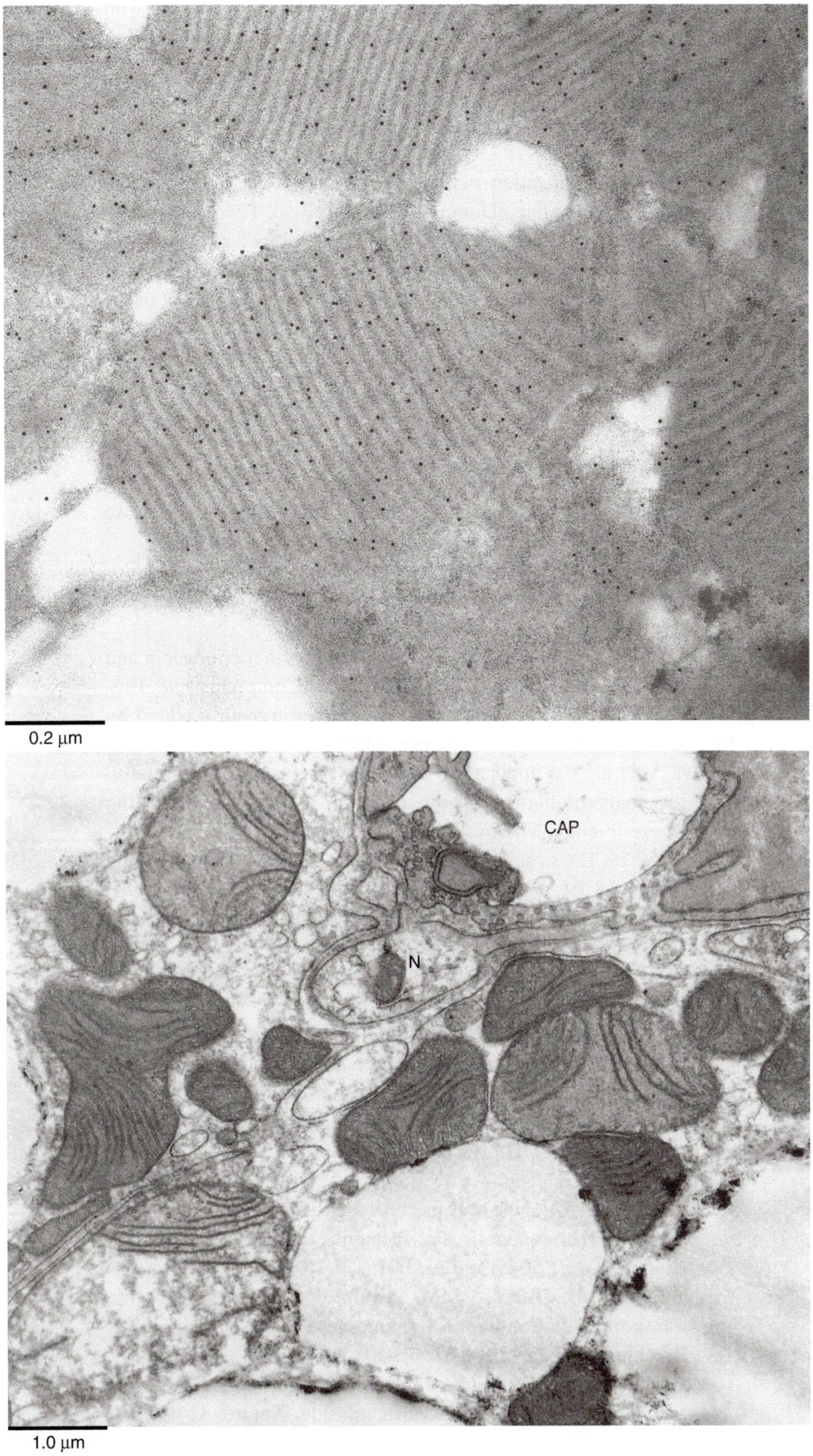

Plate 7.9 *Upper*: IBAT mitochondria of cold-acclimated adult mouse. IGS method. TEM. *Lower*: IBAT mitochondria of TFAM-KO adult mouse (from Vernochet C et al. Adipose-specific deletion of TFAM increases mitochondrial oxidation and protects mice against obesity and insulin resistance. Cell Metab. 16:765–76, 2012 with permission). CAP, capillary. N, nerve ending TEM

PLATE 7.10

Mitochondria-HRSEM

This technique allows studying organelles of cells, processed with the osmium maceration procedure, by a high-resolution scanning electron microscopy (HRSEM).

Mitochondria of BAT of a cold-exposed mouse are open by this maceration procedure allowing the observation of their internal structure.

The high magnification obtained with this HRSEM microscope allows seeing the fine 3D morphology of cristae. The laminar cristae seem to be formed or covered by aligned globular structures of about 35–40 nm of diameter (some indicated by small arrows) possibly in relation to the high number of UCP1 protein present in the mitochondria in this very activated functional state. Interestingly, mitochondria of brown adipocytes lacking UCP1 show cristae formed by very thin and irregular membranes (see Plate 2.4).

Suggested Reading

Rial E, Nicholls DG. The uncoupling protein from brown adipose tissue mitochondria. Revis Biol Celular. 11:75–104, 1987.

Klaus S, et al. The uncoupling protein UCP: a membraneous mitochondrial ion carrier exclusively expressed in brown adipose tissue. Int J Biochem 23:791–801, 1991.

Nedergaard J, Cannon B. The uncoupling protein thermogenin and mitochondrial thermogenesis. In: New Comprehensive Biochemistry: Molecular Mechanisms in Bioenergetics, edited by Ernster L. Amsterdam: Elsevier, 23:385–420, 1992.

Riva A, et al. The application of the OsO4 maceration method to the study of human bioptic material. A procedure avoiding freeze-fracture. Microsc Res Tech. 26:526–7, 1993.

Rial E, et al. The structure and function of the brown fat uncoupling protein UCP1: current status. Biofactors. 8(3–4):209–19, 1998.

Nicholls DG, Rial E. A history of the first uncoupling protein, UCP1. J Bioenerg Biomembr. 31:399–406, 1999.

Garlid KD, et al. How do uncoupling proteins uncouple? Biochim Biophys Acta. 1459:383–89, 2000.

Klingenberg M, Echtay KS. Uncoupling proteins: the issues from a biochemist point of view. Biochim Biophys Acta. 1504:128–143, 2001.

Arechaga I, et al. The mitochondrial uncoupling protein UCP1: a gated pore. IUBMB Life. 52:165–73, 2001.

Nedergaard J, Golozoubova V, Matthias A, Asadi A, Jacobsson A, Cannon B. UCP1: the only protein able to mediate adaptive non-shivering thermogenesis and metabolic inefficiency. Biochim Biophys Acta. 1504:82–106, 2001.

Rial E, Gonzalea-Barroso MM. Physiological regulation of the transport activity in the uncoupling proteins UCP1 and UCP2. Biochim Biophys Acta. 1504:70–81, 2001.

Pebay-Peyroula E, et al. Structure of mitochondrial ADP/ATP carrier in complex with carboxyatractyloside. Nature. 426:39–44, 2003.

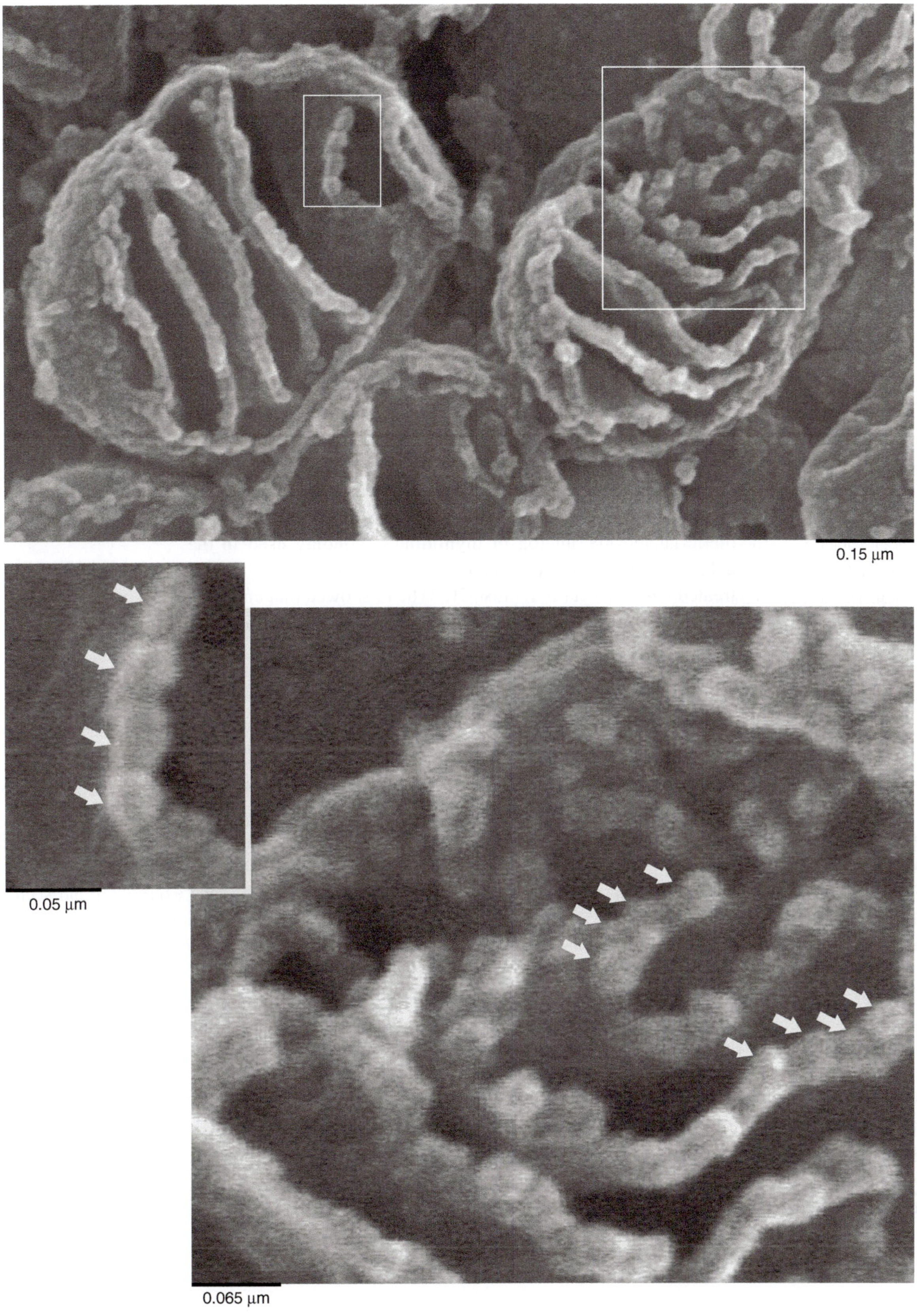

Plate 7.10 Mitochondria of brown adipocytes from BAT of adult (10 weeks old) B6 mouse exposed to 6° for 24 h. Middle and lower panels are enlargements of squared areas in the upper panel. High-resolution SEM

PLATE 7.11

Mitosis

Interscapular BAT of newborns and cold-exposed animals contains many mitotic cells. In these cells, electron microscopy recognizes the organelles, which allow the cell type undergoing mitosis to be identified. This plate shows a brown adipoblast-preadipocyte (upper panel) and an endothelial cell (lower panel) undergoing mitosis in the interscapular BAT of a cold-exposed (4 °C for 3 days) adult rat.

In the upper panel "pre-typical" mitochondria (m, some indicated) and small lipid droplets (L) are visible in the dividing cell; note the great abundance of ribosomes and polyribosomes (*) (typical of blast cells; compare with Plates 2.26–2.28).

The close relationship between the adipoblast in mitosis and two capillaries (CAP) is evident.

Our quantitative measurements in the whole adipose organ of cold-acclimated mice (B6 and Sv129) showed that interscapular BAT is the only site where there is an increase in brown adipocytes' number after cold acclimation.

The endothelial cells line the capillary lumen (CAP); thus endothelial cells in mitosis are easily recognized (lower panel). Our bromodeoxyuridine (5-bromo-2′-deoxyuridine, BrdU, a synthetic nucleoside, analog of thymidine commonly used in the detection of proliferating cells in vivo) experiments in rats treated with the beta-3 agonist CL 316243 showed that endothelial cells proliferate after the adrenergic stimulus in retroperitoneal WAT.

Suggested Reading

Cannon B, et al. In "Living in the cold", Malan and Canguilhern Eds, Libbey, 359–366, 1989.

Rehnmark S, Nedergaard J. DNA synthesis in mouse brown adipose tissue is under beta-adrenergic control. Exp Cell Res. 180:574–79, 1989.

Morroni M, et al. Immunohistochemical, ultrastructural and morphometric evidence for brown adipose tissue recruitment due to cold acclimation in old rats. Int J Obesity. 19:126–31, 1995.

Tvrdik P, et al. Cig30, a mouse member of a novel membrane protein gene family, is involved in the recruitment of brown adipose tissue. J Biol Chem. 272:31738–46, 1997.

Himms-Hagen J, et al. Multilocular fat cells in WAT of CL-316243-treated rats derive directly from white adipocytes. Am J Physiol Cell Physiol. 279:C670–81, 2000.

Murano I, et al. The adipose organ of Sv129 mice contains a prevalence of brown adipocytes and shows plasticity after cold exposure. Adipocytes. 1:121–30, 2005.

Vitali A, et al. The adipose organ of obesity-prone C57BL/6J mice is composed of mixed white and brown adipocytes. J Lip Res. 53:619–29, 2012.

Lee YH, et al. Cellular origins of cold-induced brown adipocytes in adult mice. FASEB J. 29:286–99, 2015.

Peeraully MR et al. NGF gene expression and secretion in white adipose tissue: regulation in 3T3-L1 adipocytes by hormones and inflammatory cytokines. Am J Physiol EM 287: 331–9, 2004.

Sornelli F et al. Adipose tissue-derived nerve growth factor and brain-derived neurotrophic factor: results from experimental stress and diabetes. Gen Physiol Biophys 28: 179–83, 2009.

Rosell M et al Brown and white adipose tissues: intrinsic differences in gene expression and response to cold exposure in mice. Am J Physiol EM 306: 945–64.

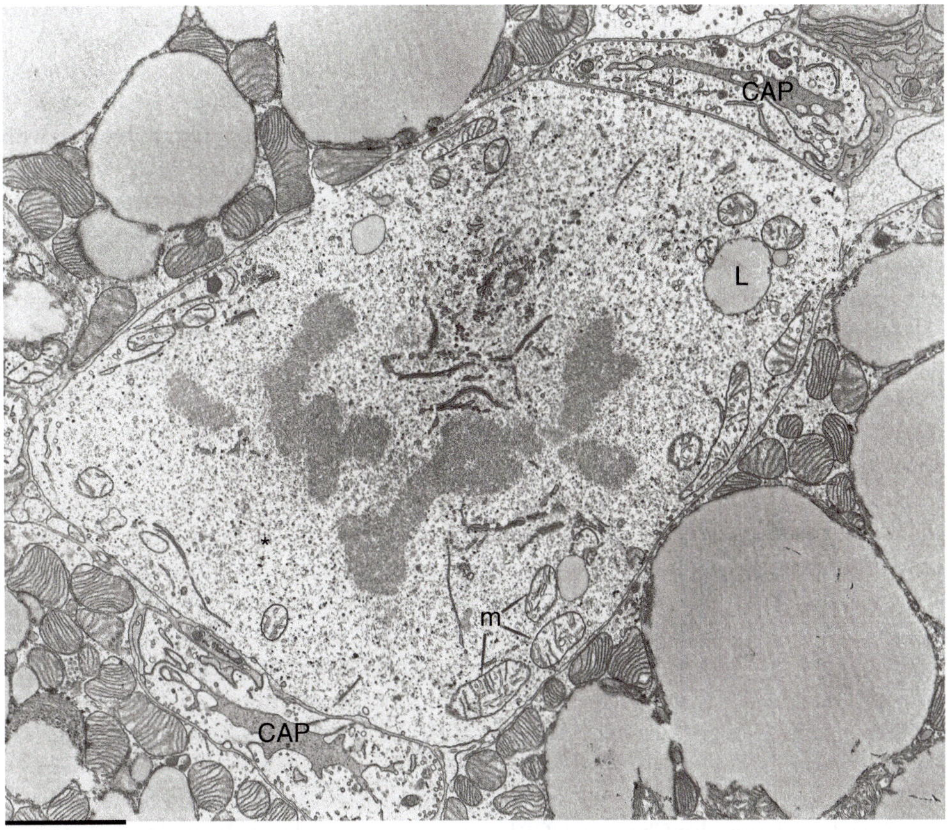

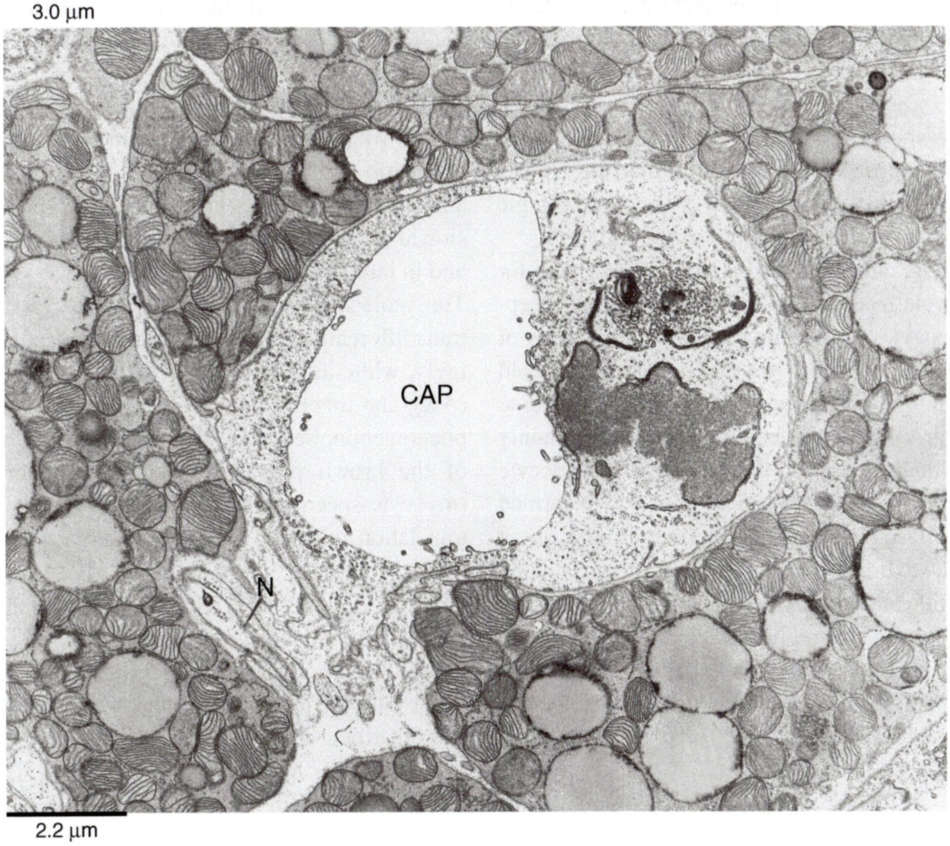

Plate 7.11 Interscapular BAT of cold-exposed (3 days at 4 °C) adult rat. *Upper*: brown adipoblast in mitosis. *Lower*: endothelial cell in mitosis. N, small parenchymal nerve. TEM

PLATE 7.12

WAT Browning

The visually evident transformation of the color of adipose organ after cold exposure (Plate 7.1) corresponds to a transformation in the cellular composition of the organ with rearrangement of the adipocyte parenchymal composition and remodeling of the tissue components including nerves and vessel supply. In this context it is important to outline the potent nerve and vascular factors produced by WAT and BAT such as NGF (nerve growth factor), VEGF (vascular endothelium growth factor), Nrg4 (Neeuregulin 4), and Sema3A (semaphorin-3A). This phenomenon is of pivotal importance because energy dissipated by BAT has been proved to be able to prevent obesity, type 2 diabetes, and atherosclerosis; thus BAT activation is nowadays regarded as one of the most realistic strategies to combat the epidemic metabolic syndrome.

Our data support the hypothesis that a large part of the white adipocytes directly transdifferentiate into brown adipocytes in all the areas of the adipose organ that change the color from white to brown. As shown in Plate 7.1, not all areas of the adipose organ undergo white-to-brown transdifferentiation because some remain white. All the intermediate morphological features linking white with brown adipocytes are visible in most WAT depots of cold-exposed mice. In browned areas of the adipose organ, we detected a very important type of paucilocular cell (see also Chap. 6): UCP1-immunoreactive paucilocular cell with predominant central lipid droplet (see Plate 7.14). This type of cell is also present in the transition areas of the adipose organ of mice maintained at room temperature (see Plate 6.3) but much more numerous in cold-exposed mice. We think that the UCP1-immunoreactive paucilocular adipocyte is the morphologic marker of white to brown adipocyte transdifferentiation.

Of note, browning is almost abolished in knockout mice for the beta-3 adrenergic receptors (AR). We found these receptors in white adipocytes (even in hypertrophic adipocytes of obese subjects), and their gene expression increases after cold exposure in both murine and human WAT. Bromodeoxyuridine experiments suggest that proliferative events are mainly restricted to endothelial cells and to a minority of adipocyte precursors (5–15%), meaning that 85–90% of newly formed brown adipocyte in WAT browning is derived from a direct conversion of white to brown adipocytes. Electron microscope excluded any significant development of pre-existing poorly differentiated precursors. Recent lineage tracing studies are in substantial agreement that at least a large population of white adipocytes are able to directly convert into brown adipocytes under adrenergic stimuli.

In this plate the white to brown transdifferentiation of inguinal fat of adult mouse is shown. In the middle panel the classic morphology of unilocular white adipocytes is shown in mice maintained at 28 °C. After prolonged fasting the same depot is mostly (about 90%) composed of slimmed cells (upper panel) demonstrating that the unilocular cells present in mice maintained at 28 °C are true white adipocytes (i.e., an adipose cell able to respond to prolonged fasting by complete delipidation). Furthermore immunohistochemistry showed that these cells are leptin and S-100B (markers of white adipocytes) immunoreactive. The same depot is mostly (about 90%) composed of multilocular UCP1-immunoreactive brown adipocytes after 10 days of cold (6 °C) acclimation (bottom panel).

Most parenchymal cells have the morphology, UCP1 immunoreactivity, and ultrastructure of brown adipocytes. Some authors denominated these newly formed multilocular adipocytes beige/brite adipocytes mainly because of the different molecular signature and developmental origin from the classic interscapular brown adipocytes. Until a different function for these cells will be found, we prefer to call these cells brown adipocytes mainly because a clear difference between classic brown adipocytes and these cells has never been shown in vivo at single cell level and we think that this cell retains the anatomy and physiology of this cell type.

WAT browning proneness depends on age (aging is accompanied by BAT whitening), strain, and surface area to volume ratio (S/V) of the animal. It is easily induced in young and small mammals (with high S/V thus high thermal dispersion and need for BAT), but it can be induced also in old rats and in humans (see Plates 7.19–7.21).

The molecular mechanisms of white to brown reversible transdifferentiation are still poorly understood, but interestingly, white adipocytes express beta-3 adrenergic receptors (AR), and this receptor is a very important mediator of this phenomenon. Several molecular pathways that are inhibitors of the brown phenotype genetic program (e.g., MEF2c (myocyte-specific enhancer factor 2C), 4EBP1 (eukaryotic translation initiation factor 4E-binding protein 1), SMAD3 (SMAD family member 3), Rb or p107 (retinoblastoma-like protein 1), RIP140 (receptor interacting protein 140), HOXC8 (homeobox protein Hox-C8), CK2 (casein kinase 2), and MR (mineralocorticoid receptor) activity) are inhibited by the signaling molecules activated by noradrenaline and other beta-3 AR agonists.

Suggested Reading

Loncar D, et al. Epididymal white adipose tissue after cold stress in rats. II. Mitochondrial changes. J Ultrastruct Res. 101:199–209, 1988.

Champigny O, et al. Beta 3-adrenergic receptor stimulation restores message and expression of brown-fat mitochondrial uncoupling protein in adult dogs. PNAS. 88: 10774–7, 1991.

Cousin B, et al. Occurrence of brown adipocytes in rat white adipose tissue: molecular and morphological characterization. J Cell Sci. 103:931–42, 1992.

Lowell BB, et al. Development of obesity in transgenic mice after genetic ablation of brown adipose tissue. Nature. 366:740–2, 1993.

Morroni M, et al. Immunohistochemical, ultrastructural and morphometric evidence for brown adipose tissue recruitment due to cold acclimation in old rats. Int J Obes Relat Metab Disord. 19:126–31, 1995.

Ghorbani M, Himms-Hagen J. Appearance of brown adipocytes in white adipose tissue during CL 316,243-induced reversal of obesity and diabetes in Zucker fa/fa rats. Int J Obes. 21:465–75, 1997.

Guerra C, et al. Emergence of brown adipocytes in white fat in mice is under genetic control. Effects on body weight and adiposity. J Clin Invest. 102:412–20, 1998.

Nisoli E, et al. Nerve growth factor, beta3-adrenoceptor and uncoupling protein 1 expression in rat brown fat during postnatal development. Neurosci Lett. 246:5–8, 1998.

Himms-Hagen J, et al. Multilocular fat cells in WAT of CL-316243-treated rats derive directly from white adipocytes. Am J Physiol Cell Physiol. 279:C670–81, 2000.

Guerra C, et al. Brown adipose tissue-specific insulin receptor knockout shows diabetic phenotype without insulin resistance. J Clin Invest. 108:1205–13, 2001.

Tsukiyama-Kohara K, et al. Adipose tissue reduction in mice lacking the translational inhibitor 4E-BP1. Nat Med. 7:1128–32, 2001.

Bachman ES, et al. betaAR signaling required for diet-induced thermogenesis and obesity resistance. Science. 297:843–5, 2002.

De Matteis R, et al. Immunohistochemical identification of the beta(3)-adrenoceptor in intact human adipocytes and ventricular myocardium: effect of obesity and treatment with ephedrine and caffeine. Int J Obes Relat Metab Disord. 26:1442–50. 2002.

Rossmeisl M, et al. Expression of the uncoupling protein 1 from the aP2 gene promoter stimulates mitochondrial biogenesis in unilocular adipocytes in vivo. Eur J Biochem. 269:19–28, 2002.

Jimenez M, et al. Beta 3-adrenoceptor knockout in C57BL/6J mice depresses the occurrence of brown adipocytes in white fat. Eur J Biochem. 270:699–705, 2003.

Giordano A, et al. Sema3A and neuropilin-1 expression and distribution in rat white adipose tissue. J Neurocytol. 32:345–52, 2003.

Granneman JG, et al. Metabolic and cellular plasticity in white adipose tissue I: effects of β3-adrenergic receptor activation. Am J Physiol Endocrinol Metab. 289:E608–16, 2005.

Christian M, et al. RIP140-targeted repression of gene expression in adipocytes. Mol Cell Biol. 25:9383–939, 2005.

Gray SL. Decreased brown adipocyte recruitment and thermogenic capacity in mice with impaired peroxisome proliferator-activated receptor (P465L PPARgamma) function. Endocrinology. 147:5708–14, 2006.

Mercader J, et al. Remodeling of white adipose tissue after retinoic acid administration in mice. Endocrinology. 147:5325–32, 2006.

Fink BD, et al. Mitochondrial proton leak in obesity-resistant and obesity-prone mice. Am J Physiol Regul Integr Comp Physiol. 293:R1773–80, 2007.

Cao Y. Angiogenesis modulates adipogenesis and obesity. J Clin Invest. 117:2362–68, 2007.

Almind K, et al. Ectopic brown adipose tissue in muscle provides a mechanism for differences in risk of metabolic syndrome in mice. Proc Natl Acad Sci USA. 104:2366–71, 2007.

Mercader J, et al. Haploinsufficiency of the retinoblastoma protein gene reduces diet-induced obesity, insulin resistance, and hepatosteatosis in mice. Am J Physiol Endocrinol Metab. 297:E184–93, 2009.

Barbatelli G, et al The emergence of cold-induced brown adipocytes in mouse white fat depots is determined predominantly by white to brown adipocyte transdifferentiation. Am J Physiol Endocrinol Metab. 298:E1244–53, 2010.

Madsen L, et al. UCP1 induction during recruitment of brown adipocytes in white adipose tissue is dependent on cyclooxygenase activity. PLoS One. 5:e11391, 2010.

Gaidhu MP, et al. Chronic AMP-kinase activation with AICAR reduces adiposity by remodeling adipocyte metabolism and increasing leptin sensitivity. J Lipid Res. 52:1702–11, 2011.

Vitali A, et al. The adipose organ of obesity-prone C57BL/6J mice is composed of mixed white and brown adipocytes. J Lip Res. 53:619–29, 2012.

Cinti S, Transdifferentiation properties of adipocytes in the adipose organ. Am J Physiol Endocrinol Metab. 297:E977–86, 2009.

Xue B, et al. Neuronal protein tyrosine phosphatase 1B deficiency results in inhibition of hypothalamic AMPK and isoform-specific activation of AMPK in peripheral tissues. Mol Cell Biol. 29:4563–73 2009.

Petrovic N, et al. Chronic peroxisome proliferator-activated receptor gamma (PPARgamma) activation of epididymally derived white adipocyte cultures reveals a population of thermogenically competent, UCP1-containing adipocytes molecularly distinct from classic brown adipocytes. J Biol Chem. 285:7153–64, 2010.

Seale P, et al. Prdm16 determines the thermogenic program of subcutaneous white adipose tissue in mice. J Clin Invest. 121:96–105, 2011.

Bartelt A, et al. Brown adipose tissue activity controls triglyceride clearance. Nat Med. 17:200–5, 2011.

Whittle AJ, et al. Using brown adipose tissue to treat obesity – the central issue. Trends Mol Med. 17:405–11, 2011.

Yadav H, et al. Protection from obesity and diabetes by blockade of TGF-β/Smad3 signaling. Cell Metab. 14:67–79, 2011.

Wu J, et al. Beige adipocytes are a distinct type of thermogenic fat cell in mouse and human. Cell. 150:366–76, 2012.

Bostrom P, et al. A PGC1-α-dependent myokine that drives brown-fat-like development of white fat and thermogenesis. Nature. 481:463–8, 2012.

Mori M, et al. Essential role for miR-196a in brown adipogenesis of white fat progenitor cells. PLoS Biol. 10:e1001314, 2012.

Kornfeld JW, Brüning JC. MyomiRs-133a/b turn off the heat. Nat Cell Biol. 14:1248–9, 2012.

Trajkovski M, Ahmed K, Esau CC, Stoffel M. MyomiR-133 regulates brown fat differentiation through Prdm16. Nat Cell Biol. 14:1330–35, 2012.

Rosenwald M, et al. Bi-directional interconversion of brite and white adipocytes. Nat Cell Biol. 15:659–67, 2013.

Wang QA, et al. Tracking adipogenesis during white adipose tissue development, expansion and regeneration. Nat Med. 19:1338–44, 2013.

Stanford KI, et al. Brown adipose tissue regulates glucose homeostasis and insulin sensitivity. J Clin Invest. 123:215–23, 2013.

Barneda D, et al. Dynamic changes in lipid droplet-associated proteins in the "browning" of white adipose tissues. Biochim Biophys Acta. 1831:924–33, 2013.

Rajakumari S, et al. EBF2 determines and maintains brown adipocyte identity. Cell Metab. 17:562–574, 2013.

Lee YH, et al. Adipose tissue plasticity from WAT to BAT and in between. Biochim Biophys Acta. 1842:358–69, 2014.

Rosenwald M, Wolfrum C. The origin and definition of brite versus white and classical brown adipocytes. Adipocyte 3: 4–9, 2014.

Rosen ED, Spiegelman BM. What we talk about when we talk about fat. Cell. 156:20–44, 2014.

Nedergaard J, Cannon B. The browning of white adipose tissue: some burning issues. Cell Metab. 20:396–407, 2014.

Chechi K, et al. Brown adipose tissue as an anti-obesity tissue in humans. Obesity Rev. 15:92–106, 2014.

Sun K, et al. Brown adipose tissue derived VEGF-A modulates cold tolerance and energy expenditure. Mol Metab. 3:474–83, 2014.

Gao H, et al. Early B cell factor 1 regulates adipocyte morphology and lipolysis in white adipose tissue. Cell Metab. 19:981–92, 2014.

Kiskinis E, et al. RIP140 represses the "brown-in-white" adipocyte program including a futile cycle of triacylglycerol breakdown and synthesis. Mol Endocrinol. 28:344–56, 2014.

Cohen P, et al. Ablation of PRDM16 and beige adipose causes metabolic dysfunction and a subcutaneous to visceral fat switch. Cell. 156:304–16, 2014.

Berbee JF, et al. Brown fat activation reduces hypercholesterolaemia and protects from atherosclerosis development. Nat Commun. 6:6356, 2015.

Shinoda K, et al. Phosphoproteomics identifies CK2 as a negative regulator of beige adipocyte thermogenesis and energy expenditure. Cell Metab. 22:997–1008, 2015.

Pisani DF, et al. The K+ channel TASK1 modulates β-adrenergic response in brown adipose tissue through the mineralocorticoid receptor pathway. FASEB J. 30:909–22, 2015.

Colaianni G, et al. The myokine irisin increases cortical bone mass. Proc Natl Acad Sci USA. 112:12157–62, 2015.

Hallenborg P, et al. p53 regulates expression of uncoupling protein 1 through binding and repression of PPARγ coactivator-1α. Am J Physiol Endocrinol Metab. 310:E116–28, 2016.

Pisani DF, et al. The K+ channel TASK1 modulates b-adrenergic response in brown adipose tissue through the mineralocorticoid receptor pathway. FASEB J. 30:909–22, 2016.

Yang H, et al. Adipose-specific deficiency of fumarate hydratase in mice protects against obesity, hepatic steatosis and insulin resistance. Diabetes. pii:db160136, 2016.

Reis FC, et al. Fat-specific Dicer deficiency accelerates aging and mitigates several effects of dietary restriction in mice. Aging (Albany NY). 8:1201–22, 2016.

Giordano A, et al. Convertible visceral fat as a therapeutic target to curb obesity. Nat Rev Drug Discov. 15:405–24, 2016.

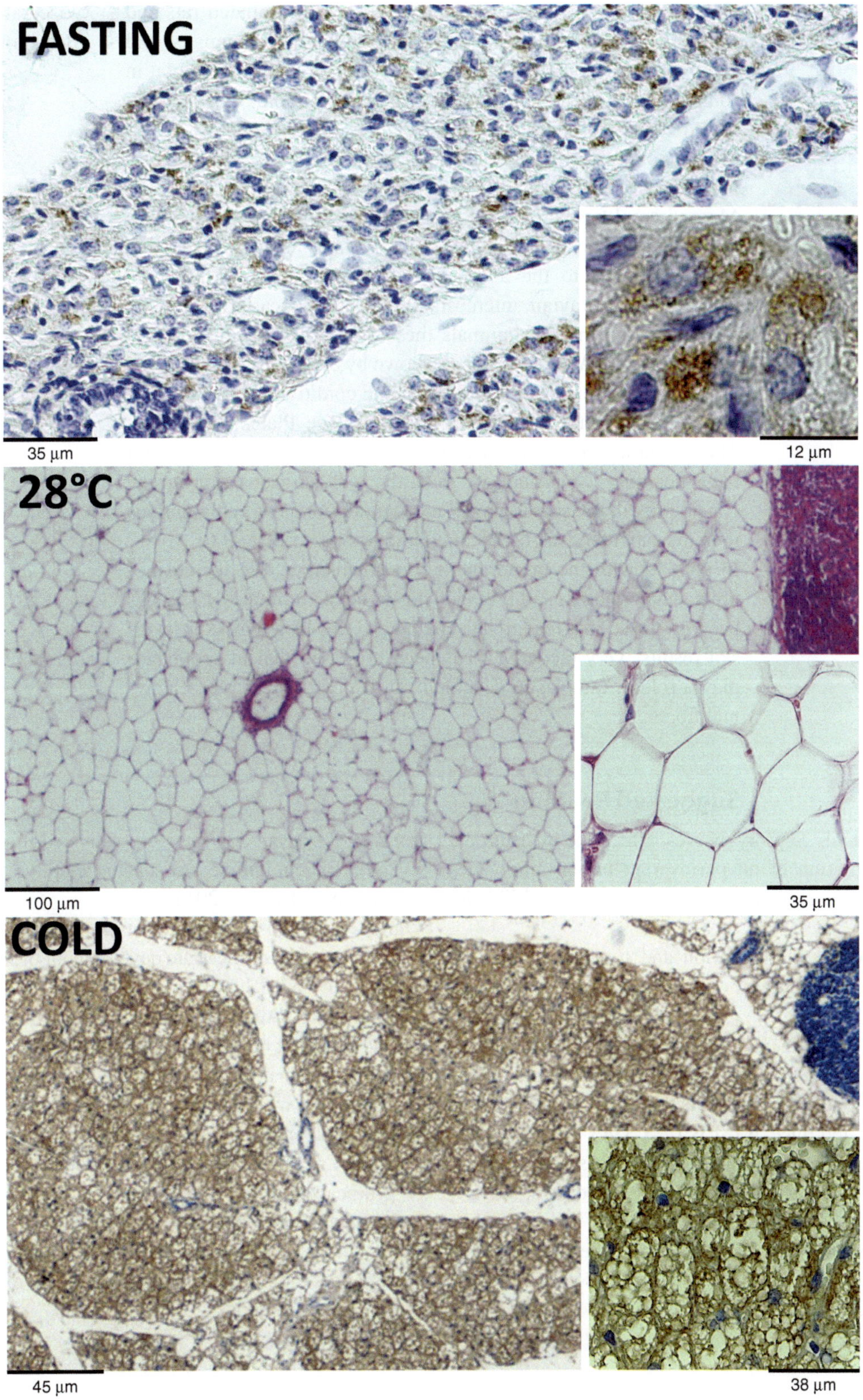

Plate 7.12 Inguinal fat of adult female Sv129 mouse. *Top*: 48 h of fasting. Most unilocular adipocytes disappear. Elongated slimmed (delipidated) adipocytes with small lipid droplets immunostained by perilipin1 are present in the cytoplasm of slimmed cells (enlarged in inset). Immunohistochemistry: perilipin1 ab (1:300). Kindly provided by Andy Greenberg. *Middle*: mouse maintained at 28 °C for 10 days. Most adipocytes are unilocular (enlarged in inset). On the right a small part of the inguinal lymph node is visible. H&E. *Bottom*: 10 days of cold acclimation (6 °C). Most adipocytes are multilocular UCP1 immunoreactive (enlarged in inset). Immunohistochemistry: UCP1 ab (1: 500 Abcam). On the right upper corner, a small part of the inguinal lymph node is visible

PLATE 7.13

Visceral WAT
Browning

Also visceral WAT transdifferentiates in cold-acclimated rats and mice. In this plate histology, UCP1 immunohistochemistry and electron microscopy of periovarian fat (predominantly white fat in room temperature maintained rats; see Plates 6.5–6.6) of a rat acclimated at 4 °C for 2 weeks is shown.

We did not find any morphological difference between the subcutaneous and visceral transdifferentiation phenomenon.

Most visceral fat seems more prone to browning than the subcutaneous fat probably because most of brown fat is naturally located in close proximity to the aorta and its main branches (anonyma, carotid, left subclavian, intercostal, renal, and iliac arteries), i.e., in visceral areas. In adult animals these areas convert into visceral WAT prone to BAT conversion as shown by data in cold-acclimated animals. Omentum, retroperitoneum, and epididymal fat are examples of visceral fat resistant to browning (see Plates 7.16–7.18). These data are important because the visceral conversion should have healthier consequences than the subcutaneous conversion considering that visceral white fat accumulation is more dangerous than the subcutaneous fat accumulation (see also Plate 9.6).

In parallel with the noradrenergic mechanism, a role for eosinophils, macrophages, and lymphocytes of innate immune system has been proposed, but recent data challanged this idea with controversial results. Very recently it has been proposed that macrophages play a role in the plastic development of noradrenergic parenchymal fibers.

Suggested Reading

Giordano A, et al. Sensory nerves affect the recruitment and differentiation of rat periovarian brown adipocytes during cold acclimation. J Cell Sci. 111:2587–94, 1998.

Cinti S. Adipocyte differentiation and transdifferentiation: plasticity of the adipose organ. J Endocrinol Invest. 25:823–35, 2002.

Armani A, et al. Mineralocorticoid receptor antagonism induces browning of white adipose tissue through impairment of autophagy and prevents adipocyte dysfunction in high-fat-diet-fed mice. FASEB J. 28:3745–57, 2014.

Giordano A, et al. Convertible visceral fat as a therapeutic target to curb obesity. Nat Rev Drug Discov. 15:405–24, 2016.

Wu D et al. Eosinophils sustain adipose alternatively activated macrophages associated with glucose homeostasis. Science. 332:243-7, 2011.

Nguyen KD et al. Alternatively activated macrophages produce catecholamines to sustain adaptive thermogenesis. Nature 480:104-8, 2011

Qiu Y et al. Eosinophils and type 2 cytokine signaling in macrophages orchestrate development of functional beige fat. Cell 157: 1292-308, 2014.

Lee MW et al. Activated type 2 innate lymphoid cells regulate beige fat biogenesis. Cell 160: 74-87, 2015.

Brestoff JR et al. Group 2 innate lymphoid cells promote beiging of white adipose tissue and limit obesity. Nature 519: 242-6, 2015.

Fischer K et al. Alternatively activated macrophages do not synthesize catecholamines or contribute to adipose tissue adaptive thermogenesis. Nat Med 23: 623-30, 2017.

Wolf Y et al. Brown-adipose-tissue macrophages control tissue innervation and homeostatic energy expenditure. Nat Immunol 18: 665-74, 2017.

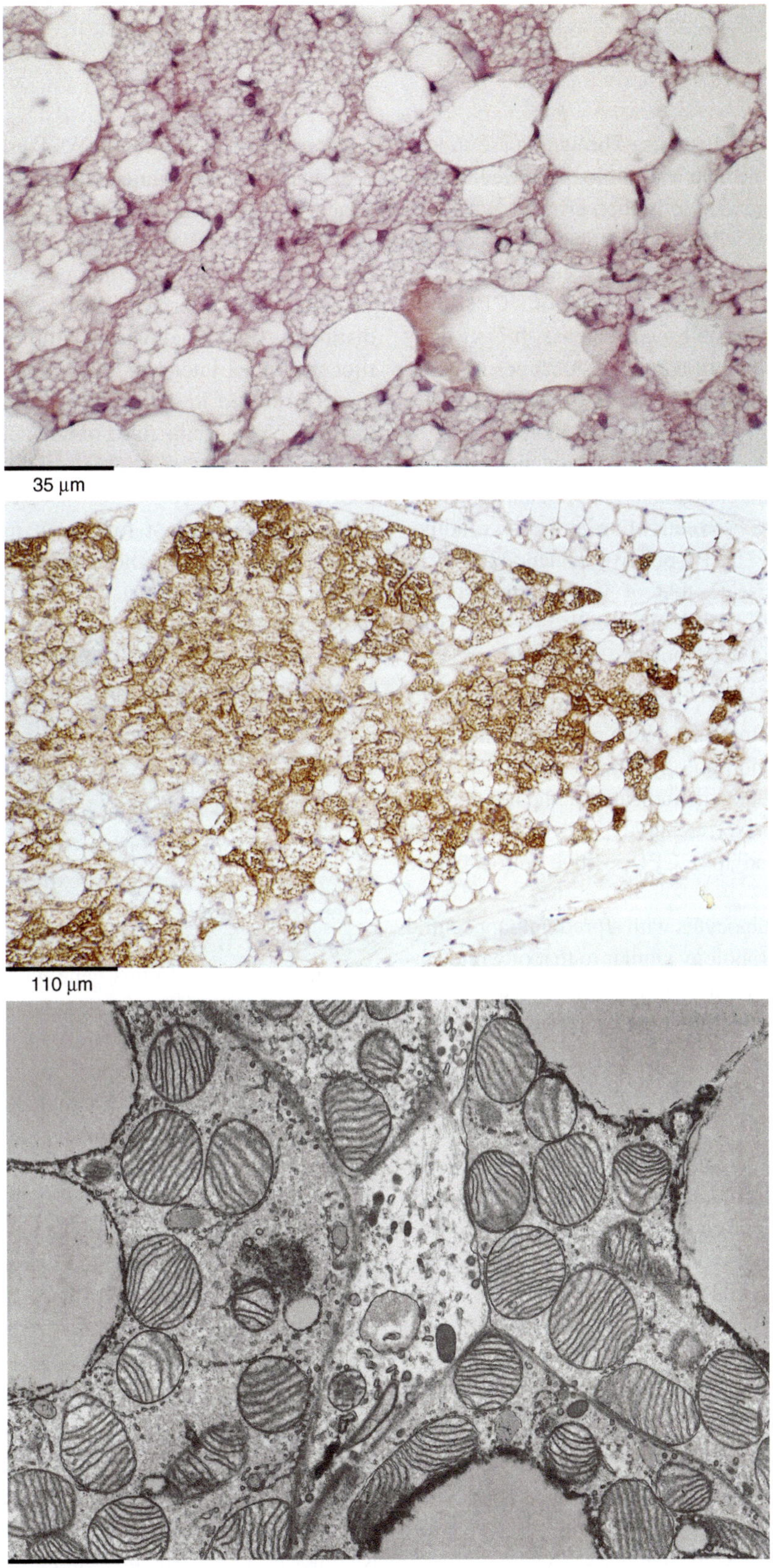

Plate 7.13 Periovarian adipose tissue of an adult rat acclimated at 4 °C for 14 days. *Top*: several multilocular cells are visible among the unilocular adipocytes. LM. H&E. *Middle*: multilocular cells are UCP1 immunoreactive. IHC: UCP1 ab (1:10,000). *Bottom*: multilocular cells show the typical ultrastructure of brown adipocytes. TEM

PLATE 7.14

Paucilocular
UCP1-immunoreactive
Adipocytes

In this plate some cytological details of browning are shown. Several cells with intermediate morphology between white and brown adipocytes are visible in the perirenal WAT during browning. Only a few cells are unilocular UCP1-negative adipocytes (white adipocytes); most of the cells in this plate are UCP1 immunoreactive, but the intensity of UCP1 staining is variable from very weak to very intense. It is visually evident that the morphology of adipocytes changes in parallel with the UCP1 immunoreactivity: the more adipocytes approach to the classic multilocular brown morphology, the more they increase the intensity of UCP1 immunostaining.

Thus, several UCP1-immunoreactive paucilocular cells are in an intermediate stage between white and brown adipocytes: from the weakly UCP1-positive paucilocular cells with a morphology close to that of white adipocytes to intensely UCP1-positive multilocular cells. At least four morphological stages of UCP1-positive adipocytes are visible in this plate:

1. Large paucilocular adipocytes with a predominant central lipid vacuole and a morphology similar to that of white adipocytes. Note that the one indicated in the lower panel seems to be immunoreactive mainly in cytoplasmic dots that likely correspond to UCP1-positive mitochondria (arrows).
2. Small paucilocular adipocytes with a predominant central lipid vacuole and morphology similar to that of white adipocytes but size close to that of brown adipocytes.
3. Small paucilocular adipocytes with large vacuoles of similar size.
4. Typical multilocular adipocyte with several small lipid droplets (brown adipocytes).

The ultrastructure of these cells, identical to that shown in Plates 6.7–6.8, fully confirms the intermediate morphology between classic white and classic brown adipocytes, with numerous mitochondria with intermediate morphology between that of classic white and that of classic brown mitochondria.

Gene expression profiles of WAT browning show an aspect different from both white and brown profiles in line with the idea of the presence of a tissue with cells expressing intermediate organelles. We propose to restrict the term of beige/brite adipocytes to these intermediate forms between classic white and classic brown adipocytes, at least until a specific distinctive functional feature will be discovered for the multilocular UCP1 intensely immunoreactive adipocytes such as those presented in this and in previous plates. Furthermore the term beige seems to be quite appropriate to these cells if we look at their color obtained by immunostaining with UCP1.

Some authors suggest to restrict the definition of classic brown adipocytes for those contained in the interscapular area of the adipose organ, considered classic BAT. However the definition of classic BAT seems quite questionable. If BAT derived from Myf-5 precursors is classic, then we should consider classic also the perirenal brown adipocytes that derive from Myf-5-expressing precursors like those in the interscapular fat. Of note, perirenal fat is not composed only of brown adipocytes but is a mixed depot (see Chap. 6 and in particular Plates 6.5–6.6).

BAT of anterior subcutaneous depot is the only anatomical site where brown adipocytes express the zinc finger protein of the cerebellum (ZIC1). If we consider this gene marker to define classic BAT, we should first discover which differential function is due to this gene with respect to the thermogenic function of a brown adipocyte.

If we consider the persistence in the adipose organ with aging as an important aspect for the definition of classic BAT, then we need more systematic studies in different areas of the body, because in our experience the periaortic and perirenal sites seem to be the areas where BAT persists in old-aged persons (see Plates 3.1, 5.4, and 6.10).

Interestingly β-less mice (see Plate 2.25) under chronic stress show browning of IBAT and upregulation of beige/brite genes in inguinal fat in the absence of any evidence of multilocular transformation of adipocyte morphology.

Suggested Reading

Mattson MP. Does brown fat protect against diseases of aging? Ageing Res Rev. 9:69–76, 2010.

Kajimura S, et al. Brown and beige fat: physiological roles beyond heat generation. Cell Metab. 22:546–59, 2015.

de Jong JM, et al. A stringent validation of mouse adipose tissue identity markers. Am J Physiol Endocrinol Metab. 308:E1085–105, 2015.

Razzoli M, et al Stress-induced activation of brown adipose tissue prevents obesity in conditions of low adaptive thermogenesis. Mol Metab. 5:19–33, 2015.

Cinti S. UCP1 protein: the molecular hub of adipose organ plasticity. Biochimie. 2016, in press.

Ricquier D. UCP1, the mitochondrial uncoupling protein of brown adipocyte: a personal contribution and a historical perspective. Biochimie. 2016, in press.

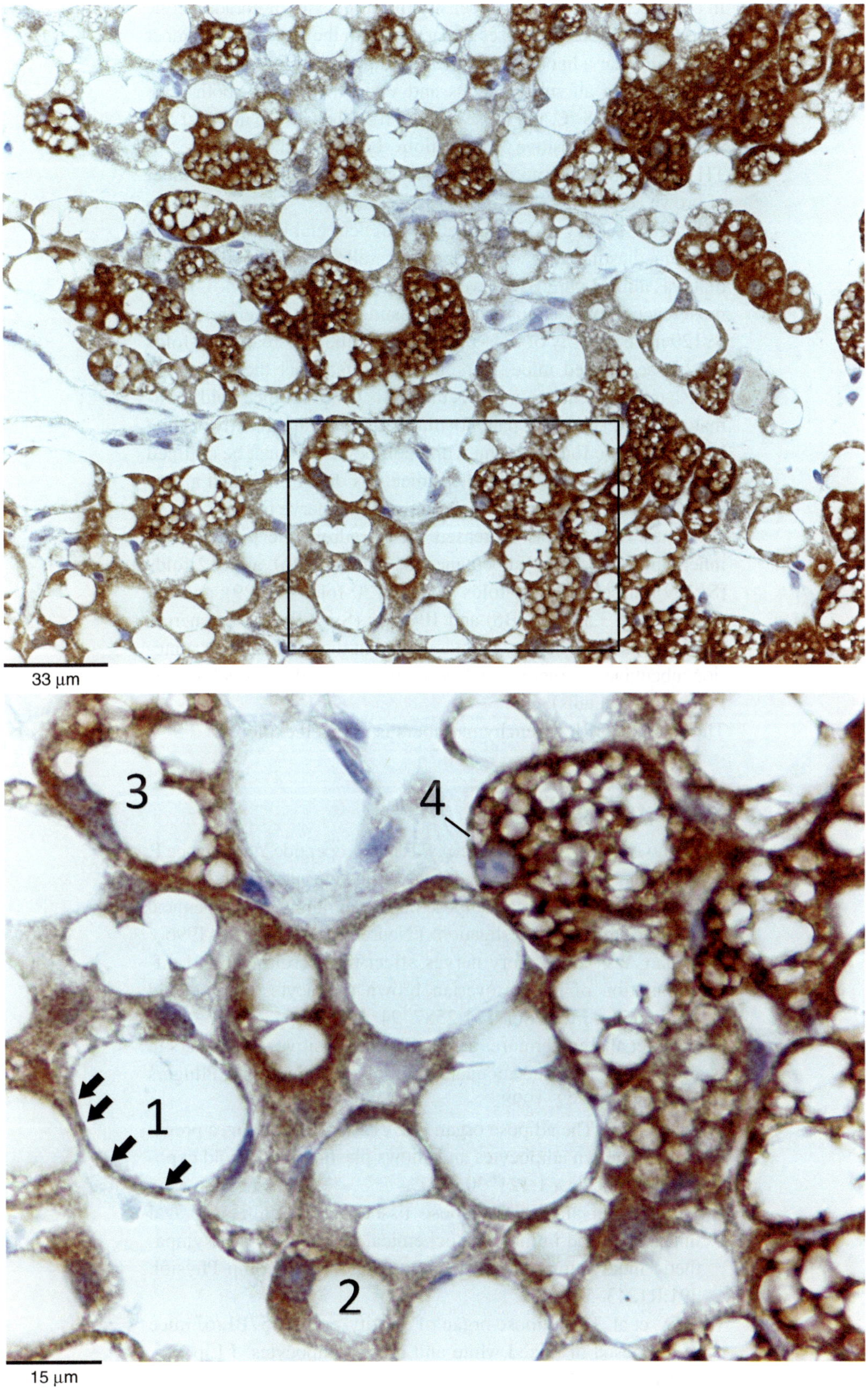

Plate 7.14 Perirenal fat of adult female mouse maintained at 6 °C for 10 days. *Lower*: enlargement of squared area in the *upper panel*. IHC. UCP1 ab (1:3,000). LM

PLATE 7.15

WAT Nerves

In cold-acclimated mice, the density (n°/adipocyte) of noradrenergic parenchymal fibers increases in parallel with the increase in number of paucilocular adipocytes and brown adipocytes. Considering these phenomena in all subcutaneous and visceral depots in both mice maintained at 28 °C and those at 6 °C for 10 days (B6 and Sv129), we found a positive correlation between the density of TH-immunoreactive (noradrenergic) parenchymal fibers and number of brown adipocytes.

The higher density of noradrenergic parenchymal fibers was found in the mediastinal-periaortic depot in parallel with its composition that was almost pure BAT (even in mice maintained at 28 °C). The most reactive WAT depot to cold exposure was the mesenteric fat in Sv129 mice (density of TH+ parenchymal fibers increased 20-folds in cold-acclimated mice), in spite of the fact that there were no UCP1-immunoreactive multilocular cells (even in mice cold acclimated at 6 °C) and only paucilocular UCP1-immunoreactive beige/brite cells were found among white adipocytes. It must be outlined anyway that in warm-acclimated mice this depot presented a very scarce amount of noradrenergic parenchymal nerve fibers.

All other WAT depots increased the noradrenergic parenchymal innervation: posterior subcutaneous, 3-folds (B6) and 12-folds (Sv129); mesenteric, 1.5-folds (B6) and 20-folds (Sv129); and retroperitoneal, 3.5-folds (B6) and 10-folds (Sv 129). Noradrenergic parenchymal fiber density increased also in the mixed depots: anterior subcutaneous, mediastinal-periaortic, and abdominopelvic (see Plate 7.3 for details).

The role of CGRP parenchymal fibers is not well explored.

Suggested Reading

Giordano A, et al. Tyrosine hydroxylase, neuropeptide Y, substance P, calcitonin gene-related peptide and vasoactive intestinal peptide in nerves of rat periovarian adipose tissue: an immunohistochemical and ultrastructural investigation. J Neurocytol. 25:125–36, 1996.

Giordano A, et al. Sensory nerves affect the recruitment and differentiation of rat periovarian brown adipocytes during cold acclimation. J Cell Sci. 111:2587–94, 1998.

Osaka T, et al. Temperature- and capsaicin-sensitive nerve fibers in brown adipose tissue attenuate thermogenesis in the rat. Pflugers Arch. 437:36–42, 1998.

Murano I, et al The adipose organ of Sv129 mice contains a prevalence of brown adipocytes and shows plasticity after cold exposure. Adipocytes. 1:121–30, 2005.

Giordano A, et al. White adipose tissue lacks significant vagal innervation and immunohistochemical evidence of parasympathetic innervation. Am J Physiol Regul Integr Comp Physiol. 291:R1243–55, 2006.

Vitali A, et al. The adipose organ of obesity-prone C57BL/6J mice is composed of mixed white and brown adipocytes. J Lip Res. 53:619–29, 2012.

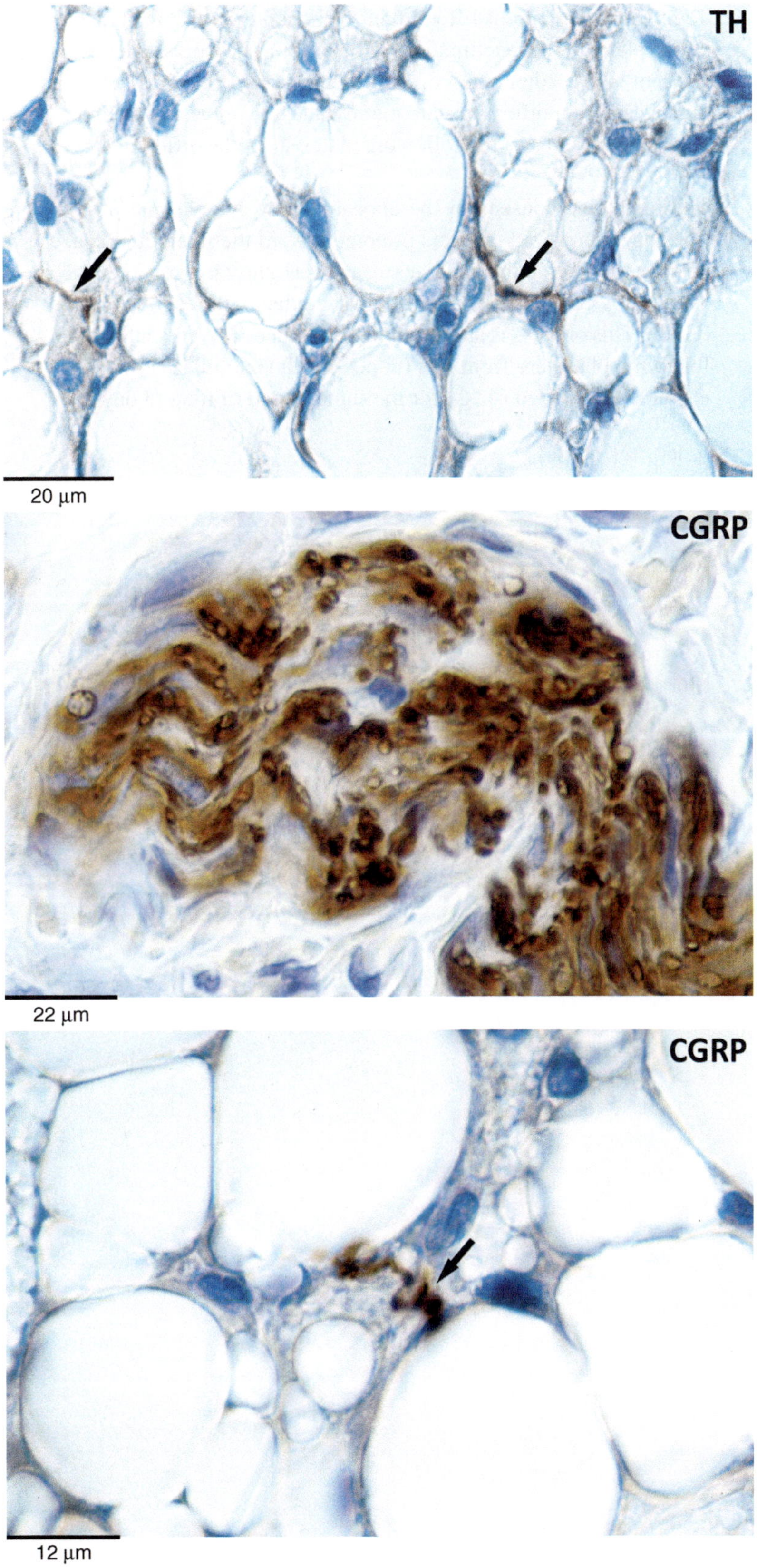

Plate 7.15 Periovarian depot of adult rats maintained at 4 °C for 14 days. TH-immunoreactive (noradrenergic) fibers (*upper*) and CGRP-immunoreactive fibers (*middle* and *lower*). In the middle panel, a high magnification of a nerve at the periphery of a WAT lobule is visible. In the upper and lower figures, parenchymal fibers (*arrows*) are visible among multilocular and unilocular adipocytes. LM. IHC: TH ab (1:300), CGRP ab (1:2,000)

PLATE 7.16

EM Lipolysis I

Together with the transdifferentiation phenomena described in previous plates, cold acclimation induces morphological modifications in white adipocytes of poorly innervated areas of adipose organ. These modifications are mainly due to a process of delipidation. The present and the following plates show the different stages of this process.
The first stage consists in the appearance of cytoplasmic projections devoid of lipid droplets oriented toward the interstitial space (arrows). Note that the cellular surface is slightly irregular.
These projections are usually in close contact with capillary walls (CAP). This process is similar in rats and mice. The present and the following plates are from rats (upper panels) and mice (lower panels) cold acclimated (4 °C) for the same period of time (3 days).

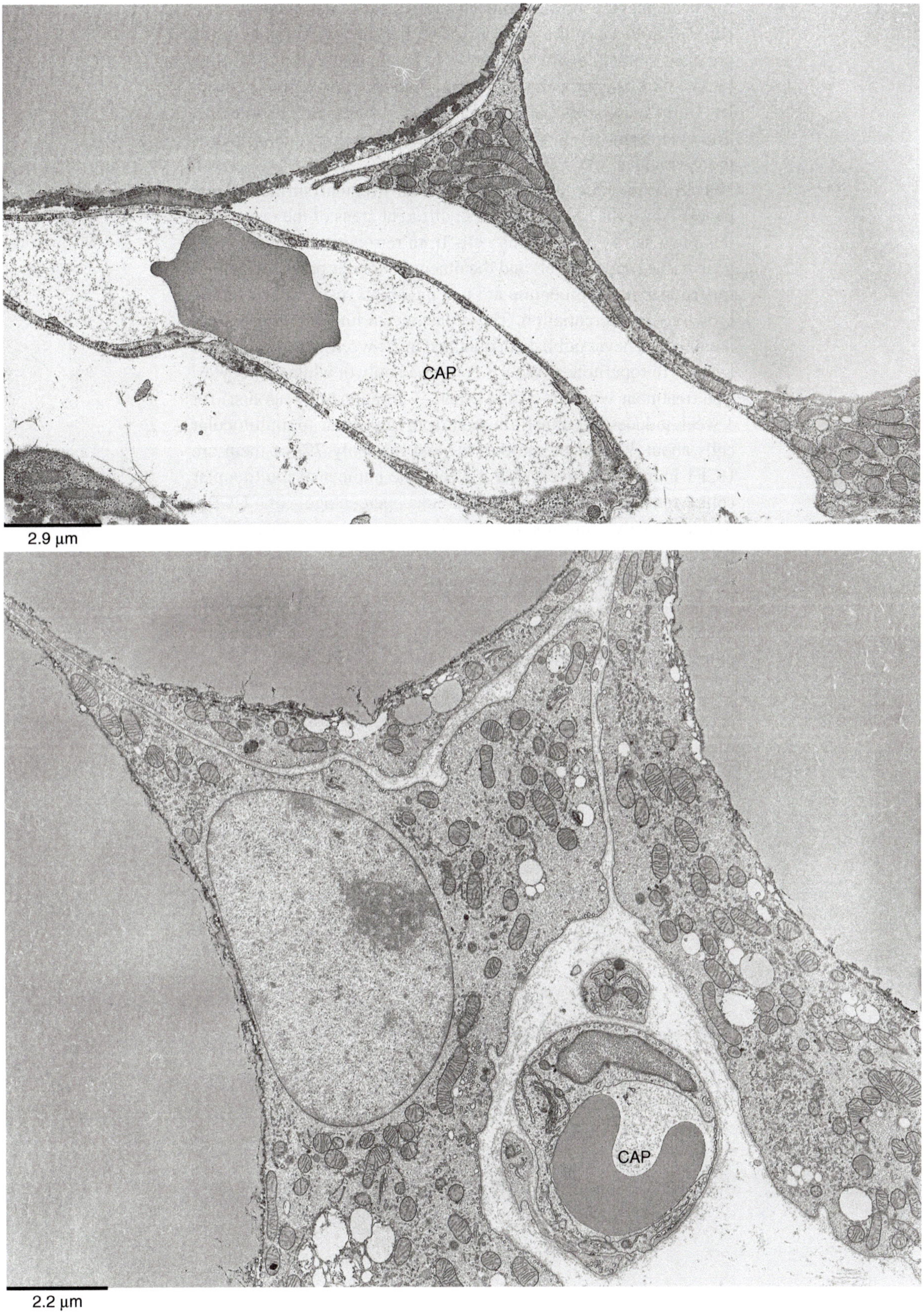

Plate 7.16 Retroperitoneal WAT of an adult rat (*lower*, mouse) acclimated at 4 °C for 3 days. CAP, capillary. TEM

PLATE 7.17

EM Lipolysis II

These adipocytes show a more advanced stage of delipidation compared with those in the previous plate, but they were found in the organ of animals maintained at 4 °C for the same period of time (3 days). Cells are much smaller and lipids are now stored in droplets of different sizes. Several very small droplets are also visible. The cytoplasm is rich in mitochondria and the cellular surface is more irregular.

Not all delipidizing adipocytes show an irregular surface (lower panel). This process takes place in different areas of the organ, and this plate shows delipidizing cells from retroperitoneal white adipose tissue (upper panel) and the omentum (lower panel). Thus retroperitoneum and omentum are two fat depots resistant to white to brown transdifferentiation. These data are in line with our experimental data, never published, obtained in 20-week-old rats. In these animals retroperitoneal WAT is composed only of white adipocytes. The treatment with CL 316243 (beta-3 noradrenergic agonist) for 1 week induces the transformation from unilocular to multilocular cells about 30% of the adipocytes and that only 7% of them are UCP1 immunoreactive. After 2 weeks the number of multilocular cells remains unchanged, but the percentage of UCP1-immunoreactive multilocular adipocytes goes up to 30%. These data suggest that in this depot only 30% of adipocytes are prone to transdifferentiate into brown adipocytes.

On the other end the resistance to transdifferentiation in omentum could be related to its immunologic implications as suggested by morphologic data presented in Plate 4.12.

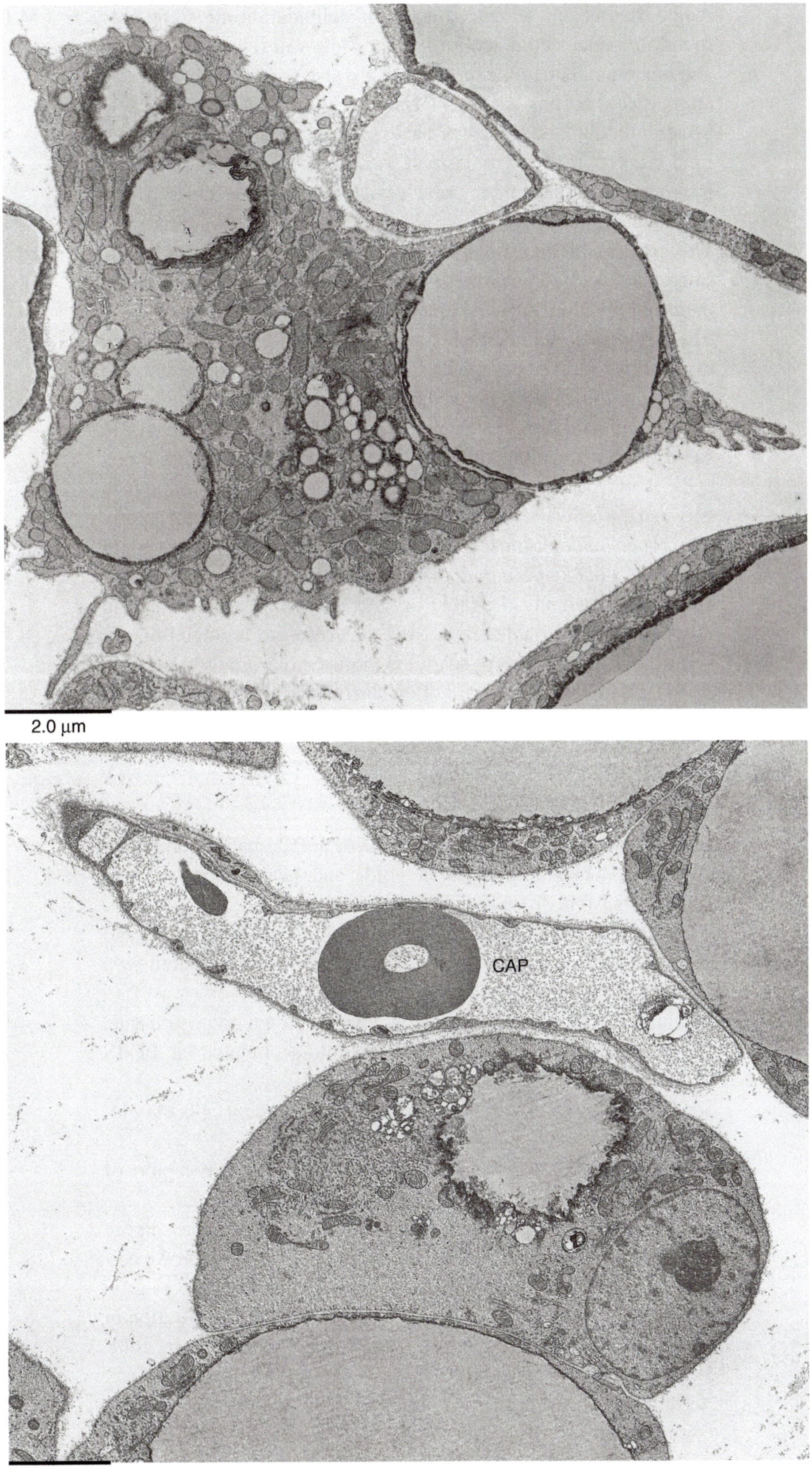

Plate 7.17 Retroperitoneal WAT of an adult rat (*lower*: mouse omentum) acclimated at 4 °C for 3 days. TEM

PLATE 7.18

EM Lipolysis III

Adipocytes at this advanced stage of delipidation are frequently found in animals cold acclimated for 7 days in retroperitoneal fat and omentum, but cells in this stage are also occasionally found in animals cold acclimated for 3 days.

Most delipidizing adipocytes have an elongated shape and small lipid droplets in the cytoplasm. The cellular surface is sometimes irregular and many pinocytotic vesicles are visible close to the plasma membrane.

This process of lipolysis does not occur in all adipocytes at the same time, and adipocytes in different stages of delipidation are therefore found in the same area of the tissue (middle panel).

The cytoplasm of adipocytes undergoing lipolysis due to cold exposure is rich in organelles. Mitochondria are numerous, but their morphology does not differ from that found in white adipocytes of animals kept in standard conditions (bottom left panel). In some depots of young mice, some mitochondria of delipidizing cells acquire a morphology that can be considered intermediate between that of white and brown mitochondria (bottom right panel). The rough endoplasmic reticulum (RER) is often organized in stacks, and the smooth endoplasmic reticulum (SER) is abundant and scattered among the other organelles. Lipids are arranged in droplets (L) of variable sizes. SER cisternae are arranged on the surface of lipid droplets or scattered in the cytoplasm (bottom right panel). Capillaries (CAP) are often surrounded by the cytoplasmic projections of adipocytes (also see Plate 7.15).

Suggested Reading

Kuroshima A, et al. Calorigenic effects of noradrenaline and glucagon on white adipocytes in cold- and heat-acclimated rats. Pflugers Arch. 381:113–7, 1979.

Portet R, et al. Prostaglandins E2 and F alpha levels in white and brown adipose tissues of cold acclimated rats as measured by a new micromethod. Biochimie. 61:429–31, 1979.

Trayhurn P. Fatty acid synthesis in vivo in brown adipose tissue, liver and white adipose tissue of the cold-acclimated rat. FEBS Lett. 104:13–6, 1979.

Senault C, et al. Beta-adrenergic receptors in white fat cells of cold-acclimated rats. Biochimie. 65:301–6, 1983.

Uehara A, et al. Effect of cold acclimation on glucagon receptors of rat white adipocytes. Jpn J Physiol. 36:891–903, 1986.

Loncar D, et al. The effect of intermittent cold treatment on the adipose tissue of the cat. Apparent transformation from white to brown adipose tissue. J Ultrastruct Mol Struct Res. 97:119–29, 1986.

Habara Y, Effects of cold exposure on cyclic AMP concentration in plasma, liver, and brown and white adipose tissues in cold-acclimated rats. Int J Biometeorol. 33:95–100, 1989.

Herpin P, et al. Adipose tissue lipolytic activity and urinary catecholamine excretion in cold-acclimated piglets. Can J Physiol Pharmacol. 69:362–68, 1991.

Himms-Hagen J, et al. Multilocular fat cells in WAT of CL-316243-treated rats derive directly from white adipocytes. Am J Physiol Cell Physiol. 279:C670–81, 2000.

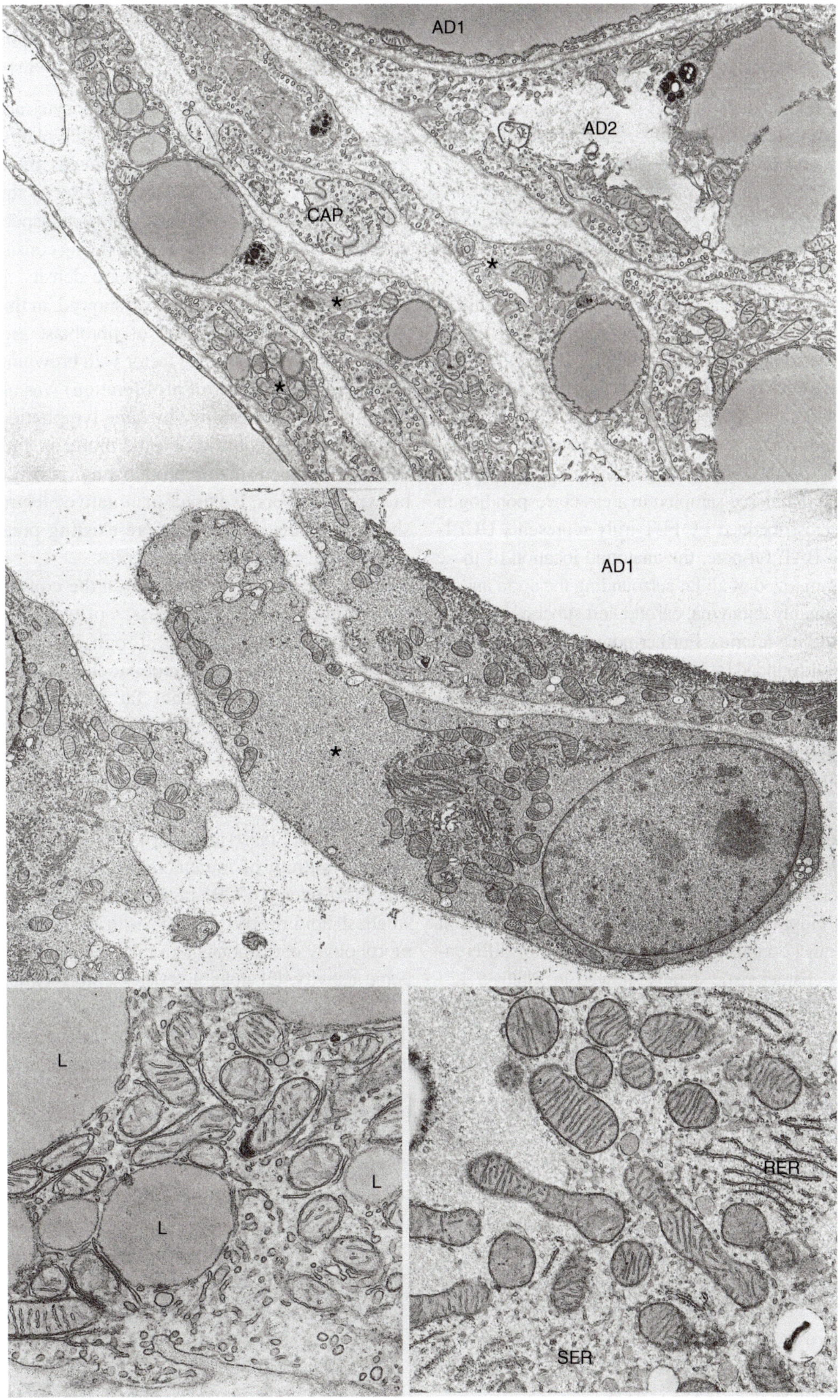

Plate 7.18 Retroperitoneal WAT of an adult rat (*middle*: mouse omentum) acclimated at 4 °C for 7 days. Different stages of delipidation are visible: AD1 (early), AD2 (*middle*), *asterisk* (late). CAP, capillary. *Bottom*: retroperitoneal WAT of a rat (*left*) and mouse (*right*) mesenteric depot. Animals acclimated at 4 °C for 7 days. TEM

PLATE 7.19

Transdifferentiation in Adipose Organ of Humans

In previous plates the details of WAT to BAT transdifferentiation in murine adipose organ have been shown in details. Here the morphology and immunohistochemistry of WAT to BAT transdifferentiation in humans is presented. Pheochromocytoma is a benign tumor of adrenal glands that must be surgically treated because of its intense production of adrenalin and noradrenalin dangerous for the cardiovascular system. For decades it is well known that these patients develop a variable amount of BAT mainly in the peri-adrenal part of the adipose organ. Positron emission tomography (PET) allows detecting tissue with high uptake of marked glucose and is usually performed to detect tumor metastasis. PET analyses of subjects suffering from pheochromocytoma revealed a strong uptake of marked glucose in areas of the adipose organ supposed to contain BAT. We showed that tissue sampled in areas corresponding to the positive images obtained by PET truly represents UCP1-immunoreactive BAT. Of note, the anatomic location of these areas can be summarized as all fat surrounding the aorta and its main branches, mainly anonyma, carotid, left subclavian, intercostal, renal, and iliac arteries. Furthermore many of their collaterals are also surrounded by BAT. This distribution of BAT is easy to understand from a finalistic point of view: the heat produced by BAT can easily be distributed to the rest of the body via arterial blood. Interestingly, just after removal of the tumor, PET becomes silent, suggesting that only adrenergically stimulated BAT can be detected with this technique. Murine omentum is one of the most resistant fat areas in the adipose organ for conversion in BAT (see previous plates), and rarely pheochromocytoma patients show PET-positive signals from this depot. Our analyses of bioptic specimen from the omentum of several patients (data from 12 published) showed signs of transdifferentiation, with all characteristic details showed in Plates 7.12–7.14. In half of the cases, we found a variable amount of well-differentiated UCP1-immunoreactive multilocular adipocytes (brown adipocytes) that were absent in 20 controls. All the intermediate forms between white adipocytes and brown adipocytes (similar to those presented in this plate), including the transdifferentiation marker represented by UCP1-positive paucilocular cells, were found (* in inset of the upper panel). Importantly, together with the cytological aspects of adipocyte conversion, we proved a tissue remodeling consisting in increase of noradrenergic parenchymal nerve density and increase of capillary density. Furthermore we showed, in this converted tissue, a significant expression of fibroblast growth factor 21 (FGF21) that is a hormonal factor with browning properties.

Of note, Ki67 (marker of proliferation) was always negative on adipocytes but positive in some lymphatic cells in lymph nodes (internal control). Furthermore, in order to exclude any development from pre-existing poorly differentiated brown precursors, we used quantitative electron microscopy showing no development of pre-existing preadipocytes and no differences with control samples.

Thus, these data suggest that even the conversion-resistant omentum can undergo processes of transdifferentiation in humans under appropriate stimuli. In these three Plates 7.18–7.21, UCP1 immunohistochemistry and electron microscopy of peri-adrenal fat removed from a patient with pheochromocytoma are shown.

Unilocular cells are UCP1 negative. Note the extremely variable UCP1 immunoreactivity in multilocular cells. Paucilocular UCP1-negative (** some indicated) and paucilocular UCP1-positive cells (* inset) are shown. Multilocular adipocytes show all the spectrum of immunoreactivity from weak to intense. The most intense UCP1-immunoreactive adipocytes have the smallest lipid droplets in line with the general rule that this morphology corresponds to a high level of functional thermogenic activity. Of note, a series of biopsies taken from peri-adrenal fat in patients surgically treated for incidentalomas (benign tumors of adrenal glands without any endocrine activity) revealed a WAT histology of this tissue in most patients.

Suggested Reading

Lean ME, et al. Brown adipose tissue in patients with phaeochromocytoma. Int J Obes. 10:219–27, 1986.

Zingaretti MC, et al. The presence of UCP1 demonstrates that metabolically active adipose tissue in the neck of adult humans truly represents brown adipose tissue. FASEB J. 23:3113–20, 2009.

Kuji I, et al. Brown adipose tissue demonstrating intense FDG uptake in a patient with mediastinal pheochromocytoma. Ann Nucl Med. 22:231–5, 2008.

Cheng W, et al. Intense FDG activity in the brown adipose tissue in omental and mesenteric regions in a patient with malignant pheochromocytoma. Clin Nucl Med. 37:514–15, 2012.

Fisher FM, et al. FGF21 regulates PGC-1α and browning of white adipose tissues in adaptive thermogenesis. Genes Dev. 26:271–81, 2012.

Frontini A, et al. White-to-brown transdifferentiation of omental adipocytes in patients affected by pheochromocytoma. Biochim Biophys Acta. 1831:950–9, 2013.

Dong A, et al. Hypermetabolic mesenteric brown adipose tissue on dual-time point FDG PET/CT in a patient with benign retroperitoneal pheochromocytoma. Clin Nucl Med. 39:e229–32, 2014.

Hondares E, et al. Fibroblast growth factor-21 is expressed in neonatal and pheochromocytoma-induced adult human brown adipose tissue. Metabolism. 63:312–7, 2014.

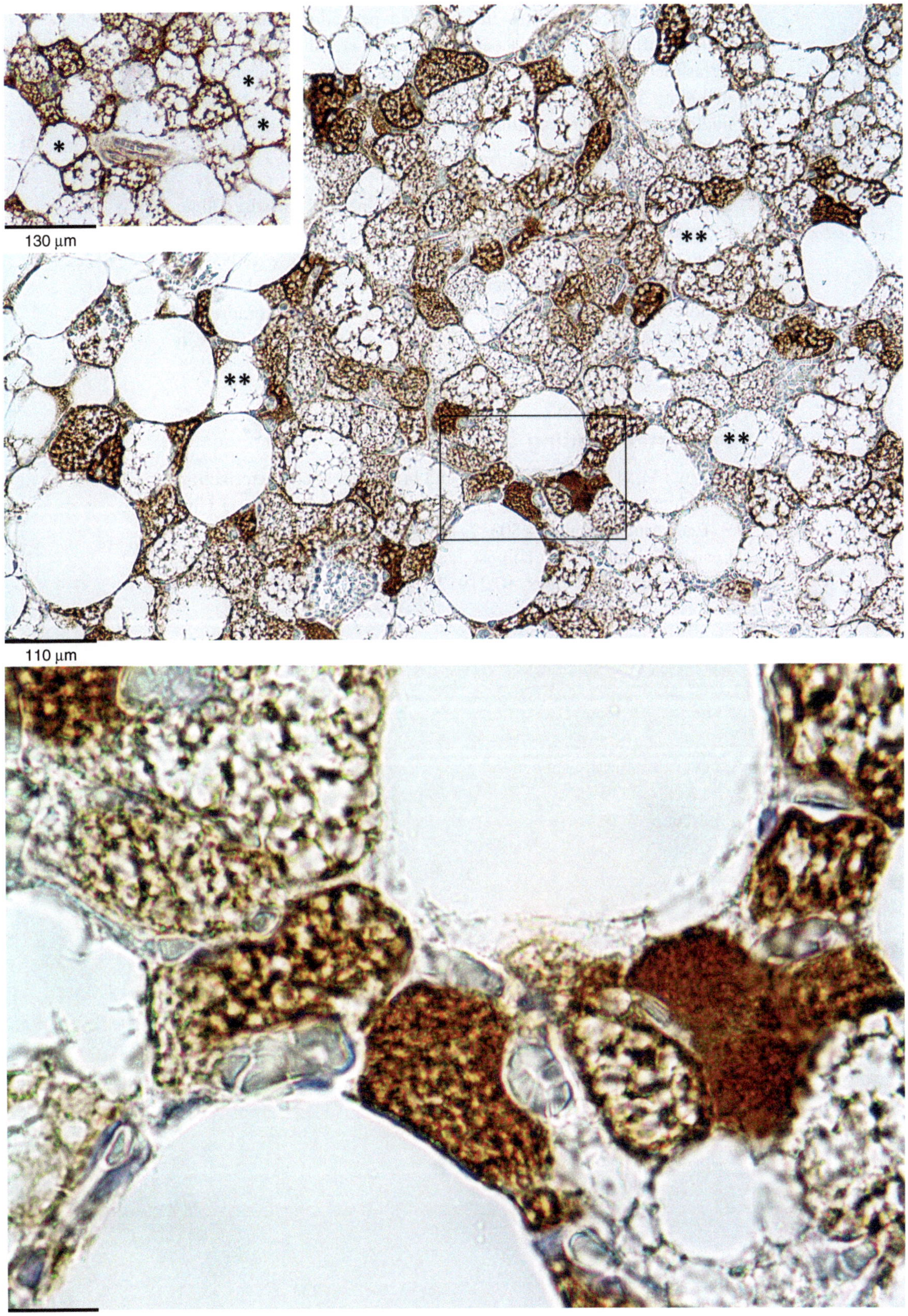

Plate 7.19 Peri-adrenal fat from a subject suffering for pheochromocytoma. Multilocular UCP1-immunoreactive adipocytes. Inset: area of the same tissue containing UCP1-immunoreactive paucilocular adipocytes (*asterisk*). *Lower*: enlargement of squared area in the upper panel. Note the variable immunostaining in relationship with morphology. IHC. UCP1 ab (1:3,000). LM

PLATE 7.20

EM of Transdifferentiated Human Adipocytes

Human brown adipocytes in converted peri-adrenal fat from a patient suffering from pheochromocytoma are shown here. The ultrastructure of the tissue is quite similar to that of murine BAT including the high density of capillaries (CAP), the roundish nucleus, the numerous quite regular small lipid droplets, and the abundant mitochondria. Note the absence of parenchymal nerve fibers.

In line with the blood source of adrenaline and noradrenaline, browned areas of the adipose organ in pheochromocytoma patients are usually poorly innervated. In this case only rare TH-immunoreactive parenchymal fibers were detected. In the middle panel, a parenchymal TH-immunoreactive (noradrenergic) fiber is shown (left arrow) together with some TH+ fibers in the perivascular connective interstitium (right arrow).

Suggested Reading

Ricquier D, et al. Ultrastructural and biochemical characterization of human brown adipose tissue in pheochromocytoma. J Clin Endocrinol Metab. 54:803–7, 1982.

Lean ME, et al. Brown adipose tissue in patients with phaeochromocytoma. Int J Obes. 10:219–27, 1986.

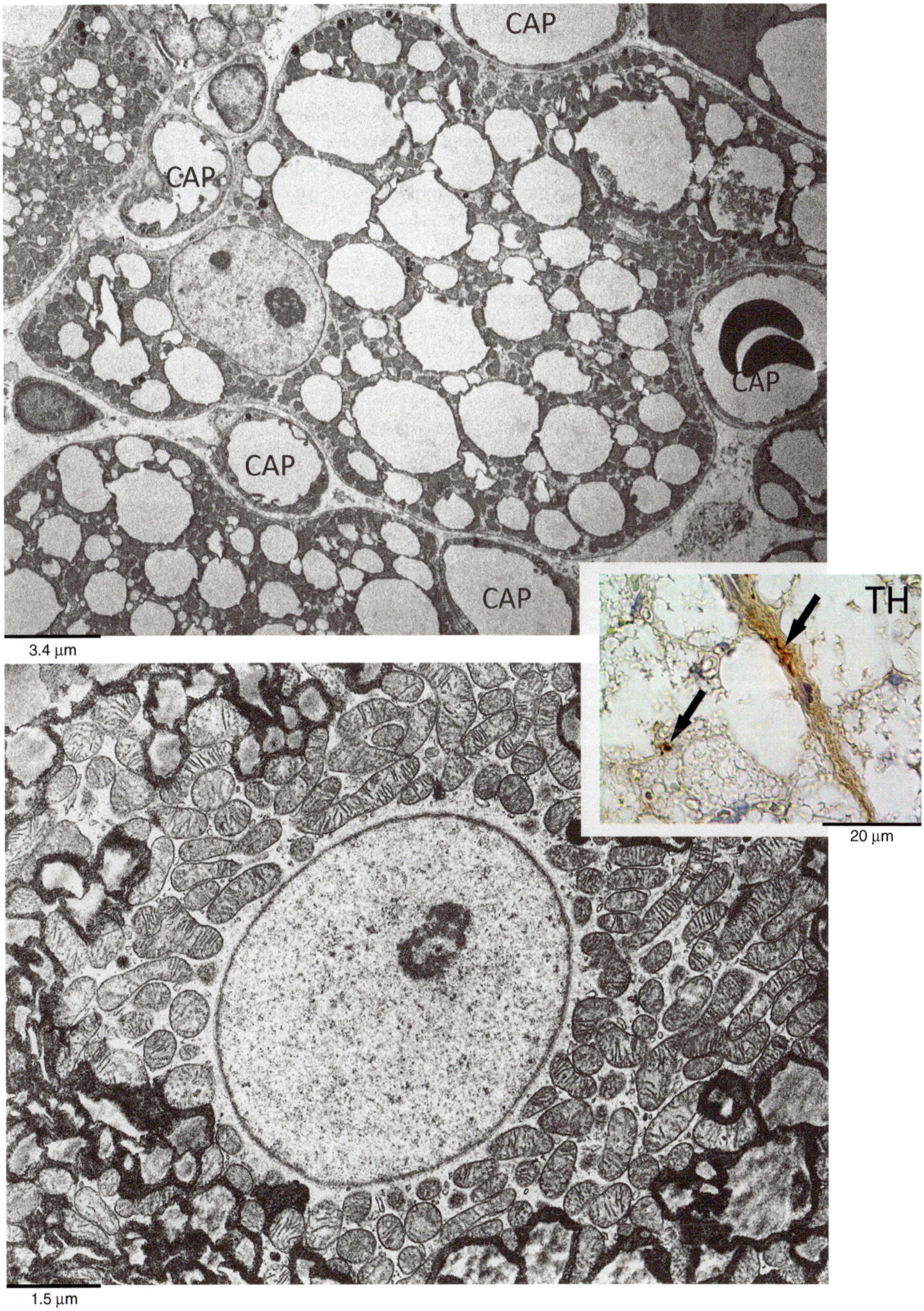

Plate 7.20 Ultrastructure of brown adipocytes from browned peri-adrenal fat of a subject suffering for pheochromocytoma (same subject of Plate 7.19). CAP, capillary. TEM. *Middle*: same tissue. IHC: TH ab (1:300). LM

PLATE 7.21

EM of Mitochondria

The morphology of mitochondria in brown adipocytes of browned peri-adrenal fat in pheochromocytoma patients is quite variable. In some adipocytes (upper panel), they tended to be mainly elongated and with short randomly oriented cristae.

In the cell presented in the middle panel, mitochondria are still predominantly elongated, but the cristae are more laminar.

In the cell presented in the bottom panel, mitochondria are more roundish approaching the typical morphology of BAT mitochondria found in cold-exposed or acclimated rats or mice (see Plates 7.7–7.9).

Our interpretation is that the three examples shown in this plate are an expression of progressive (up to down) stages of mitochondrial transdifferentiation, in line with the variable UCP1 density shown in Plate 7.19.

Suggested Reading

Cigolini M, et al. Human brown adipose cells in culture. Exp Cell Res. 159:261–66, 1985.

Frontini A, et al. White-to-brown transdifferentiation of omental adipocytes in patients affected by pheochromocytoma. Biochim Biophys Acta. 1831:950–9, 2013.

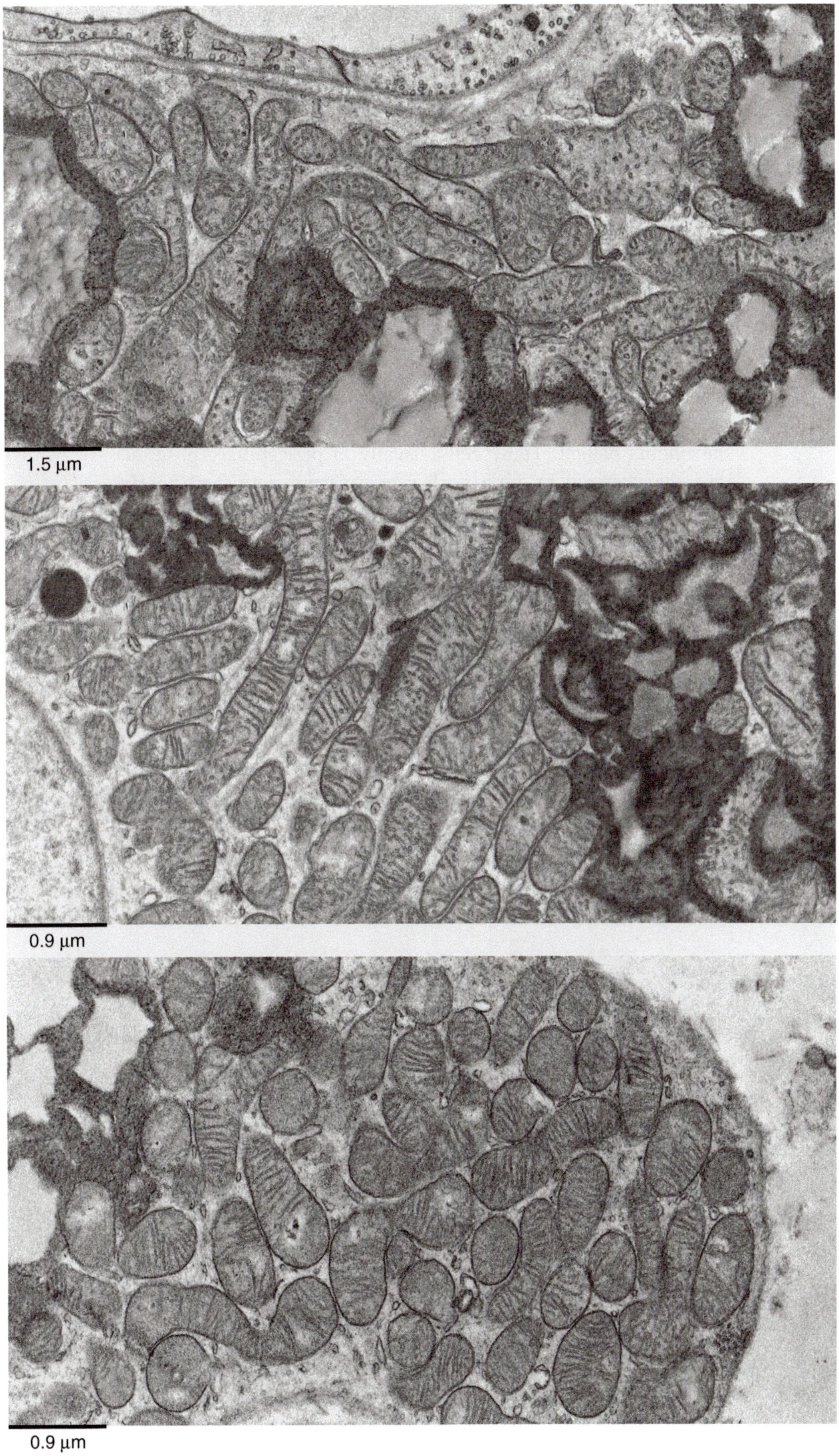

Plate 7.21 Mitochondrial ultrastructure of brown adipocytes from browned peri-adrenal fat of a subject suffering for pheochromocytoma (same subject of Plates 7.18–7.19). TEM

PLATE 7.22

Unilocular Adipocytes and Preadipocytes

Frequently, unilocular cells with abundant "pre-typical" mitochondria are present among brown adipocytes in the peri-adrenal fat sampled from pheochromocytoma patients (upper panel).

These cells could represent a first step of conversion of white adipocytes to brown adipocytes and are very similar to those found in mixed areas of adipose organ (see Plates 6.8 and 6.11) and in WAT of cold-exposed rats or mice. The morphology of mitochondria does not exclude the possibility that even at this early stage of conversion, UCP1 protein is present in these types of mitochondria (see also below). In fact almost all unilocular adipocytes (presumably with this type of mitochondria) resulted in UCP1 immunostained in cold-exposed mice (see Panel 7.14) and in the perirenal fat of a patient (see Plate 6.10).

Poorly differentiated cells with the general characteristics of an adipoblast are also identified in this peri-adrenal fat from pheochromocytoma patient. These cells, usually in pericapillary position, are characterized by high nucleus/cytoplasmic ratio and poorly developed organelles and are surrounded by a distinct external lamina (EL). Some of them show pre-typical mitochondria, but not in this case (bottom panel), although one mitochondrion (arrow) seems to be larger than the others. The absence of pre-typical mitochondria can be explained by an early stage of differentiation.

In the middle panel an adipoblast from the omentum of a pheochromocytoma patient is shown. Note the external lamina (EL) and the large and numerous pre-typical mitochondria (arrows, some indicated). The morphology of these organelles is similar to that of mitochondria found in brown adipoblast in fetal BAT (see Chap. 12). These last mitochondria resulted immunoreactive for UCP1 by immuno-gold ultrastructural cytochemistry. These data prove that mitochondria with this ultrastructure can be UCP1 positive.

Note the extreme variability in mitochondrial morphology of the multilocular adipocyte on the right of the lower panel.

Suggested Reading

Ricquier D, et al. Ultrastructural and biochemical characterization of human brown adipose tissue in pheochromocytoma. J Clin Endocrinol Metab. 54:803–7, 1982.

Lean ME, et al. Brown adipose tissue in patients with phaeochromocytoma. Int J Obes. 10:219–27, 1986.

Frontini A, et al. White-to-brown transdifferentiation of omental adipocytes in patients affected by pheochromocytoma. Biochim Biophys Acta. 1831:950–9, 2013.

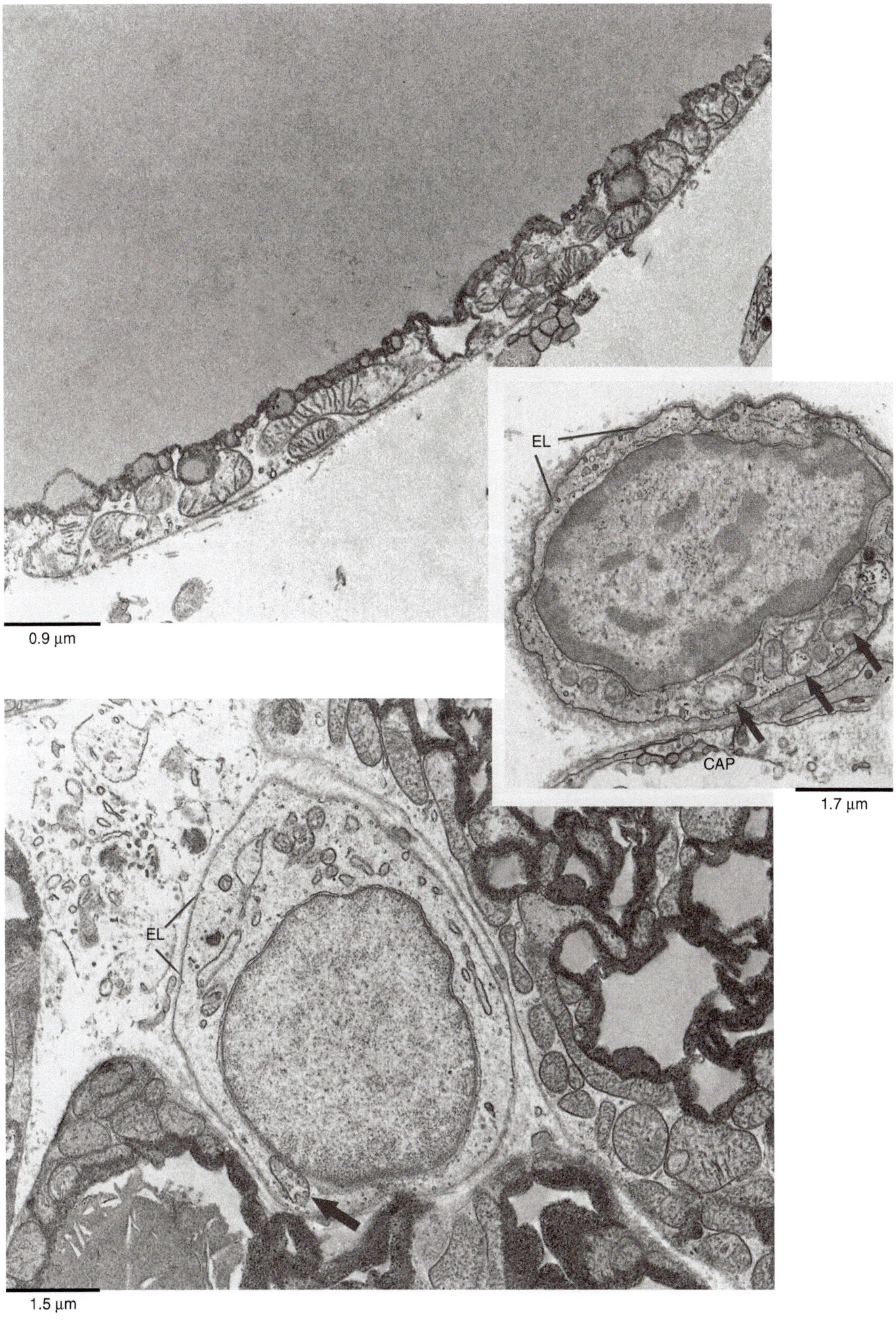

Plate 7.22 *Upper*: cytoplasmic rim of a unilocular cell in peri-adrenal fat of a subject suffering from pheochromocytoma (same subject of Plates 7.18–7.20). *Lower*: bona fide adipoblast from the same tissue and from omentum of a pheochromocytoma patient (*middle panel*, from: Frontini et al. White-to-brown transdifferentiation of omental adipocytes in patients affected by pheochromocytoma. Biochimica et Biophysica Acta 1831 (2013) 950–9, with permission). CAP, capillary. TEM

8 Warm-Acclimated Adipose Organ

S. Cinti, *Obesity, Type 2 Diabetes and the Adipose Organ*, https://doi.org/10.1007/978-3-319-40522-3_8

8.1 Warm-Acclimated Adipose Organ

PLATE 8.1

Gross Anatomy

The adipose organ anatomy of animals maintained in warm conditions (28–29 °C) is similar to that observed in animals living in standard conditions (19–22 °C in our laboratory) except for the color intensity of the areas of the organ constituted of brown adipose tissue (BAT), which appear paler in the former animals.

Suggested Reading

Rabi T, et al. Lipolysis in brown adipose tissue of cold- and heat-acclimated hamsters. J Appl Physiol. 43:1007–11, 1977.

Kuroshima A, et al. Thermogenic responses of brown adipocytes to noradrenaline and glucagon in heat-acclimated and cold-acclimated rats. Jpn J Physiol. 29:683–90, 1979.

Murano I, et al. The adipose organ of Sv129 mice contains a prevalence of brown adipocytes and shows plasticity after cold exposure. Adipocytes. 1:121–30, 2005.

Vitali A, et al. The adipose organ of obesity-prone C57BL/6J mice is composed of mixed white and brown adipocytes. J Lip Res. 53:619–29, 2012.

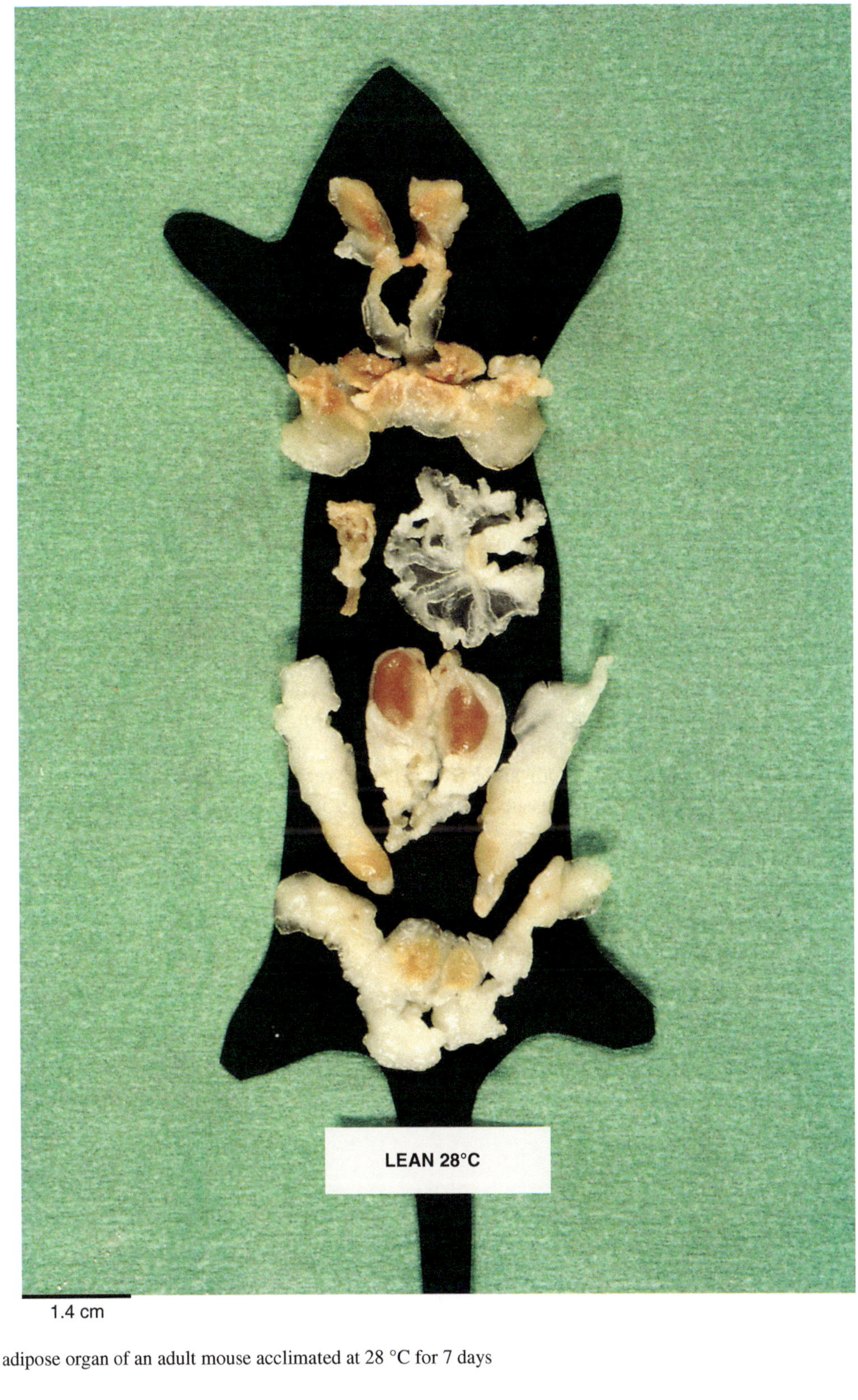

Plate 8.1 The adipose organ of an adult mouse acclimated at 28 °C for 7 days

PLATE 8.2

IHC: UCP1-Leptin

The paler appearance of BAT in warm-acclimated animals (see the previous plate) is accompanied by a dramatic change in its morphology. Many (in rats) or most (in mice) BAT adipocytes show a unilocular appearance. They are therefore similar to white adipocytes except for their smaller size (about 20–50 μm vs 80–100 μm in diameter) and their usually thicker cytoplasmic rim. The reduction in noradrenergic BAT stimulation in warm-acclimated animals induces the inhibition of the activity of the gene/s responsible for multilocularity and of other thermogenic genes. In this condition, UCP1 is still found (weak immunostaining) in these unilocular brown adipocytes (lower left), but leptin can also be detected (lower right). Classic multilocular brown adipocytes of mice maintained in standard conditions (19 °C in this case) or cold exposed do not express leptin (also see Plate 4.4).

Suggested Reading

Dechamma PA, Shetty P. Changes in brown adipocyte morphology and cellularity in response to acute starvation. Indian J Exp Biol. 25:627–31, 1987.

Sakurada S, et al. Shivering and nonshivering thermogenic responses of rats subjected to different patterns of heat acclimation. Can J Physiol Pharmacol. 71:576–81, 1993.

Cinti S, et al. Immunohistochemical localization of leptin and uncoupling protein in white and brown adipose tissue. Endocrinology. 138:797–804, 1997.

Cancello R, et al. Leptin and UCP1 genes are reciprocally regulated in brown adipose tissue. Endocrinology. 139:4747–50, 1998.

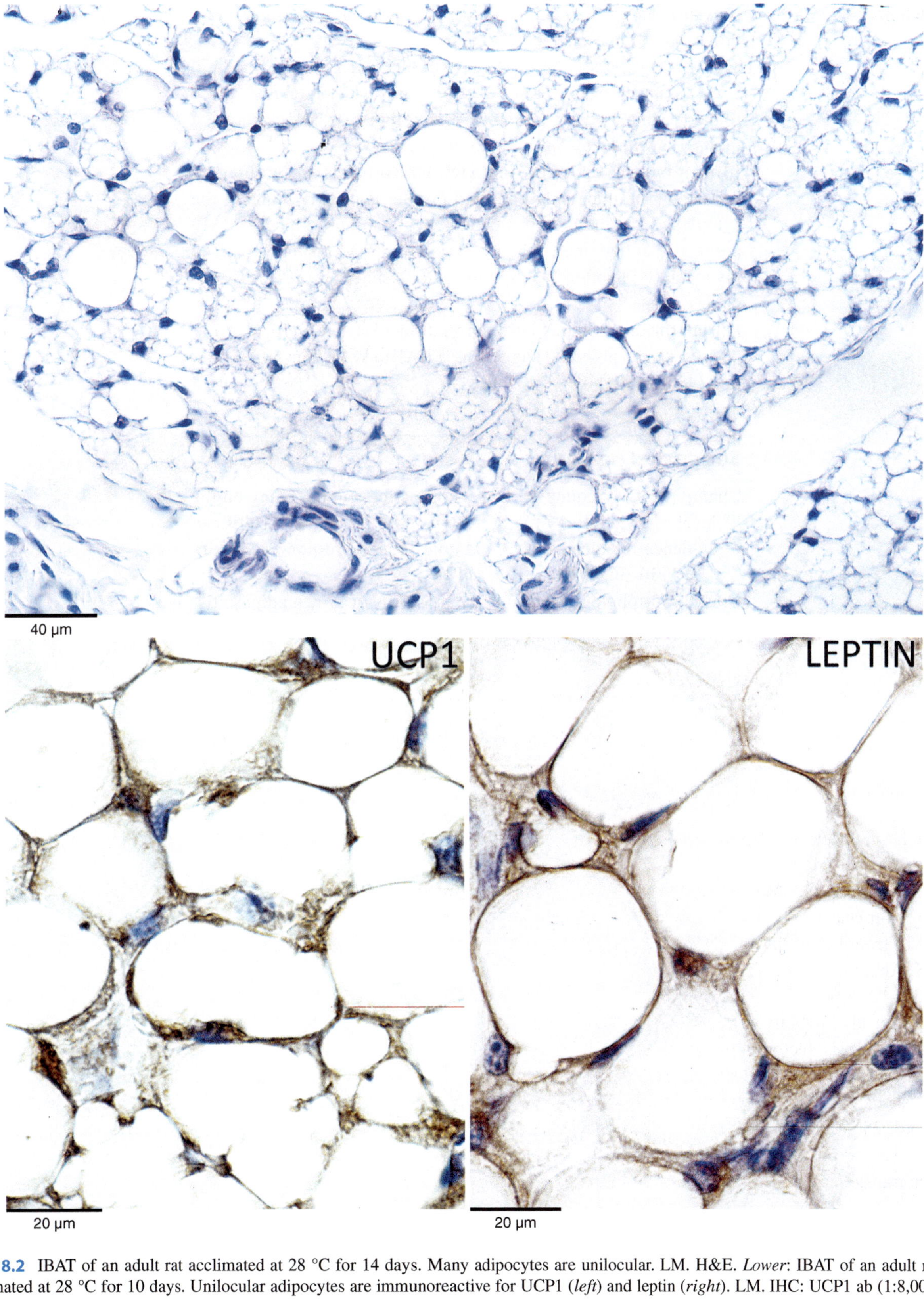

Plate 8.2 IBAT of an adult rat acclimated at 28 °C for 14 days. Many adipocytes are unilocular. LM. H&E. *Lower*: IBAT of an adult mouse, acclimated at 28 °C for 10 days. Unilocular adipocytes are immunoreactive for UCP1 (*left*) and leptin (*right*). LM. IHC: UCP1 ab (1:8,000) and leptin ab (1:1,000)

PLATE 8.3

EM Lipid Droplets

In warm-acclimated animals, the ultrastructure of multilocular brown adipocytes changes.
They become larger mainly because of increased cytoplasmic lipid content (upper panel). Lipid droplets are also larger than those found in animals kept in standard conditions or cold-acclimated (compare with Plates 2.2 and 7.6, respectively).
In many brown adipocytes, only a few lipid droplets can be observed in rats, and in mice only one lipid droplet is usually found in the cytoplasm (see the previous plate). Most capillary lumens (CAP) are nearly closed due to the hypertrophy of endothelial cells, and glycogen (G) is often found in the cytoplasm of adipocytes (lower panel).
All intermediate figures between multilocular and unilocular adipocytes can be observed suggesting a BAT to WAT transdifferentiation (whitening).

Suggested Reading

Champigny O, Ricquier D. Effects of fasting and refeeding on the level of uncoupling protein mRNA in rat brown adipose tissue: evidence for diet-induced and cold-induced responses. J Nutr. 120:1730–36, 1990.

Cinti S. Morphologic and functional aspects of brown adipose tissue. Pediatric Adolesc Med. 2:125–32, 1992.

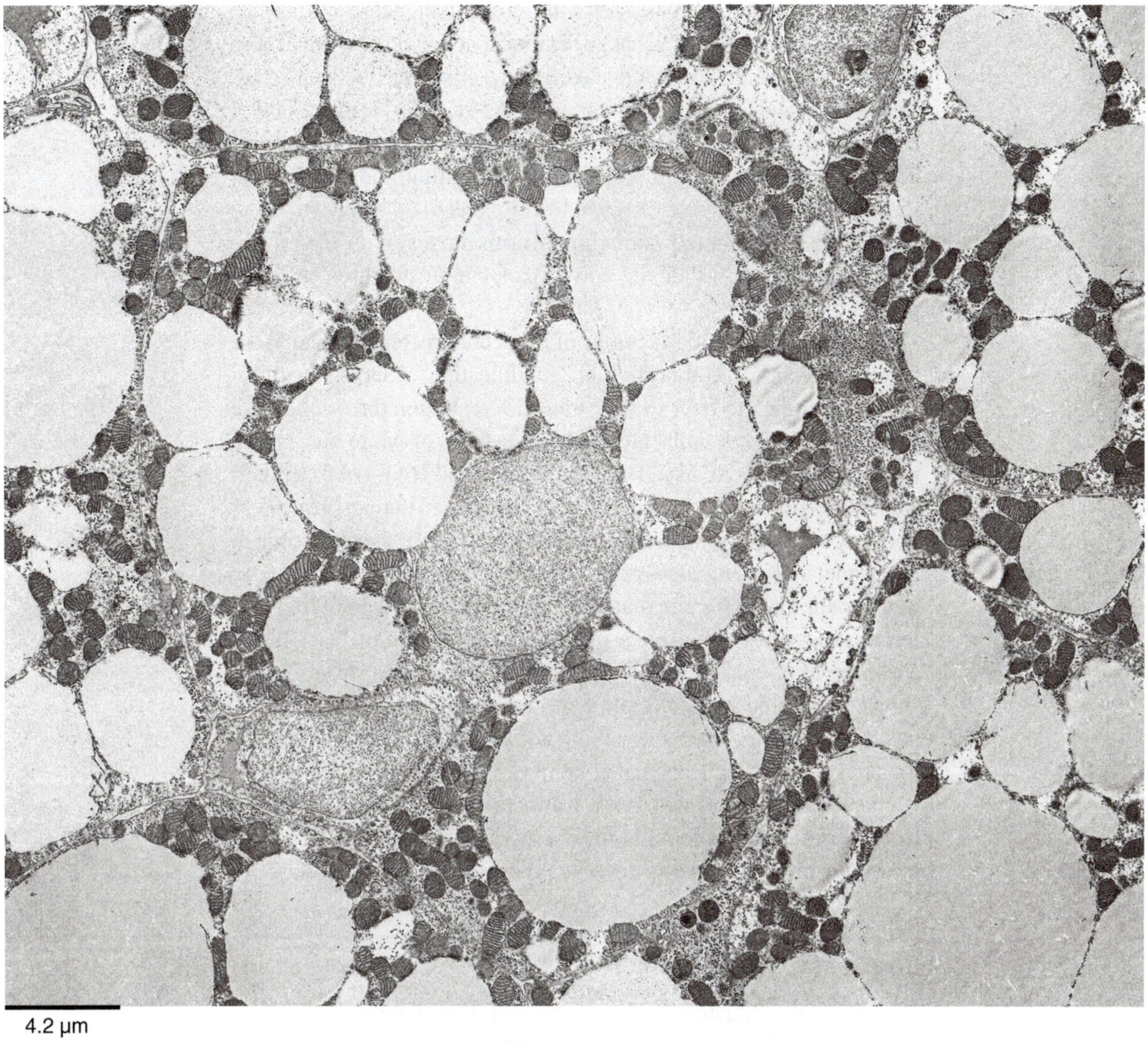

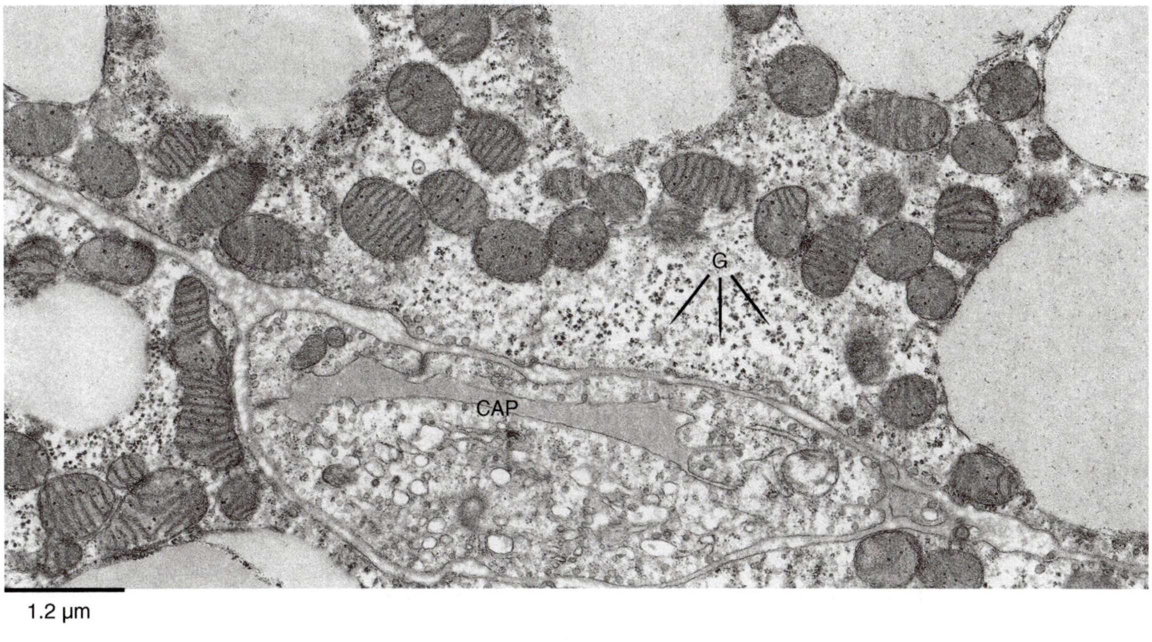

Plate 8.3 IBAT of a young rat acclimated at 25 °C for 10 days. *Lower*: enlargement of the cytoplasm of a brown adipocyte from the same depot shown in the upper figure. TEM

PLATE 8.4

EM Mitochondria

In warm-acclimated animals, one of the most striking features of brown adipocyte ultrastructure is a change in mitochondrial morphology. These organelles are small, often elongated, and the cristae are less numerous, less laminar, and less packed (compare with Plates 7.6–7.9).

The extension of the internal membrane (cristae) varies from almost complete absence (*) to complete differentiation and distribution throughout the organelle (arrows, lower panel).

The internal membrane sometimes forms honeycomb-like structures. Curved arrows in the lower panel indicate three possible phases of division.

These morphologic modifications of mitochondria recapitulate in the inverse direction the morphologic modification observed in mitochondria during the WAT to BAT transdifferentiation (browning). We found mitochondria with intermediate features of white and brown mitochondria in both WAT-BAT (browning) and BAT-WAT (whitening) bidirectional transdifferentiations. In cultured human brown adipocytes, cells with white and brown mitochondria at the same time in the same cell were also observed (see Plate 3.5). Furthermore mitochondria with intermediate features were found also in transdifferentiating white adipocytes (browning) in omentum from pheochromocytoma patients and in cultured adipocytes from fat of subjects suffering from multiple symmetric lipomatosis (MSL). MSL is a rare disease primarily involving adipose tissue, characterized by the presence of not encapsulated fat masses, symmetrically disposed at characteristic body sites (neck, trunk, proximal parts of upper and lower limbs). MSL is thought to be a disease in which brown adipocytes undergo a benign proliferative process of whitened cells.

Suggested Reading

Cinti S, et al. Ultrastructural features of cultured mature adipocyte precursors from adipose tissue in multiple symmetric lipomatosis. Ultrastruct Pathol. 5:145–52, 1983.

Rothwell NJ, et al. Brown fat activity in fasted and refed rats. Biosci Rep. 4:351–57, 1984.

Desautels M, et al. Effects of fasting and food restriction on brown adipose tissue composition in normal and dystrophic hamsters. Can J Physiol Pharmac. 64:970–75, 1986.

Trayhurn P, Jennings G. Nonshivering thermogenesis and the thermogenic capacity of brown fat in fasted and/or refed mice. Am J Physiol. 254:R11–6, 1988.

Puerta M. Brown adipose tissue thermogenesis above the lower critical temperature. Rev Esp Physiol. 45:331–5, 1989.

Zancanaro C, et al. Multiple symmetric lipomatosis. Ultrastructural investigation of the tissue and preadipocytes in primary culture. Lab Invest. 63:253–8, 1990.

Frontini A, et al. White-to-brown transdifferentiation of omental adipocytes in patients affected by pheochromocytoma. Biochim Biophys Acta. 1831:950–9, 2013.

Enzi G, et al. Multiple symmetric lipomatosis: a rare disease and its possible links to brown adipose tissue. Nutr Metab Cardiovasc Dis. 25:347–53, 2015.

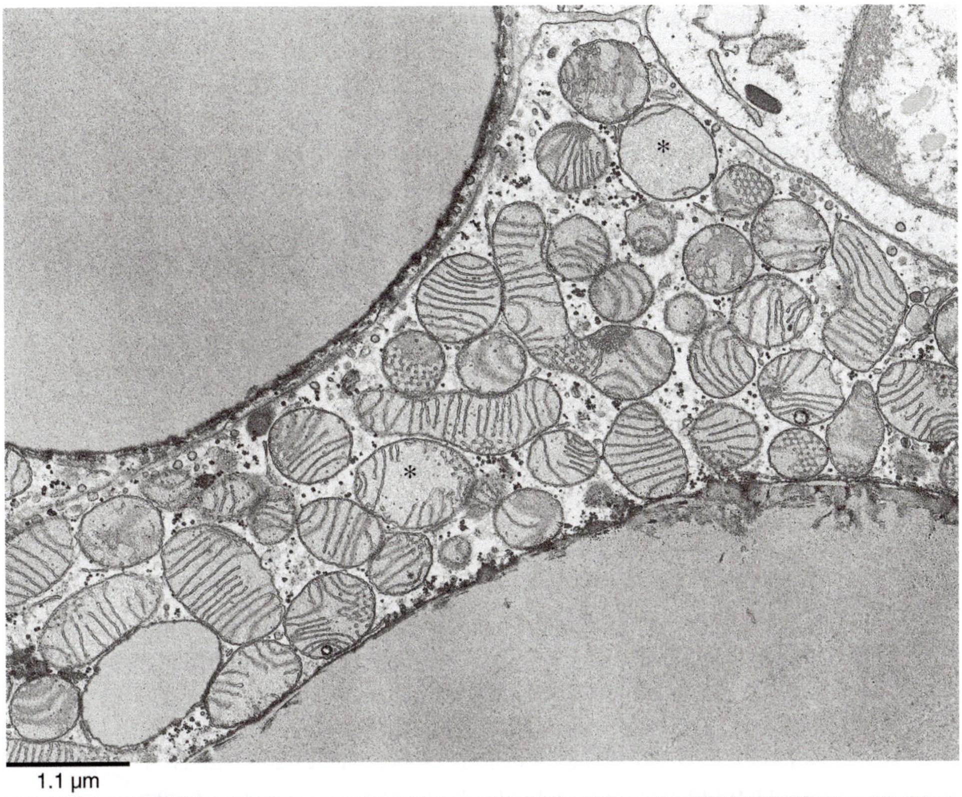

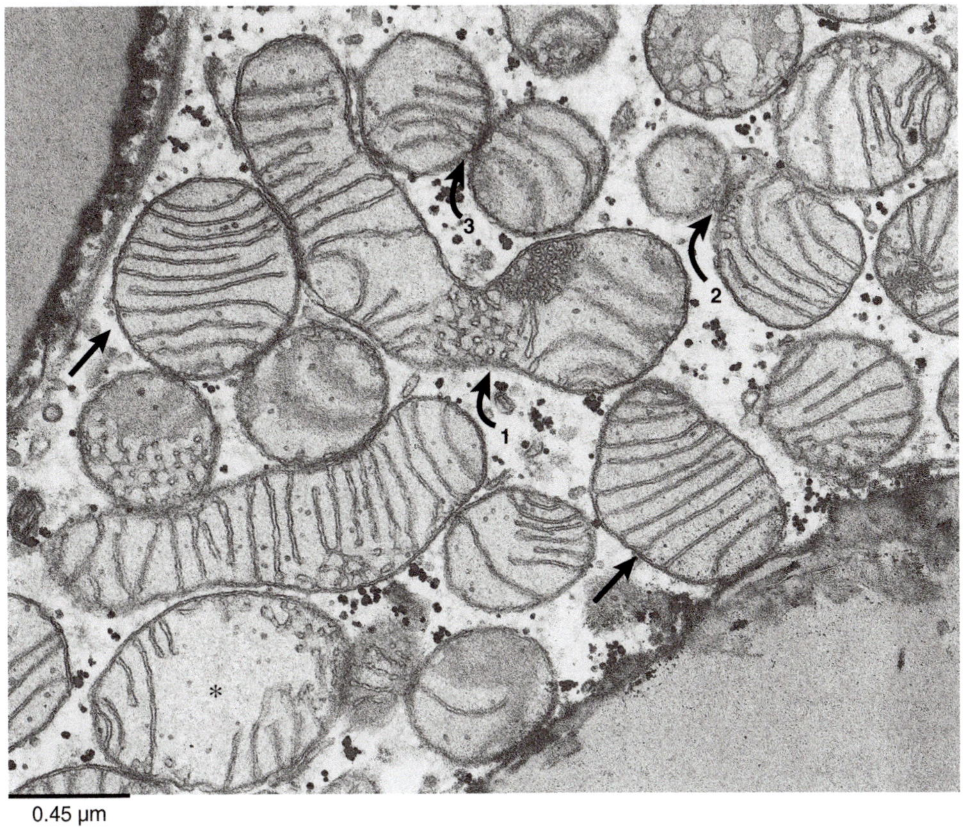

Plate 8.4 Brown adipocytes of IBAT from adult rat acclimated at 25 °C for 14 days. *Lower*: enlargement of the mitochondria shown in the upper figure. TEM

PLATE 8.5 Unilocular white adipocytes of warm-acclimated mice of Sv129 and B6 mice are enlarged in all white depots. The number and size of mitochondria reduce. Macrophage content of WAT increases, and crown-like structures can be visible (see Plate 9.6). All these modifications can be explained by the reduced afflux of noradrenaline to the tissues. Murine and human white adipocytes express the beta-3 adrenoceptor that is the most important receptor for the WAT-BAT transdifferentiation (see Plate 7.12). The size reduction of white adipocytes in cold-exposed animals and humans could be considered as an early step of white to brown conversion, at least for a subpopulation of white adipocytes prone to this conversion. These early stages of white to brown transdifferentiation were obtained also in subcutaneous fat of ferrets by beta-carotene diet supplementation and in mice treated with n-3 fatty acid diet supplementation. WAT

Suggested Reading

De Matteis R, et al. Immunohistochemical identification of the beta(3)-adrenoceptor in intact human adipocytes and ventricular myocardium: effect of obesity and treatment with ephedrine and caffeine. Int J Obes Relat Metab Disord. 26:1442–50, 2002.

Murano I, et al. Morphology of ferret subcutaneous adipose tissue after 6-month daily supplementation with oral beta-carotene. Biochim Biophys Acta. 1740:305–12, 2004.

Kuda O, et al. n-3 fatty acids and rosiglitazone improve insulin sensitivity through additive stimulatory effects on muscle glycogen synthesis in mice fed a high-fat diet. Diabetologia. 52:941–51, 2009.

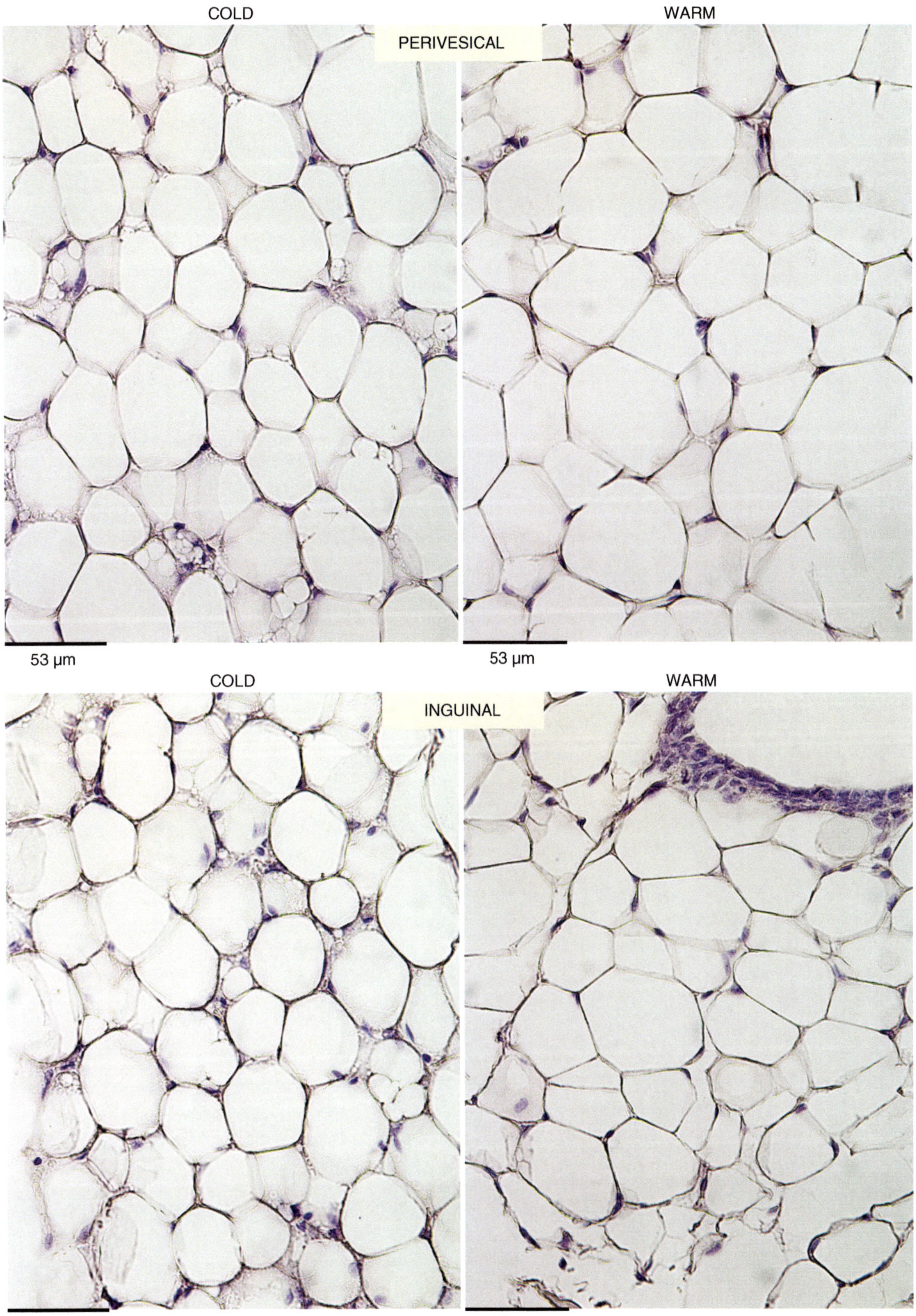

Plate 8.5 Perivesical and inguinal WAT of adult female B6 mice acclimated at 6 °C (*left panels*) or 28 °C (*right panels*). H&E. LM

9 The Obese Adipose Organ

S. Cinti, *Obesity, Type 2 Diabetes and the Adipose Organ*, https://doi.org/10.1007/978-3-319-40522-3_9

9.1 The Obese Adipose Organ

PLATE 9.1

In genetically obese db/db and ob/ob adult mice, the weight of the adipose organ is three times that of lean animals. All subcutaneous and visceral depots are hypertrophic, and about 70% of the total weight of the organ is represented by the two subcutaneous depots. Brownish areas nearly disappear in genetically obese mice.

Genetic Obesity Gross Anatomy

Suggested Reading

Faust IM, et al. Diet-induced adipocyte number increase in adult rats: a new model of obesity. Am J Physiol. 235:E279–86, 1978.

Lowell BB, et al. Development of obesity in transgenic mice after genetic ablation of brown adipose tissue. Nature. 366:740–42, 1993.

Spiegelman BM, Flier JS. Adipogenesis and obesity: rounding out the big picture. Cell. 87:377–89, 1996.

Calderan L, et al. In vivo phenotyping of the ob/ob mouse by magnetic resonance imaging and 1H-magnetic resonance spectroscopy. Obesity (Silver Spring). 14:405–14, 2006.

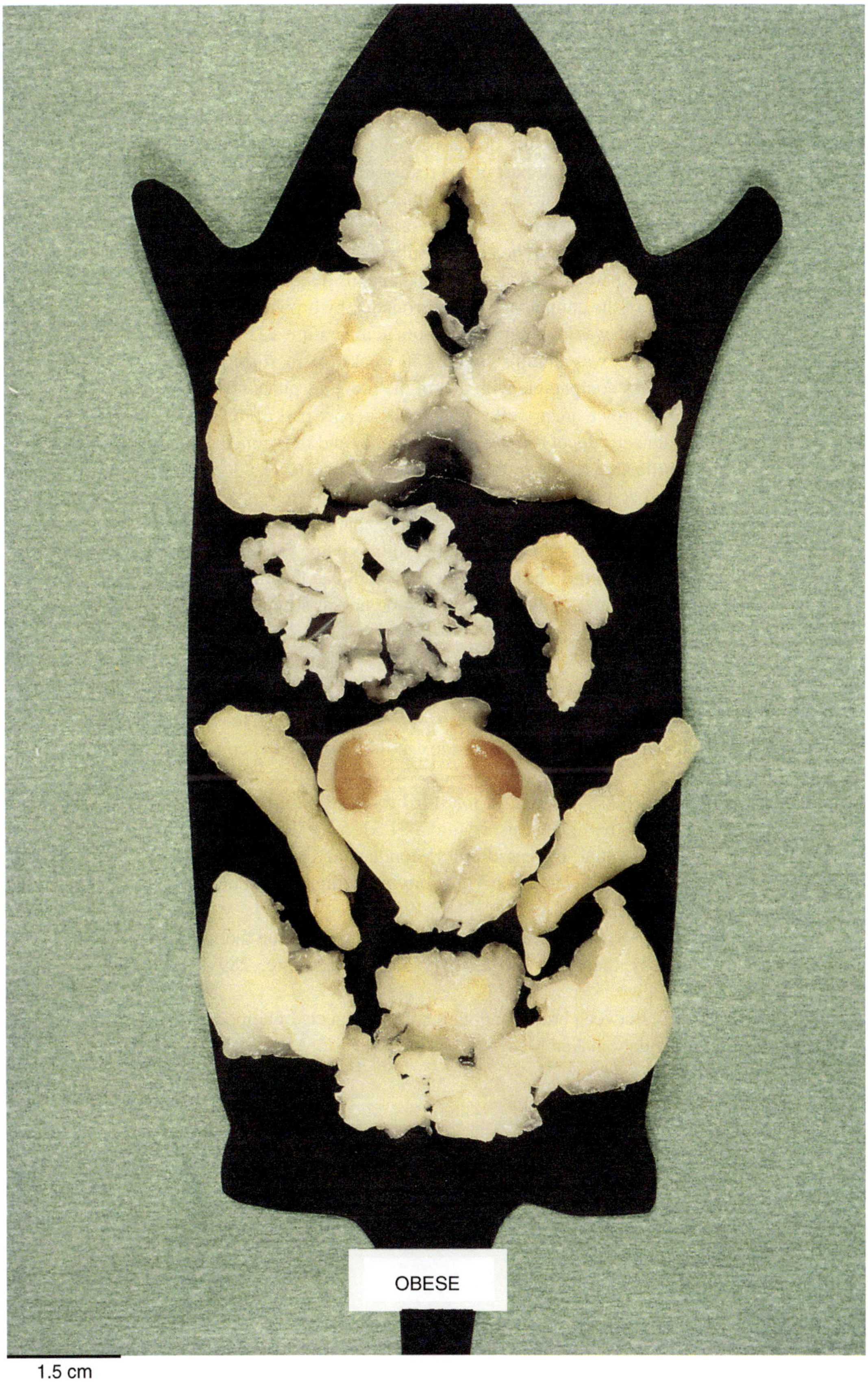

Plate 9.1 The adipose organ of an adult obese db/db mouse

PLATE 9.2

Diet-Induced Obesity
Gross Anatomy

The obese adipose organ in diet-induced obesity is shown in this plate. Dissection shows its unitary structure (i.e., anatomic continuity among all subcutaneous and visceral depots as also shown for the lean adipose organ in Chap. 1). The organ is shown as it appears after removal, as a unitary structure, from the body of the animal: the left panel shows the dorsal part of the anterior subcutaneous depot and the ventral part of the rest of the organ. The right panel shows the ventral surface of the anterior subcutaneous depot and the dorsal surface of the rest of the organ. This is due to the prevalent dorsal location of the anterior subcutaneous depot. The hole in the central part of the anterior subcutaneous depot corresponds to the neck of the animal, and it is surrounded by brownish fat.
The animal was maintained at room temperature (22 °C) and a high-fat diet was administered for 30 weeks. At sacrifice the body weight was comparable with that of the previous plate: 50 grams.
Note the brown areas well visible in the deeper part of the anterior subcutaneous depot (brown in the scheme) and in the mediastinal-periaortic area (beige in the scheme) of the organ. The dorsal part of the abdominopelvic depot is darker than the rest of the depot (pale beige in the scheme). The specific anatomical sites of brown and beige areas are indicated in the right scheme. The presence of visible BAT in this obese mouse could be due to the environmental temperature and to diet-induced noradrenergic stimuli to the adipose organ.

Suggested Reading

Rothwell NJ, Stock MJ. A paradox in the control of energy intake in the rat. Nature. 273:146–7, 1978.

Rothwell NJ, Stock MJ. A role for brown adipose tissue in diet-induced thermogenesis. Nature. 281:31–5, 1979.

Brooks SL, et al. Increased proton conductance pathway in brown adipose tissue mitochondria of rats exhibiting diet-induced thermogenesis. Nature. 286:274–6, 1980.

Perkins MN, et al. Activation of brown adipose tissue thermogenesis by the ventromedial hypothalamus. Nature. 289:401–2, 1981.

Cinti S. Between brown and white: novel aspects of adipocyte differentiation. Ann Med. 43:104–15, 2011.

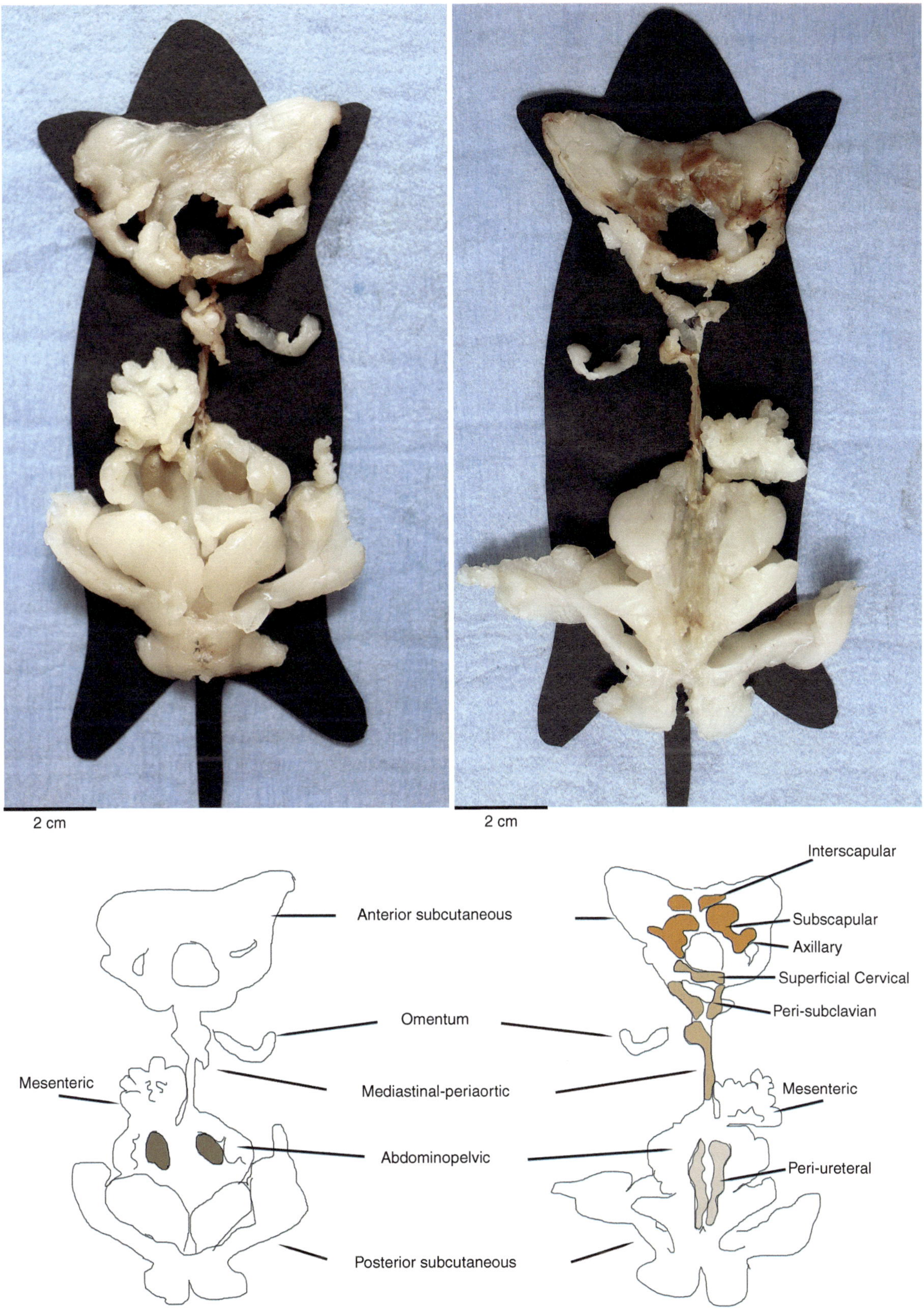

Plate 9.2 The adipose organ of an adult B6 mouse maintained in high-fat diet for 30 weeks. *Left*: anterior view. *Right*: posterior view. In this dissection the anatomic continuity among all depots (with the exception of omentum) is preserved. In schemes the different depots are indicated. Some areas are brown, beige, or pale beige as indicated. Kidneys are in their normal sites for orientation

PLATE 9.3

BAT Histology, IHC UCP1

In genetically obese animals, interscapular BAT (IBAT) is mainly constituted of unilocular adipocytes (upper panel). Their morphology is therefore similar to that of adipocytes found in IBAT of warm-acclimated animals (Plate 8.2). These cells can be distinguished from white adipocytes by their smaller size (20–50 μm vs. 80–100 μm in diameter) and their immunoreactivity for UCP1 (lower panel). UCP1 immunoreactivity was prevalent in areas containing also multilocular cells. Multilocular brown adipocytes are present as single elements or as foci of variable extension (arrows, upper figure) and are also UCP1 immunoreactive (lower panel).

Leptin administration in fasted mice increases interscapular BAT noradrenaline turnover. The absence of leptin or its receptor in genetically obese animals could be responsible for the reduced noradrenergic input to interscapular BAT and for the consequent transformation of brown adipocytes into unilocular cells. In fact, unilocular brown adipocytes can be found in lean animals in the physiological conditions known to induce a reduction of the noradrenergic input to IBAT: warm acclimation (Plate 8.2) and fasting (Plate 10.2).

In diet-induced obese animals, interscapular BAT is usually more activated than that in genetically obese mice, as is evident from its gross appearance (see the previous plate).

Suggested Reading

Trayhurn P, et al. Thermogenic defect in pre-obese ob/ob mice. Nature. 266:60–2, 1977.

Trayhurn P, et al. Effects of overfeeding on energy balance and brown fat thermogenesis in obese (ob/ob) mice. Nature. 295:323–5, 1982.

Rothwell NJ, Stock MJ. In "Brown Adipose Tissue", Trayhurn and Nicholls Eds, Arnold, 269–98, 1986.

Trayhurn P. In "Brown Adipose Tissue", Trayhurn and Nicholls Eds, Arnold, 299–338, 1986.

Collins S, et al. Role of leptin in fat regulation. Nature. 380:677, 1996.

Cinti S, et al. Immunohistochemical localization of leptin and uncoupling protein in white and brown adipose tissue. Endocrinology. 138:797–804, 1997.

Cancello R, et al. Leptin and UCP1 genes are reciprocally regulated in brown adipose tissue. Endocrinology. 139:4747–50, 1998.

Nisoli E, et al. Tumor necrosis factor alpha mediates apoptosis of brown adipocytes and defective brown adipocyte function in obesity. Proc Natl Acad Sci U S A. 97:8033–8, 2000.

Vijgen GHEJ, et al. Increase in brown adipose tissue activity after weight loss in morbidly obese subjects. J Clin Endocrinol Metab. 97:E1229–33, 2012.

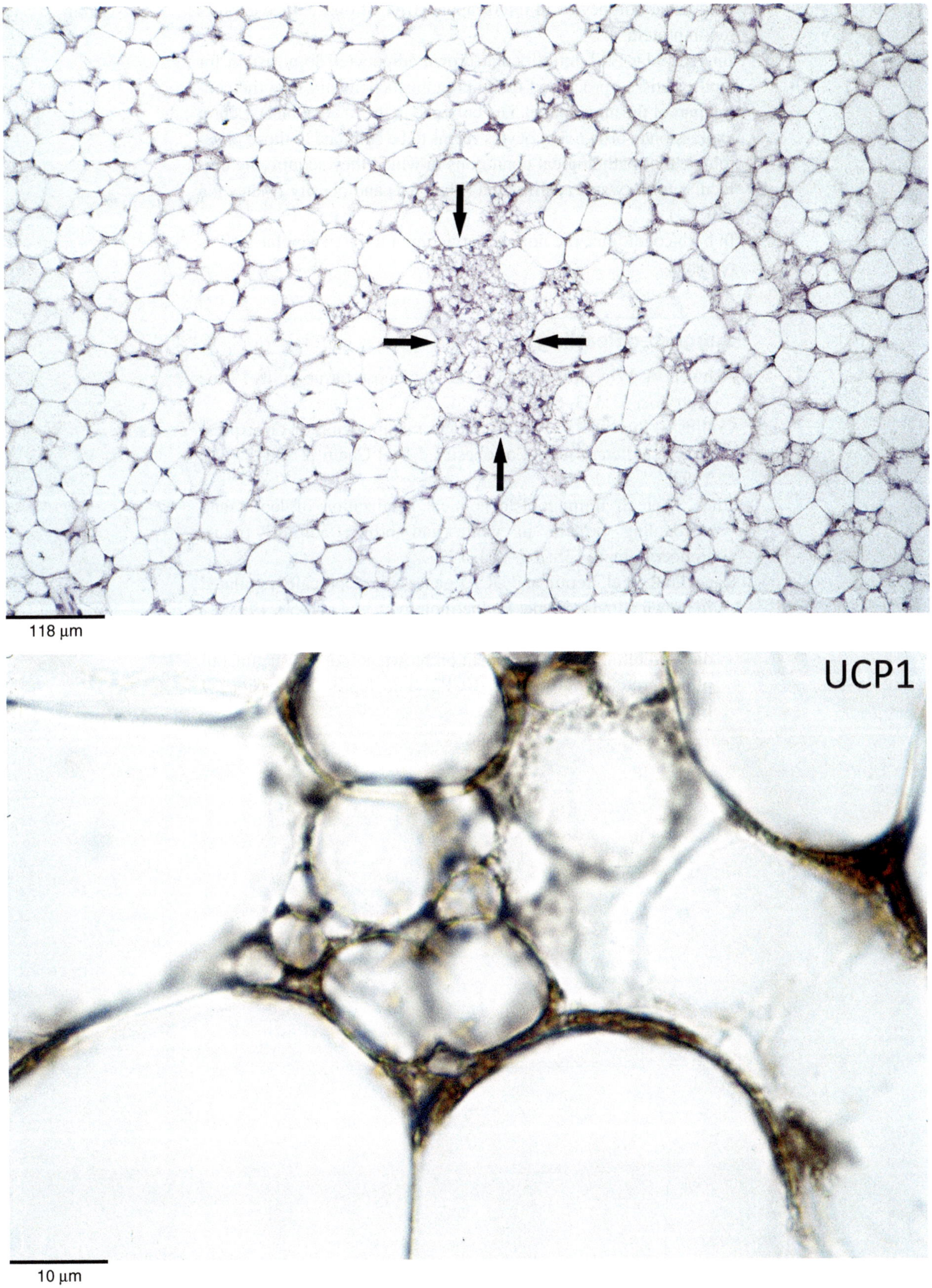

Plate 9.3 IBAT of adult obese mouse (db/db). LM. H&E. *Lower*: IBAT of adult obese mouse (db/db). Multilocular and some unilocular adipocytes are immunoreactive for UCP1. LM. IHC: UCP1 ab (1:8,000)

PLATE 9.4

IHC-Leptin

Unilocular adipocytes in interscapular BAT of obese mice express leptin protein.

Interscapular BAT multilocular brown adipocytes do not stain for leptin in tissue processed for immunohistochemistry (see the central part of the upper panel, i.e., enlarged in the lower panel). Leptin expression in brown adipocytes seems to be confined to those physiological or pathological conditions in which they acquire the unilocular form: warm acclimation (Plate 8.2) and obesity (Plates 9.3 and 9.4).

In both conditions, the noradrenergic input to interscapular BAT is reduced.

Suggested Reading

Ashwell M. Why do people get fat: is adipose tissue guilty? Proc Nutr Soc. 51:353–65, 1992.

Collins S, Surwit RS. Pharmacologic manipulation of ob expression in a dietary model of obesity. J Biol Chem. 271:9437–40, 1996.

Cinti S, et al. Immunohistochemical localization of leptin and uncoupling protein in white and brown adipose tissue. Endocrinology. 138:797–804, 1997.

Cancello R, et al. Leptin and UCP1 genes are reciprocally regulated in brown adipose tissue. Endocrinology. 139:4747–50, 1998.

Bonet ML, et al. Opposite effects of feeding a vitamin A-deficient diet and retinoic acid treatment on brown adipose tissue uncoupling protein 1 (UCP1), UCP2 and leptin expression. J Endocrinol. 166:511–7, 2000.

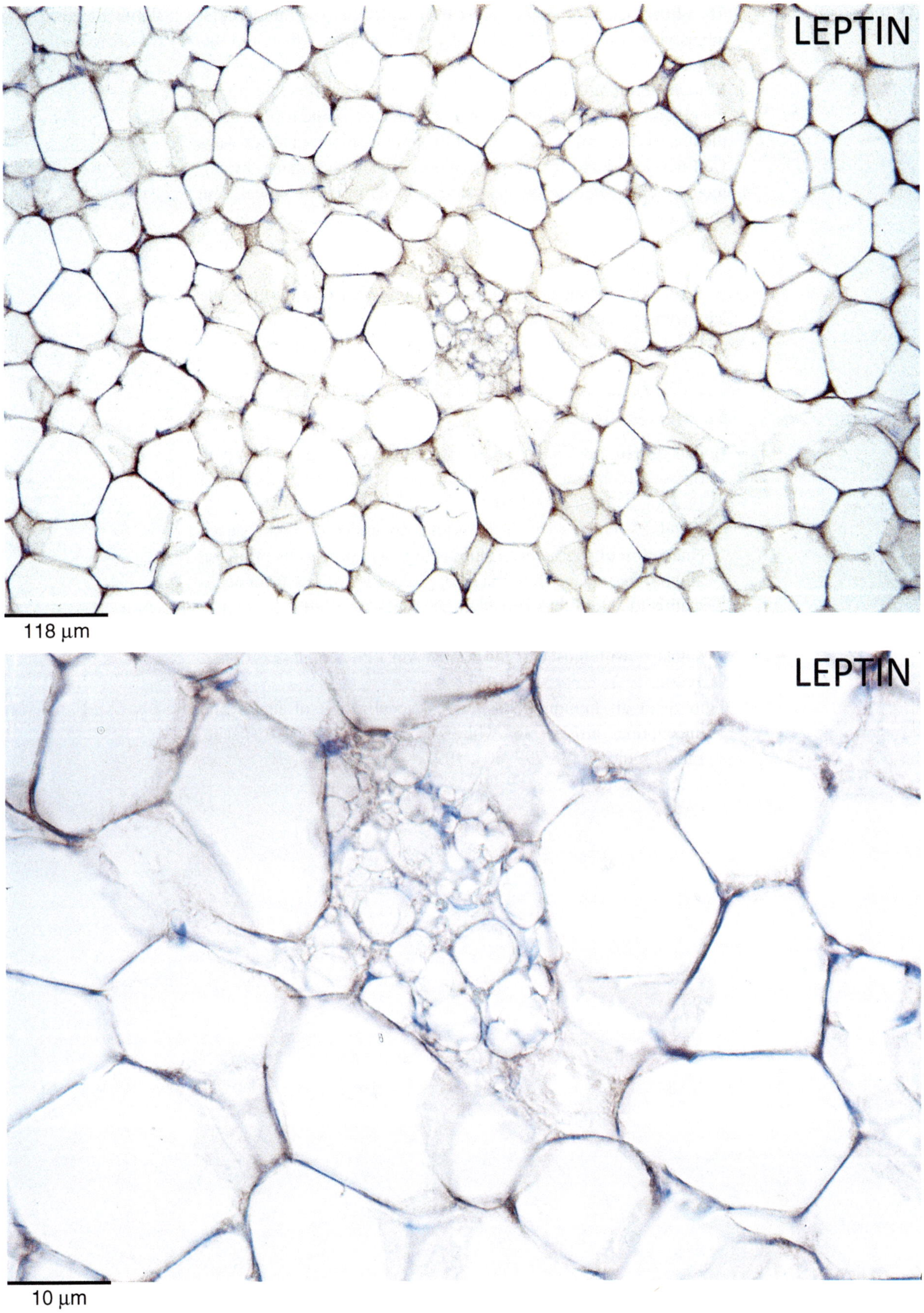

Plate 9.4 IBAT of adult obese (db/db) mouse. *Lower*: enlargement of the central part of the upper figure. LM. IHC leptin ab (1:1000)

PLATE 9.5

IBAT Electron Microscopy

The ultrastructure of interscapular BAT unilocular and multilocular adipocytes from an adult genetically obese mouse is shown in this plate.

Mitochondrial morphology is quite different in multilocular (upper panel) and unilocular (lower panel) adipocytes. In the former cells, their size is extremely variable, but the internal membrane is always well developed and forms densely packed laminar cristae. In unilocular cells their size is also variable, even in the same cell, but smaller mitochondria are much more frequent. The larger ones usually have a well-developed internal membrane with dense laminar cristae. Small mitochondria contain few cristae.

A nerve fiber (N) in a cytoplasmic invagination of a multilocular adipocyte is shown in the upper figure. Nerve fiber density is usually higher in interscapular BAT's multilocular cell foci.

Suggested Reading

Hogan S, Himms-Hagen J. Abnormal brown adipose tissue in obese (ob/ob) mice: response to acclimation to cold. Am J Physiol. 239:E301–9, 1980.

Desautels M, Himms-Hagen J. Parallel regression of cold-induced changes in ultrastructure, composition, and properties of brown adipose tissue mitochondria during recovery of rats from acclimation to cold. Can J Biochem. 58:1057–68, 1980.

Himms-Hagen J, Gwilliam C. Abnormal brown adipose tissue in hamsters with muscular dystrophy. Am J Physiol. 239:C18–22, 1980.

Cinti S, et al. Immunohistochemical localization of leptin and uncoupling protein in white and brown adipose tissue. Endocrinology. 138:797–804, 1997.

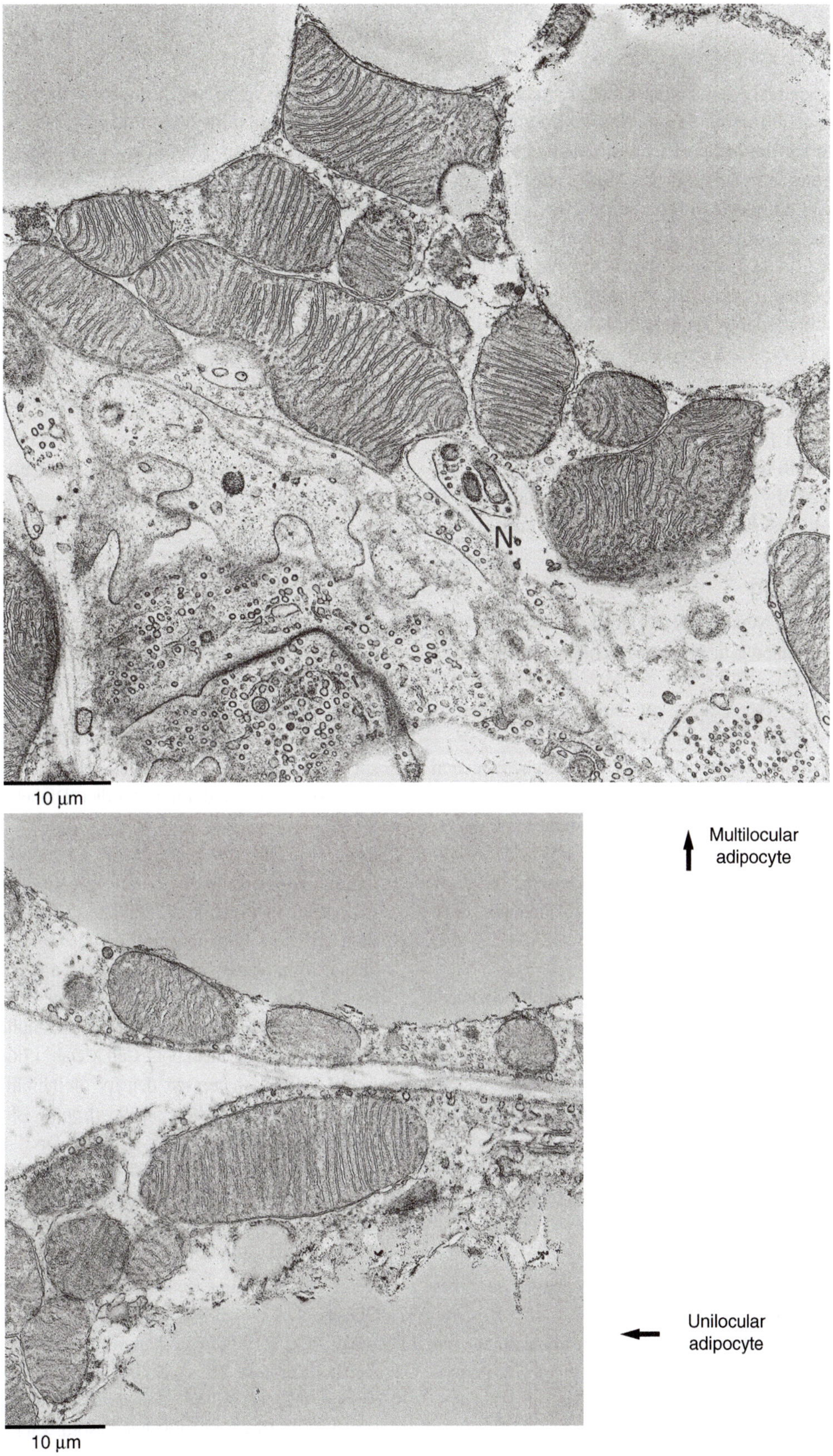

Plate 9.5 IBAT of adult obese (db/db) mouse. TEM

PLATE 9.6

WAT Histology IHC
MAC2

WAT of obese mice and humans is infiltrated by macrophages causing a low-grade chronic inflammation that seems to play an important role for the onset of insulin resistance, a major component of the metabolic syndrome and a step preceding T2 diabetes. White adipocytes in the adipose organ of obese murine and human adipose organ are hypertrophic. Our calculations in genetically obese mice (db/db) showed that in visceral areas adipocytes increase their size of about six times. Adipocytes of subcutaneous fat resulted seven times larger than controls. In ob/ob mice the increase was less pronounced, but again subcutaneous adipocytes were larger than visceral adipocytes. Mice lacking the adipocyte-specific peroxisome proliferator-activated receptor-gamma2 isoform have larger white adipocytes both in visceral and subcutaneous fat.
Adipocyte hypertrophy seems to play an important role in the development of insulin resistance, and in this context it is interesting that mice and humans with hyperplastic obesity do not develop insulin resistance.
A positive correlation between macrophage infiltration and adipocyte size has been found. We showed that about 90% of MAC2 (galectin-3)-immunoreactive macrophages (active) are organized to form characteristic crown-like structures (CLS) shown in this plate (some indicated by *). CLS were not exclusive of obese fat, but their frequency was about 30 times higher in obese than in lean fat. The size of CLS is quite variable, the largest corresponds to the size of hypertrophic adipocytes and the smallest has the central hole almost invisible (* in lower panel). MAC2-immunoreactive macrophages are sometimes aggregated in a syncytium (M, multinucleated giant cells) (lower panel* and upper panel of Plate 9.7).

Suggested Reading

Bjorntorp P, Sjostrom L. Number and size of adipose tissue fat cells in relation to metabolism in human obesity. Metabolism. 20:703–13, 1971.

Hirsch J, Batchelor B. Adipose tissue cellularity in human obesity. Clin Endocrinol Metab. 5:299–311, 1976.

Bosello O, et al. Adipose tissue cellularity and weight reduction forecasting. Am J Clin Nutr. 33:776–82, 1980.

Kubota N, et al. PPARγ mediates high-fat diet–induced adipocyte hypertrophy and insulin resistance. Mol Cell. 4:597–609, 1999.

Valet P, et al. Expression of human alpha 2-adrenergic receptors in adipose tissue of beta 3-adrenergic receptor-deficient mice promotes diet-induced obesity. J Biol Chem. 275:34797–802, 2000.

Xu X et al. Obesity activates a program of lysosomal-dependent lipid metabolism in adipose tissue macrophages independently of classic activation. Cell Metab 18: 816–30, 2013.

Chiellini C, et al. Obesity modulates the expression of haptoglobin in the white adipose tissue via TNFalpha. J Cell Physiol. 190:251–8, 2002.

Arner P. The adipocyte in insulin resistance: key molecules and the impact of the thiazolidinediones. Trends Endocrinol Metab. 14:137–45, 2003.

Yang X, et al. Reduced expression of FOXC2 and brown adipogenic genes in human subjects with insulin resistance. Obes Res. 11:1182–91, 2003.

Medina-Gomez G, et al. The link between nutritional status and insulin sensitivity is dependent on the adipocyte-specific peroxisome proliferator-activated receptor-gamma2 isoform. Diabetes. 54:1706–16, 2005.

Cinti S, et al. Adipocyte death defines macrophage localization and function in adipose tissue of obese mice and humans. J Lip Res. 46:2347–55, 2005.

Murano I, et al. Dead adipocytes, detected as crown-like structures, are prevalent in visceral fat depots of genetically obese mice. J Lipid Res. 49:1562–8, 2008.

Tchoukalova YD, et al. Subcutaneous adipocyte size and body fat distribution. Am J Clin Nutr. 2008, 87:56–63.

Kuda O, et al. n-3 fatty acids and rosiglitazone improve insulin sensitivity through additive stimulatory effects on muscle glycogen synthesis in mice fed a high-fat diet. Diabetologia. 52:941–51, 2009.

Zoico E, et al. In vitro aging of 3T3-L1 mouse adipocytes leads to altered metabolism and response to inflammation. Biogerontology. 11:111–22, 2009.

Neuhofer A, et al. Impaired local production of proresolving lipid mediators in obesity and 17-HDHA as a potential treatment for obesity-associated inflammation. Diabetes. 62:1945–56, 2013.

Tchkonia T, et al. Mechanisms and metabolic implications of regional differences among fat depots. Cell Metab. 17:644–56, 2013.

Giannulis I, et al. Increased density of inhibitory noradrenergic parenchymal nerve fibers in hypertrophic islets of Langerhans of obese mice. Nutr Metab Cardiovasc Dis. 24:384–92, 2014.

Lackey DE, et al. Contributions of adipose tissue architectural and tensile properties toward defining healthy and unhealthy obesity. Am J Physiol Endocrinol Metab. 306:E233–46, 2014.

Kranendonk ME, et al. Human adipocyte extracellular vesicles in reciprocal signaling between adipocytes and macrophages. Obesity. 22:1296–308, 2014.

Febbraio MA. Role of interleukins in obesity: implications for metabolic disease. Trends Endocrinol Metab. 25(6):312–9, 2014.

Kammoun HL, et al. Adipose tissue inflammation in glucose metabolism. Rev Endocr Metab Disord. 15(1):31–44, 2014.

Vishvanath L, et al. Pdgfrβ+ mural preadipocytes contribute to adipocyte hyperplasia induced by high-fat-diet feeding and prolonged cold exposure in adult mice. Cell Metab. 23:350–9, 2016.

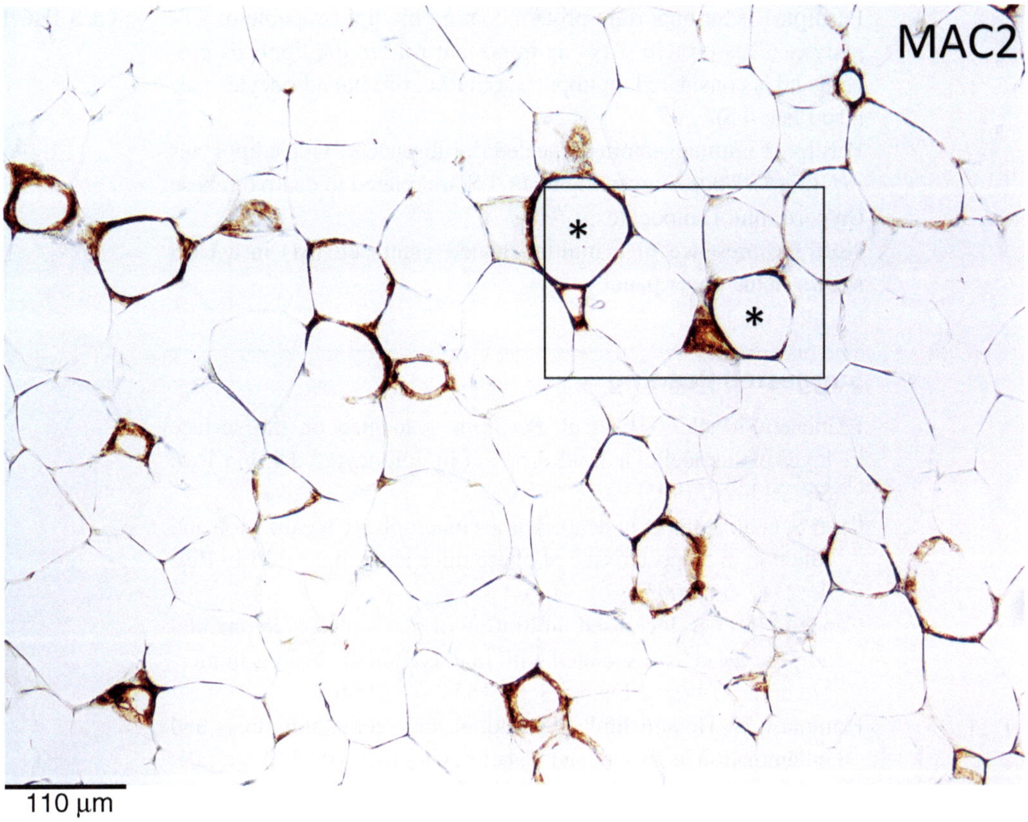

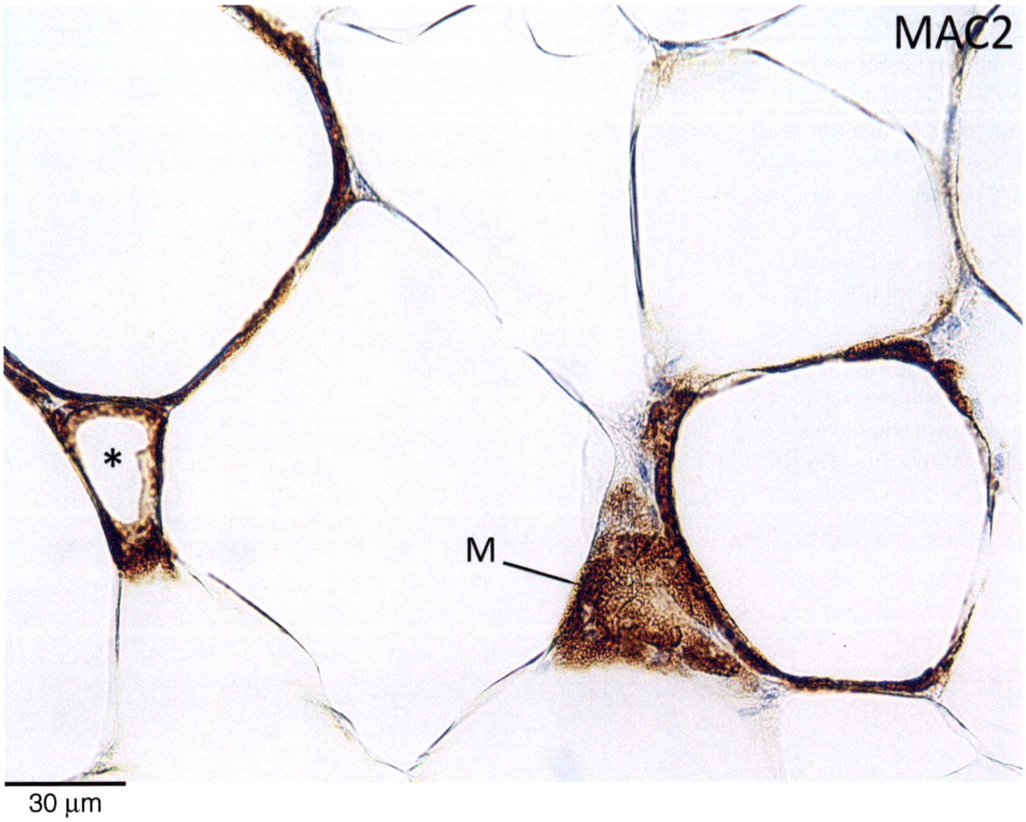

Plate 9.6 Mesenteric fat of obese mouse (db/db). Several crown-like structures (CLS) are visible among hypertrophic adipocytes. *Lower*: enlargement of the framed area showing two large CLS and one very small (*asterisk*) that could represent a very late stage of lipid reabsorption. LM. IHC MAC2 ab (1.3,000)

PLATE 9.7

CLS IHC Perilipin1

Perilipin1 is an important protein coating the lipid vacuole of adipocytes. This protein plays an important role in the lipolysis process and is considered an important marker of vital adipocytes (see also Plate 4.5).

Perilipin1 immunostaining revealed the absence of vital adipocytes in CLS (*). Thus, suggesting that CLS are related to death of obese (hypertrophic) adipocytes.

Note the presence of a multinucleated giant cell (M) in a CLS shown in the upper panel.

Suggested Reading

Blanchette-Mackie EJ, et al. Perilipin is located on the surface layer of intracellular lipid droplets in adipocytes. J Lipid Res. 36:1211–26, 1995.

Cinti S, et al. Adipocyte death defines macrophage localization and function in adipose tissue of obese mice and humans. J Lip Res. 46:2347–55, 2005.

Cancello R, et al. Increased infiltration of macrophages in omental adipose tissue is associated with marked hepatic lesions in morbid human obesity. Diabetes. 55:1554–61, 2006.

Hummasti S, Hotamisligil GS. Endoplasmic reticulum stress and inflammation in obesity and diabetes. Circ Res. 107:579–91, 201.

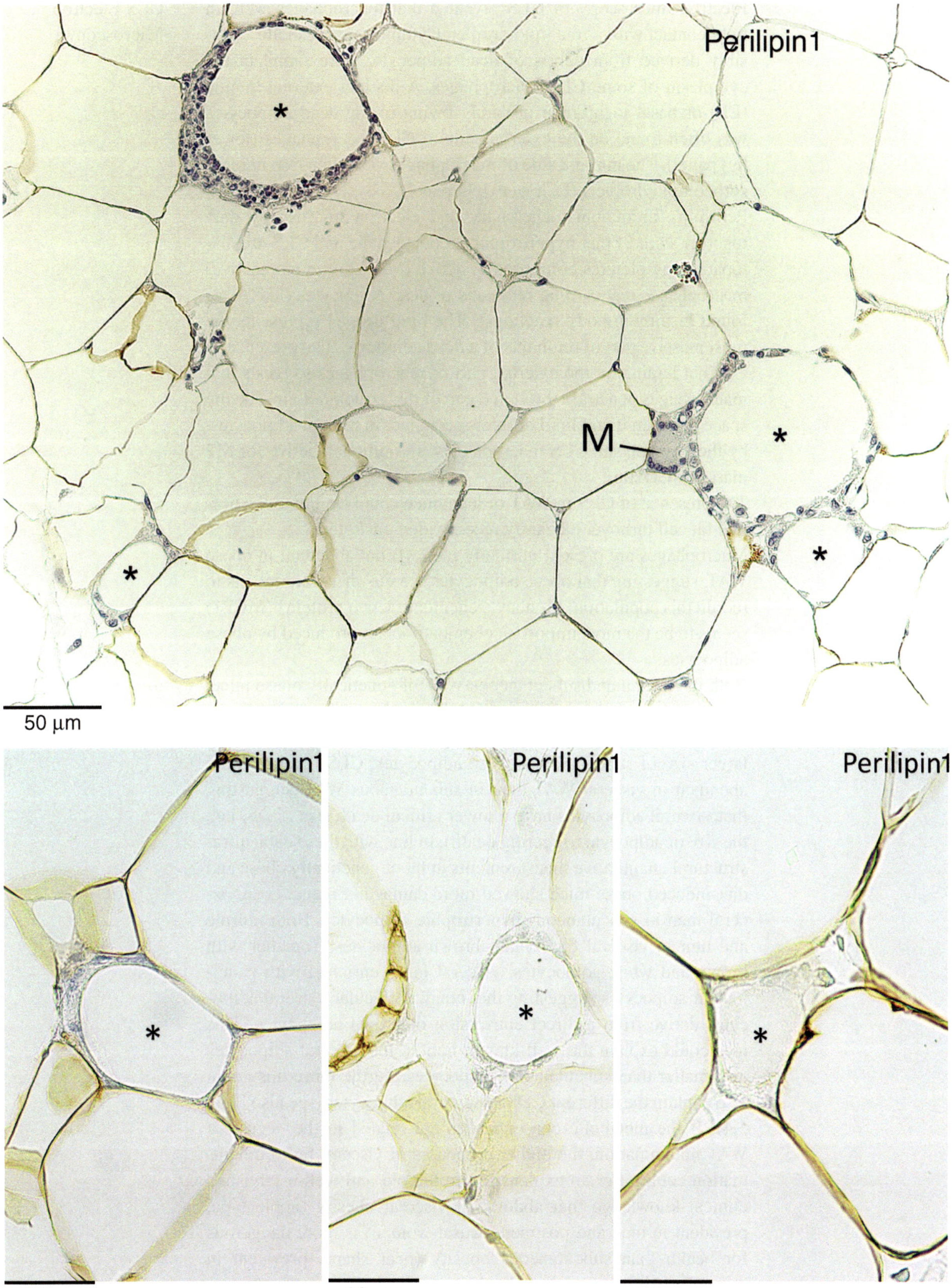

Plate 9.7 Mesenteric fat of obese mouse (db/db). CLS are always perilipin1 negative among perilipin1-immunoreactive adipocytes. LM. IHC perilipin1 ab (1:300)

PLATE 9.8

CLS Electron Microscopy I

Electron microscopy of CLS revealed that macrophages were in tight contact with a free lipid droplet. Cytoplasmic organelles, possibly derived from debris of dead adipocyte, were found in the cytoplasm of some CLS macrophages. A distinct external lamina (EL) or basal membrane probably owing to the dead adipocytes was often found on the external side of CLS macrophages (lower left panel). The internal side of macrophages was often rich in reabsorbed lipid droplets (L, lower right panel).

Perilipin1 immunohistochemistry and electron microscopy data together suggest that hypertrophic adipocytes die and CLS are histopathology pictures composed of active (MAC2 immunoreactive) macrophages reabsorbing remnants of dead adipocytes (like those found in foreign body reactions). The lipid droplet represents the most massive part of remnants of a dead adipocyte. The presence of external lamina on the external part of macrophages suggests that macrophages penetrate through a gap of this structure to invade the space between it and lipid droplets occupied, in normal adipocytes, by their cytoplasm. CLS macrophages are immunoreactive for M2 markers (CD206).

The presence of CLS in WAT of lean mice could be due to the normal fat cell turnover elegantly recently demonstrated.

Macrophages are present normally in WAT, but abundant in obese WAT, suggesting that obese adipocytes secrete chemoattractants to recruit this population. Monocyte chemoattractant protein1 (MCP1) seems to be the most important chemoattractant produced by obese adipocytes.

Both in visceral and subcutaneous WAT of genetically obese mice, a positive correlation between CLS density (number of CLS/number of adipocytes) and size of adipocytes was found. In spite of the larger size of subcutaneous obese adipocytes, CLS resulted more abundant in visceral WAT than in subcutaneous WAT, suggesting that visceral adipocytes have a lower critical death size (CDS, i.e., the size of adipocyte triggering death). In line with these data, ultrastructural quantitative measurements in fat of genetically obese and diet-induced obese mice showed more damaged organelles in visceral than in subcutaneous hypertrophic adipocytes. Both murine and human visceral fat contain brown adipocytes. Together with brown and white adipocytes, visceral fat is enriched with paucilocular adipocytes suggesting that many unilocular visceral adipocytes derive from a direct conversion of brown adipocytes. This idea could explain the well-known notion that visceral adipocytes are smaller than subcutaneous adipocytes. Furthermore this could also explain the different CDS of visceral adipocytes (see also Plate 5.4). If the metabolic consequences are related to the degree of WAT inflammation, the higher proneness of visceral fat to inflammation could offer an explanation to the old and well-established clinical knowledge that abdominal visceral obesity (apple type, prevalent in men and postmenopausal women) is more dangerous for health than subcutaneous obesity (pear shape, prevalent in women).

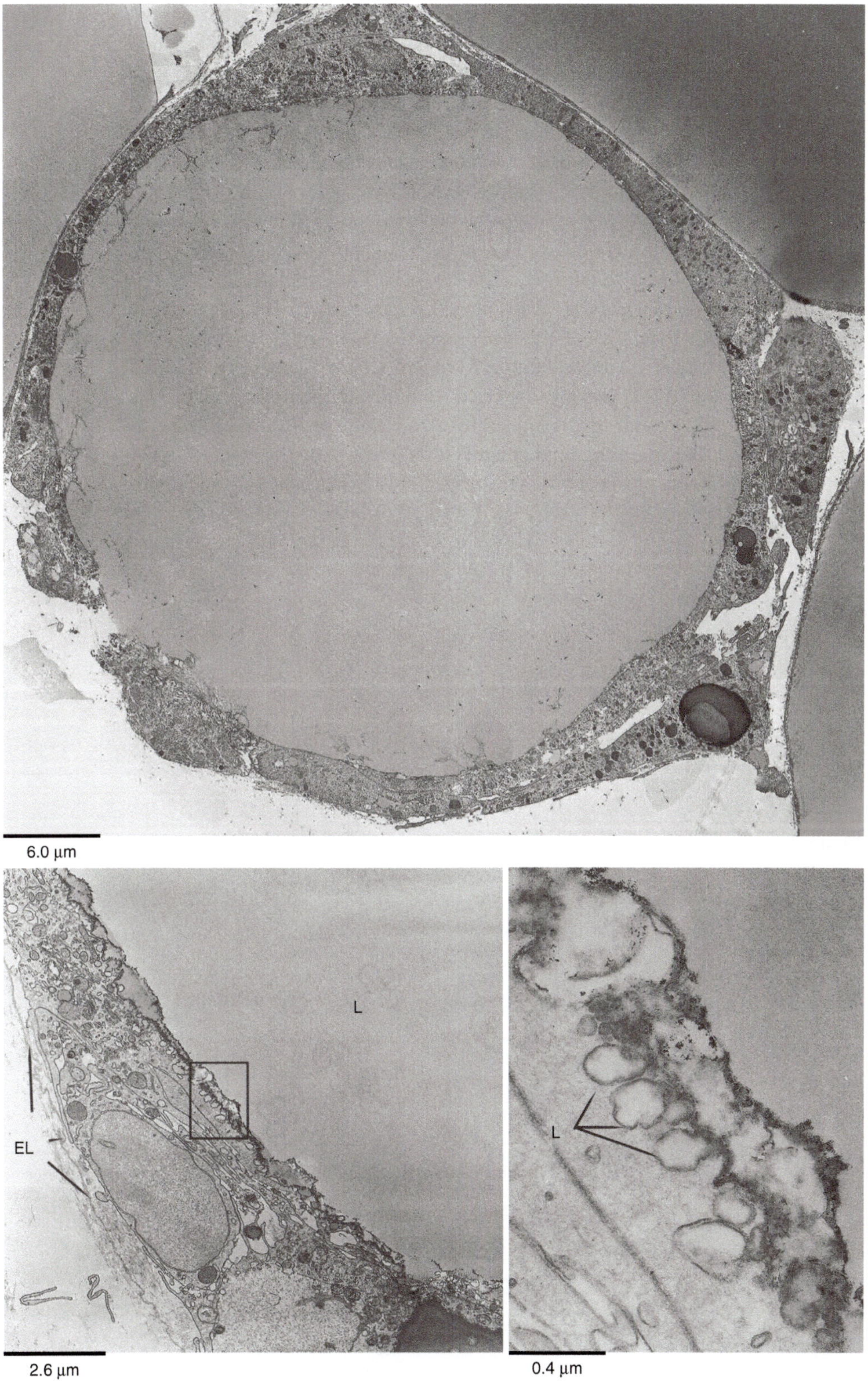

Plate 9.8 Mesenteric fat of obese mouse (db/db). *Upper*: ultrastructure of a CLS. Macrophages surround a free lipid droplet. *Lower left*: ultrastructure of the wall of a CLS; tightly apposed and interdigitated macrophages occupy the space between the external lamina (EL) and the lipid droplet (L) remnants of a dead adipocyte. *Lower right*: enlargement of the squared area showing lipid droplets reabsorption (L) by the macrophage in contact with the residual central lipid droplet of dead adipocyte (*upper right corner*). TEM. (*Lower panels* from: Cinti S. Morphology of the inflammatory state of the adipose organ in obese mice and humans. Obesity and Metabolism 2:95–103, 2006 with permission)

PLATE 9.9

CLS Electron Microscopy II

In this plate (upper panel) an enlargement of macrophages-lipid contact in a CLS is shown. Lipid reabsorption of the residual lipid vacuole of dead adipocyte is not evident in this case (compare with lower panels in previous plate), suggesting an early stage of CLS activity. Note the presence of residual discontinuous external lamina (EL). The cytoplasm of dead adipocyte is not visible (compare with the cytoplasm of a hypertrophic adipocyte visible in the upper part of the panel). Macrophages are arranged in a multilayer, as it is also apparent at light microscopy level in the upper panel of Plate 9.7.

In the lower panel three adipocytes and a macrophage, rich in primary and secondary lysosomes (Ly), are visible. The adipocyte at the bottom part of the panel shows clear signs of degeneration (cytoplasm is dense, compact, with no visible organelles), and lipid material is apparently extruded from the moribund adipocyte. This lipid material is surrounded by cytoplasmic projections of macrophage suggesting lipid phagocytosis (arrows) by the macrophage. Note the presence of a cholesterol crystal in the hypertrophic adipocyte on the left (see also Plate 9.15 for explanations).

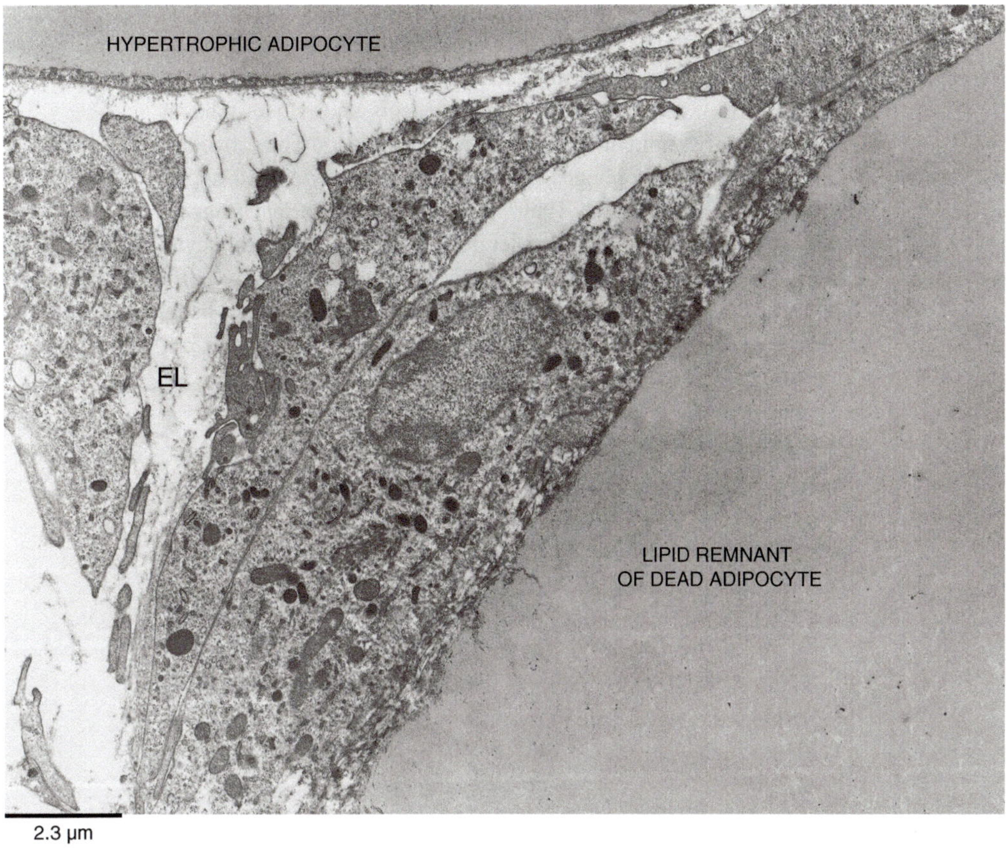

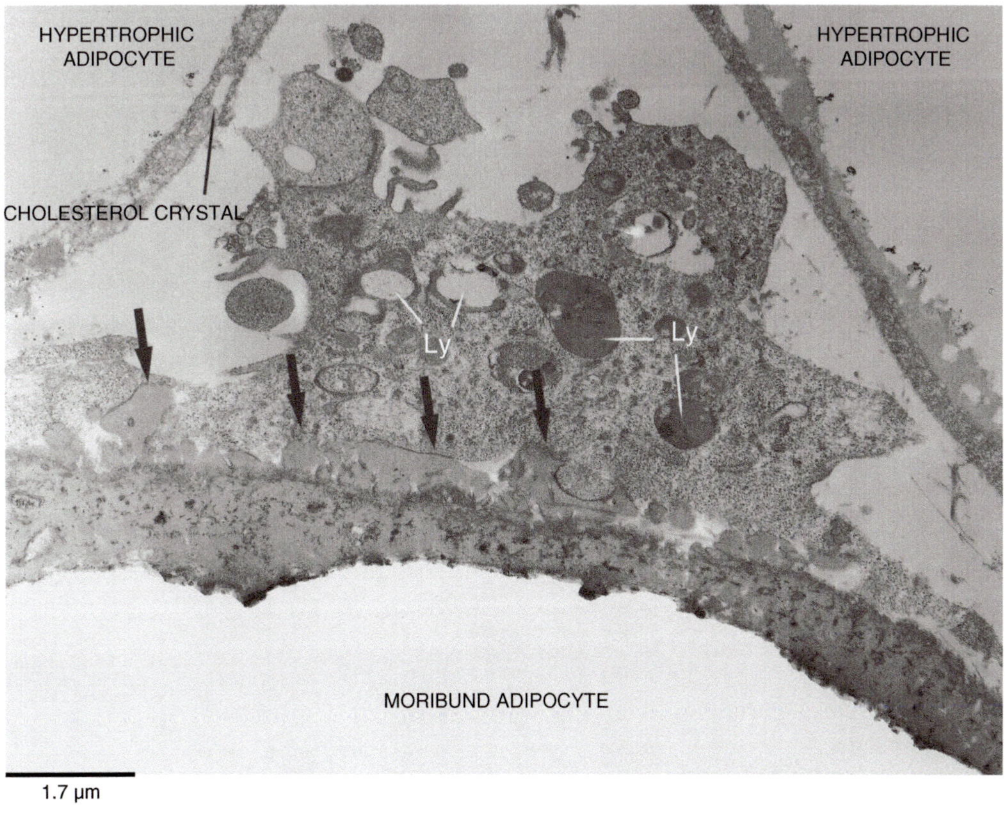

Plate 9.9 Retroperitoneal fat of obese mouse (db/db). Ultrastructure of a CLS near a hypertrophic adipocyte. *Lower*: a macrophage among three adipocytes. Morphology suggesting reabsorption of lipids extruded from a moribund adipocyte. TEM

PLATE 9.10

CLS Electron Microscopy III

This plate shows macrophages engulfed with lipid droplets further supporting the lipid phagocytosis by CLS macrophages. The top panel shows a macrophage in a CLS with a large lipid droplet in the cytoplasm (L). The middle and lower panels show macrophages with a very large lipid droplet (L) in their cytoplasm. These two last panels refer to macrophages found among adipocytes and apparently not related to CLS. They could represent the last stage of reabsorption of a free lipid droplet derived from a dead adipocyte. Their size corresponds to the smallest MAC2-immunoreactive CLS visible at the light microscopy level (compare with the lower panel in Plate 9.6).

Suggested Reading

Spalding KL, et al. Dynamics of fat cell turnover in humans. Nature. 453:783–7, 2008.

Gregor MF, Hotamisligil GS. Inflammatory mechanisms in obesity. Annu Rev Immunol. 29:415–45, 2011.

Sun K, et al. Fibrosis and adipose tissue dysfunction. Cell Metab. 18:470–7, 2013.

Giordano A, et al. Obese adipocytes show ultrastructural features of stressed cells and die of pyroptosis. J Lipid Res. 54:2423–36, 2013.

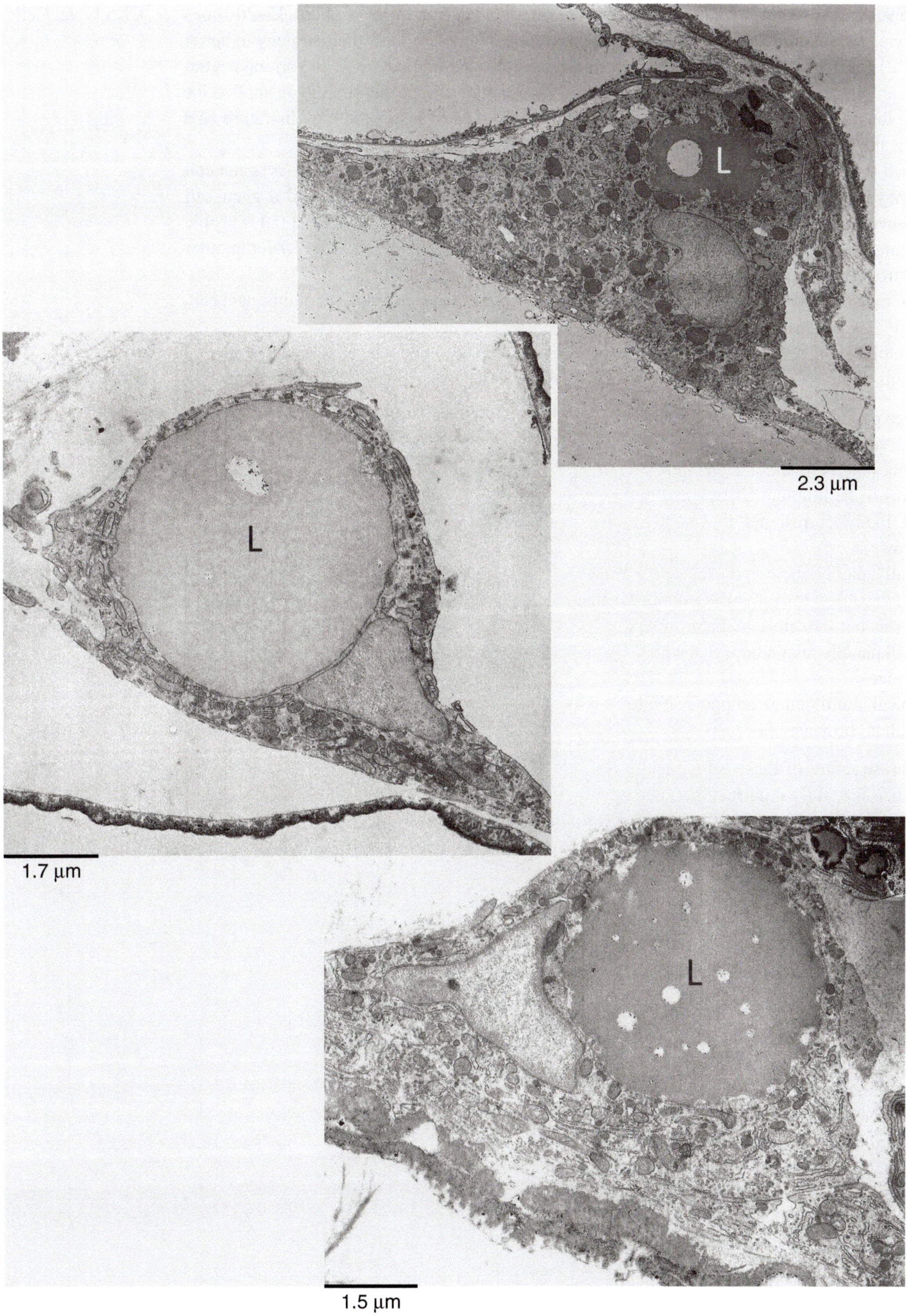

Plate 9.10 Retroperitoneal fat of obese mouse (db/db). Ultrastructure of macrophages of CLS (*top*) and in the interstitial space (*middle* and *bottom*) with large lipid droplets (L) in their cytoplasm. TEM

PLATE 9.11

CLS Giant Cells

The normal size of a macrophage in WAT is about 15–20 times smaller than a hypertrophic adipocyte. Thus their strategy to better reabsorb the giant debris of dead adipocytes is to form syncytial multinucleated cells. As a matter of fact this strategy is applied for any similar need and well known in histopathology literature as a "foreign body reaction."
In this plate a MAC2-immunoreactive multinucleated (N) giant cell adjacent to a CLS is shown in the upper panel, and a giant cell ultrastructure in close apposition to a free lipid droplet (L) is visible in the lower panel. See also the upper panel in Plate 9.7 for another example of multinucleated giant cell in CLS.
Abundant lipid droplets are present in the cytoplasm of this giant cell.

Suggested Reading

Coleman DL, et al. The foreign body reaction: a chronic inflammatory response. J Biomed Mater Res. 8(5):199–211, 1974.

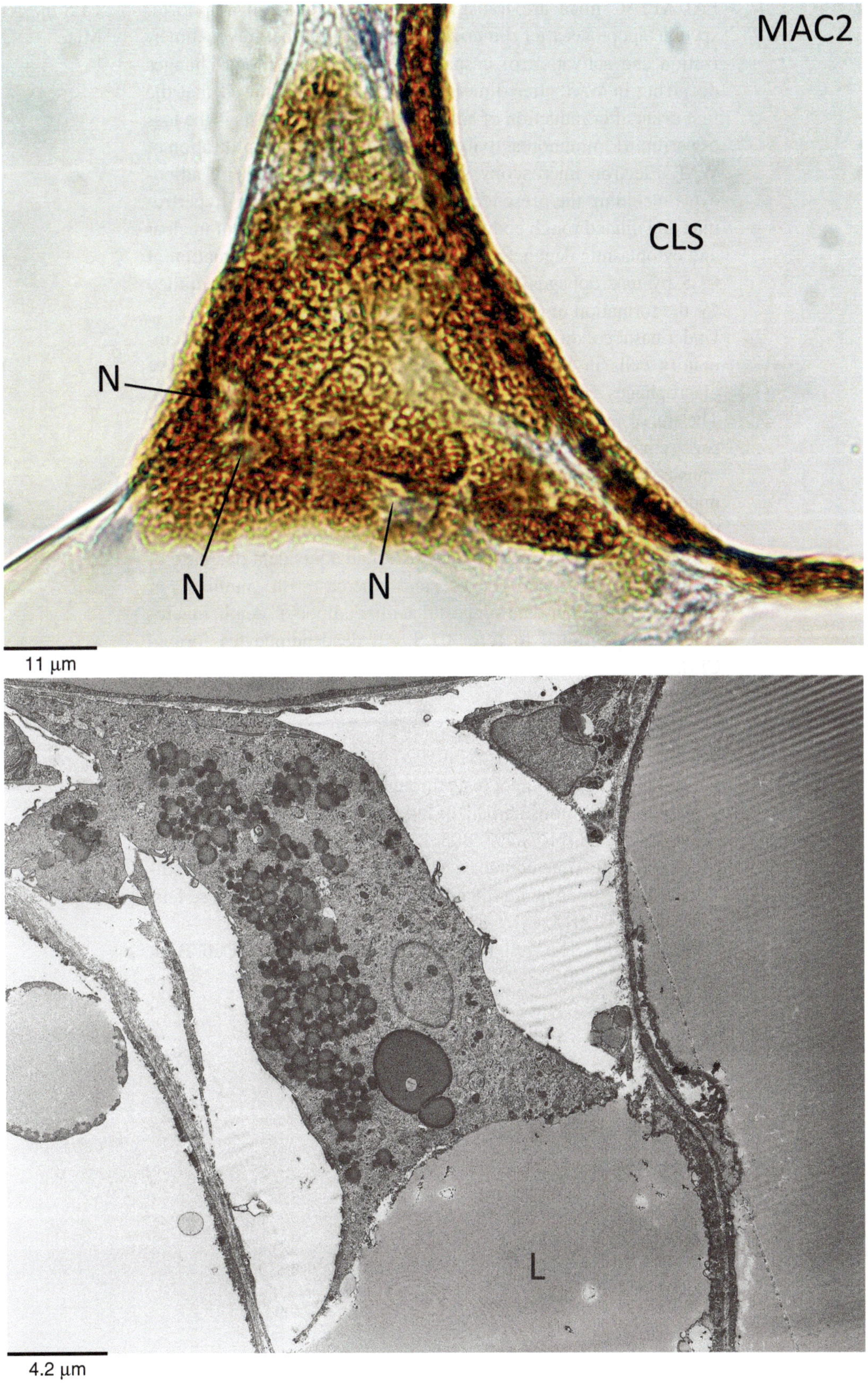

Plate 9.11 Mesenteric fat of obese mouse (db/db). *Upper*: a MAC2-immunoreactive multinucleated giant cell associated to a CLS. IHC. MAC2 ab (1: 3,000). *Lower*: ultrastructure of a giant cell. TEM

PLATE 9.12

CLS in FAT-ATTAC Mice

FAT-ATTAC mice are transgenic mice that undergo adipocyte-specific apoptosis after dimerizer administration that forces dimerization and activation of caspase-8. The histopathology changes occurring in WAT after dimerizer administration showed that the first event after induction of adipocyte-specific apoptosis is the loss of perilipin1 immunoreactivity and inflammatory cell infiltration of WAT. Electron microscopy showed several alterations in adipocytes including the presence of abnormal mitochondria, hypertrophic and dilated rough endoplasmic reticulum, and signs of nuclear and cytoplasmic degeneration. The second step is the formation of CLS by macrophages suggesting that macrophages are recruited for the formation of CLS upon adipocyte death.

Under basal conditions, nearly 90% of the small number of inflammatory cells in WAT is largely represented by MAC2-negative macrophages (inactive), and neutrophils are completely absent. The initial infiltration of neutrophils appears concurrent with the early emergence of dead adipocytes. Neutrophil populations are transient. Over time, lymphocyte numbers also reduced. The vast majority of the inflammatory cells were, at all stages studied, identified as macrophages. MAC2-positive macrophages (active) progressively increased in coincidence with an equivalent decrease of MAC2-negative macrophages and increase in number of CLS. Altogether our data suggest that after adipocyte death, macrophages are recruited to form CLS. All dead adipocytes formed CLS.

Suggested Reading

Pajvani UB, et al. Fat apoptosis through targeted activation of caspase 8: a new mouse model of inducible and reversible lipoatrophy. Nat Med. 11(7):797–803, 2005.

Murano I, et al. Time course of histomorphological changes in adipose tissue upon acute lipoatrophy. Nutr Metab Cardiovasc Dis. 23:723–31, 2013.

Rutkowski JM. The cell biology of fat expansion. J Cell Biol. 208:501–12, 2015.

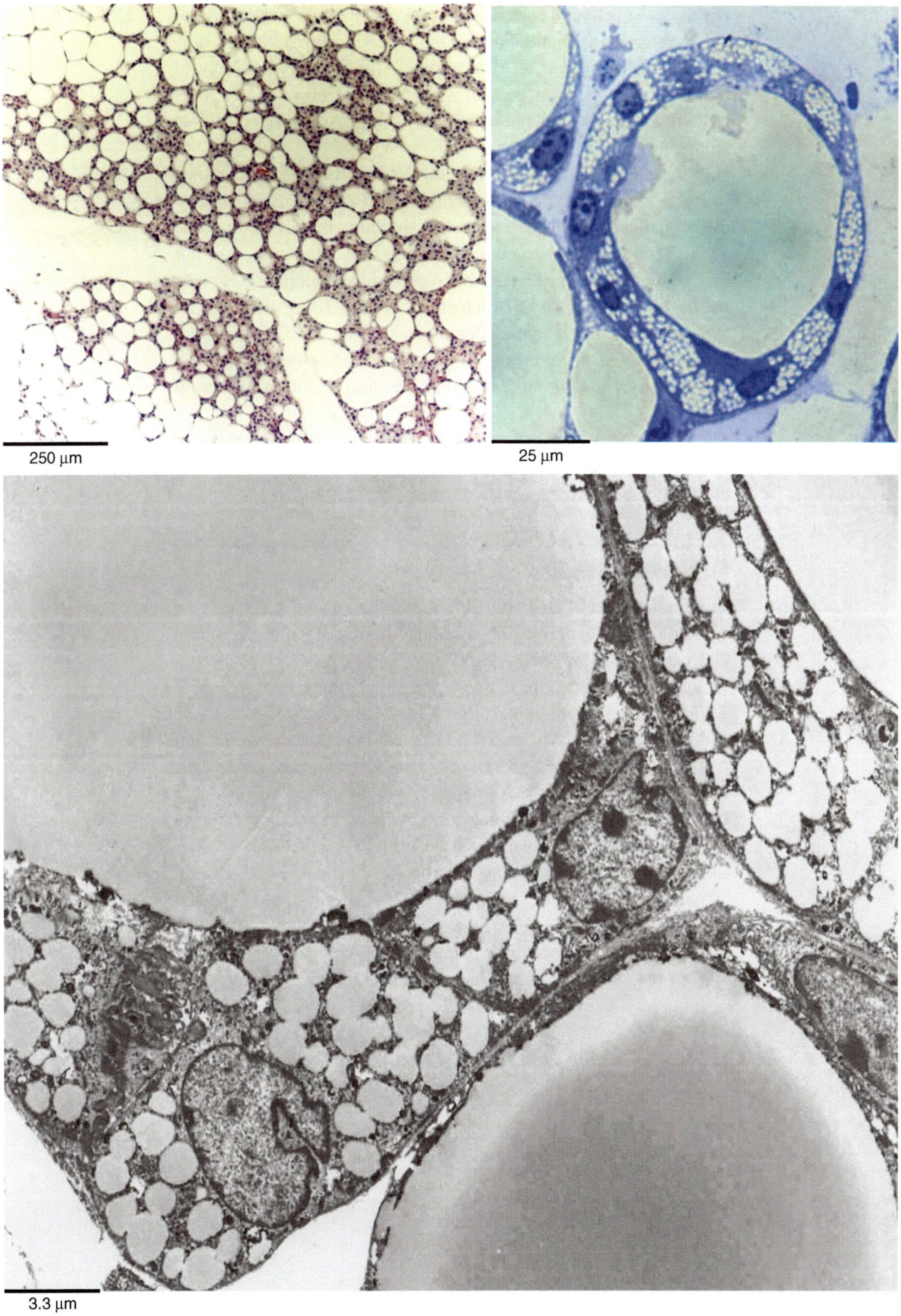

Plate 9.12 FAT-ATTAC transgenic mouse. Mesenteric fat after 10 days of dimerizer treatment. All dead adipocytes form classic CLS with lipid-laden macrophages. *Upper left*: LM. H&E. *Upper right*: classic CLS. LM. Resin embedded tissue. Toluidine blue. *Lower*: classic CLS. TEM

PLATE 9.13

HSL-KO CLS

Hormone-sensitive lipase (HSL) is a major lipase in mature adipocytes, and HSL abrogation results in increased adipocyte lipid storage and, thus, adipocyte hypertrophy. Adipocyte hypertrophy in HSL-KO mice is not associated with increased adipose mass; thus HSL-KO mice are lean, but their WAT is composed of hypertrophic adipocytes similar to those found in obese mice.

A representative example of visceral WAT of these HSL-KO mice is shown in this plate. Note the abundance of F4/80 (mature macrophage marker) immunoreactive CLS, similar to that found in obese WAT. Thus the CLS structures, i.e., death of adipocytes, are not linked to obesity per se but to the hypertrophic condition.

In the lower panel an enlargement of a CLS from the same fat shown in the upper panel demonstrates that macrophages are immunoreactive for perilipin2 (a lipid droplet-associated protein that increases in cells in response to the accumulation of neutral lipid).

Macrophages of CLS are immunoreactive for several markers of active macrophages: MAC2, F4/80, perilipin2, and CD64. In humans CLS macrophages stain mainly for CD64.

Suggested Reading

Brasaemle D, et al. Adipose differentiation related protein is an ubiquitously expressed lipid storage droplet-associated protein. J Lipid Res. 38:2249–63, 1997.

Wang SP, et al. The adipose tissue phenotype of hormone-sensitive lipase deficiency in mice. Obes Res. 9:119–28, 2001.

Cinti S, et al. Adipocyte death defines macrophage localization and function in adipose tissue of obese mice and humans. J Lip Res. 46:2347–55, 2005.

Lumeng CN, et al. Obesity induces a phenotypic switch in adipose tissue macrophage polarization. J Clin Invest. 117:175–84, 2007.

Lumeng CN, et al. Increased inflammatory properties of adipose tissue macrophages recruited during diet-induced obesity. Diabetes. 56:16–23, 2007.

Shaul ME, et al. Dynamic, M2-like remodeling phenotypes of CD11c+ adipose tissue macrophages during high-fat diet–induced obesity in mice. Diabetes. 59:1171–81, 2010.

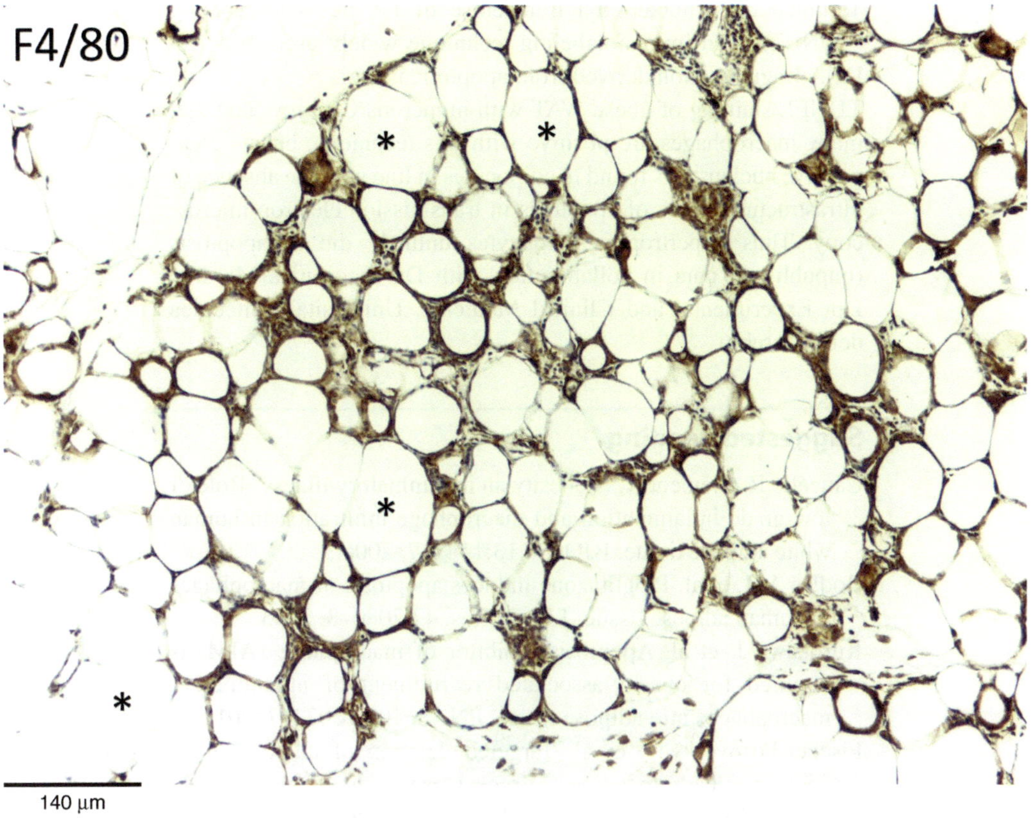

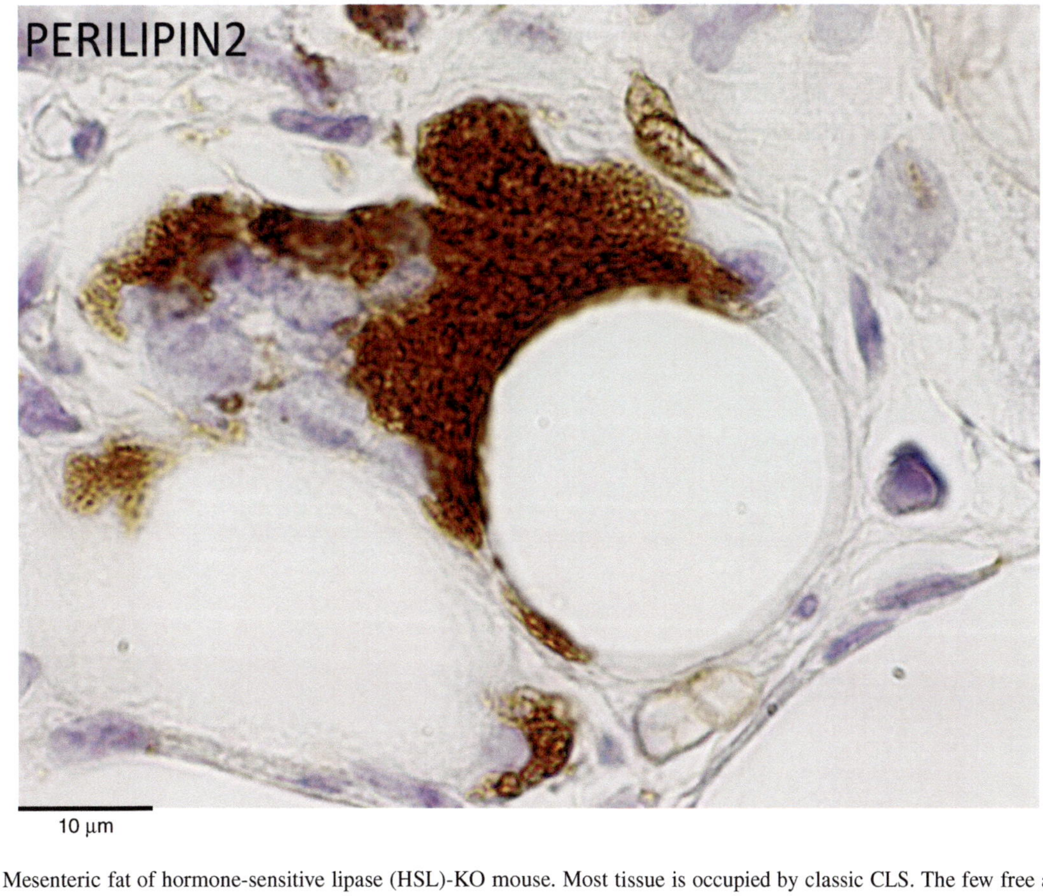

Plate 9.13 Mesenteric fat of hormone-sensitive lipase (HSL)-KO mouse. Most tissue is occupied by classic CLS. The few free adipocytes are hypertrophic (*asterisk*, some indicated). LM. IHC F4/80 ab (1:150). *Lower*: a CLS partially formed by perilipin2-immunoreactive macrophages. LM. IHC perilipin2 ab (1:300)

PLATE 9.14

CLS TUNEL

Terminal deoxynucleotidyl transferase dUTP nick end labeling (TUNEL) is an immunolabeling technique widely used to detect DNA fragmentation derived from apoptotic nuclei.

TUNEL staining of obese WAT with numerous CLS revealed that many macrophages are positive with this technique, but no clear positive nucleus was found in adipocytes in line with the absence of ultrastructural signs of apoptosis in transmission electron microscopy. Thus hypertrophic adipocytes unlikely die of apoptosis (unpublished data in collaboration with Dr. Incoronata Murano, Dpt Experimental and Clinical Medicine, Università Politecnica delle Marche).

Suggested Reading

Cancello R, Clément K. Is obesity an inflammatory illness? Role of low-grade inflammation and macrophage infiltration in human white adipose tissue. BJOG. 113:1141–7, 2006.

Bodles AM, et al. Pioglitazone induces apoptosis of macrophages in human adipose tissue. J Lipid Res. 47:2080–8, 2006.

Kurokawa J, et al. Apoptosis inhibitor of macrophage (AIM) is required for obesity-associated recruitment of inflammatory macrophages into adipose tissue. PNAS. 108:12072–7, 2011.

Fischer-Posovszky P, et al. Targeted deletion of adipocytes by apoptosis leads to adipose tissue recruitment of alternatively activated M2 macrophages. Endocrinology. 152:3074–81, 2011.

Dalmas E, et al. Defining macrophage phenotype and function in adipose tissue. Trends Immunol. 32:307–14, 2011.

Kyrylkova K, et al. Detection of apoptosis by TUNEL assay. Methods Mol Biol. 887:41–7, 2012.

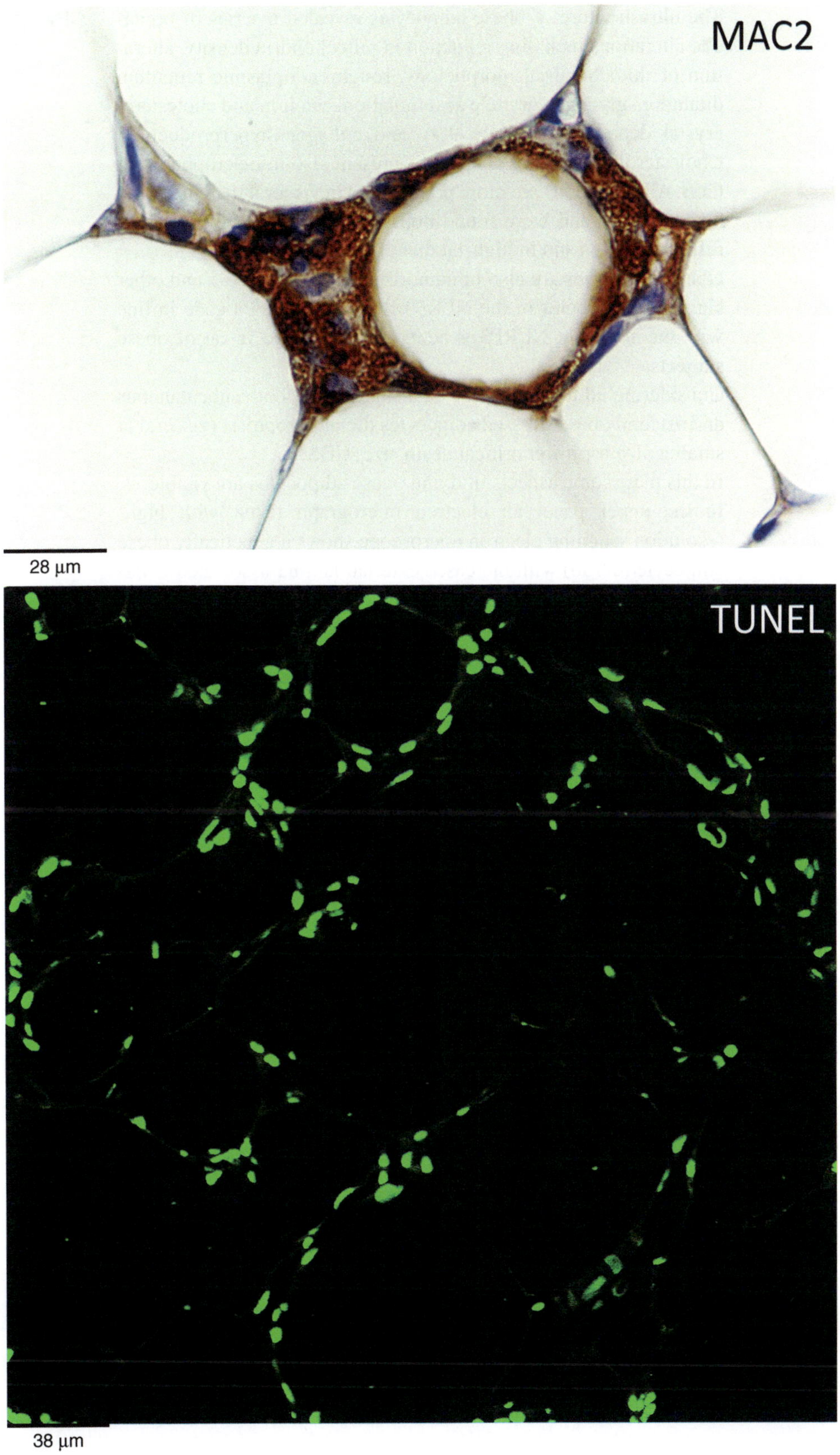

Plate 9.14 *Upper*: epididymal fat of diet-induced obese mouse. Classic CLS. LM. IHC MAC2 ab (1.3,000). *Lower*: mesenteric fat of HSL-KO mouse. Many classic CLS (compare with the *upper panel*) are present. Positive nuclei are very likely to own to macrophages. LM (immunofluorescence). IHC TUNEL method

PLATE 9.15

Pyroptosis

The ultrastructure of obese adipocytes revealed a series of organelle alterations including reduction in mitochondria density, alteration of mitochondrial morphology, rough endoplasmic reticulum dilatation, glycogen granule accumulation, calcium and cholesterol crystal deposits (see Plate 9.9), and collagen hyperproduction. Cholesterol crystals are sometimes present also in macrophages of CLS. All alterations are more pronounced in visceral than in subcutaneous WAT and were found both in genetically obese mice of different strains and in high-fat diet obese mice.

Obese adipocytes are also immunoreactive for caspase-1 and other signaling molecules of the NLRP3 inflammasome cascade in line with the abundant NLRP3 gene expression found in fat of obese subjects.

Considering all together these data suggest that both subcutaneous and visceral obese stressed adipocytes die of pyroptosis (visceral at smaller size for lower critical death size, CDS).

In this plate some aspects of dying obese adipocytes are visible.

In the upper panel an electron micrograph taken with high-resolution scanning electron microscope shows a genetically obese adipocyte (db/db) with increased external lamina-associated collagen fibrils and protruding lipid droplets (arrows, some indicated). One of the larger lipid droplets (white arrow) possibly derived from this adipocyte is surrounded by macrophages (Mac), in line with the idea that macrophages act on debris derived from dead or dying adipocytes.

The corresponding ultrastructure observed with transmission electron microscopy is visible in the lower panel: two dying adipocytes (L, their main lipid droplet) with degenerating electron-dense cytoplasmic rim are shown. Note the lipid droplets protruding from the cells (arrows). A macrophage (Mac) in the interstitium is surrounding the protruded lipid material with its cytoplasmic projections, and a phagocytized big lipid droplet (L) is visible in its cytoplasm.

Suggested Reading

Vandanmagsar B, et al. The NLRP3 inflammasome instigates obesity-induced inflammation and insulin resistance. Nat Med. 17:179–88, 2011.

Giordano A, et al. Obese adipocytes show ultrastructural features of stressed cells and die of pyroptosis. J Lipid Res. 54:2423–36, 2013.

Gautheron J, et al. The necroptosis-inducing kinase RIPK3 dampens adipose tissue inflammation and glucose intolerance. Nat Commun. 7:11869, 2016.

Vitale G, et al. Oxidative stress and the ageing endocrine system. Nat Rev Endocrinol. 9:228–40, 2013.

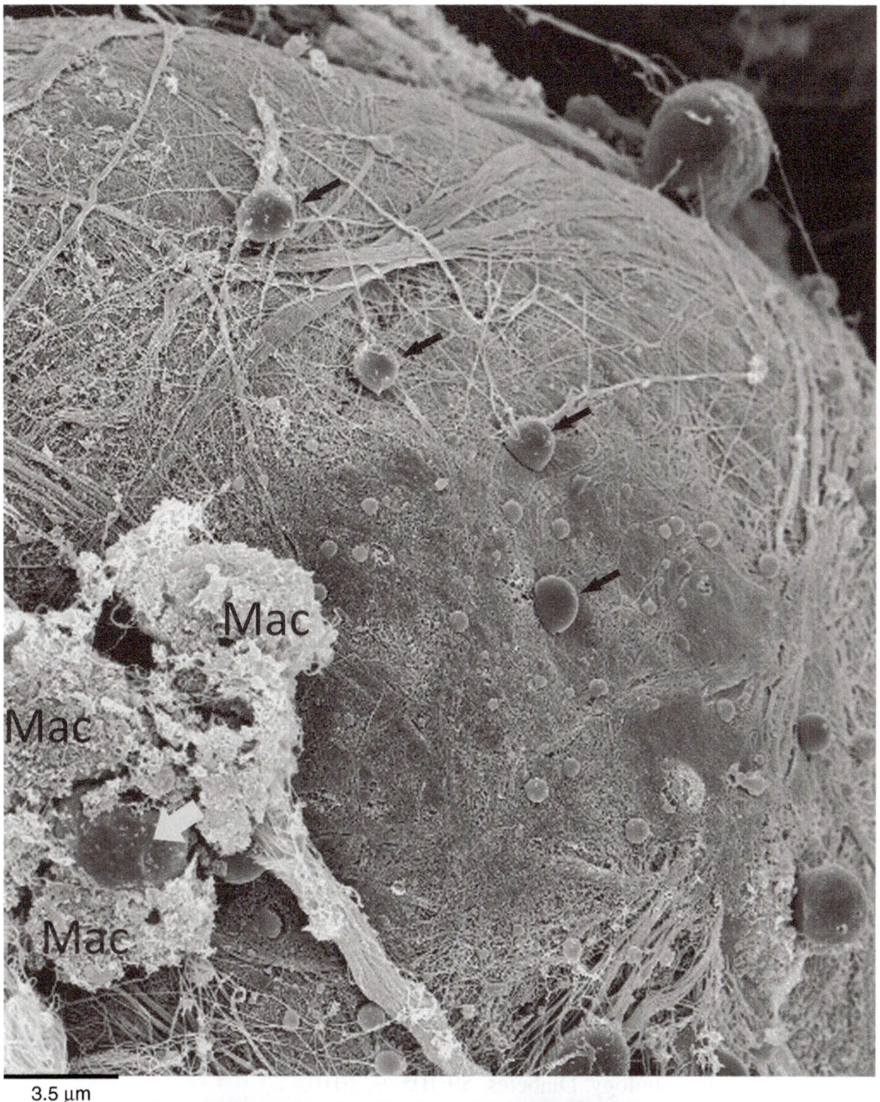

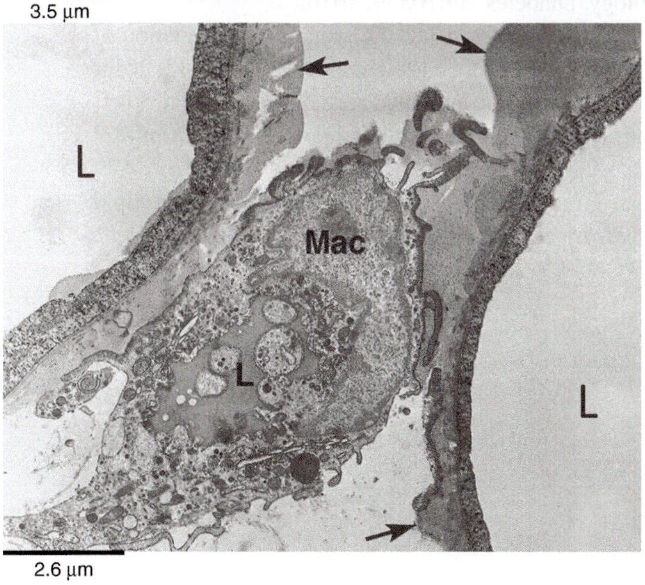

Plate 9.15 Mesenteric fat of obese mouse (db/db). Obese "moribund" adipocytes extruding lipid droplets and with thickened collagen coating, observed by high-resolution SEM (*upper*) and TEM (*lower*). (From Fig. 7 in Giordano A et al. Obese adipocytes show ultrastructural features of stressed cells and die of pyroptosis. J Lipid Res. 54:2423–36, 2013 with permission)

PLATE 9.16

Human Hypertrophic Adipocyte TEM

Human hypertrophic adipocytes can show a well-preserved ultrastructure (compare with Plate 9.17). The adipocyte shown in this plate is from the intermuscular fat of an overweight patient. The framed area is enlarged in the lower panel. The enlargement shows the very thin cytoplasmic rim in which only a small mitochondrion (M) and few membrane-bound organelles (pinocytotic vesicles and short cisternae of smooth endoplasmic reticulum) are visible. The organelle reduction is quite evident, and in particular no RER, Golgi complex, and microvesicles are visible (compare with normal human adipocyte shown in Plate 5.5). Note the regular dense line (DL) running at the border between the lipid droplet (L) and cytoplasmic rim of the cell. This dense line is the location of lipid-droplet-related proteins. On the external side of the cytoplasmic membrane, a dense external lamina (EL) is visible. Numerous collagen fibrils (CF) associated with the external lamina and free in the interstitium (C) are visible.

In the upper left side of the top panel, a venule (V in lumen) is present.

Suggested Reading

Blanchette-Mackie EJ, et al. Perilipin is located on the surface layer of intracellular lipid droplets in adipocytes. J Lipid Res. 36:1211–26, 1995.

Puri V, et al. Fat-specific protein 27, a novel lipid droplet protein that enhances triglyceride storage. J Biol Chem. 282:34213–8, 2007.

Murphy S, et al. Lipid droplet-organelle interactions; sharing the fats. Biochim Biophys Acta. 1791:441–7, 2009.

Pasarica M, et al. Adipose tissue collagen VI in obesity. J Clin Endocrinol Metab. 94:5155–62, 2009.

Arner E, et al. Adipocyte turnover: relevance to human adipose tissue morphology. Diabetes. 59:105–9, 2010.

Fujimoto T, Parton RG. Not just fat: the structure and function of the lipid droplet. Cold Spring Harb Perspect Biol. 3:1–17, 2011.

Christian M. Nuclear receptor-mediated regulation of lipid droplet-associated protein gene expression in adipose tissue. Horm Mol Biol Clin Investig. 14:87–97, 2013.

Wilfling F, et al. Triacylglycerol synthesis enzymes mediate lipid droplet growth by relocalizing from the ER to lipid droplets. Dev Cell. 24:384–99, 2013.

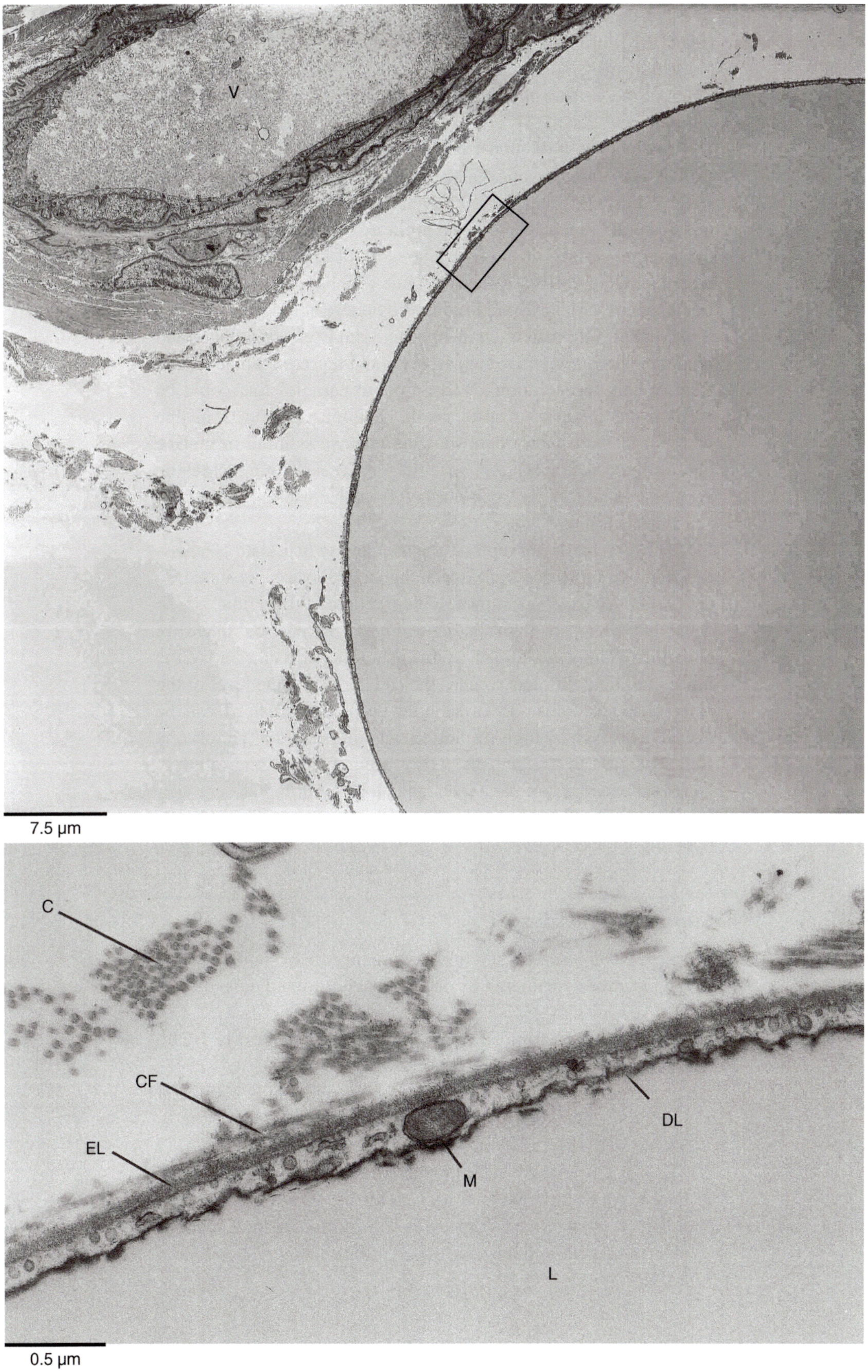

Plate 9.16 Intermuscular adipocyte from adult overweight subject. *Lower*: enlargement of squared area. TEM

PLATE 9.17

Human Obese Adipocytes TEM

Most of the abnormalities described in murine obese adipocytes (Plate 9.15) are also present in subcutaneous and visceral fat of obese humans.

Some of these abnormalities are shown here (compare with previous plate and Plate 5.5).

In the adipocyte of the upper left panel, the cytoplasmic rim is still visible with some organelles such as the small mitochondria (m, some indicated). Small lipid droplets (SL) seem to gem from the main central lipid droplet (L) and infiltrate the cytoplasmic rim. On the external surface of the cell, a network of microfibrils with the size of amyloid fibrils are present in line with our previous observation that amyloid fibrils are produced by obese adipocytes.

In the upper right panel, the cytoplasmic rim is electron dense and no organelles are visible. This aspect could represent an advanced level of cell degeneration. Electron-dense particles that could be calcium precipitates are also visible. This observation is in line with our histochemistry data showing positive staining in murine obese adipocytes by calcium-specific von Kossa staining. Note the abundant and dense collagen fibrils (C) on the external side of the cell (see also Plate 9.15).

In the lower panel a cell representing an intermediate state of stress-degenerative ultrastructural aspects between those represented by the two upper panels is shown. Note the lipid "infiltration" of the dense line (compare with the dense line in the previous plate) in both obese adipocytes shown in this panel. In particular one of the infiltrating lipid droplets reaches the cell surface at the level of the external lamina (arrow). These lipid droplet protrusions can be directly observed by high-resolution scanning electron microscopy (see Plate 9.15). Glycogen (Gly) accumulation and slightly increased external lamina-associated collagen fibrils (CF) are visible (compare with the massive increase of collagen fibrils in the upper right panel (C)).

Suggested Reading

Poitou C, et al. Serum amyloid A: production by human white adipocyte and regulation by obesity and nutrition. Diabetologia. 48(3):519–28, 2005.

Pasarica M, et al. Adipose tissue collagen VI in obesity. J Clin Endocrinol Metab. 94:5155–62, 2009.

Heinonen S, et al. Adipocyte morphology and implications for metabolic derangements in acquired obesity. Int J Obes (Lond). 38(11):1423–31, 2014.

Gao H, et al. Early B cell factor 1 regulates adipocyte morphology and lipolysis in white adipose tissue. Cell Metab. 19:981–92, 2014.

Giordano A, et al. Obese adipocytes show ultrastructural features of stressed cells and die of pyroptosis. J Lipid Res. 54:2423–36, 2013.

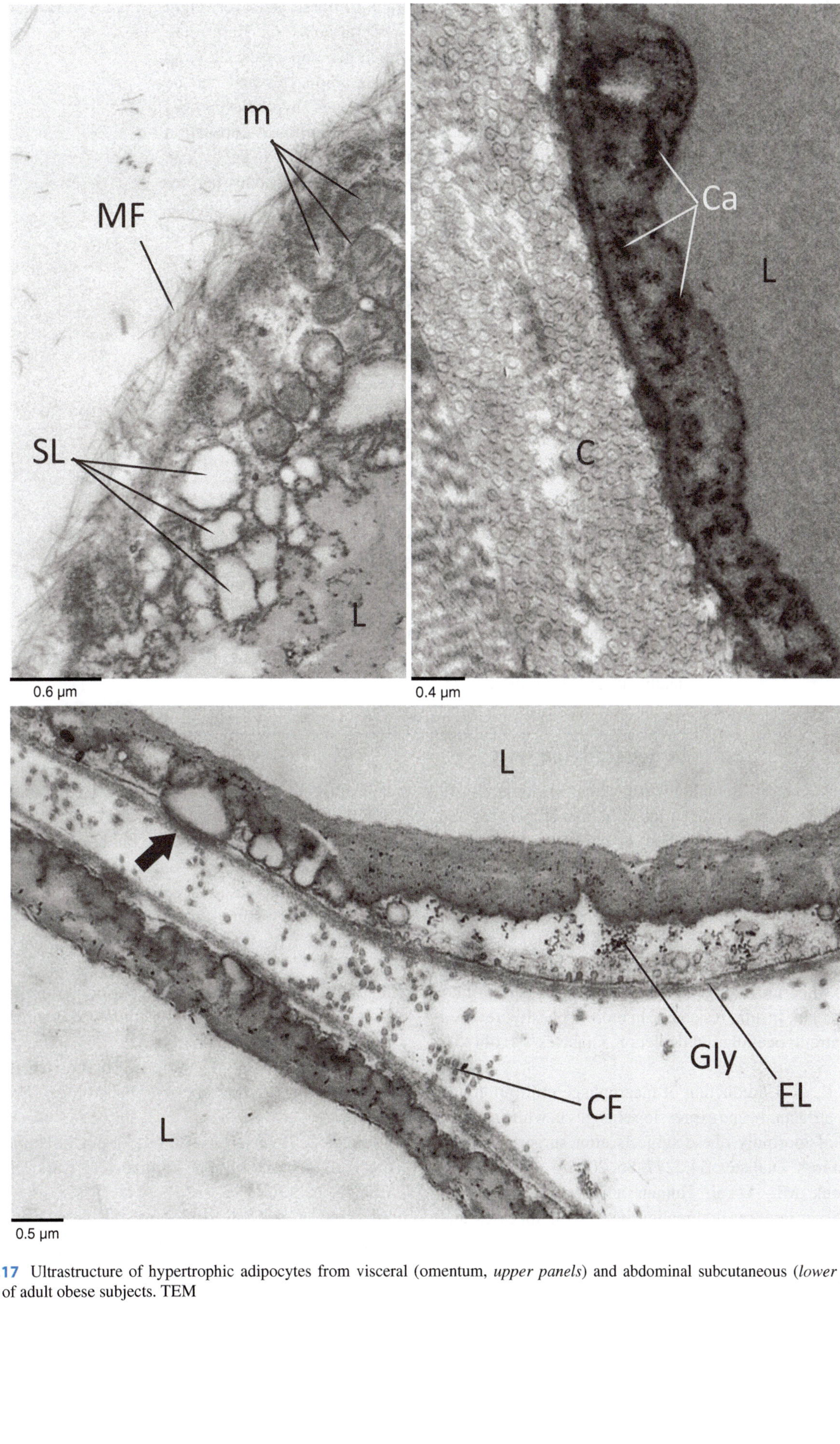

Plate 9.17 Ultrastructure of hypertrophic adipocytes from visceral (omentum, *upper panels*) and abdominal subcutaneous (*lower panel*) fat samples of adult obese subjects. TEM

PLATE 9.18

CLS in Human WAT

We found CLS in human adipose organ of obese and overweight subjects both in subcutaneous and visceral areas. CLS are more frequently found in obese subjects with larger adipocytes. CLS can be observed in lean subjects with large adipocytes and can be absent in obese subjects with small adipocytes (hyperplastic obesity). These data are in line with those supporting a correlation between size of adipocytes and insulin resistance even in lean patients. The high density of CLS in human subcutaneous fat presented in this plate is a rare event. The biopsy specimen of subcutaneous fat shown here is from an obese subject that received surgical treatment (sleeve gastrectomy) 7 weeks before the biopsy. During this period the weight loss was about 10 kg (unpublished results in collaboration with Dr Eric Ravussin Pennington Biomedical Research Center, Baton Rouge).

Enlargement in the middle left panel is from the same specimen shown in the top panel. Macrophages of CLS resulted CD68 immunoreactive (middle right panel).

Two CLS in visceral (perirenal) fat biopsy from an obese patient undergoing nephrectomy for kidney neoplasia are visible in the bottom panel.

Human white adipocytes are immunoreactive for beta-3 adrenoceptors both in lean and obese subjects. This opens the possibility for treatment with agonists that in rodents allow a direct transformation of white to brown adipocytes (see Plates 7.12–7.14 and 7.19–7.21 for details). Even an induction of early steps of white to brown transdifferentiation could be relevant for health because it implies a size reduction. Size of adipocytes is positively correlated to cell death and CLS formation.

Suggested Reading

De Matteis R, et al. Immunohistochemical identification of the beta(3)-adrenoceptor in intact human adipocytes and ventricular myocardium: effect of obesity and treatment with ephedrine and caffeine. Int J Obes Relat Metab Disord. 26:1442–50, 2002.

Camastra S, et al. Relationship between muscle and adipose tissue morphology, insulin sensitivity and beta-cell function in diabetic and nondiabetic obese patients: effects of bariatric surgery. Scientific Rep 2017 in print.

Greco AV, et al. Insulin resistance in morbid obesity: reversal with intramyocellular fat depletion. Diabetes. 51:144–51, 2002.

Cancello R, et al. Reduction of macrophage infiltration and chemoattractant gene expression changes in white adipose tissue of morbidly obese subjects after surgery-induced weight loss. Diabetes. 54:2277–86, 2005.

Kranendonk ME, et al. Human adipocyte extracellular vesicles in reciprocal signaling between adipocytes and macrophages. Obesity. 22:1296–308, 2014.

Lackey DE, et al. Contributions of adipose tissue architectural and tensile properties toward defining healthy and unhealthy obesity. Am J Physiol Endocrinol Metab. 306:E233–46, 2014.

Conti G, et al. The post-adipocytic phase of the adipose cell cycle. Tissue Cell. 46:520–6, 2014.

Acosta JR, et al. Increased fat cell size: a major phenotype of subcutaneous white adipose tissue in non-obese individuals with type 2 diabetes. Diabetologia. 59:560–70, 2016.

Pellegrinelli V, et al. Adipose tissue plasticity: how fat depots respond differently to pathophysiological cues. Diabetologia. 59:1075–88, 2016.

Boutens L, Stienstra R. Adipose tissue macrophages: going off track during obesity. Diabetologia. 59:879–94, 2016.

Kohlgruber A, Lynch L. Adipose tissue inflammation in the pathogenesis of type 2 diabetes. Curr Diab Rep. 15:92–103, 2015.

Giordano A, et al. Convertible visceral fat as a therapeutic target to curb obesity. Nat Rev Drug Discov. 15:405–24, 2016.

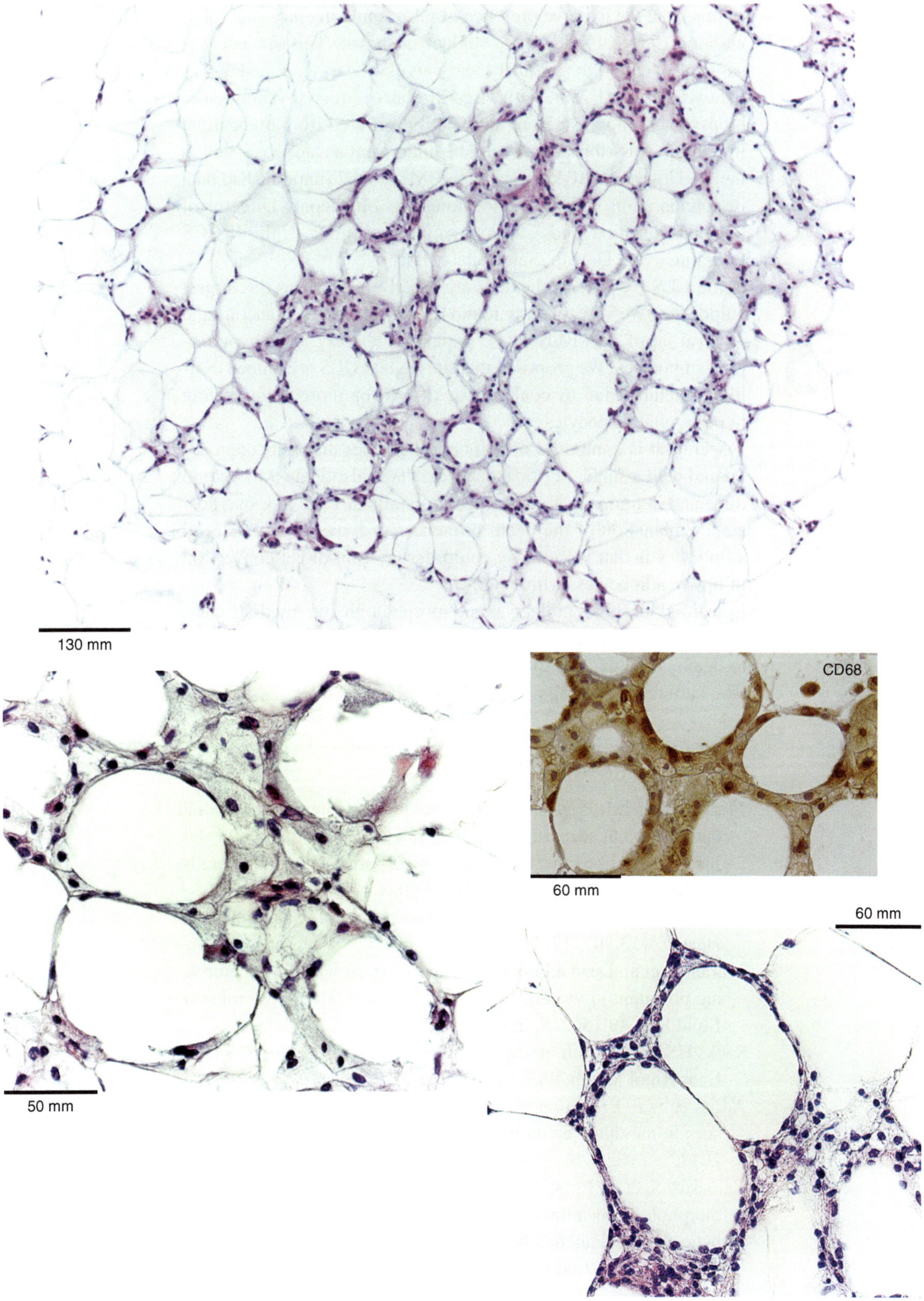

Plate 9.18 Massively inflamed abdominal subcutaneous fat from an obese subject 7 weeks after sleeve gastrectomy intervention. LM. H&E. *Middle left*: enlargement of CLS from tissue shown in the *top panel*. *Middle right*: same bioptic specimen shown in the *upper panel*. LM. IHC CD68 ab (1:200). *Bottom*: CLS in perirenal fat of an obese patient. LM. H&E

PLATE 9.19

Human Visceral CLS

In this plate the massive presence of CLS found in epicardial fat of an adult (78 years old) male subject is shown. This subject was surgically treated for coronary and valvular heart disease. He was overweight (BMI 28.4, with visceral obesity) for 10 years before biopsy and 3 months before intervention suffered from myocardial infarction. After this acute event, he underwent a calorie restriction diet and lost about 10 kg reaching a BMI of 24.2 (unpublished data in collaboration with Dr Lelio Francesco Morricone, Director of Clinical Nutrition and Cardiovascular Prevention Unit; IRCCS Policlinico San Donato, San Donato, Italy).

Some CLS (*, some indicated) are clearly larger than the largest adipocytes. We very recently found this aspect in subcutaneous and visceral fat of massively obese patients with very large hypertrophic adipocytes. We proposed that these giant CLS are indeed cyst-like structures due to coalescence of two or more degenerating hypertrophic adipocytes.

Visceral fat is composed of adipocytes smaller than subcutaneous fat and with a smaller critical death size (see also Plate 9.8) both in mice and in humans. As described in details in Plate 9.8, one possible explanation of the death proneness of hypertrophic visceral adipocytes is that visceral fat could derive from direct conversion of brown adipocytes (whitening).

Epicardial fat shows molecular and morphologic intermediate characteristics between classic WAT and classic BAT, and its proneness to death could explain the massive CLS infiltration in this patient who suffered chronically from visceral obesity.

Suggested Reading

Marchington JM, Pond CM. Site-specific properties of pericardial and epicardial adipose tissue: the effects of insulin and high-fat feeding on lipogenesis and the incorporation of fatty acids in vitro. Int J Obes. 14:1013–22, 1990.

Sacks HS, Fain JN. Human epicardial adipose tissue: a review. Am Heart J. 153:907–17, 2007.

Murano I, et al. Dead adipocytes, detected as crown-like structures, are prevalent in visceral fat depots of genetically obese mice. J Lipid Res. 49:1562–8, 2008.

Sacks HS, et al. Adult epicardial fat exhibits beige features. J Clin Endocrinol Metab. 98:E1448–55, 2013.

Adliss P, et al. Browning the cardiac and peri-vascular adipose tissues to modulate cardiovascular risk. Int J Cariol. 228:265–74, 2017.

Camastra S, et al. Relationship between muscle and adipose tissue morphology, insulin sensitivity and beta-cell function in diabetic and nondiabetic obese patients: effects of bariatric surgery. Scientific Rep. 7:9007, 2017

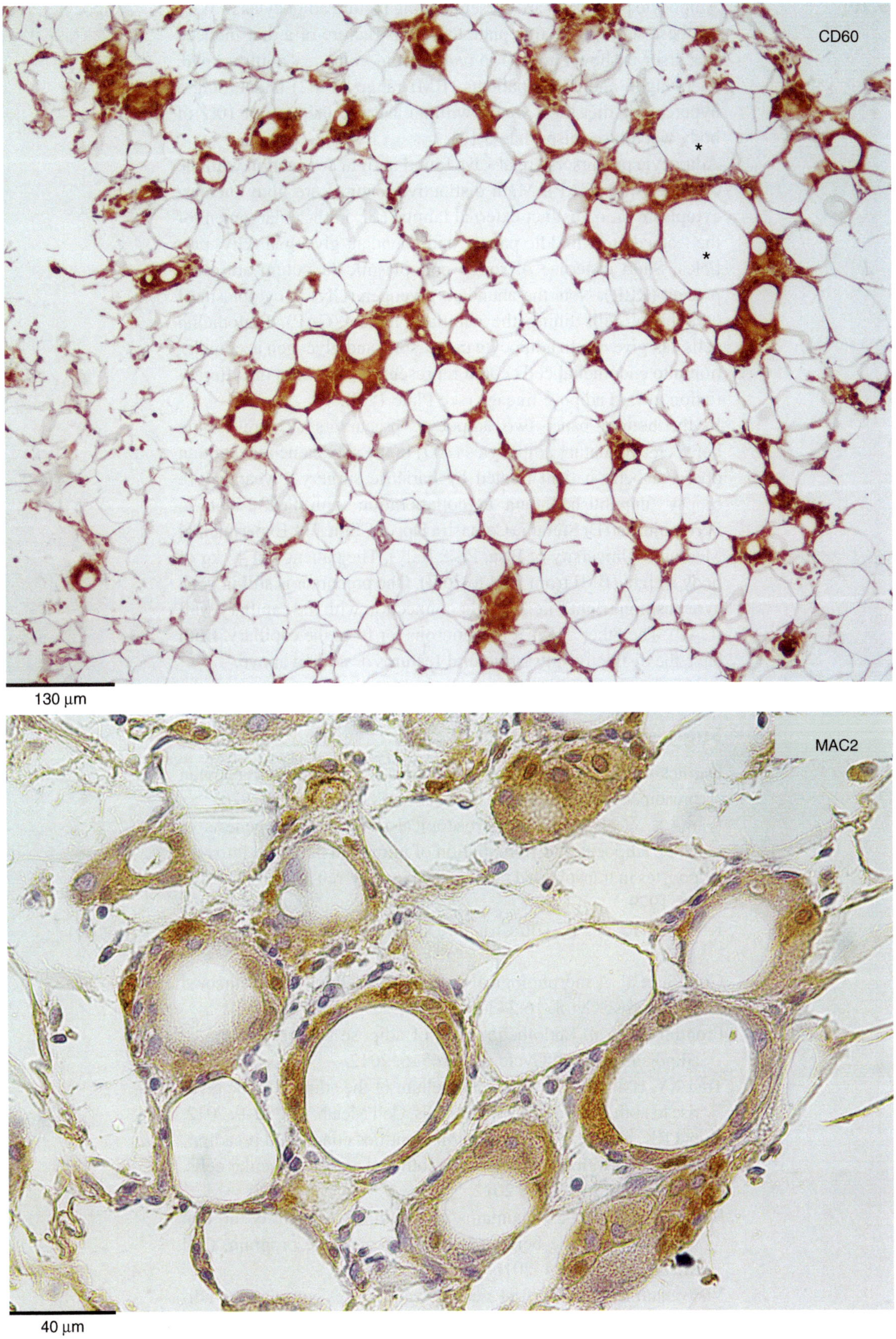

Plate 9.19 Massive CLS density in human epicardial fat. *Upper*, LM. IHC CD68 ab (1:200). *Bottom*, same biopsy: LM. IHC MAC2 (1:1,500)

PLATE 9.20

Adipocyte Precursors

Adipocyte precursors are present among mature adipocytes in WAT of obese subjects. In this plate the ultrastructure of a diet-induced precursor is shown in the top panel (from voluntary adult normal, overweight, and obese patients (BMI range 22–32) undergoing a hypercaloric diet for 8 weeks with an average increase of 10% of body weight, see also Plate 5.10).

Adipocyte precursors are always found in tight connection with the capillary wall (CAP). Main distinctive features are high nucleus/cytoplasm ratio, distinct external lamina (EL in the enlargement of the framed area: middle panel), and abundant glycogen (Gly) particles. Short cisternae of rough endoplasmic reticulum are often present (RER). Note the abundant glycogen (Gly) in cytoplasm of endothelial cells lining the capillary lumen (CAP). Endothelial cells can give rise to adipocyte precursors, and glycogen accumulation into endothelial cells could represent the first sign of differentiation toward adipose lineage (see Plate 12.8).

In the bottom panel two adipocyte precursors (P) are visible between two mature adipocytes (AD) in the subcutaneous fat of an obese diabetic patient treated by bariatric surgery 1 year before biopsy (unpublished data in collaboration with Prof Eleuterio Ferrannini and Dr Stefania Camastra Dpt of Clinical & Experimental Medicine, University of Pisa, Pisa, Italy). The patient lost 43 kg of body weight (BMI from 55.4 to 36.7). One precursor is still in pericyte position (right), i.e., in tight connection with the capillary wall (CAP). The other one is a few microns far from the capillary. Both have the distinctive ultrastructural features described above.

Suggested Reading

Dardick I, et al. Ultrastructural observations on differentiating human preadipocytes cultured in vitro. Tissue Cell. 8:561–71, 1976.

Iyama K, et al. Electron microscopical studies on the genesis of white adipocytes: differentiation of immature pericytes into adipocytes in transplanted preadipose tissue. Virch Arch B. 31:143–55, 1979.

Kim YH, Reiner L. Ultrastructure of lipoma. Cancer. 50:102–6, 1982.

Cinti S, et al. A morphological study of the adipocyte precursor. J Submicrosc Cytol. 16:243–51, 1984.

Frontini A, et al. Endothelial cells of adipose tissues: a niche of adipogenesis. Cell Cycle. 11:2765–6, 2012.

Tran KV, et al. The vascular endothelium of the adipose tissue gives rise to both white and brown fat cells. Cell Metab. 15:222–9, 2012.

Gupta RK, et al. Zfp423 expression identifies committed preadipocytes and localizes to adipose endothelial and perivascular cells. Cell Metab. 15:230–9, 2012.

Shao M, et al. Zfp423 maintains white adipocyte identity through suppression of the beige cell thermogenic gene program. Cell Metab. 23:1167–84, 2016.

Vishvanath L, et al. Pdgfrβ+ mural preadipocytes contribute to adipocyte hyperplasia induced by high-fat-diet feeding and prolonged cold exposure in adult mice. Cell Metab. 23:350–9, 2016.

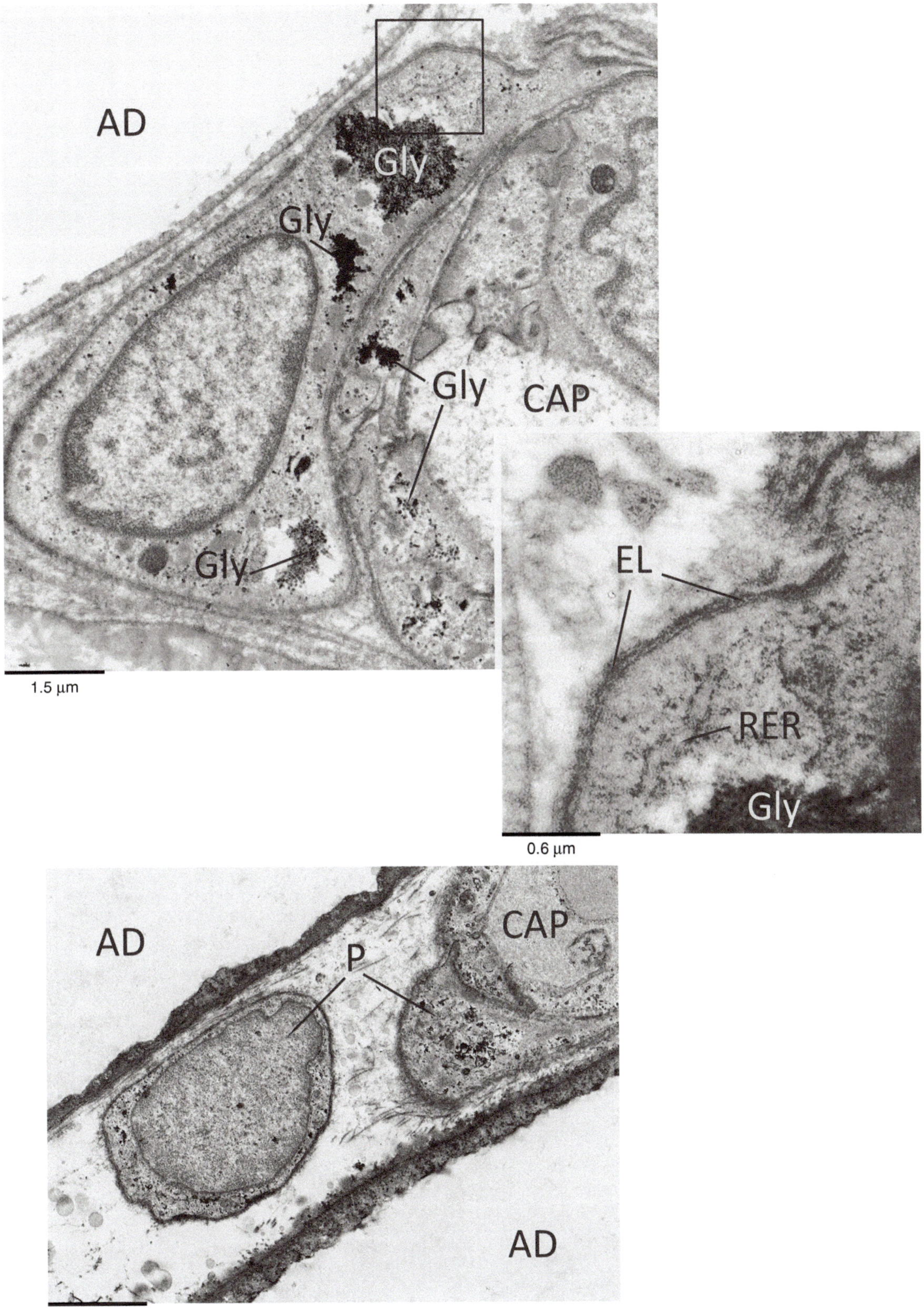

Plate 9.20 Human adipocyte precursor ultrastructure. *Upper*: abdominal subcutaneous fat from a voluntary subject that gained 8 kg of body weight after 8 weeks of hypercaloric diet (unpublished data in collaboration with Dr Eric Ravussin, Pennington Biomedical Research Center, Baton Rouge). *Lower*: subcutaneous abdominal fat of diabetic obese subject 1 year after bariatric surgery and a weight loss of 43 kg (unpublished data in collaboration with Prof Eleuterio Ferrannini and Dr Stefania Camastra Dpt of Clinical & Experimental Medicine, University of Pisa, Pisa, Italy). TEM

10 The Fasted Adipose Organ

S. Cinti, *Obesity, Type 2 Diabetes and the Adipose Organ*, https://doi.org/10.1007/978-3-319-40522-3_10

10.1 The Fasted Adipose Organ

PLATE 10.1

Gross Anatomy

In fasted animals, the adipose organ undergoes modifications, which depend on the duration of fasting and on environmental temperature. After 48 h of fasting, the adipose organ of an adult mouse is almost unchanged if the animal is maintained at 28 °C, but it changes dramatically if the animal is kept at 10 °C.

In the former condition, the only visible modification of the adipose organ is in the color of brownish areas, which appear paler due to warm acclimation, as described in Plate 8.2. In animals kept at 10 °C, nearly all the white areas of the organ disappear: the upper subcutaneous depot consists only of intensely brownish-red brown adipose tissue, and in all other depots brownish areas expanded.

These modifications clearly indicate that the allocation of energy expenditure privileges thermogenesis over the other metabolic requirements in these experimental conditions.

Suggested Reading

Sheldon H, et al. Observations on the morphology of adipose tissue. I. The fine structure of cells from fasted and diabetic rats. Diabetes. 11:378–87, 1962.

Sarzani R, et al. Fasting inhibits natriuretic peptides clearance receptor expression in rat adipose tissue. J Hypertens. 13:1241–6, 1995.

Giordano A, et al. Regional-dependent increase of sympathetic innervation in rat white adipose tissue during prolonged fasting. J Histochem Cytochem. 53:679–87, 2005.

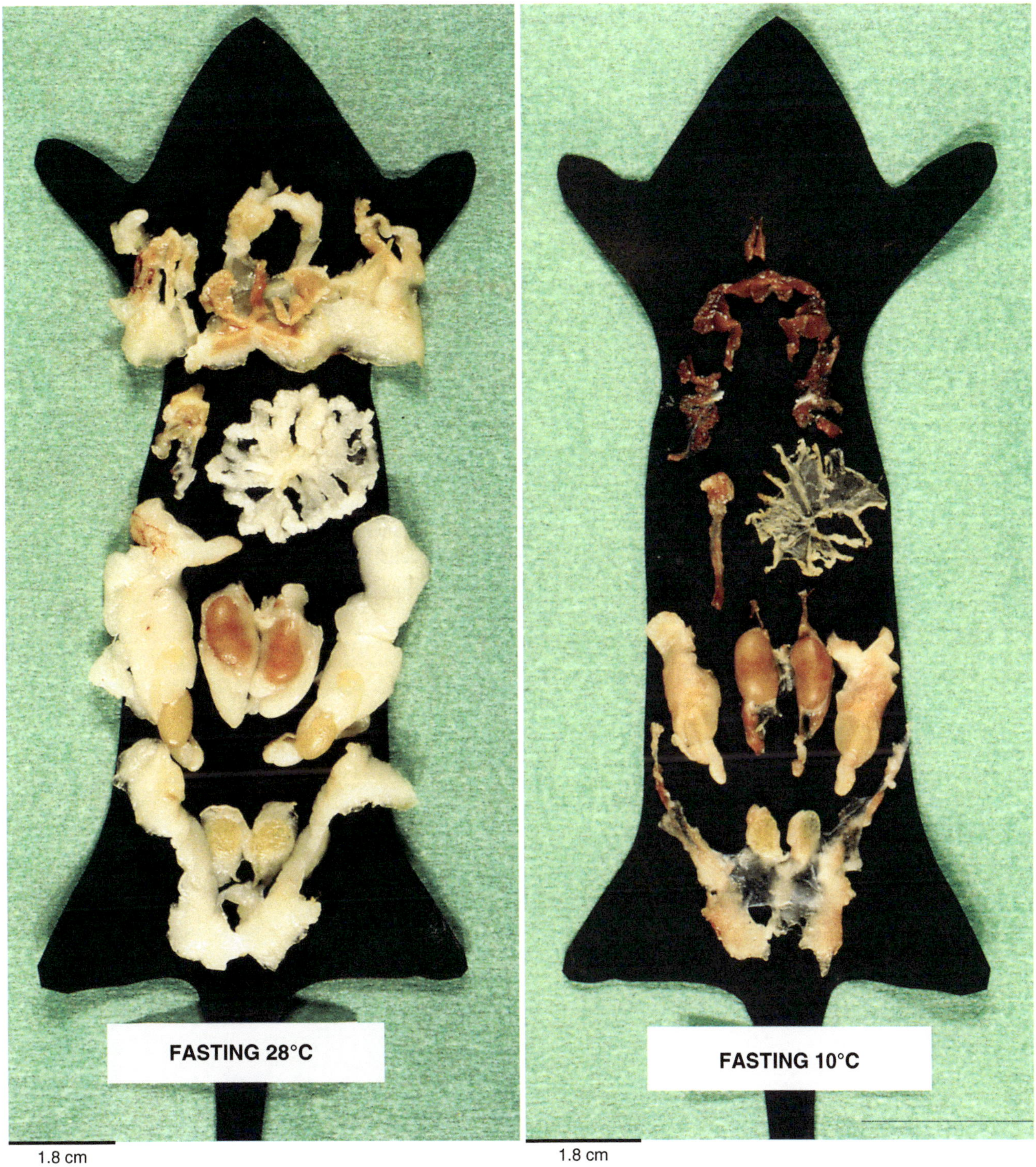

Plate 10.1 The adipose organ of adult mice after 48 h of fasting at 28 °C (*left*) and at 10 °C (*right*)

PLATE 10.2

BAT Histology IHC-UCP1-Leptin

Plate 8.2 shows the transformation of brown adipocytes from multilocular into unilocular cells in warm-acclimated fasted animals. Since fasting reduces noradrenergic input to IBAT, the transformation into unilocular cells can be obtained at lower temperatures in fasted animals. Therefore, the morphology of brown adipocytes in warm-acclimated and fasted animals is unilocular. In both conditions, unilocular cells express UCP1, but whereas in feeding animals acclimated at 28 °C the same adipocytes also express leptin, in fasting animals they do not (compare lower panels of Plates 8.2 and 10.2).

This suggests that leptin expression in unilocular brown adipocytes does not completely depend on their morphology.

Suggested Reading

Muralidhara DV, Desautels M. Changes in brown adipose tissue composition during fasting and refeeding of diet-induced obese mice. Am J Physiol. 266:R1907–15, 1994.

Bornstein SR, et al. Immunohistochemical and ultrastructural localization of leptin and leptin receptor in human white adipose tissue and differentiating human adipose cells in primary culture. Diabetes. 49:532–8, 2000.

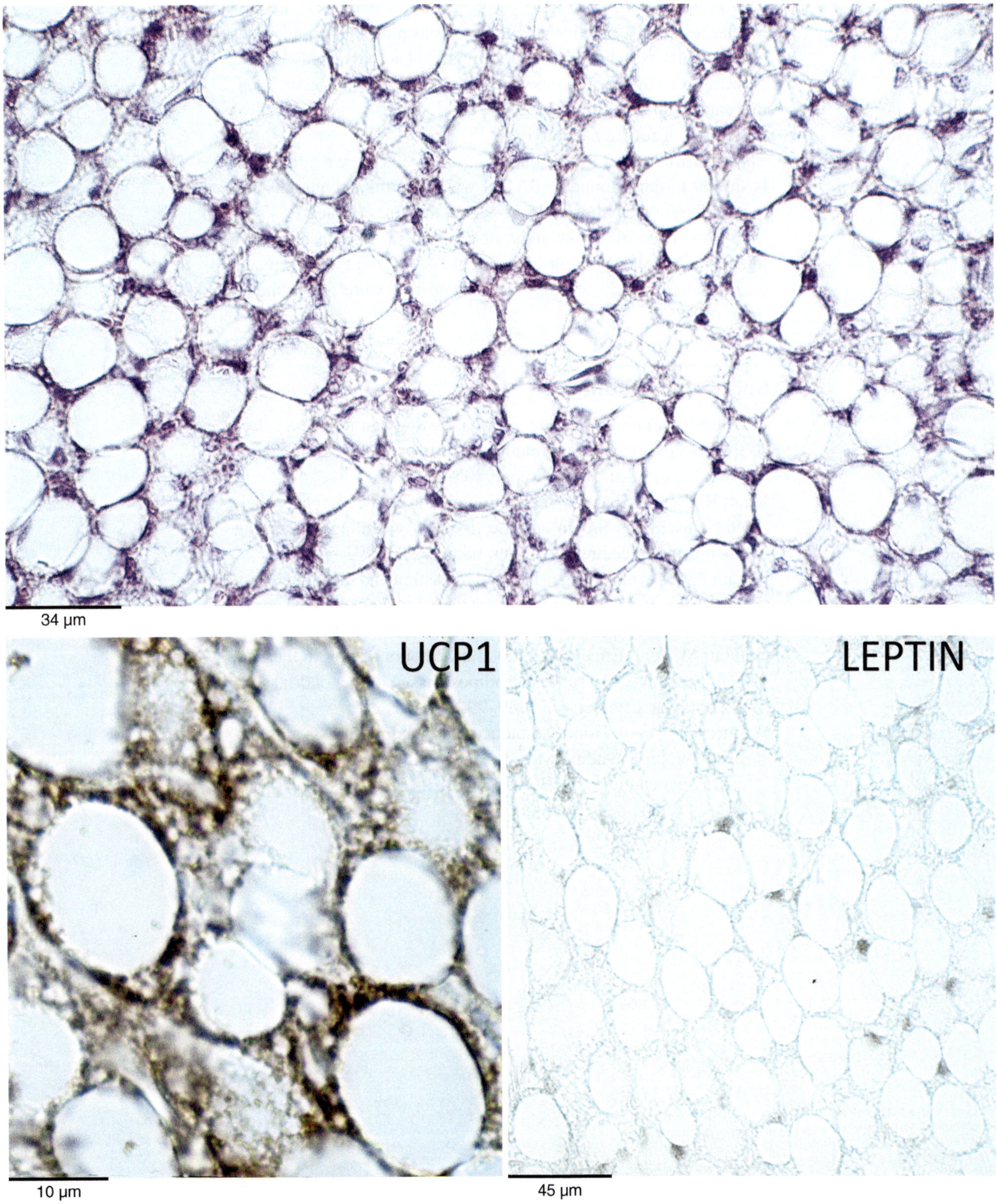

Plate 10.2 IBAT of an adult mouse after 2 days of fasting at 25 °C. LM. H&E. These adipocytes resulted UCP1 immunoreactive (*lower left*) but leptin negative (*lower right*). LM. IHC: UCP1 ab (1:8,000) and leptin ab (1:1,000)

PLATE 10.3

BAT TEM

The brown adipocytes of fasting mice maintained at 25 °C are unilocular and UCP1 positive (see the previous plate). The unilocular aspect, which is indicative of poor functional activity, is also found in warm-acclimated animals (see Plate 8.2). On the other hand, the expression of UCP1 in these cells suggests the theoretical possibility of functional activity.

The ultrastructure of mitochondria in unilocular brown adipocytes is similar to those found in BAT of warm-acclimated animals and quite different from those of cold-acclimated ones (Plates 7.6–7.9). Many mitochondria show signs of division (arrows in the lower figure), but the honeycomb-like structures described in brown adipocyte mitochondria of warm-acclimated rats were not found in these mice.

Suggested Reading

Trayhurn P, Jennings G. Evidence that fasting can induce a selective loss of uncoupling protein from brown adipose tissue mitochondria of mice. Biosci Rep. 6:805–10, 1986.

Knott RM, et al. Changes in insulin-receptor mRNA levels in skeletal muscle and brown adipose tissue of weanling rats during fasting and refeeding. Br J Nutr. 68:583–92, 1992.

Matamala JC, et al. Changes induced by fasting and dietetic obesity in thermogenic parameters of rat brown adipose tissue mitochondrial subpopulations. Biochem J. 15:529–34, 1996.

Gianotti M, et al. Effect of 12, 24 and 72 hours fasting in thermogenic parameters of rat brown adipose tissue mitochondrial subpopulations. Life Sci. 62: 1889–99, 1998.

Wikstrom JD, et al. Hormone-induced mitochondrial fission is utilized by brown adipocytes as an amplification pathway for energy expenditure. EMBO J. 33:418–36, 2014.

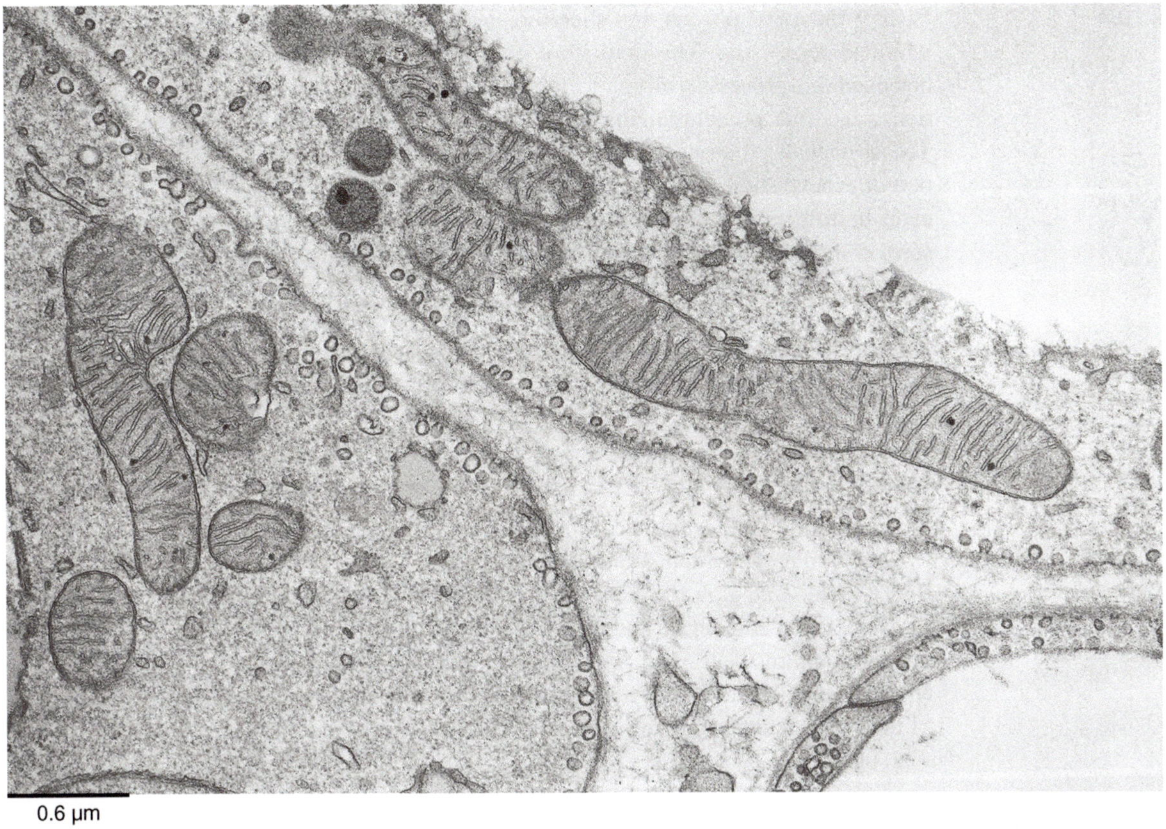

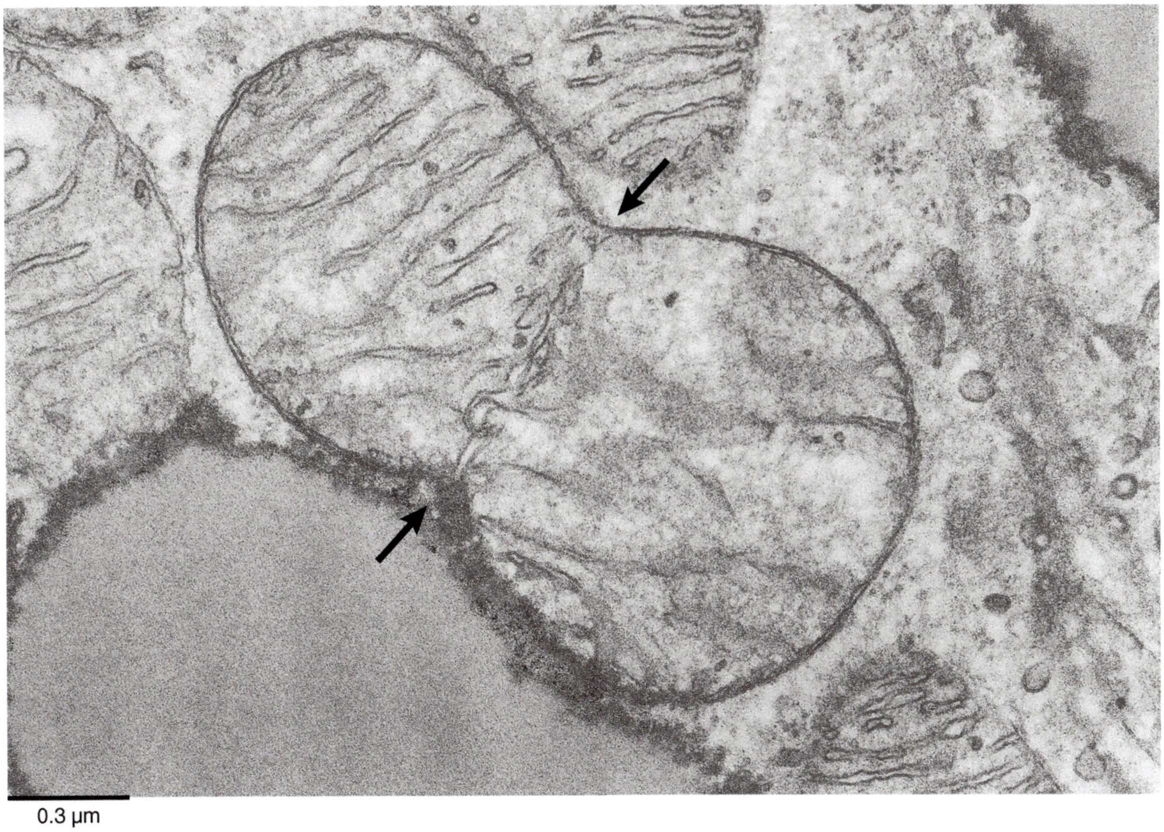

Plate 10.3 IBAT. Mitochondria of unilocular brown adipocytes of an adult mouse after 2 days of fasting at 25 °C. Dividing mitochondria (*lower panel, arrows*). TEM

PLATE 10.4

WAT Histology

Fasting induces lipolysis and therefore modifications mainly in white adipose tissue. The lipid store of adipocytes is mobilized; however, this process is not uniform in acute experimental conditions, and foci of delipidizing adipocytes can be found among almost unchanged white adipocytes. These lipolytic foci (central part of panels) show well-developed capillary networks and adipocytes in different stages of delipidation. Many cells in these areas seem completely devoid of lipids and are not recognizable as true adipocytes at the light microscopy level.

Murine and human subcutaneous and visceral white adipocytes produce ZAG (Zync-alpha2-glycoprotein), a lipid-mobilizing factor, which is upregulated in mice with cancer cachexia.

Suggested Reading

Williamson JR. Adipose tissue. Morphological changes associated with lipid mobilization. J Cell Biol. 20: 57–74, 1964.

Bing C, et al. Zinc-alpha2-glycoprotein, a lipid mobilizing factor, is expressed in adipocytes and is up-regulated in mice with cancer cachexia. Proc Natl Acad Sci U S A. 101:2500–5, 2004.

Nisoli E, et al. White adipocytes are less prone to apoptotic stimuli than brown adipocytes in rodent. Cell Death Differ. 13:2154–6, 2006.

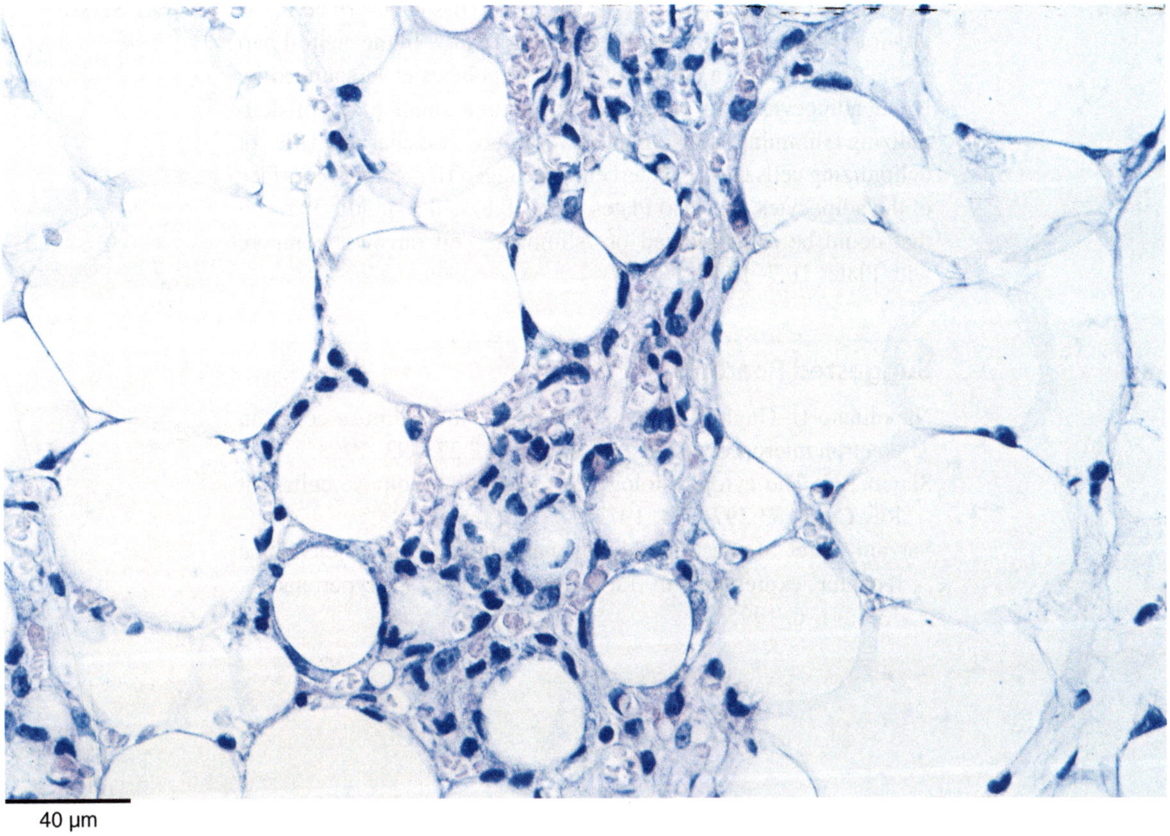

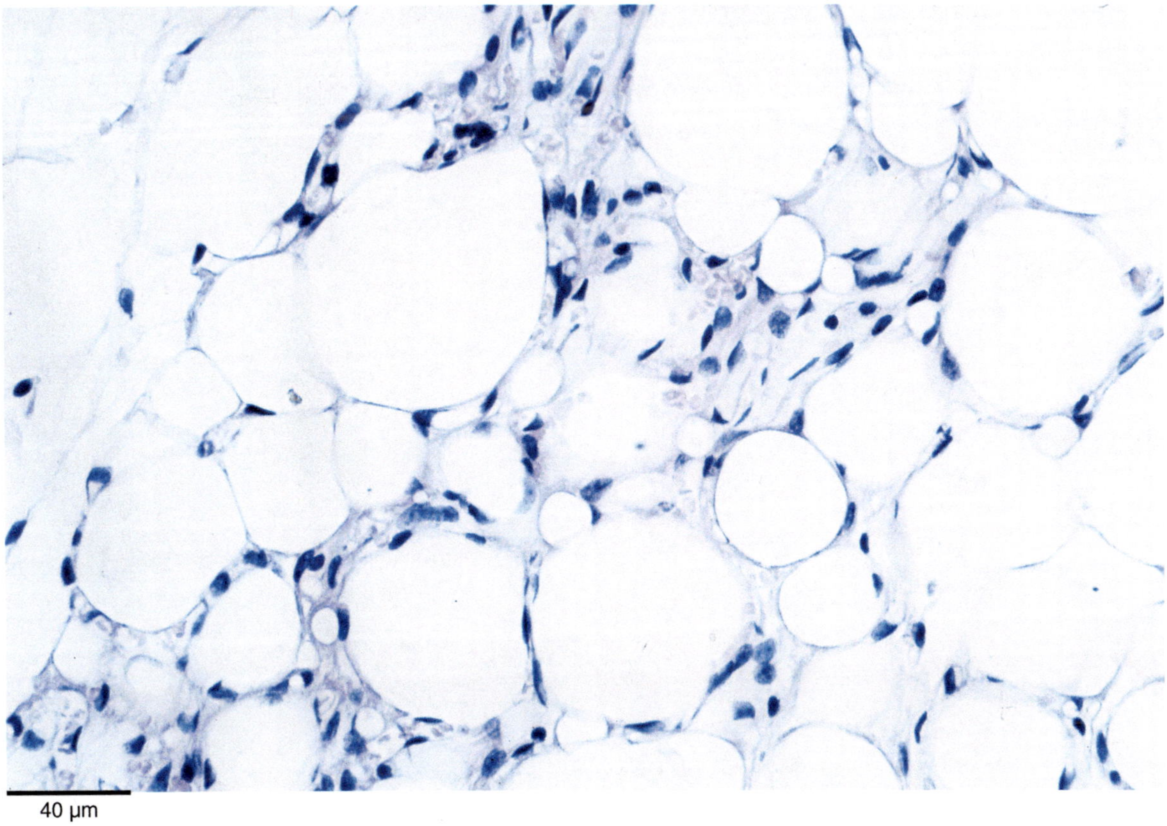

Plate 10.4 Peri-epididymal white adipose tissue of an adult mouse fasted for 48 h at 20 °C. Adipocytes in different stages of delipidation (slimming) process. LM. H&E

PLATE 10.5

WAT SEM

SEM allows the lipolytic foci of the adipose tissue described in the previous plate to be viewed three-dimensionally. In the central part of the upper figure, a cluster of small adipocytes is surrounded by larger adipocytes and probably represents a small focus of delipidizing (slimming) cells. In the lower figure, two characteristics of delipidizing cells can also be seen: the rugged (large arrow) surface of the adipocytes (see also Plates 10.7–10.8) and a spindle-like cell that could be a delipidized or "slimmed" cell (arrows, compare with Plates 10.7–10.8).

Suggested Reading

Napolitano L, Gagne HT. Lipid depleted white adipose cells: an electron microscope study. Anat Rec. 147:273–93, 1963.

Slavin BG. The cytophysiology of mammalian adipose cells. Int Rev Cytol. 33:297–334, 1972.

Sarzani R, et al. Fasting inhibits natriuretic peptides clearance receptor expression in rat adipose tissue. J Hypertension. 13:1241–6, 1995.

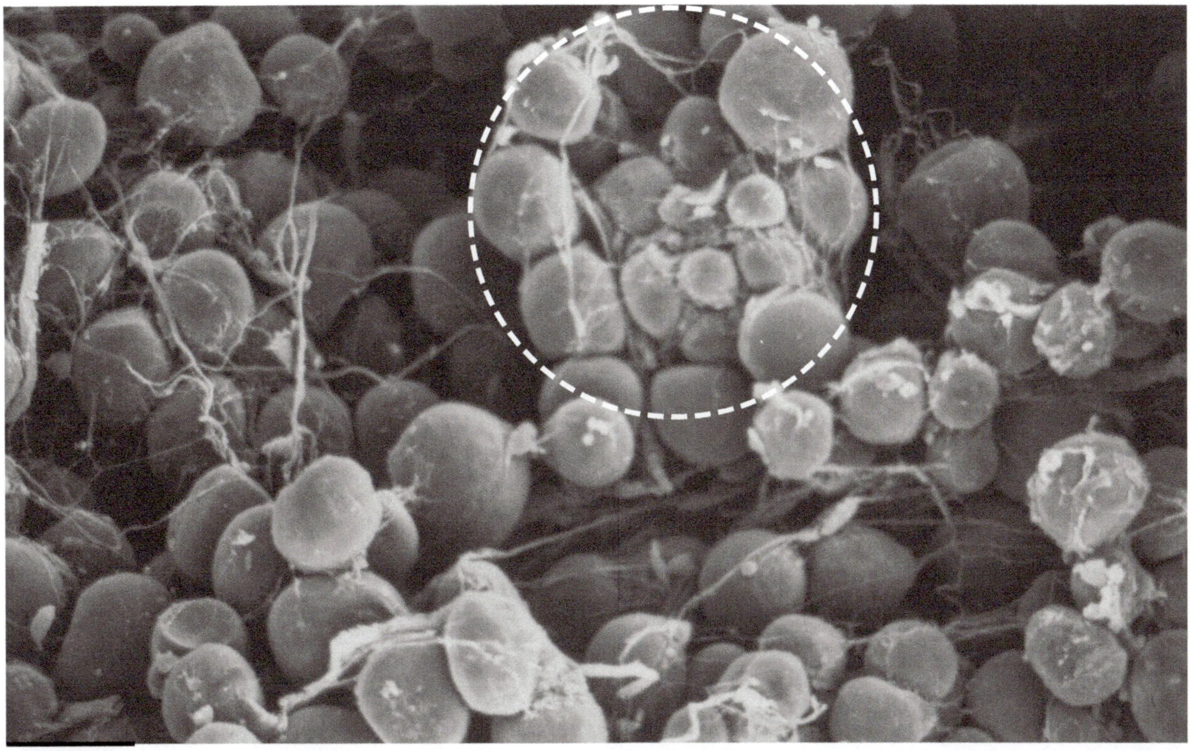

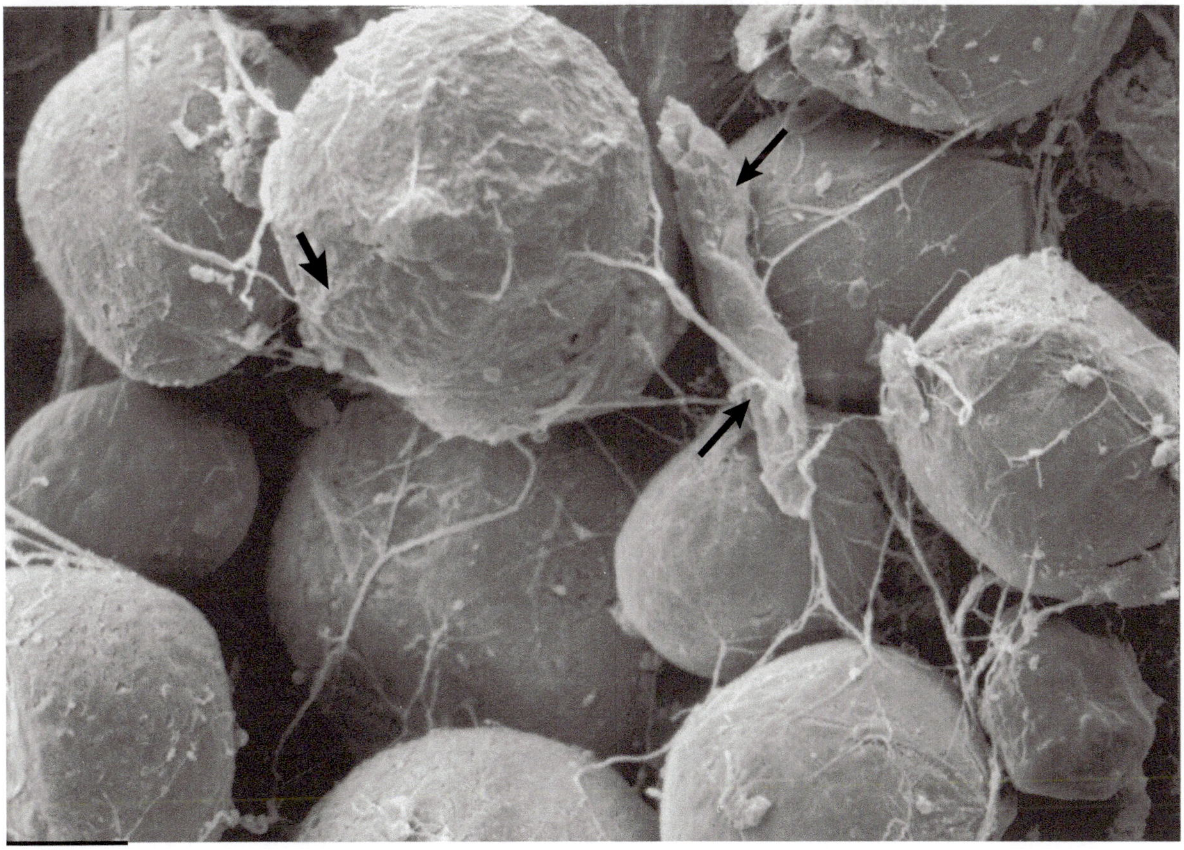

Plate 10.5 Omental depot of an adult rat fasted at 20 °C for 3 days. *Lower*: enlargement of the same depot shown in the upper panel. SEM

PLATE 10.6

The Slimmed White Adipocytes EM I

The morphology of adipocytes undergoing delipidation in fasting animals is similar to that observed in delipidizing cells from cold-acclimated animals (Plates 7.16–7.18).
Here we show that in adipocytes undergoing the lipolytic process, the residual cytoplasmic lipids are usually stored in a single main vacuole (L in large yellow areas) throughout the delipidation phases. In the same cell, small lipid droplets are also visible (L, some indicated). The adipocyte in the central part of the figure has a vacuole about 9 μm in diameter, which is clearly its remaining lipid droplet. The cytoplasmic projections of this cell are closely connected with two capillaries (CAP). A slimmed cell with small lipid droplets (L, some indicated) is visible in the upper left corner, and one adipocyte in a very early stage of delipidation is visible in the lower part of the figure. Note the abundance of capillaries and the "edematous" appearance of the interstitial space (IS), i.e., the absence of any specific structure typical of interstitial space, such as collagen fibrils.

Suggested Reading

Wassermann F, McDonald TF. Electron microscopic investigation on the surface membrane structures of the fat-cell and of their changes during depletion of the cell. Z Zellforsch Mikrosk Anat. 52:778–880, 1960.

Tavassoli M. In vivo development of adipose tissue following implantation of lipid-depleted cultured adipocyte. Exp Cell Res. 137:55–62, 1982.

Ochi M, et al. Adipocyte dynamics in hypothalamic obese mice during food deprivation and refeeding. J Nutr Sci Vitaminol. 37:479–91, 1991.

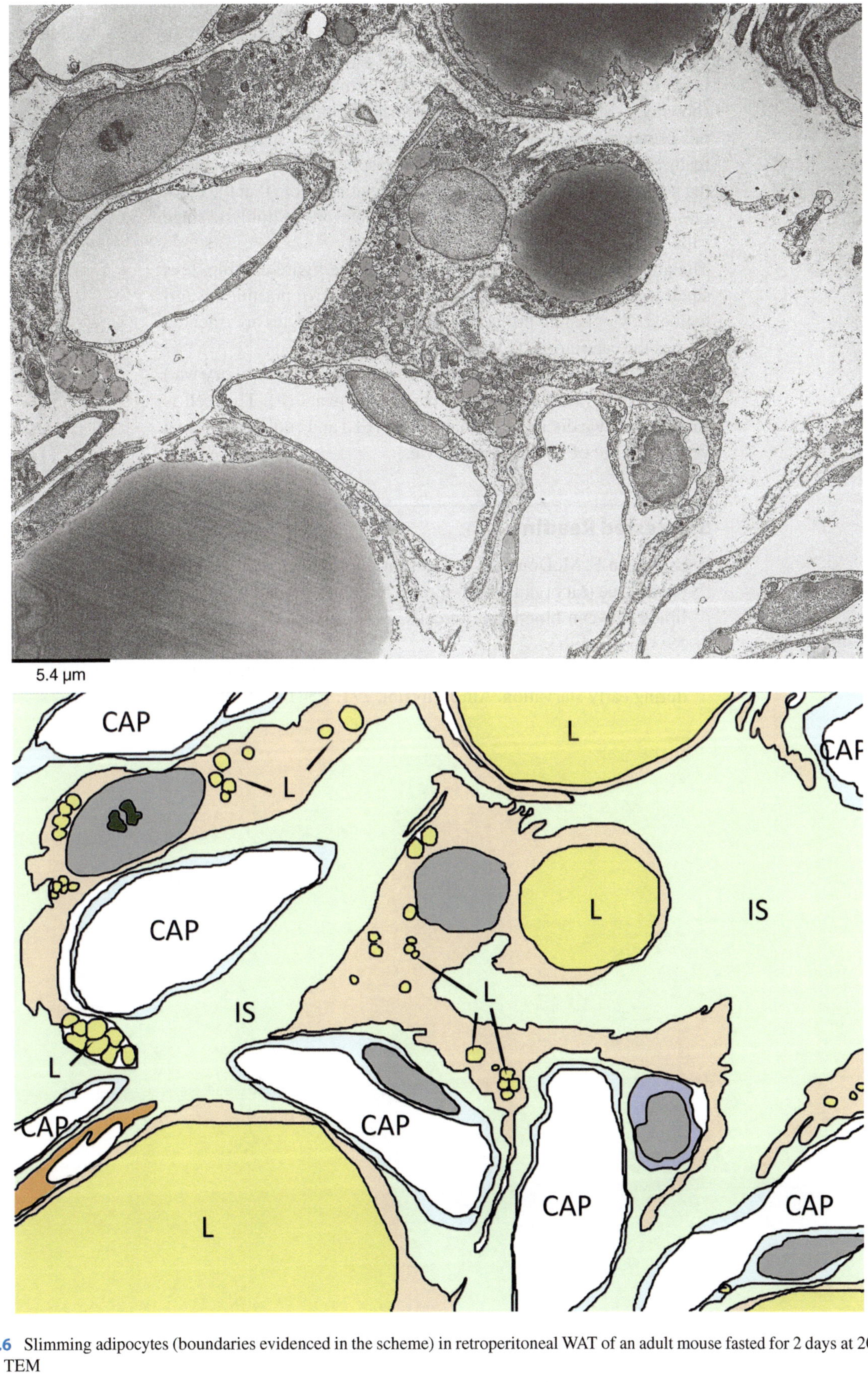

Plate 10.6 Slimming adipocytes (boundaries evidenced in the scheme) in retroperitoneal WAT of an adult mouse fasted for 2 days at 20 °C. CAP: capillary. TEM

PLATE 10.7

The Slimmed White Adipocytes EM II

This plate shows two adipocytes in the early and final phases of the slimming process. The adipocyte on the upper right side is at an early stage of delipidation, as indicated by the presence of a single large lipid vacuole (L) and of a cytoplasmic projection (arrow) showing an ultrastructural feature typical of slimming cells: numerous pseudopod-like cytoplasmic evaginations. This morphological feature can also be interpreted as cytoplasmic invaginations, and in the next plates we adopt the latter interpretation. Note that the cytoplasmic projection of this adipocyte and therefore its lipolytic stage cannot be seen in other planes of the section.

The adipocyte visible in the lower part of the figure exhibits few, small lipid droplets (L) and numerous villous cytoplasmic invaginations. Cytoplasmic projections from both adipocytes are oriented toward the capillaries (CAP).

A poorly differentiated cell in close association to the capillary wall is also visible in the middle left part of the panel (P). This cell is surrounded by a distinct external lamina (EL) and could represent a very late stage of slimmed adipocyte.

Suggested Reading

Wassermann F, McDonald TF. Electron microscopic study of adipose tissue (fat organs) with special reference to the transport of lipids between blood and fat cells. Z Zellforsch Mikrosk Anat. 59:326–57, 1963.

Samra JS, et al. Regulation of lipid metabolism in adipose tissue during early starvation. Am J Physiol. 271: E541–6, 1996.

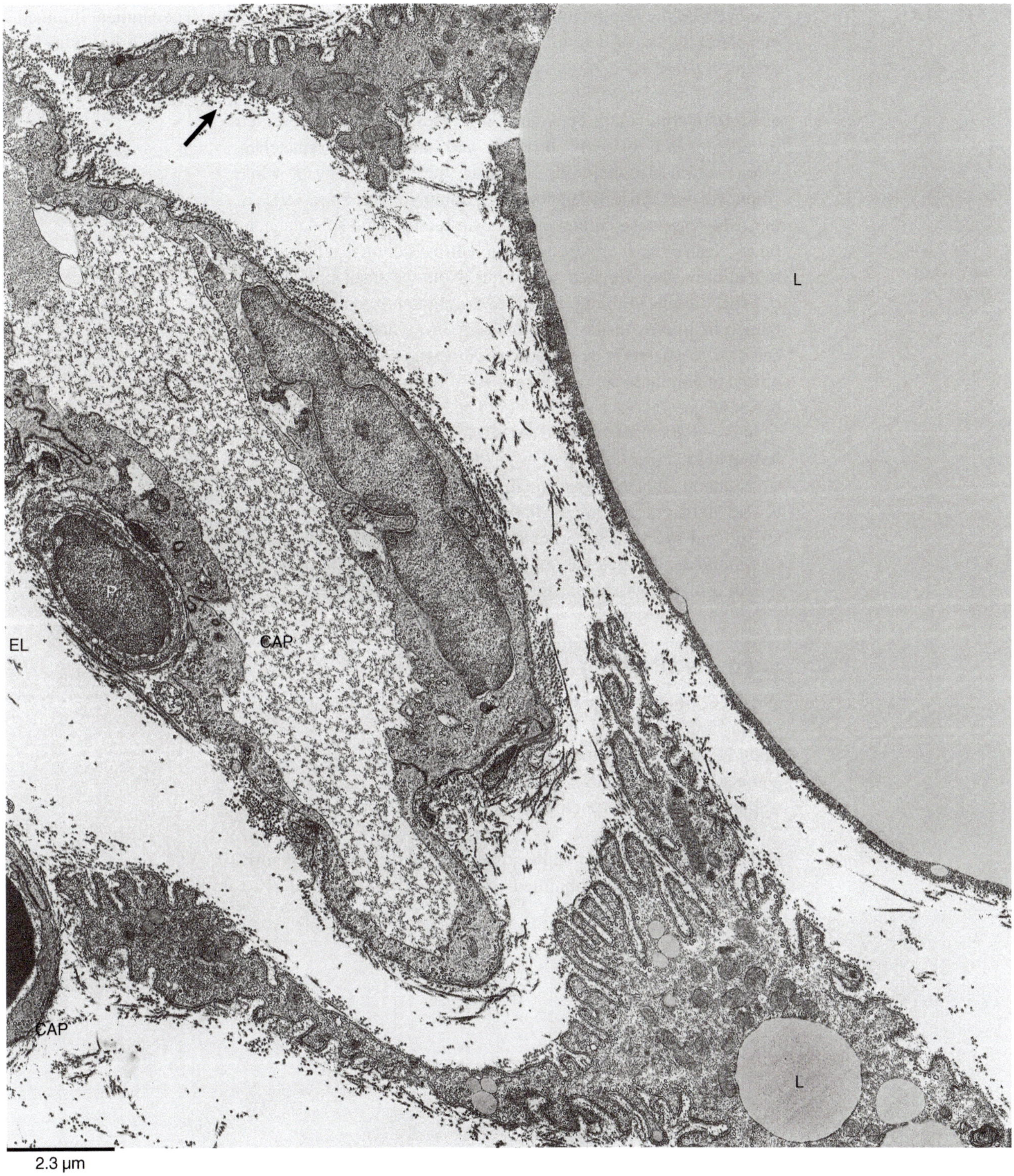

Plate 10.7 Retroperitoneal WAT of an adult rat fasted at 20 °C for 3 days. TEM

PLATE 10.8

The Human Slimmed White Adipocytes EM

The cytoplasmic invaginations (see explanation in the text of previous plate) typical of delipidizing adipocytes (see also next plates) exhibit a dense concentration of pinocytotic vesicles, although it has been claimed that their overall number does not change. Smooth endoplasmic reticulum apparently increases and can be observed on the surface of lipid droplets and among the organelles. Mitochondria are numerous and show the morphology of white adipocyte mitochondria (upper panel, compare with Plate 4.9).

In the lower panel a slimmed adipocyte found in the subcutaneous fat of a lean human subject is shown. Ultrastructure is quite similar to that of murine slimmed adipocytes. Note the small lipid droplet (L) still present in the elongated and irregular cytoplasm and the numerous microvilli-like structures (or invaginations, some indicated). The reason for the presence of this type of cell in subcutaneous fat of normal patients is unknown although the period of fasting before biopsy (about 12–15 h) should be taken into account. On the right is a unilocular adipocyte (AD). The interstitial space shows an "edematous" aspect (compare with Plate 10.6).

Considering all data shown and described in the last three plates, it is evident that the slimmed adipocyte has an ultrastructure characteristic and specific. In particular the old concept that delipidized (or slimmed) adipocytes assume a fibroblast-like phenotype is confounding and should be abandoned (see also Plate 10.14).

Suggested Reading

Wirsen C. Studies in lipid mobilization. Acta Physiol Scand. 65:1–46, 1965.

Jarett L, Smith RM. Ultrastructural localization of insulin receptors on adipocytes. PNAS. 72:3526–30, 1975.

Carpentier J, et al. Morphological changes of the adipose cell plasma membrane during lipolysis. J Cell Biol. 72:104–17, 1977.

Maurizi G, et al. Human white adipocytes convert into "rainbow" adipocytes in vitro. Submitted.

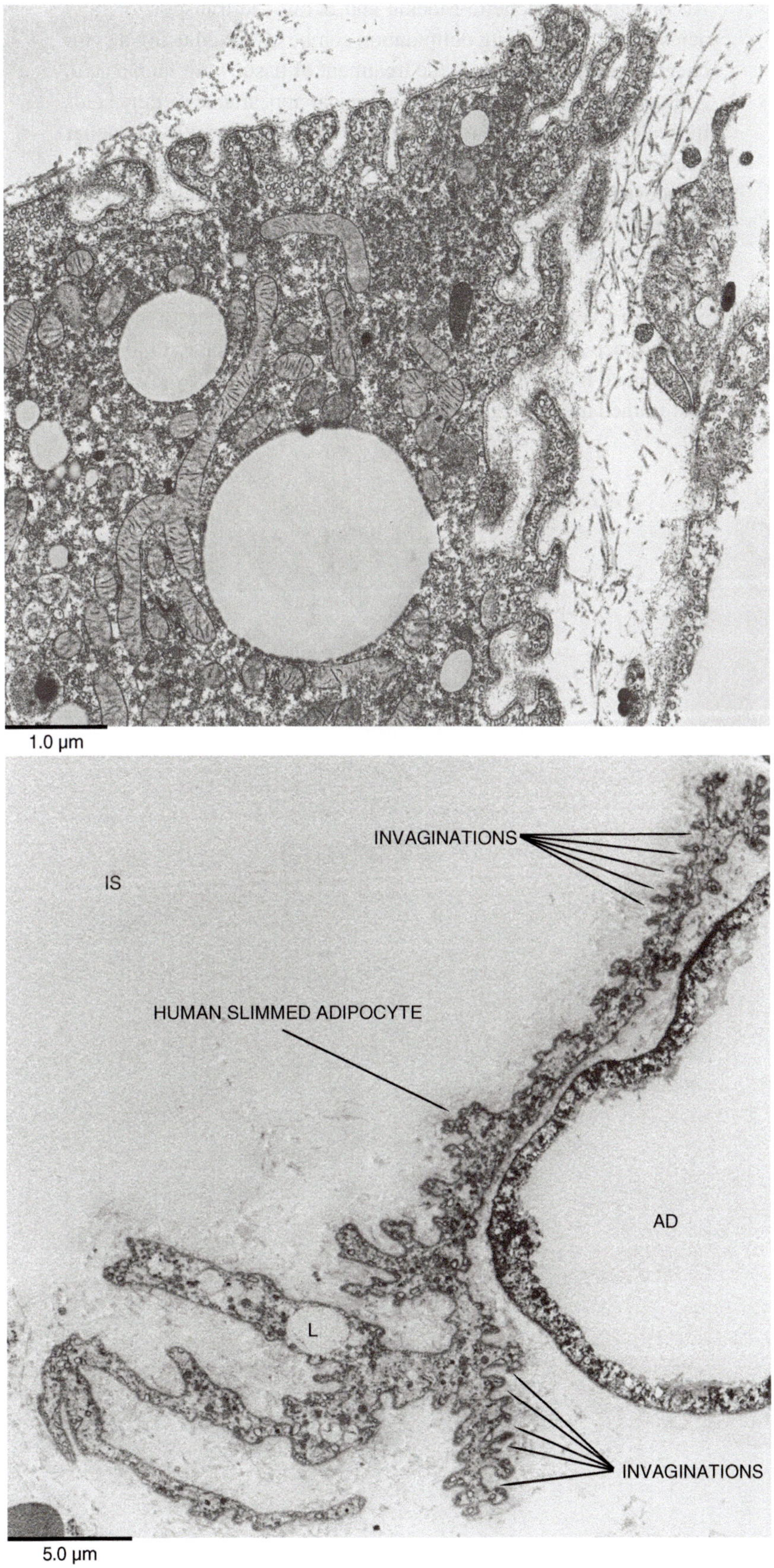

Plate 10.8 *Upper*: enlargement of the cytoplasm of a slimming adipocyte similar to that shown in the *bottom* part of the Plate 10.7. *Lower*: abdominal subcutaneous WAT from an adult lean male subject. IS: interstitial space. TEM

PLATE 10.9

Morphology of Lipolysis I

According to Blanchette-Mackie and Scow, the transport of fatty acids that occurs during delipidation can be observed using a cytochemical method based on the treatment of tissue with tannic acid. At high magnification, the morphological appearance of fatty acids in treated tissue is that of electron-dense material with a lamellar configuration (lamellar whorls; LW). This plate shows a slimming adipocyte in an advanced stage of delipidation between a vein and a unilocular adipocyte. Structures representing mobilized fatty acids (LW, some indicated) can be observed in the cytoplasm of the slimming cell and in the interstitial space.

Note that LW are mainly localized in correspondence to the interstitial space invaginated in the cytoplasm. The interstitial areas invaginated in the slimming cell are not all occupied by LW.

The framed areas are enlarged in the next two plates.

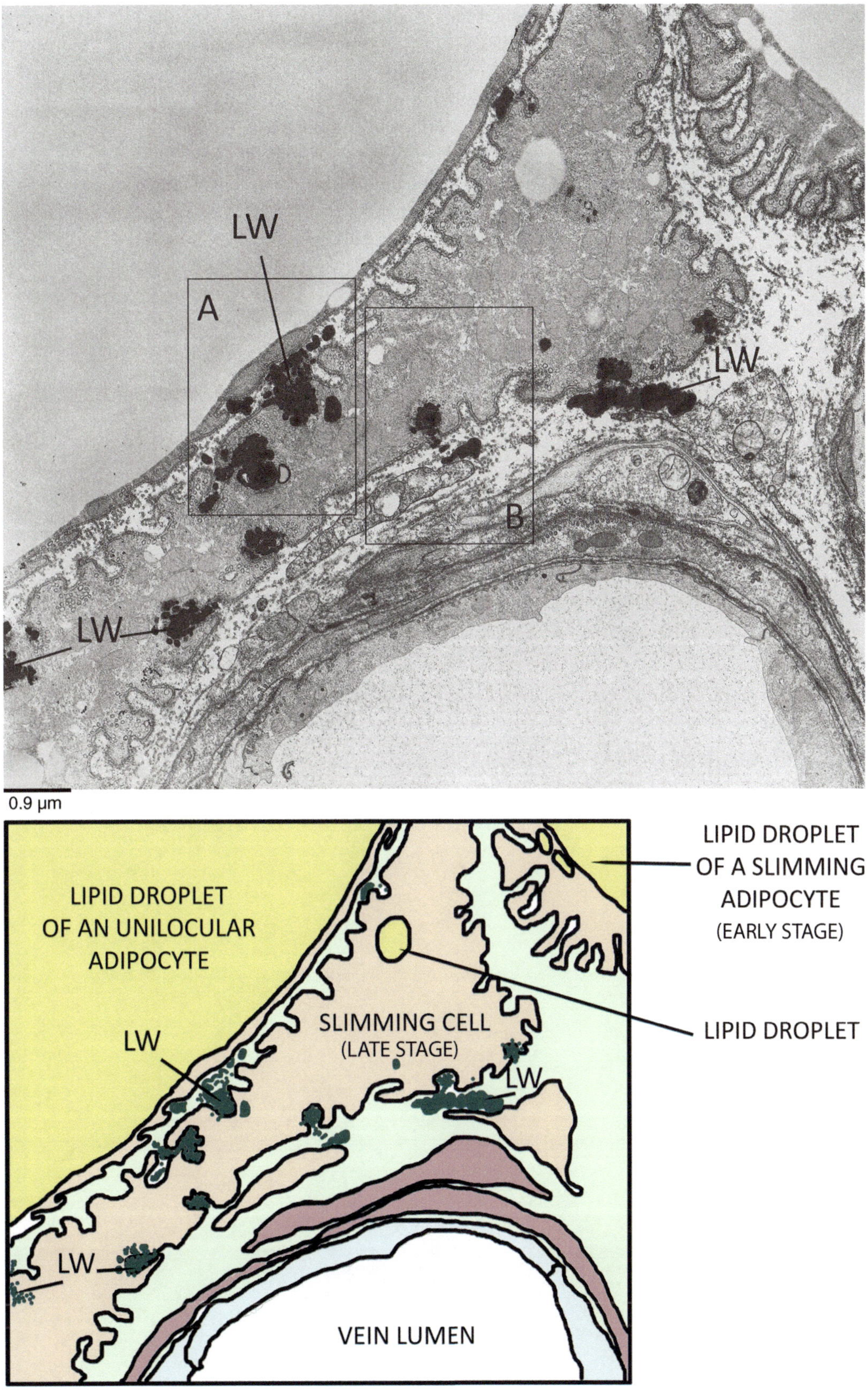

Plate 10.9 Retroperitoneal WAT of an adult rat fasted at 20 °C for 3 days. Frames A and B enlarged in the next plates. TEM. Tannic acid method

PLATE 10.10

Morphology of Lipolysis II

The enlargement of framed area A of Plate 10.9 shows lamellar whorls (LW, some indicated) occupying most of the space in the cytoplasmic invaginations of slimming adipocyte. In correspondence to LW, the plasma membrane of the cell and the underlying external lamina (EL) are not visible, and LW appear to be located in a space forming a continuum between the cytoplasm and extracellular interstitium. Note the small lipid droplets (L) surrounded by dense membranous material that can be interpreted as an early step in the formation LW (also see Plate 10.12).

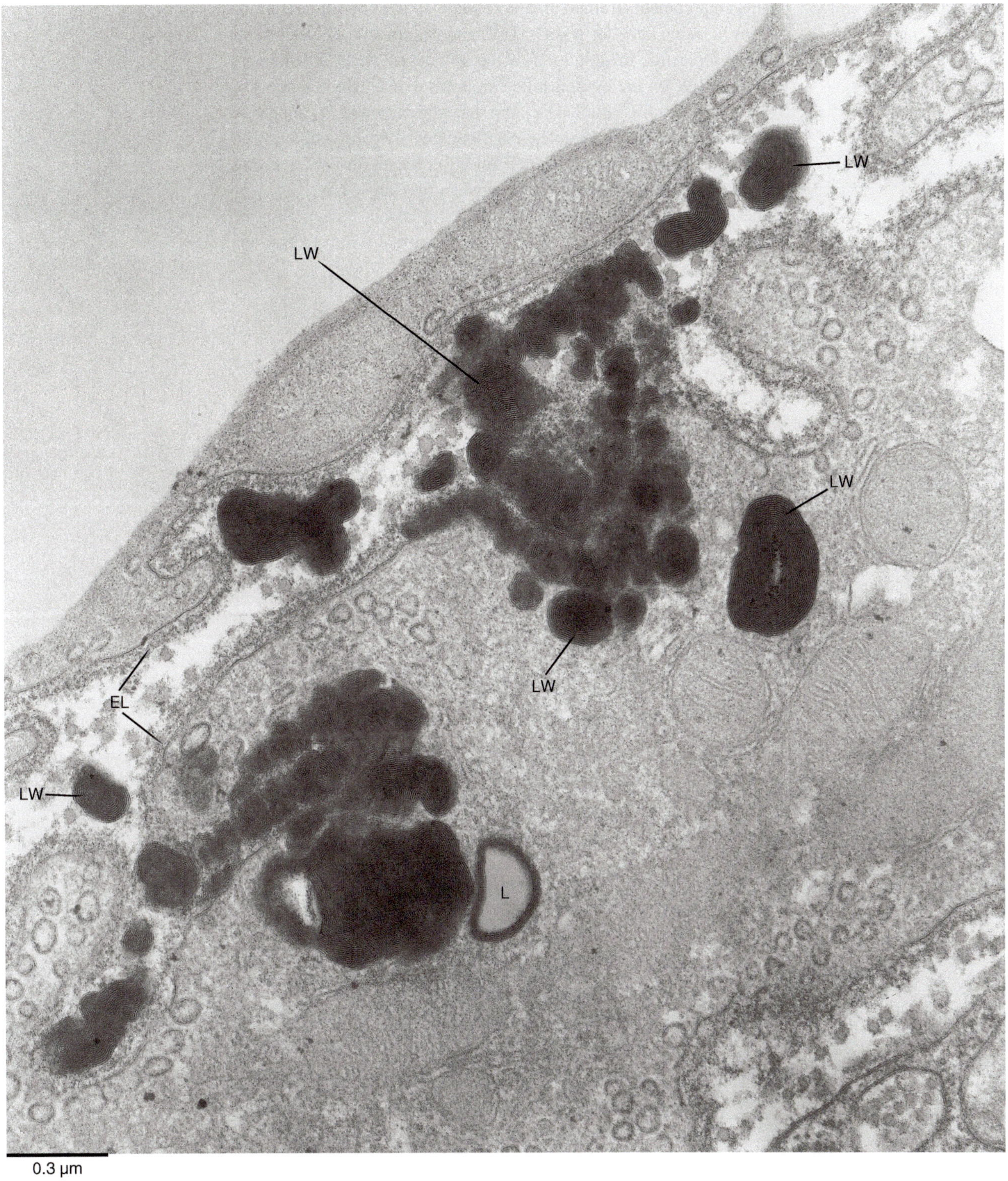

Plate 10.10 Enlargement of the frame A in Plate 10.9. TEM. Tannic acid method

PLATE 10.11

Morphology of Lipolysis III

This enlargement (framed area B of Plate 10.9) shows the relationships between lamellar whorls (LW) and the pinocytotic vesicles in one cytoplasmic invagination of the adipocyte. Note that the surfaces of LW on the cytoplasmic side form extroflexions similar in size to pinocytotic vesicles (V) and that some of them (*) appear to be contained into the vesicles. An elongated LW are visible in the interstitial space (IS) near the cell among collagen fibrils (C). Small LW form a chain-like continuity between two larger LW.

These data suggest a specific role of cytoplasmic invagination of adipocytes for the process of fatty acid extrusion during fasting-induced lipolysis.

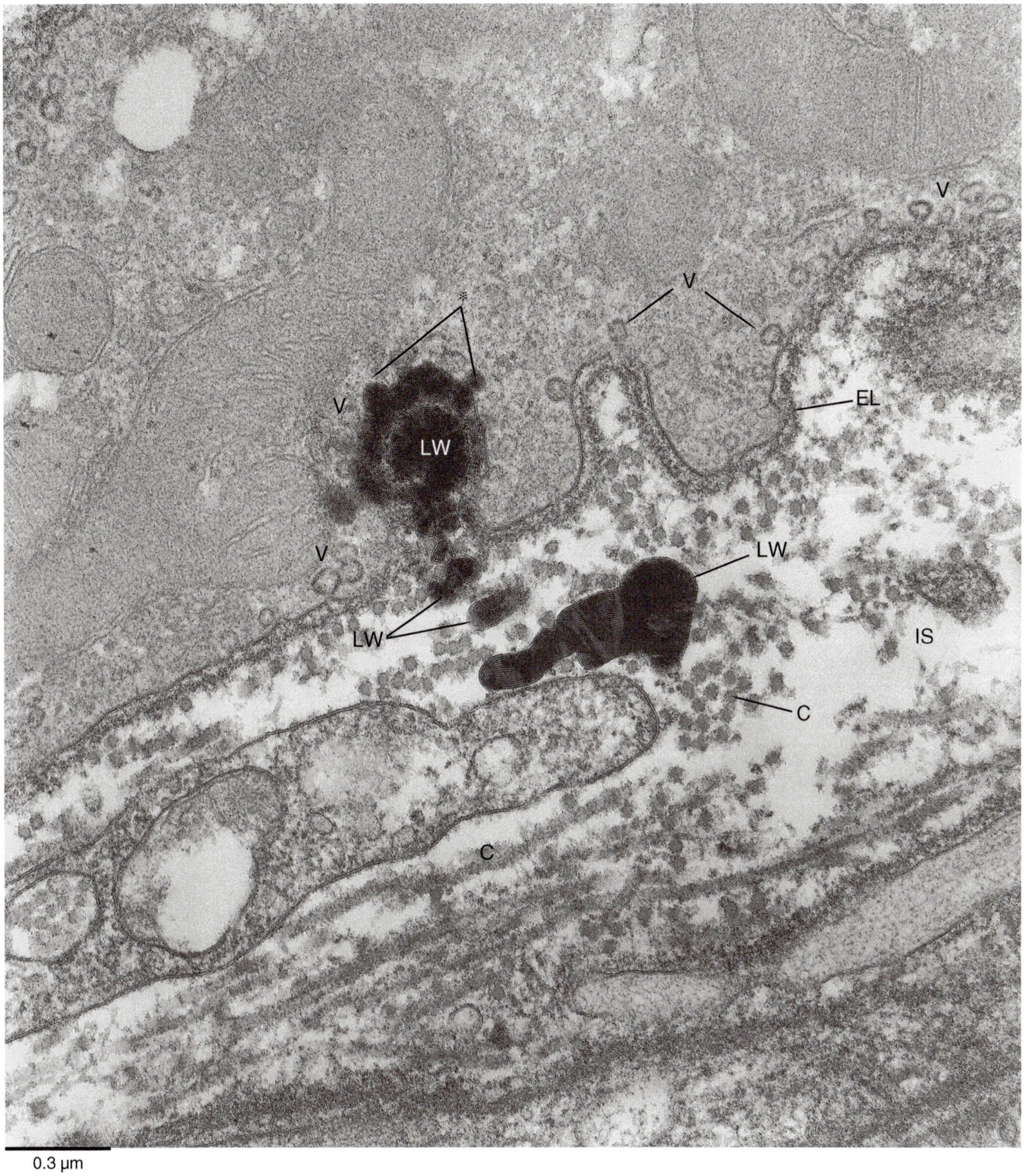

Plate 10.11 Enlargement of the frame B in Plate 10.9.TEM. Tannic acid method

PLATE 10.12

Morphology of Lipolysis IV

Plates 10.9–10.11 show the morphology of delipidizing adipocytes in fasting animals. Similar features can be seen in animals treated with the ß3 agonist CL 316,423, an agent that induces adipose tissue lipolysis. This plate shows an adipocyte from the retroperitoneal fat of an adult rat treated with CL 316,423 for 14 days. Three different stages of lipid extrusion from the cells are visible in this plate.

1. Early step (LW formation). A dense structure with the lamellar ultrastructural aspect identical to that of LW is visible on a portion of the surface of a cytoplasmic lipid droplet (L). This dense structure could represent the consequence of the early stage of lipolysis, in line with the well-known notion that this site corresponds to theoretical anatomical site for the first steps of lipolysis.
2. Intermediate step (fatty acids extrusion). LW are located at the cellular surface in correspondence to an invagination.
3. Late step (fatty acids extruded). LW are visible also in the interstitial space (IS) among collagen fibrils (C). Note three distinct LW at varying distance from the cell suggesting a movement of fatty acids in the interstitial space toward the capillary wall. The plasma membrane is not recognizable as a distinct structure at the level of the LW apposed to the cell surface. In addition, the external lamina (EL) is not visible in the area where the LW are being expelled.

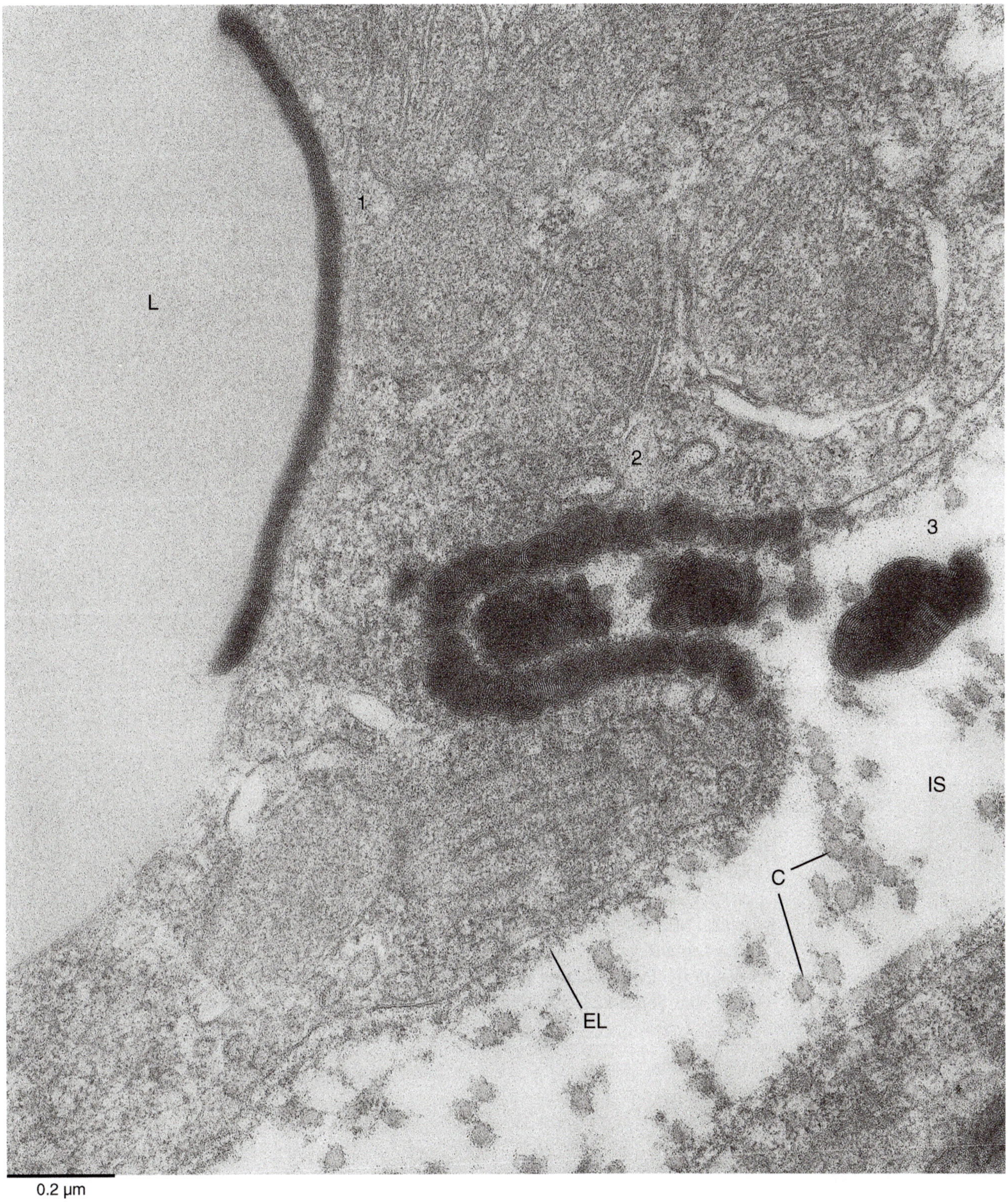

Plate 10.12 Retroperitoneal WAT of adult rat treated for 14 days with the CL 316,423 (ß3 agonist). TEM. Tannic acid method

PLATE 10.13

Morphology of Lipolysis V

According to the hypothesis of Blanchette-Mackie and Scow, fatty acids in adipocytes are transported by lateral diffusion in an interfacial plasma-intracellular membrane continuum.

In fasting condition, the free fatty acids produced by hormone-sensitive lipase from cellular triglycerides are believed to enter the interfacial continuum and flow to capillaries for transport to other tissues or to mitochondria to meet energetic requirements.

According to this hypothesis, the lamellar whorls described in Plates 10.9–10.13 are mainly associated with cellular membranes, including those of mitochondria (upper figure), but we also observed them apparently free in the hyaloplasm (lower panel), even though we cannot exclude the presence of the membranes of other organelles not included in the section, which could be in connection with these structures.

Suggested Reading

Blanchette-Mackie EJ, Scow RO. Membrane continuities within cells and intercellular contacts in white adipose tissue of young rats. J Utrastruct Res. 77:277–94, 1981.

Blanchette-Mackie EJ, Scow RO. Lipolysis and lamellar structures in white adipose tissue of young rats: lipid movement in membranes. J Ultrastruct Res. 77:295–318, 1981.

Blanchette-Mackie EJ, Scow RO. Continuity of intracellular channels with extracellular space in adipose tissue and liver: demonstrated with tannic acid and lanthanum. Anat Rec. 203:205–19, 1982.

Blanchette-Mackie EJ, Scow RO. Movement of lipolytic products to mitochondria in brown adipose tissue of young rats: an electron microscope study. J Lipid Res. 24:229–44, 1983.

Scow RO, Blanchette-Mackie EJ. Why fatty acids flow in cell membranes. Prog Lipid Res. 24:197–241, 1985.

Blanchette-Mackie EJ, et al. Cytochemical studies of lipid metabolism: immunogold probes for lipoprotein lipase and cholesterol. Am J Anat. 185: 255–63, 1989.

Rosenthal MD. Fatty acid metabolism of isolated mammalian cells. Prog Lipid Res. 26:87–124, 1987.

Veerkamp JH. Fatty acid transport and fatty acid-binding proteins. Prog Nutr Soc. 54:23–37, 1995.

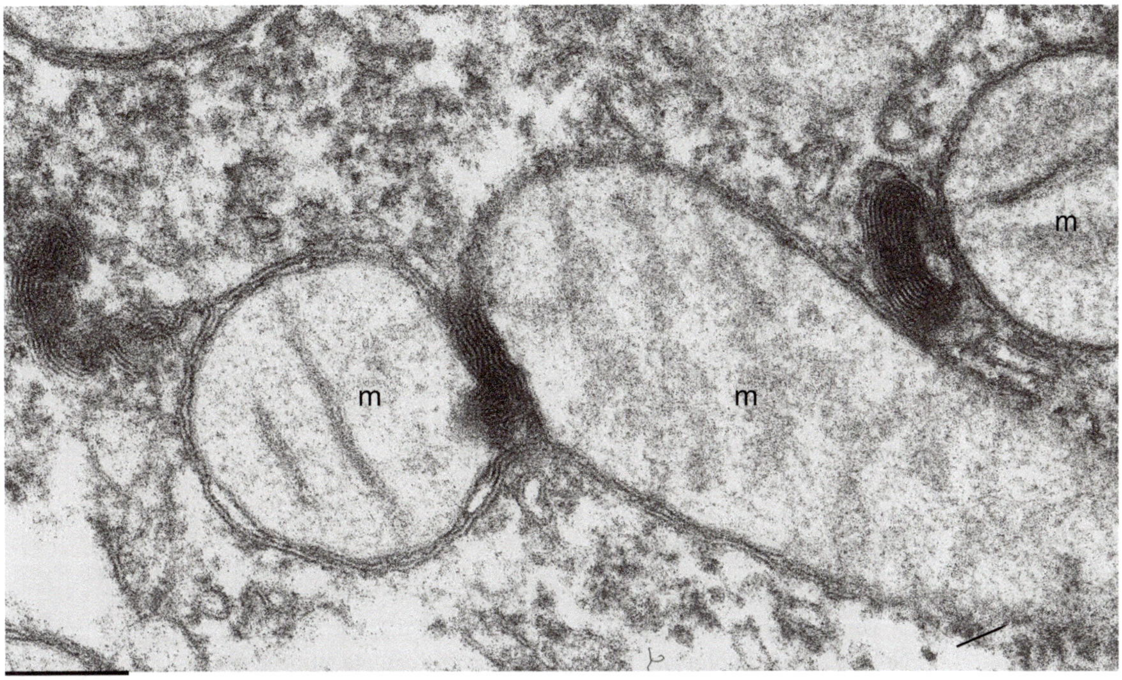

0.12 µm

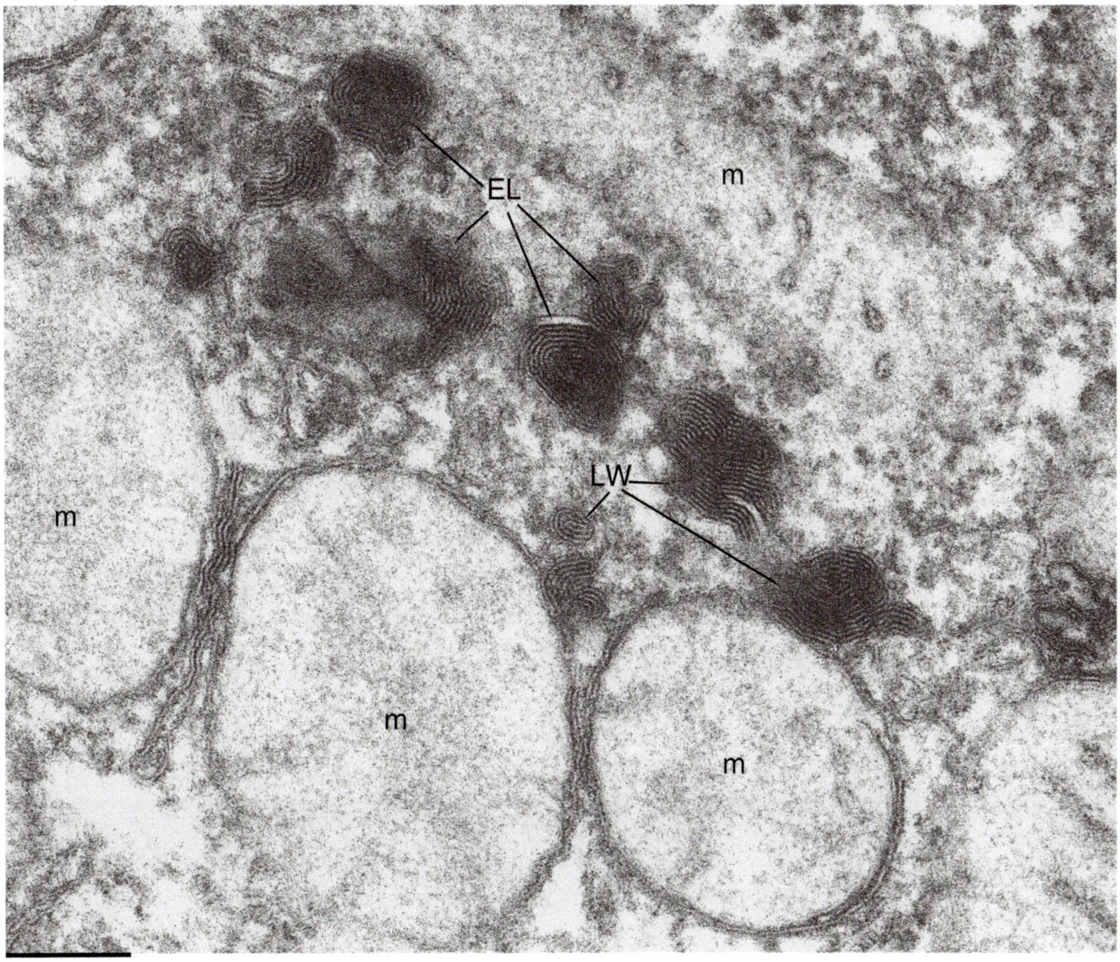

0.12 µm

Plate 10.13 Retroperitoneal WAT of an adult rat fasted for 3 days at 20 °C. Lamellar whorls (LW) in tight connection with the mitochondria (m) membrane and apparently free in the hyaloplasm. TEM. Tannic acid method

PLATE 10.14

Nerves EM

Schwann cells (SC) and perineural cells (P) observed in the nerves of the white adipose tissue of fasting animals often contain a number of lipid droplets (L). Note the adipocytes in a late stage of delipidation (slimming cells, S), and compare them with the fibroblast in the upper right corner (F). The morphology of an adipocyte in an advanced stage of delipidation differs from that of fibroblasts mainly in the much thinner, elongated, and undulated cytoplasmic processes of the former. Furthermore, the rough endoplasmic reticulum appears more abundant in the cytoplasm of fibroblasts. Moreover, fibroblasts lack an external membrane.

The interstitial space contains a variable amount of collagen fibrils (C), which appear scattered in a pale edematous matrix.

Our data support a regional-dependent increase of sympathetic innervation in rat WAT during prolonged fasting.

Suggested Reading

Cantu RC, Goodman HM. Effects of denervation and fasting on white adipose tissue. Am J Physiol. 212:207–12, 1967.

Nisoli E, et al. Leptin and nerve growth factor regulate adipose tissue. Nature Med. 2:130, 1996.

Giordano A, et al. Regional-dependent increase of sympathetic innervation in rat white adipose tissue during prolonged fasting. J Histochem Cytochem. 53:679–87, 2005.

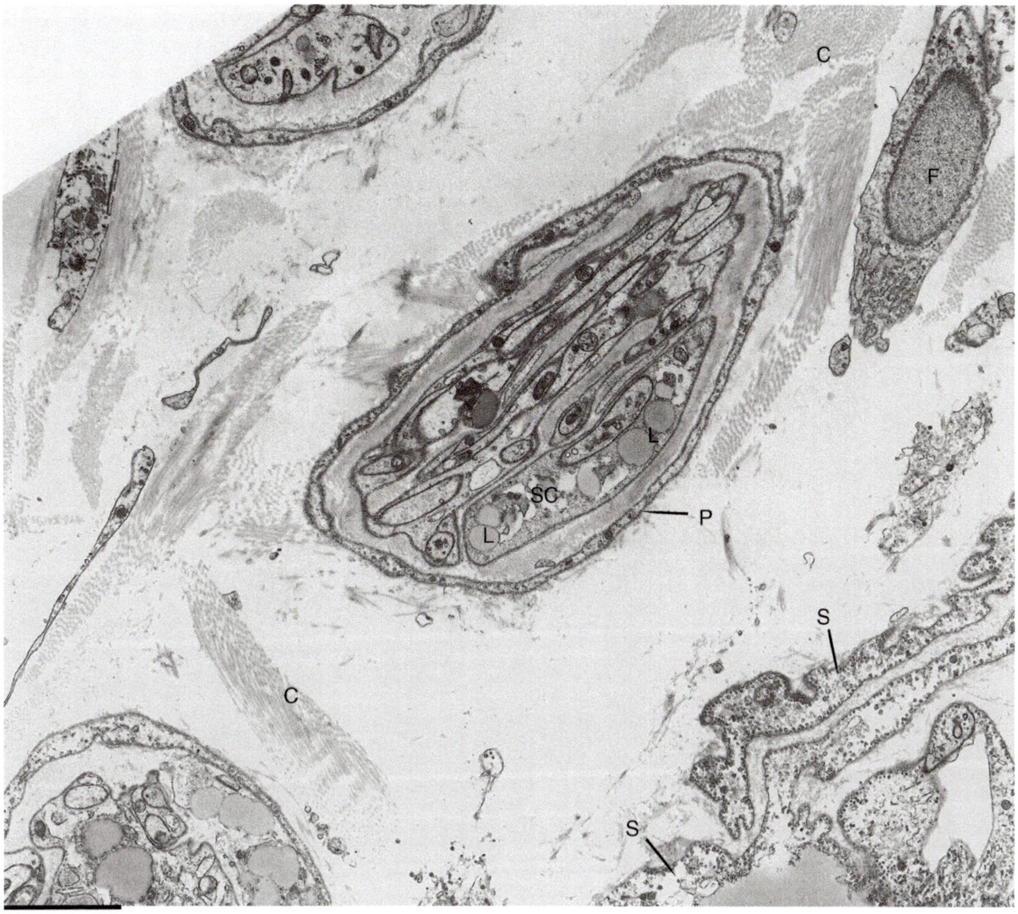

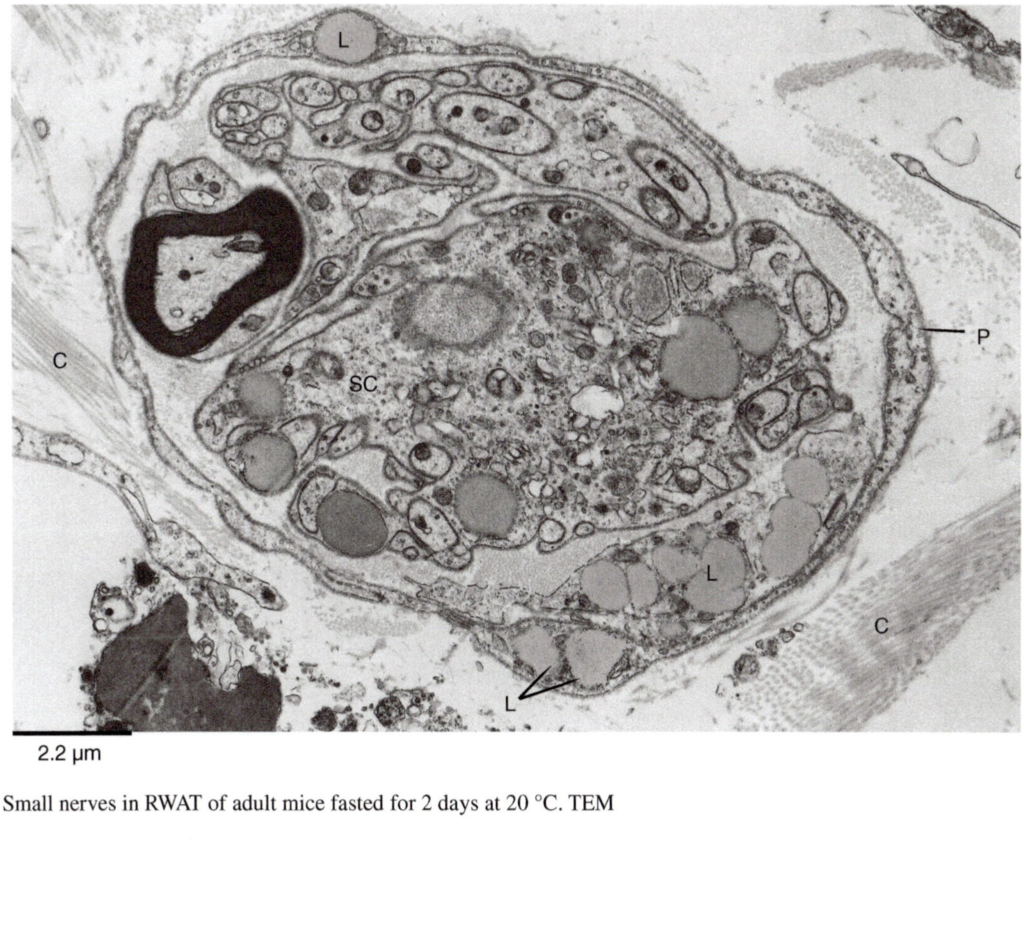

Plate 10.14 Small nerves in RWAT of adult mice fasted for 2 days at 20 °C. TEM

11 The Lactating Adipose Organ

S. Cinti, *Obesity, Type 2 Diabetes and the Adipose Organ*, https://doi.org/10.1007/978-3-319-40522-3_11

11.1 The Lactating Adipose Organ

PLATE 11.1

Gross Anatomy

The two subcutaneous depots, anterior and posterior, of the adipose organ are almost entirely replaced by brownish-pink hypertrophic mammary glands in lactating mice. Note that the upper depot lies almost entirely in dorsal position (see details in Chap. 1 and Plate 11.18). Upon dissection, the relationships between these glands and the nipples located on the axillary-inguinal axis were clearly evident (see pink circles in the lower panel). The anterior gland is connected bilaterally with the three nipples of the anterior middle part of the animal and the posterior gland with the two nipples of the posterior portion of the body.

The remaining portion (visceral depots) of the adipose organ is hypotrophic.

Thus all subcutaneous fat of adult female mice is transformed into mammary glands during pregnancy and lactation. Mice mammary glands are usually described as five bilateral glands due to the presence of ten nipples. Gross anatomy and histology show that the six nipples connected to the anterior subcutaneous depot are not owing to separate glandular structures; thus we should consider the whole glandular mass derived from anterior subcutaneous fat as a single mammary gland provided with six nipples. On the other end, the same reasoning can be applied to the posterior subcutaneous depot that should be considered as a single mammary gland provided with two bilateral nipples.

Suggested Reading

Cowie AT. Proceedings: overview of the mammary gland. J Invest Dermatol. 63:2–9, 1974.

Plagge A, et al. The imprinted signaling protein XL alpha s is required for postnatal adaptation to feeding. Nat Gen. 36:818–26, 2004.

Ercan C, et al. Mammary development and breast cancer: the role of stem cells. Curr Mol Med 11:270–85, 2011.

Bussard KM, Smith GH. The mammary gland microenvironment directs progenitor cell fate in vivo. Int J Cell Biol. 451676:1–11, 2011.

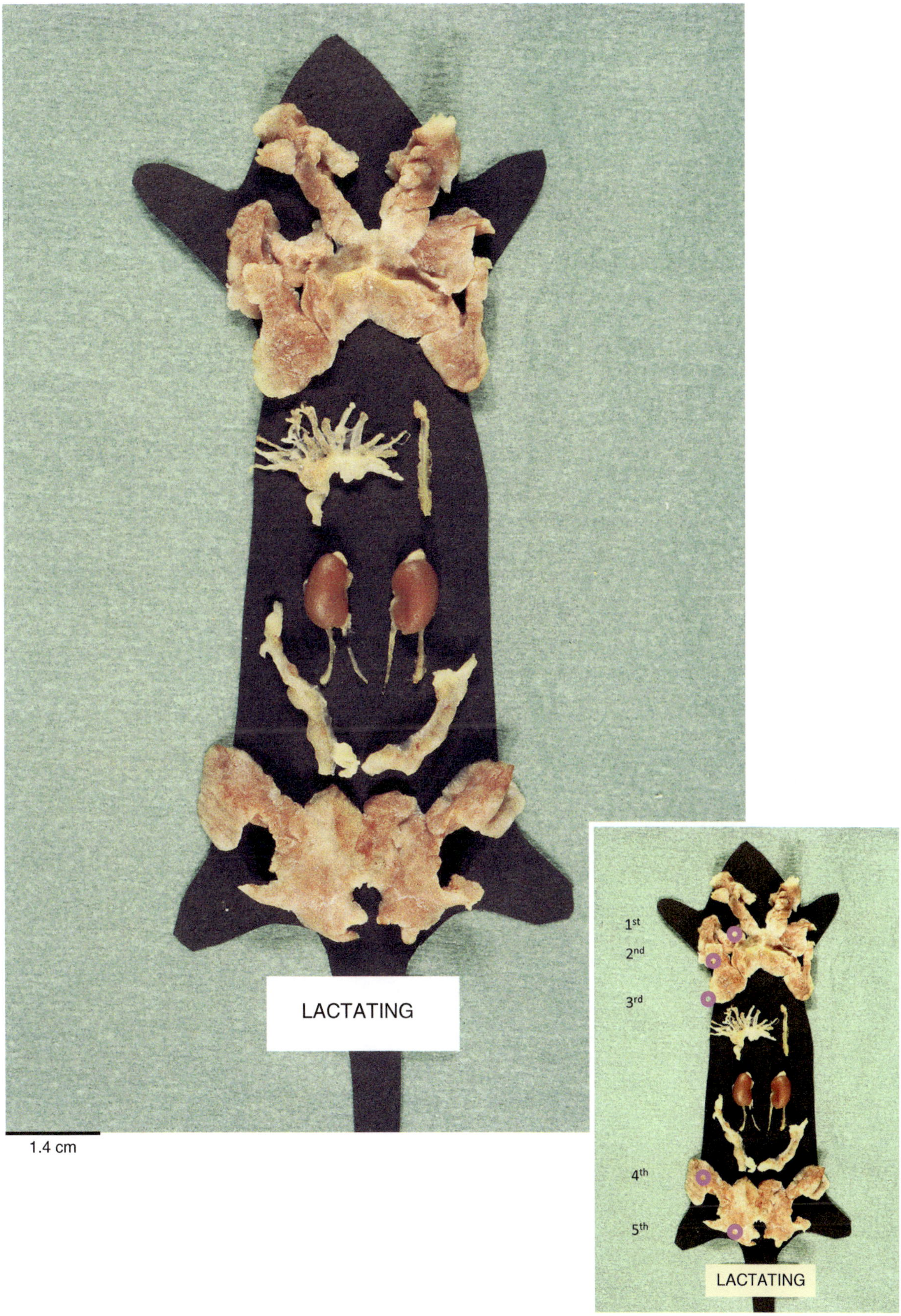

Plate 11.1 Gross anatomy of the adipose organ of a lactating mouse

PLATE 11.2

Pre-pregnancy, Pregnant, Lactating, and Post-Lactation Subcutaneous Fat Histology

The white adipose tissue of murine subcutaneous fat depots is a very plastic tissue that gradually disappears during pregnancy and lactation to reappear at post-lactation with weaning. This plate shows the histology of the inguinal portion of the posterior subcutaneous depot of an adult nonpregnant mouse (upper left), at day 18 of pregnancy (upper right), at day 14 of lactation (bottom left), and at day 10 of post-lactation (bottom right).

In the nonpregnant adult female mice, about 90% of the mammary gland (corresponding to the whole subcutaneous part of the adipose organ) is formed by adipocytes among which branched ducts ending in five bilateral nipples (total of ten mammary glands per mouse, but see details in previous plate) spread for the whole volume of the organ with the exception of the interscapular area occupied by BAT (see also Plate 11.18). In newborn mice the ductal tree is restricted to the peri-nipple area, but at sexual maturity the whole subcutaneous fat is infiltrated.

Note the progressive disappearance of adipocytes in parallel with the development of alveolar glands during pregnancy and lactation. At the apex of lactating period (in mice usually corresponding to 10th–14th day postpartum), only a few adipocytes are visible among the dilated alveolar glands (circled area in lower left panel). A few hours after the end of lactation, alveolar glands start to disappear and adipocytes reappear. At day 10 of the post-lactation period, the pre-pregnancy anatomy of the gland is usually reconstituted.

Suggested Reading

Dulbecco R, et al. Cell types and morphogenesis in the mammary gland. PNAS. 79:7346–50, 1982.

Hovey RC, Trott JF. Morphogenesis of mammary gland development. Adv Exp Med Biol. 554:219–28, 2004.

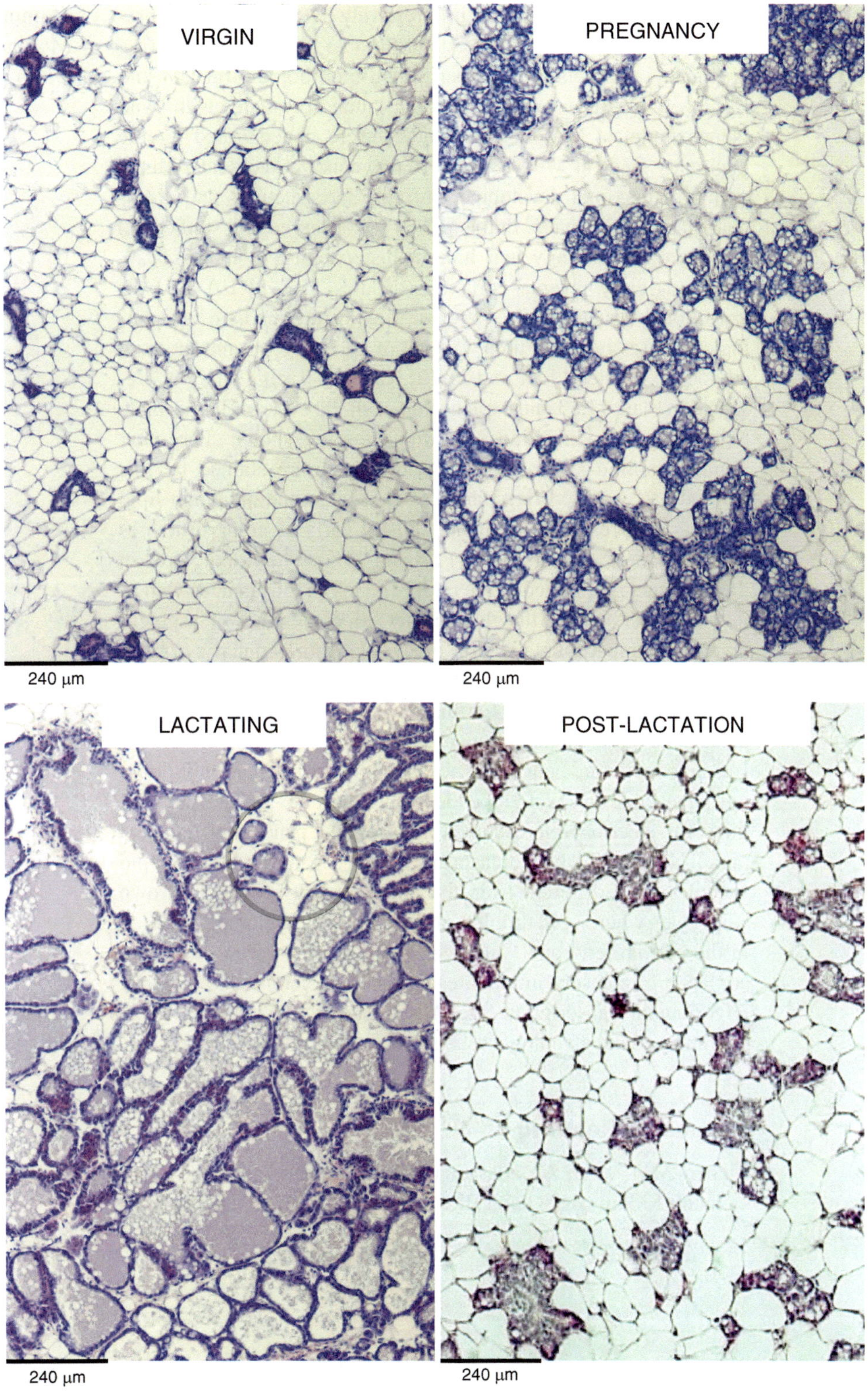

Plate 11.2 *Upper left*: subcutaneous inguinal adipose depot (or fourth mammary gland) of an adult virgin female mouse. Note the hypotrophic glands (manly ducts) among the adipocytes (*dark blue* structures). *Upper right*: fourth mammary gland (corresponding to inguinal fat outside pregnancy) of a mouse at day 18 of pregnancy; note the development of alveolar glands and disappearing of adipocytes. *Lower left*: fourth mammary gland of a mouse at day 14 of lactation; almost only mammary glands are present; few adipocytes are visible among mammary glands (*circled area*). *Lower right*: fourth mammary gland at day 10 of post-lactation; the morphology of the gland is back to the pre-pregnancy anatomy LM. H&E

PLATE 11.3

Mammary Gland Morphology and IHC During Pregnancy

During pregnancy adipocytes progressively disappear (see the previous plate). In order to understand the fate of adipocytes during pregnancy and lactation, we performed morphologic (at LM and EM level), lineage tracing, and explant studies presented in this and the next plates. Morphologic studies were concentrated on the mammary gland at 17th–18th day of pregnancy coincident with the period of maximal development of alveolar structures and disappearance of adipocytes. In this period we observed and studied (1) adipocyte morphology and immunohistochemistry (Plates 11.3–11.6), (2) early alveolar structures (Plates 11.8–11.10), and (3) transitional structures, i.e., structures with intermediate morphologic features between those typical of early alveoli and those of adipocytes (Plates 11.11 and 11.12). Lineage tracing study is presented in Plate 11.13 and explant studies in Plate 11.14. In this plate morphologic modifications of adipocytes are shown. Perilipin1 immunostaining shows that only adipocytes are stained by this antibody as expected (top panel) even if large and abundant lipid droplets are present in epithelial cells of early alveolar structures (middle panel, see also Plates 11.4 and 11.5). The framed area in the top panel is enlarged in the middle panel. In this area, as well as in many other areas of the gland, many adipocytes show a fragmentation or compartmentalization of the perilipin1-coated cytoplasmic lipid vacuole; thus adipocytes acquire a multilocular morphology quite specific for this stage of pregnancy in the subcutaneous fat of the mammary gland. Details of these compartmentalized adipocytes are better observed at higher magnification (bottom left panel) and in resin-embedded toluidine blue-stained preparations for electron microscopy (bottom right panel and the next plate). Note the thick cytoplasm and the net separation of large lipid vacuoles, well different from the multilocularity found in brown adipocytes where lipid droplets are much more regular and smaller. In the bottom left panel, nuclei of an alveolar structure (top right corner) are intensely immunoreactive for Elf5 (E74-like factor 5, ETS-domain transcription factor), a master transcription factor of mammary gland alveologenesis (see also Plate 11.5).

Suggested Reading

Richert MM, et al. An atlas of mouse mammary gland development. J Mammary Gland Biol Neoplasia. 5:227–41, 2000.

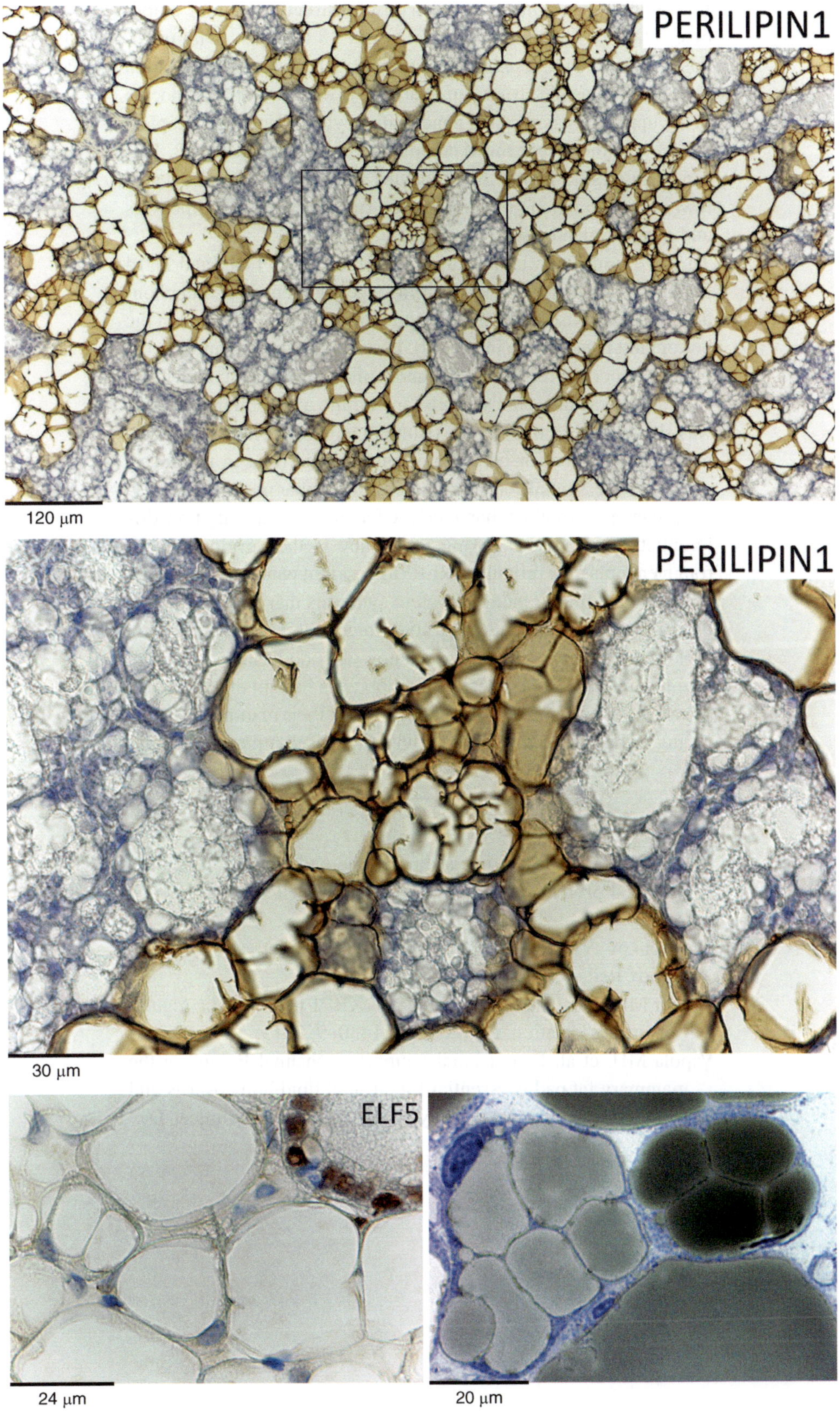

Plate 11.3 Fourth mammary gland (inguinal) of mouse at day 18 of pregnancy. LM. IHC Perilipin1 (1:400). *Lower left*: IHC ab ELF5 (1.300). *Lower right*: resin-embedded tissue. Toluidine blue

PLATE 11.4

Adipocyte Ultrastructure During Pregnancy I

In the upper panel the characteristic ultrastructure of four adipocytes (1–4) of mammary gland fat at day 18 (compare with previous plate) is shown. A partial lipid droplet (L) compartmentalization by thin cytoplasmic strips (small arrow) is evident in the adipocyte in the upper right part of the panel (adipocyte 1). Note the cytoplasmic projections (big arrows) embracing the small adipocyte 2. This aspect suggests a fusion of adipocytes 1 and 2 that could be a step toward the formation of intermediate structures between adipocytes and alveolar glands (see Plate 11.11).

These "transdifferentiating adipocytes" (see Plates 11.13 and 11.14 for further explanations) are rich in large and abundant mitochondria. Also peroxisomes are large and numerous (P) (enlarged in the bottom left panel, some indicated). Peroxisomes are organelles that play an important role in the metabolism of amphipathic molecules such as fatty acids, some steroids, and amino acids. Interestingly, it was shown that Pxmp2, a peroxisomal membrane channel of paramount importance for peroxisome physiologic role, in mammary gland fat, is essential for development of the mammary gland during pregnancy. Another characteristic feature of mammary transdifferentiating adipocytes during pregnancy is the development of rough endoplasmic reticulum RER (lower right panel), an organelle of paramount importance for protein synthesis that is poorly developed in normal adipocytes. Of note, mice lacking X-box binding protein 1 (XBP1), a central regulator of endoplasmic reticulum adaptive response, specifically in adipocytes had no effect on adipogenesis or systemic lipid metabolism, but their mammary glands during lactation had abundant fat with decreased milk production.

Suggested Reading

Ron D, Walter P. Signal integration in the endoplasmic reticulum unfolded protein response. Nat Rev Mol Cell Biol. 8:519–29, 2007.

Antonenkov VD, et al. Peroxisomes are oxidative organelles. Antiox Redox Signal. 13:525–37, 2010.

Gregor MF, et al. The role of adipocyte XBP1 in metabolic regulation during lactation. Cell Rep. 30:1430–9, 2013.

Vapola MH, et al. Peroxisomal membrane channel Pxmp2 in the mammary fat pad is essential for stromal lipid homeostasis and for development of mammary gland epithelium in mice. Dev Biol 391:66–80, 2014.

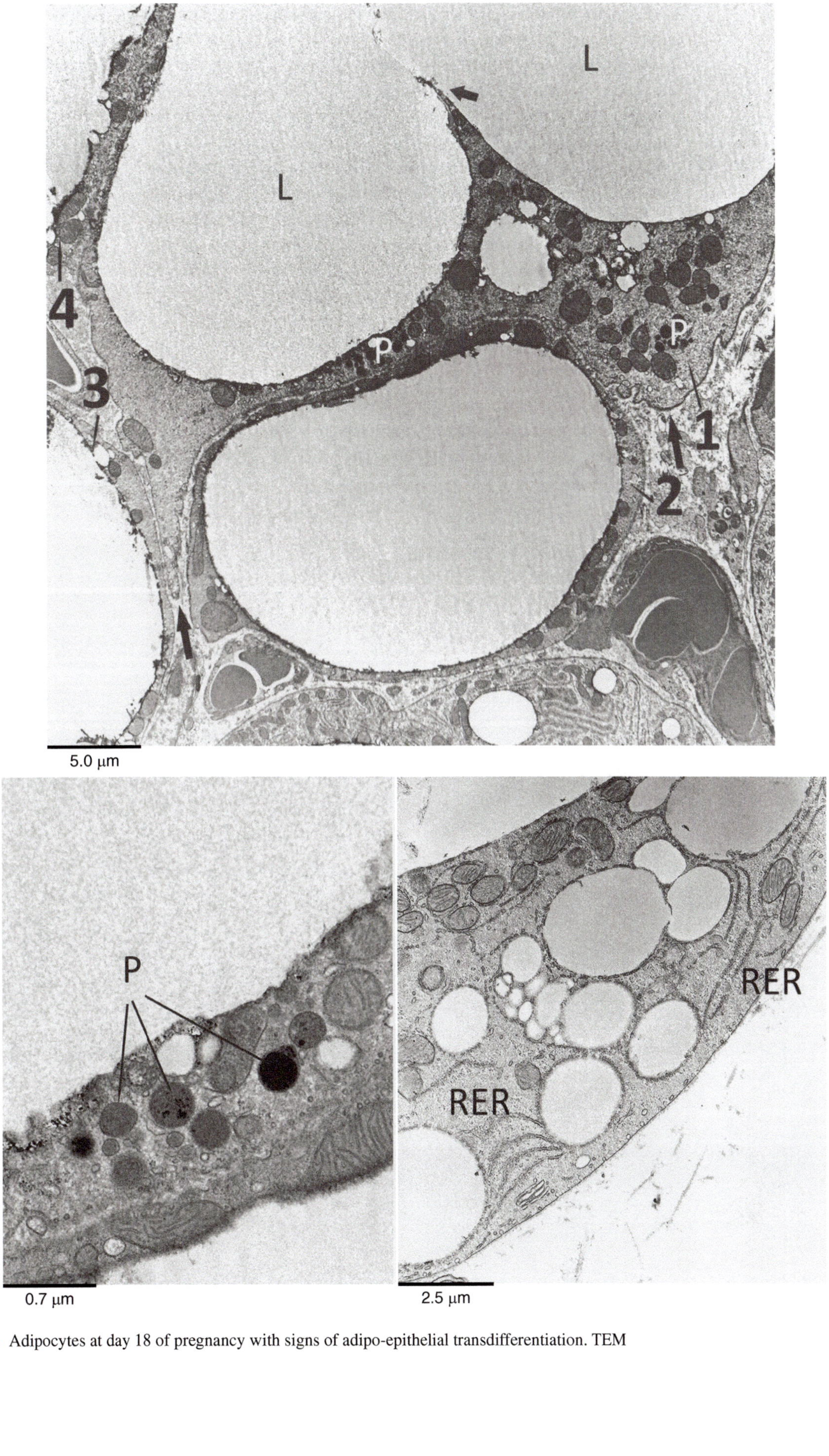

Plate 11.4 Adipocytes at day 18 of pregnancy with signs of adipo-epithelial transdifferentiation. TEM

PLATE 11.5

Adipocyte Ultrastructure During Pregnancy II

In this plate other examples of the dynamic changes occurring to adipocytes in this period of pregnancy (day 18) are shown. In the upper plate a compartmentalized adipocyte is visible on the left side. Note the thin cytoplasmic strips during early compartmentalization phase (small arrows). Two embracing adipocytes are in the center of the panel, and the embracing cytoplasmic projections are enlarged in the lower panel (arrows). The right part of the upper panel shows an early alveolus formed by glandular epithelia cells with abundant cytoplasmic lipid droplets (pink adipocytes; see Plate 11.8). Note the almost perfect correspondence in size among the compartmentalized lipid droplets of adipocytes, those in embracing adipocytes and those in pink adipocytes.

Suggested Reading

Smorlesi A, et al. The adipose organ: white-brown adipocyte plasticity and metabolic inflammation. Obes Rev. 13:83–96, 2012.

Cinti S. The adipose organ at a glance. Dis Model Mech. 5:588–94, 2012.

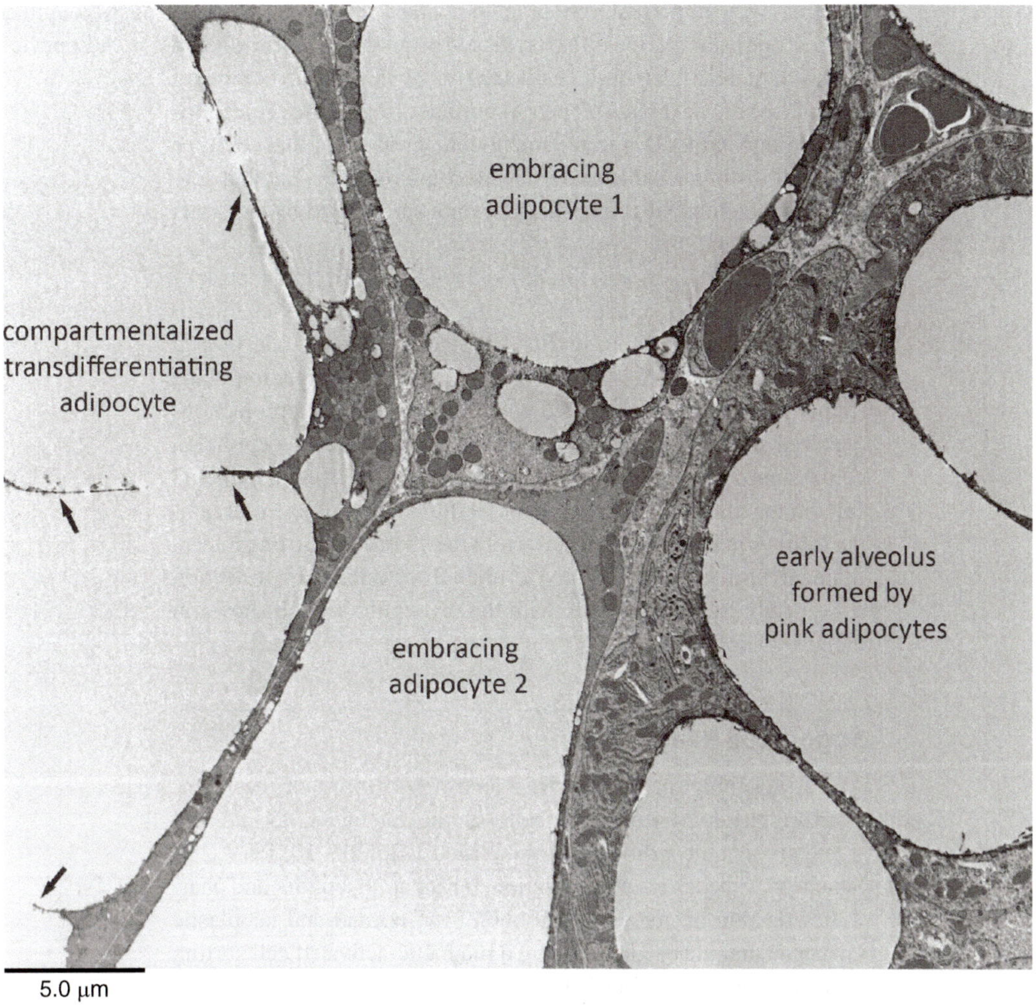

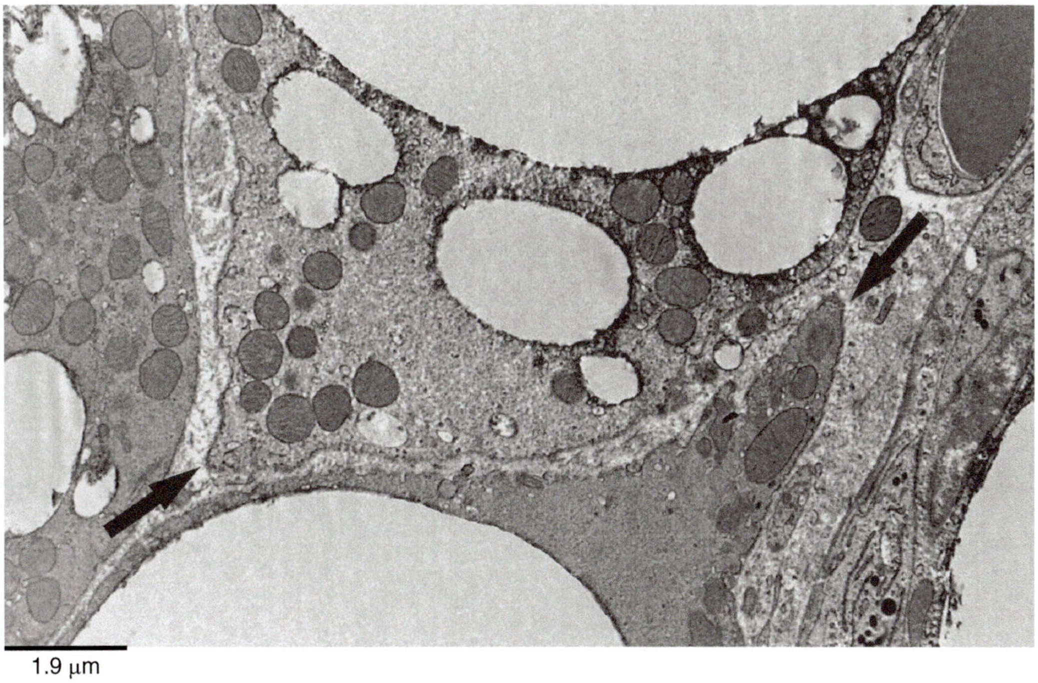

Plate 11.5 Adipocytes at day 18 of pregnancy with signs of adipo-epithelial transdifferentiation. TEM

PLATE 11.6

Myoepithelial-Adipocyte Connection

Another very important topographic feature visible by electron microscope in this period is that presented in this plate. Myoepithelial cells are stellate elements characteristic of developed mammary alveoli (see the next plate). Their fingerlike cytoplasmic projections are rich in contractile microfilament characteristic of this cell type and well distinguishable under electron microscope. Another feature of myoepithelial cells is that they are surrounded by a distinct external lamina.

In this pregnancy period (18th day) when alveoli are in the peak of their development coinciding with the peak of adipocytes, disappearance, it is possible to find isolated adipocytes with developed organelles denoting its adipo-epithelial transdifferentiation stage (upper panel) tightly connected with myoepithelial cell projections (squared area enlarged in the two lower panels). The myoepithelial cell assumes the topographic connotation typical of myoepithelial cells in the glands, i.e., inserted into a duplication of external lamina (arrows in lower right panel). Note the characteristic fine microfilament structure (F) of myoepithelial cytoplasmic projection (lower right panel). Compare with the myoepithelial cell shown in the next plate.

Suggested Reading

Abe J. Scanning electron microscopic observations of the mammary gland myoepithelial cells of the rat under normal and experimental conditions. Kurume Med J. 26:303–10, 1979.

Sánchez-Céspedes R, et al. Isolation, purification, culture and characterisation of myoepithelial cells from normal and neoplastic canine mammary glands using a magnetic-activated cell sorting separation system. Vet J. 197:474–82, 2013.

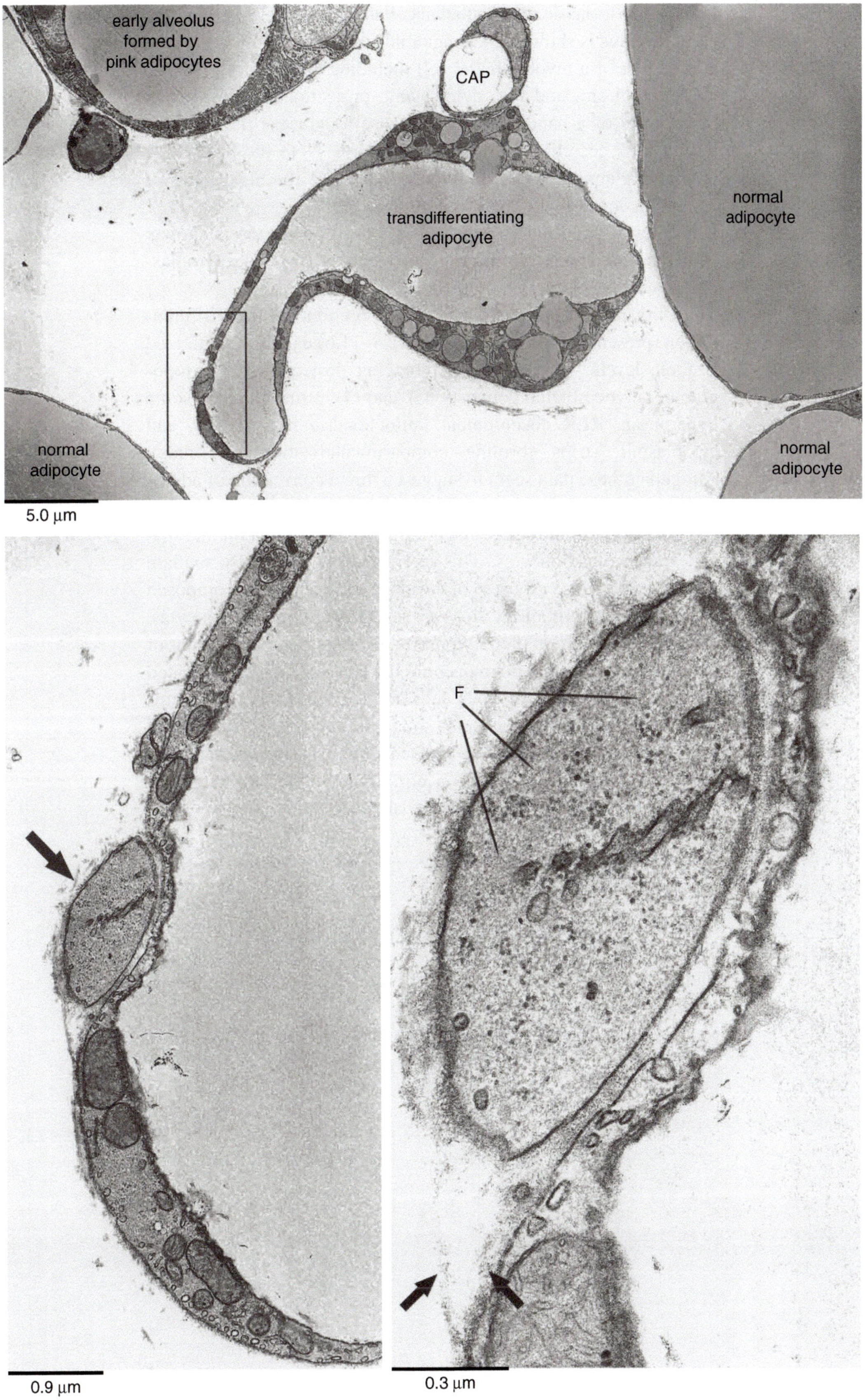

Plate 11.6 Adipocyte at day 18 of pregnancy with aspects of adipo-myoepithelial conjunction. TEM

PLATE 11.7

Myoepithelial Cell Ultrastructure

In this plate a classic myoepithelial cell at the external surface of an early alveolus is shown. The tangential section plane allows seeing a large part of a myoepithelial cell including nucleus (N), perinuclear cytoplasm, and two cytoplasmic projections (arrows) that, like fingers of a hand, have the purpose to squeeze the alveolus during milk secretion in the sucking phase. Note the lipid-filled epithelial glandular cells (pink adipocytes; see the next plate for details) in contact with the myoepithelial cell.

In the lower panel an enlargement of the framed area is shown. Note the abundant microfilaments visible in the fingerlike cytoplasmic projection of the myoepithelial cell (F).

Thus, the ultrastructural changes of adipo-epithelial transdifferentiation (present and previous plates, 11.4–11.6) can be summarized at three levels: (1) dynamic (embracing projections), (2) topographic (myoepithelial connections), and (3) intrinsic (peroxisome hyperplasia, RER development, mitochondria hypertrophy, and cytoplasmic strips forming compartmentalization of lipids). Altogether these data seem to suggest a direct conversion of adipocytes into epithelial alveolar structures during pregnancy, offering an explanation to the concomitant development of alveoli and disappearance of adipocytes. This interpretation could also explain why alveoli in this early step of development are mainly composed of cell with a morphology strongly resembling that of adipocytes. These cells contain in their cytoplasm an adipocyte-like amount of fat that is difficult to explain in epithelial cells eventually generated by a stem cell. If these alveolar cells derive from stem cells, a similar amount of cytoplasmic lipids should be considered an unusual step of development for these elements, even taking into account the fact that a lipid droplet is a normal component of secretory products in a well-developed mature alveolar cell.

Suggested Reading

Silver IA. Myoepthelial cells in the mammary and parotid glands. J Physiol Z. 125:8–9, 1954.

Radnor CJ. Myoepithelial cell differentiation in rat mammary glands. J Anat. 111: 381–98, 1972.

Moumen M, et al. The mammary myoepithelial cell. Int J Dev Biol. 55:763–71, 2011.

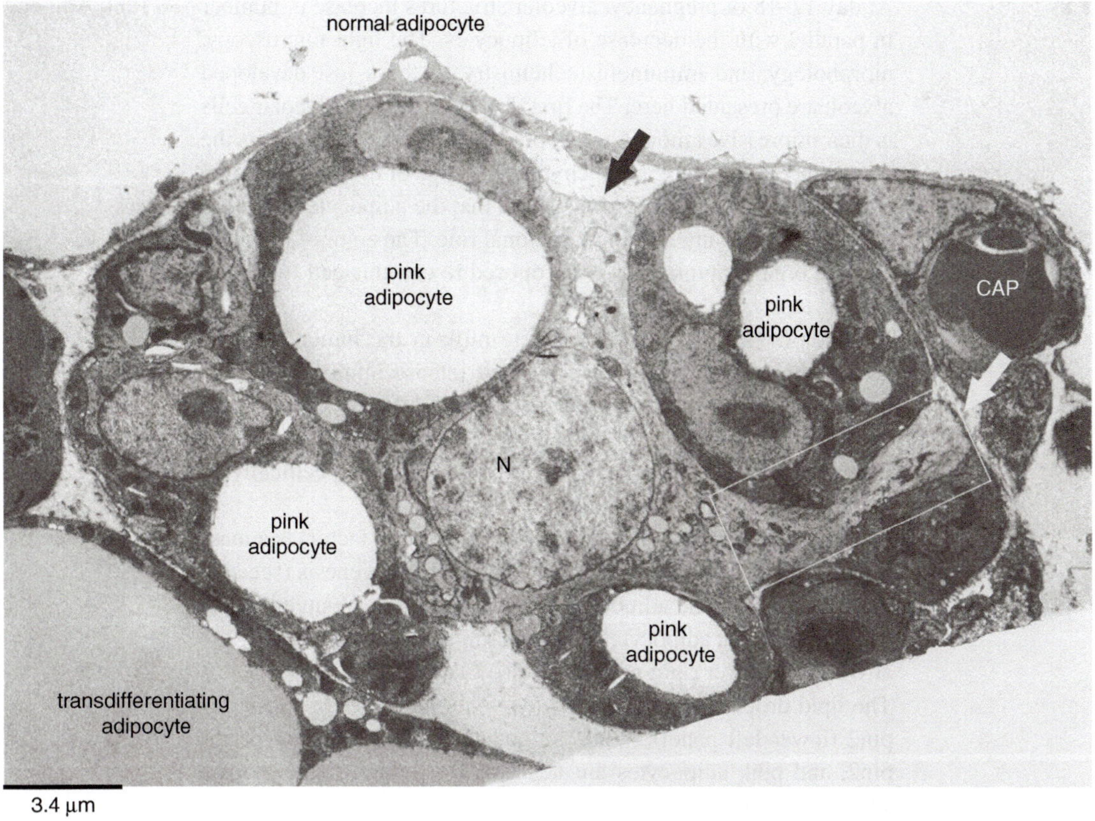

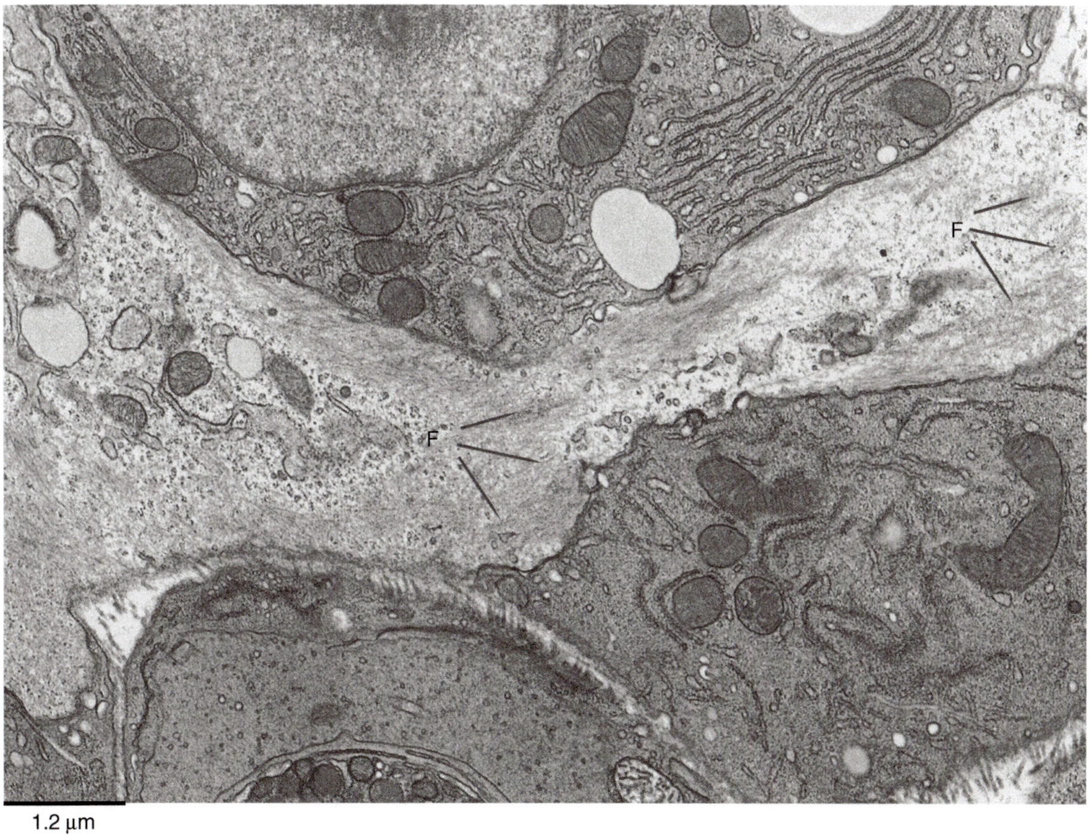

Plate 11.7 Mouse mammary gland at day 18 of pregnancy. Myoepithelial cell in tangential section of the superficial part of an alveolus. Pink adipocytes; see Plate 11.8. TEM

PLATE 11.8

Pink Adipocytes

At day 17–18 of pregnancy, alveolar structures increase in number in parallel with the decrease of adipocytes. The light microscopy, morphology, and immunohistochemistry of these just developed alveoli are presented here. The first obvious aspect of alveolar cells is their impressive amount of cytoplasmic fat. Thus, this cell fits the definition of adipocyte: parenchymal cell type of the adipose organ with relevant cytoplasmic lipids. Note that the adipocyte definition does not include any specific functional role. The color of pregnant adipose organ is pink; thus we proposed to call this cell type pink adipocyte.

Pink adipocytes produce and secrete milk in the lumen of these alveoli (upper panel) as shown by their intense immunoreactivity for the classic protein component of milk: whey acid protein (WAP).

Pink adipocytes resulted intensely immunostained specifically in their nuclei by Elf5 antibodies.

Elf5 (E74-like factor 5, ETS-domain transcription factor) is a master transcription factor of mammary gland alveologenesis (see also Plate 11.3). Note the adipocyte-like morphology of glandular epithelial cells (pink adipocytes) and in particular that indicated by the arrow in the lower right panel (see also Plate 11.14).

The lipid droplet of pink adipocytes is immunoreactive for perilipin2 (lower left panel). White adipocytes are negative for perilipin2, and pink adipocytes are negative for perilipin1 (see Plates 11.3 and 11.9).

Suggested Reading

Gordano A, et al. White, brown and pink adipocytes: the extraordinary plasticity of the adipose organ. Eur J Endocrinol. 170:R159–71, 2014.

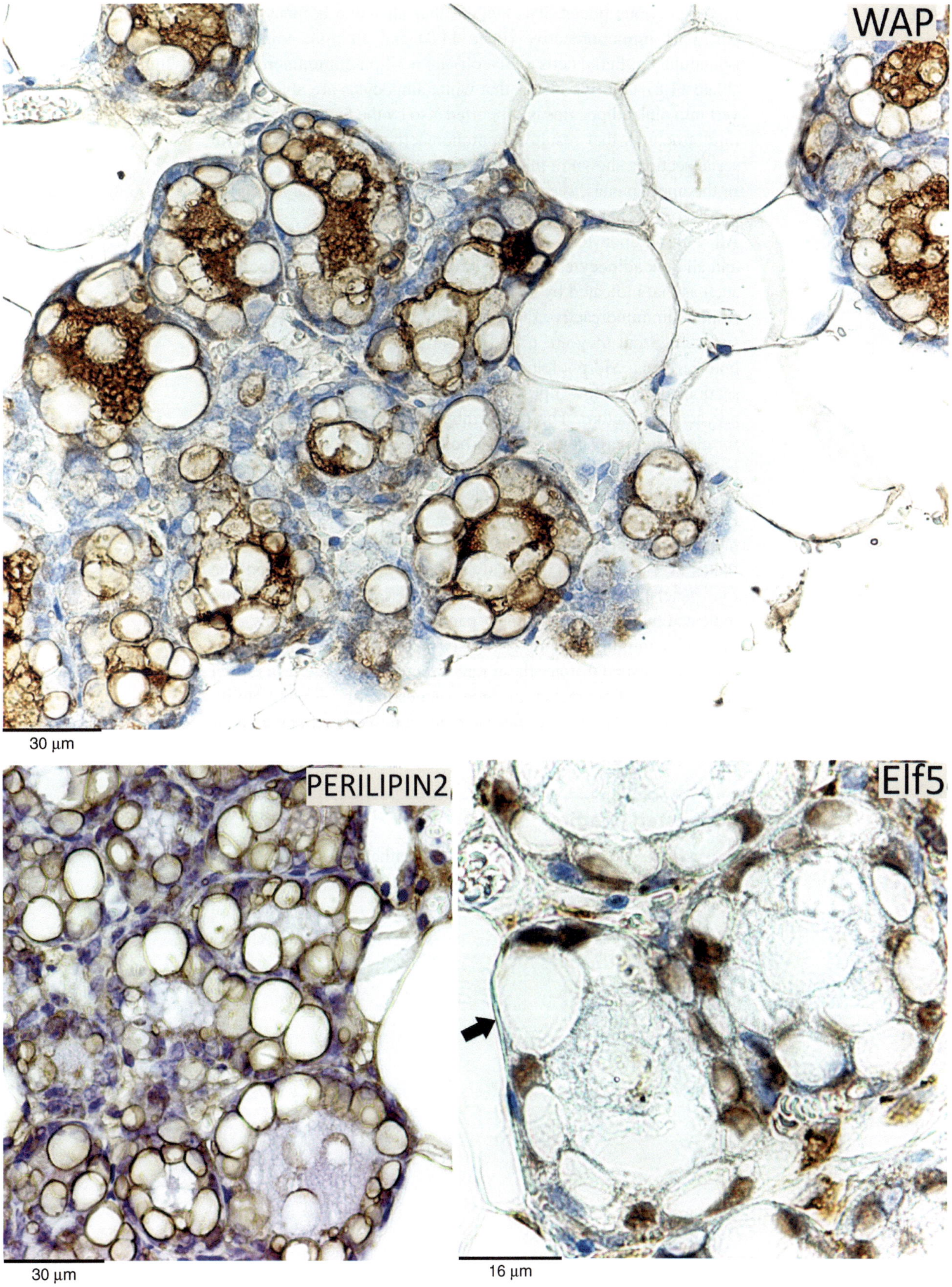

Plate 11.8 Mouse mammary gland at day 18 of pregnancy. Pink adipocytes (epithelial alveolar cells). LM. IHC ab WAP (1:400), ab perilipin2 (1:150), ab Elf5 (1:300)

PLATE 11.9

Perilipin1 and Perilipin2 Immunoreactive Structures

In the previous plates, it is evident that all white adipocytes are perilipin1 immunoreactive (Plate 11.3) and all pink adipocytes (glandular epithelial cells of alveoli) are perilipin2 immunoreactive (Plate 11.8). Our hypothesis that white adipocytes are able to convert into pink adipocytes is supported also by the fact that we found rare structures that resulted immunoreactive for both proteins in serial sections shown in this plate.

In the upper panels, serial sections of a mouse mammary gland at day 18 of pregnancy are shown.

All white adipocytes are perilipin1 immunoreactive (left panel), and all pink adipocytes resulted perilipin2 positive. Rare structures such as that indicated by an arrow and enlarged 3.6 times in insets resulted immunoreactive for both perilipin1 and perilipin2 proteins suggesting that they are transdifferentiating structures containing both proteins. Morphological details of paraffin-embedded tissue sections do not allow a precise identification of the double immunoreactive structure. The resin-embedded toluidine-stained tissue for electron microscopy allows a better detail and is shown in the lower panels. Left lower panel shows an alveolar structure lined by pink adipocytes with lipid droplets in the lumen (compare with Plates 11.10–11.12). The right lower panel shows two compartmentalized transdifferentiating white adipocytes (compare with Plates 11.3–11.5). As it is visually evident by the comparison of the four panels, the double immunoreactive serial-sectioned structure indicated by arrows in the upper panels could be both. In any case the double immunostaining obviously supports the transdifferentiation hypothesis. Of note, these rare structures become less rare at second or third pregnancy of mice, suggesting an acquired ability of mammary adipocytes (white) to convert into epithelial glandular structures (pink).

Suggested Reading

Prokesch A. Molecular aspects of adipoepithelial transdifferentiation in mouse mammary gland. Stem Cells. 32:2756–66, 2014.

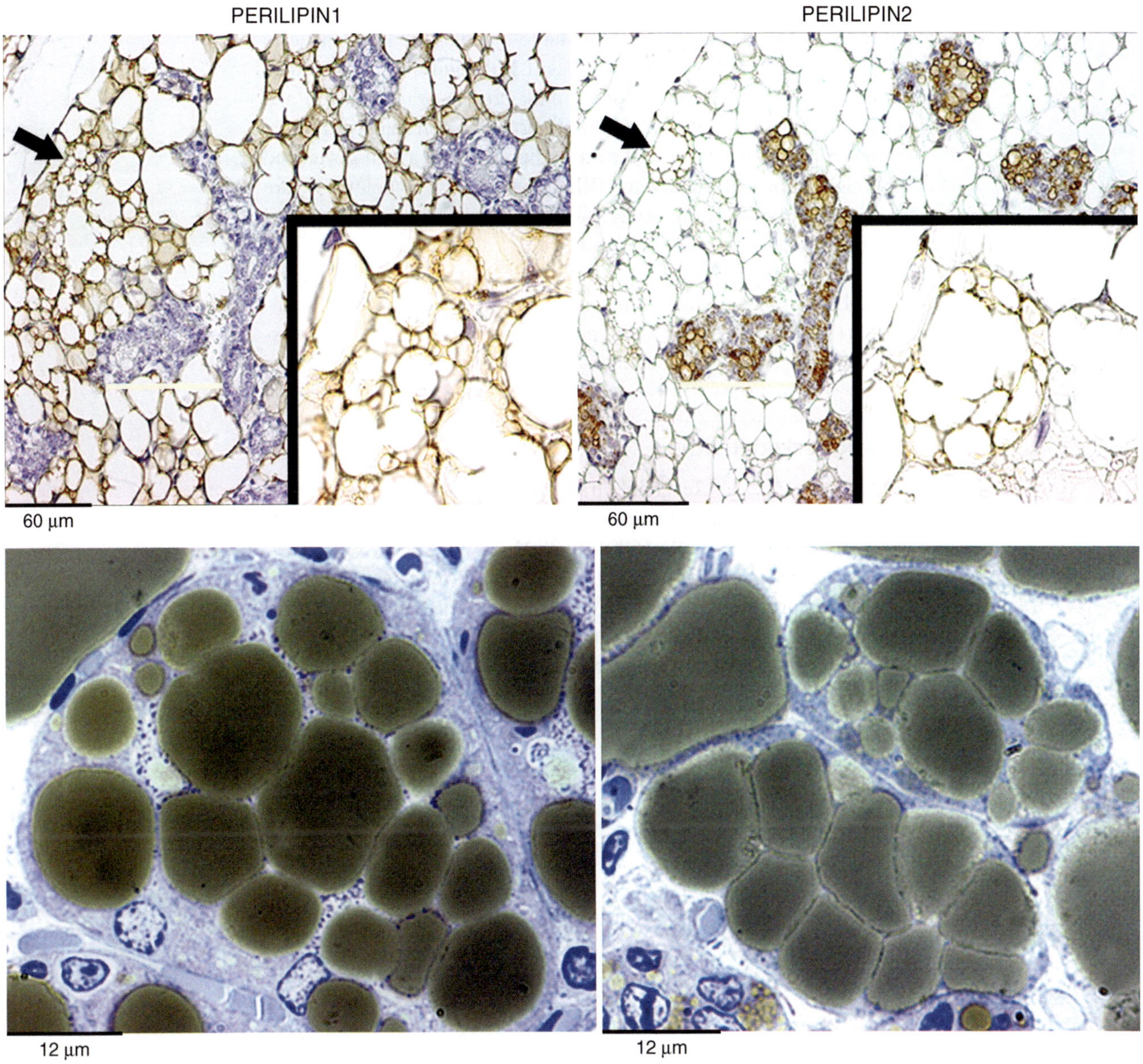

Plate 11.9 Mouse mammary gland at day 18 of pregnancy. Serial sections of same area. LM. IHC perilipin1 ab (1:400), perilipin2 ab (1:150). *Lower panels*: resin-embedded tissue from the same gland showing an early alveolus (*left*) and two compartmentalized adipocytes (*right*). Both are similar to the double-stained structure in upper panels (*arrow*). LM. Toluidine blue. (From Prokesch A. Molecular aspects of adipoepithelial trans-differentiation in mouse mammary gland. Stem Cells. 32:2756–66, 2014 with permission)

PLATE 11.10

Pink Adipocytes TEM

Pink adipocytes show the typical ultrastructure of alveolar glandular cells (upper panel). Note the large cytoplasmic lipid vacuoles (L), the large milk protein granules (LMP), and the central lumen of the gland (Lu). In the lumen milk protein granules (SG) and lipids (Li) are visible. In the basal part of alveoli (enlarged in the lower panel), the nucleus of a pink adipocyte (N), a well-developed rough endoplasmic reticulum (RER), and a Golgi complex (Go) are visible. A typical secretory granule (SG) is visible also in the Golgi complex area, but larger vacuoles rich in secretory granules are stored mainly in the apical part of pink adipocytes (upper panel, LMP) and in the lumen of the alveolus (SG). A distinct basal lamina (EL) lines the basal part of pink adipocytes, and a thin cytoplasmic projection of a myoepithelial cell (My) is also visible.

Suggested Reading

Morroni M, et al. Reversible transdifferentiation of secretory epithelial cells into adipocytes in the mammary gland. Proc Natl Acad Sci U S A. 101:16801–6, 2004.

Smorlesi A, et al. The adipose organ: white-brown adipocyte plasticity and metabolic inflammation. Obes Rev. 13:83–96, 2012.

Giordano A, et al. White, brown and pink adipocytes: the extraordinary plasticity of the adipose organ. Eur J Endocrinol. 170:R159–71, 2014.

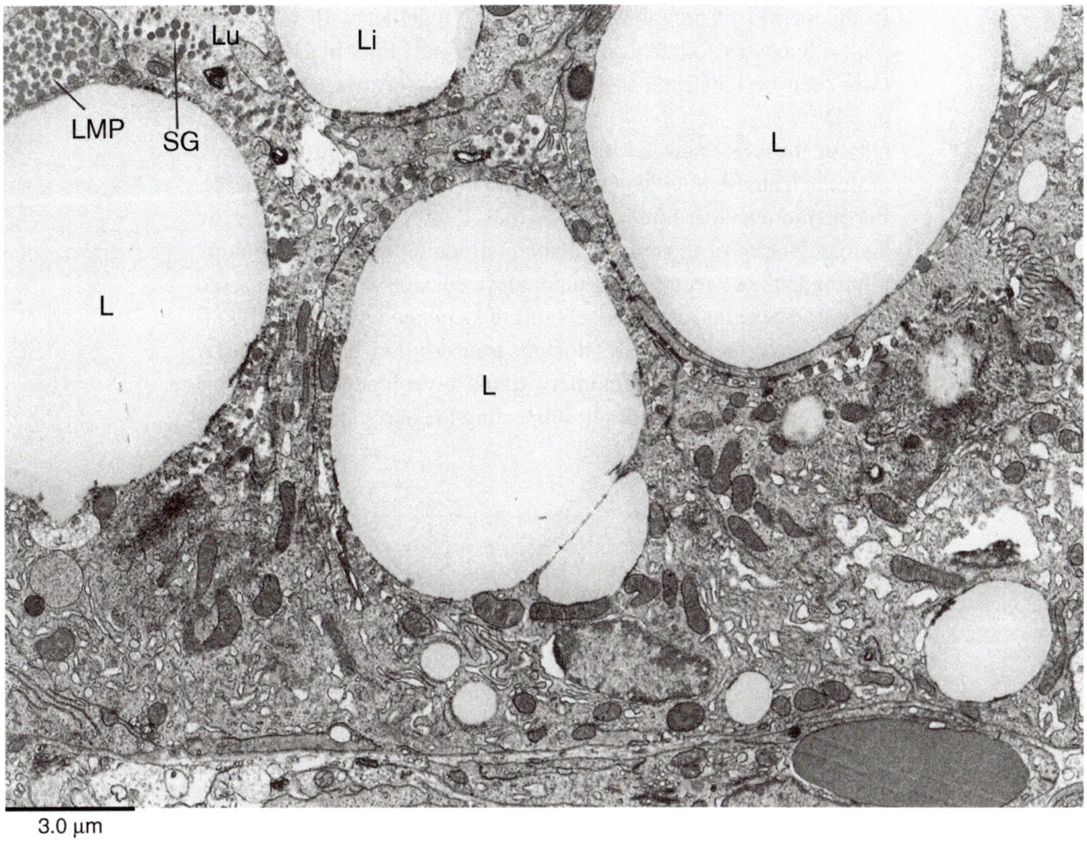

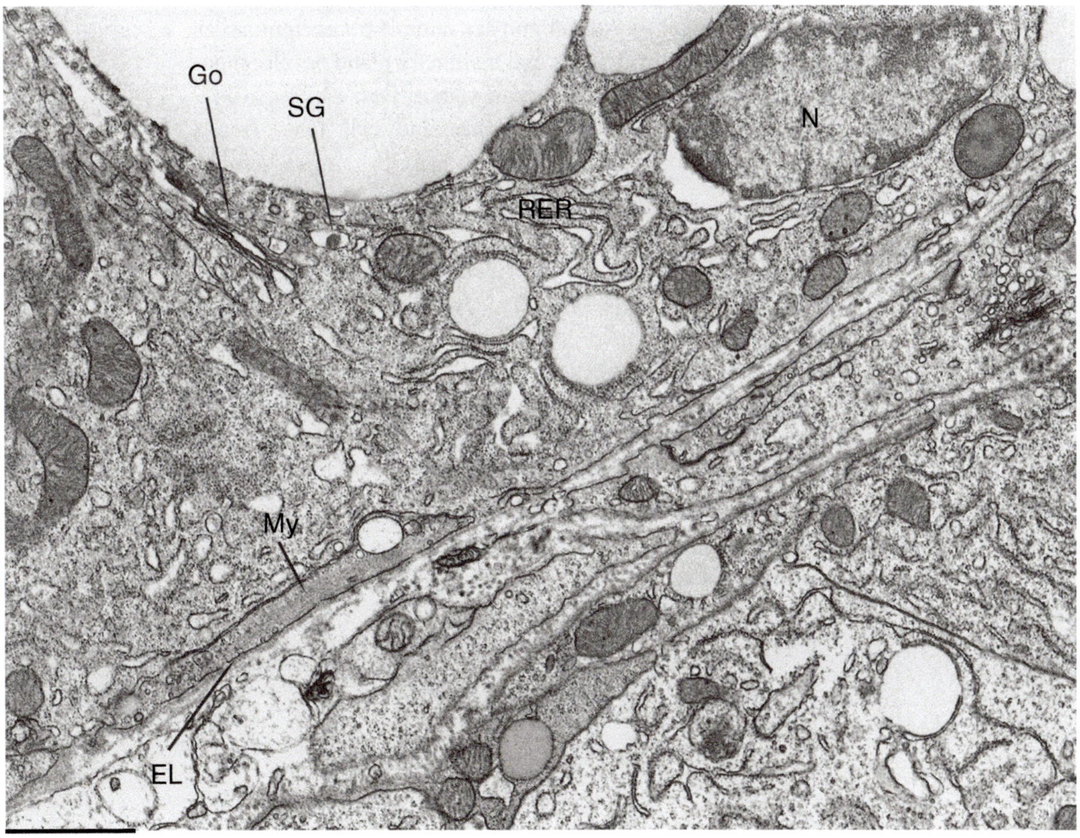

Plate 11.10 Mouse mammary gland at day 18 of pregnancy. Ultrastructure of alveolus formed by pink adipocytes. TEM

PLATE 11.11

White-Pink Intermediate Structures

In this period of pregnancy (day 17–18) together with white and pink adipocytes, other structures (white-pink intermediate structures) can be identified in mammary glands (arrows in the upper panel).

One of those is enlarged in the lower panel. These structures are multinucleated but a clear distinction between cells is not visible. Furthermore a clear lumen such as that of alveolar structures is not visible. Nuclei of these intermediate structures (with morphology intermediate between white adipocytes and early alveoli composed of pink adipocytes) are intensely immunostained with Elf5 antibodies (E74-like factor 5, ETS-domain transcription factor, a master transcription factor of mammary gland alveologenesis; see also Plates 11.3 and 11.5) strongly supporting the early alveolar epithelial nature of these structures.

Suggested Reading

Zhou J, et al. A novel transcription factor, ELF5, belongs to the ELF subfamily of ETS genes and maps to human chromosome 11p13 ± 15, a region subject to LOH and rearrangement in human carcinoma cell lines. Oncogene. 17, 2719–32, 1998.

Thomas RS, et al. The Elf group of Ets-related transcription factors. ELF3 and ELF5. Adv Exp Med Biol. 480:123–8, 2000.

Oakes SR, et al. The alveolar switch: coordinating the proliferative cues and cell fate decisions that drive the formation of lobuloalveoli from ductal epithelium. Breast Cancer Res. 8:207, 2006.

Furth PA, et al. Signal transducer and activator of transcription 5 as a key signaling pathway in normal mammary gland developmental biology and breast cancer. Breast Cancer Res. 13:220, 2011.

Lee HJ, Ormandy CJ. Elf5, hormones and cell fate. Trends Endocrinol Metab. 23:292–8, 2012.

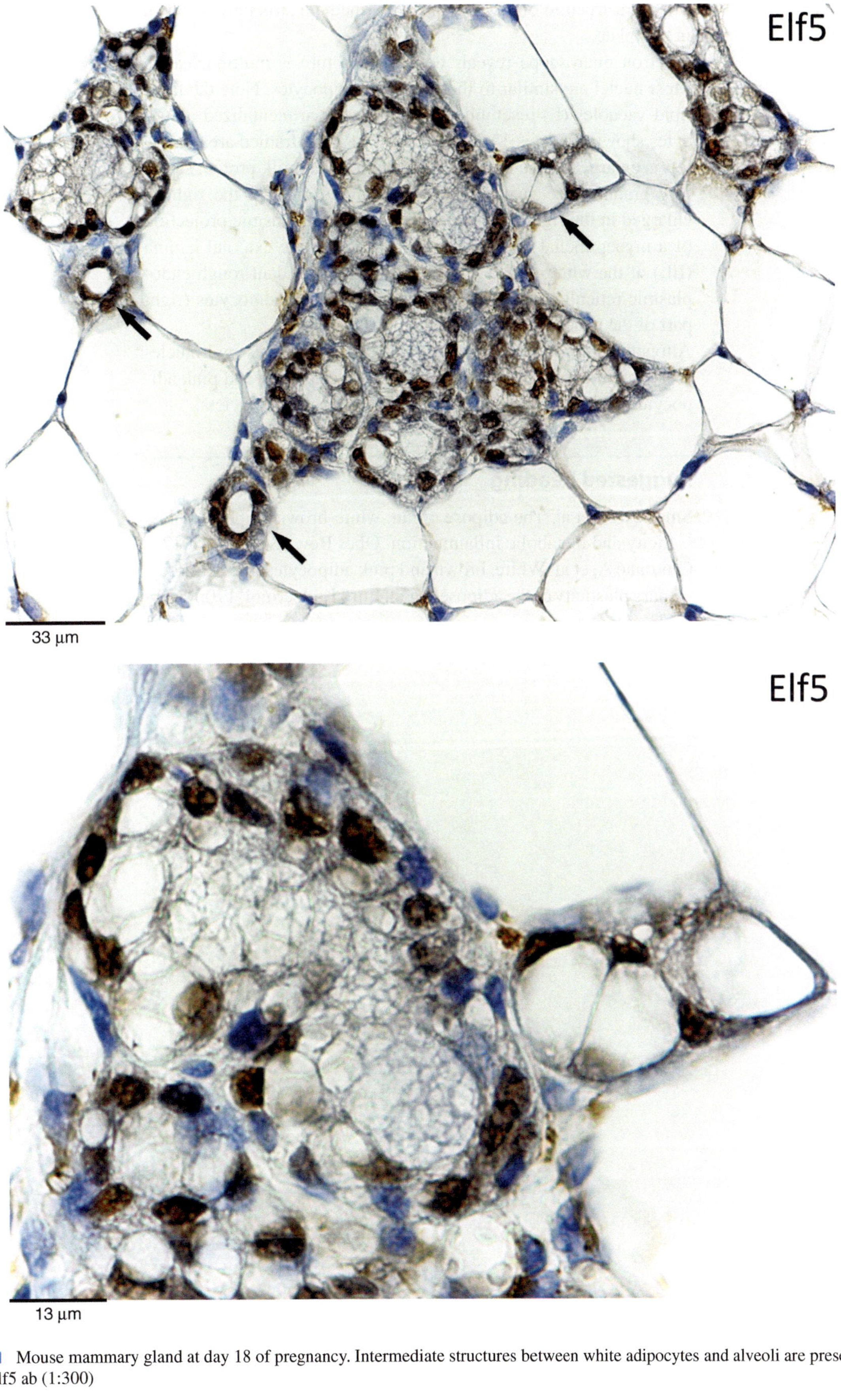

Plate 11.11 Mouse mammary gland at day 18 of pregnancy. Intermediate structures between white adipocytes and alveoli are present (*arrows*). LM. IHC Elf5 ab (1:300)

PLATE 11.12

White-Pink Adipocytes
EM

The ultrastructure of a white-pink intermediate structure is shown in this plate.

Electron microscope reveals that the structure is multinucleated. Most nuclei are similar to those of pink adipocytes. Note the large lipid vacuoles (L) resembling those in compartmentalized adipocytes shown in Plates 11.3, 11.4, and 11.9. The framed area on the left is enlarged in the bottom left panel: typical milk protein secretory granules are visible (SG). The framed area on the right is enlarged in the right bottom panel: the thin cytoplasmic projection of a myoepithelial cell (My) is visible inside the external lamina (EL) of the white-pink adipocyte. Note the abundant rough endoplasmic reticulum (RER) similar to that of pink adipocytes (right part of the panel).

Altogether these ultrastructural data suggest that this multinucleated structure is an intermediate form between white and pink adipocytes (or alveolar structure composed of pink adipocytes).

Suggested Reading

Smorlesi A, et al. The adipose organ: white-brown adipocyte plasticity and metabolic inflammation. Obes Rev. 13:83–96, 2012.

Giordano A, et al. White, brown and pink adipocytes: the extraordinary plasticity of the adipose organ. Eur J Endocrinol. 170:R159–71, 2014.

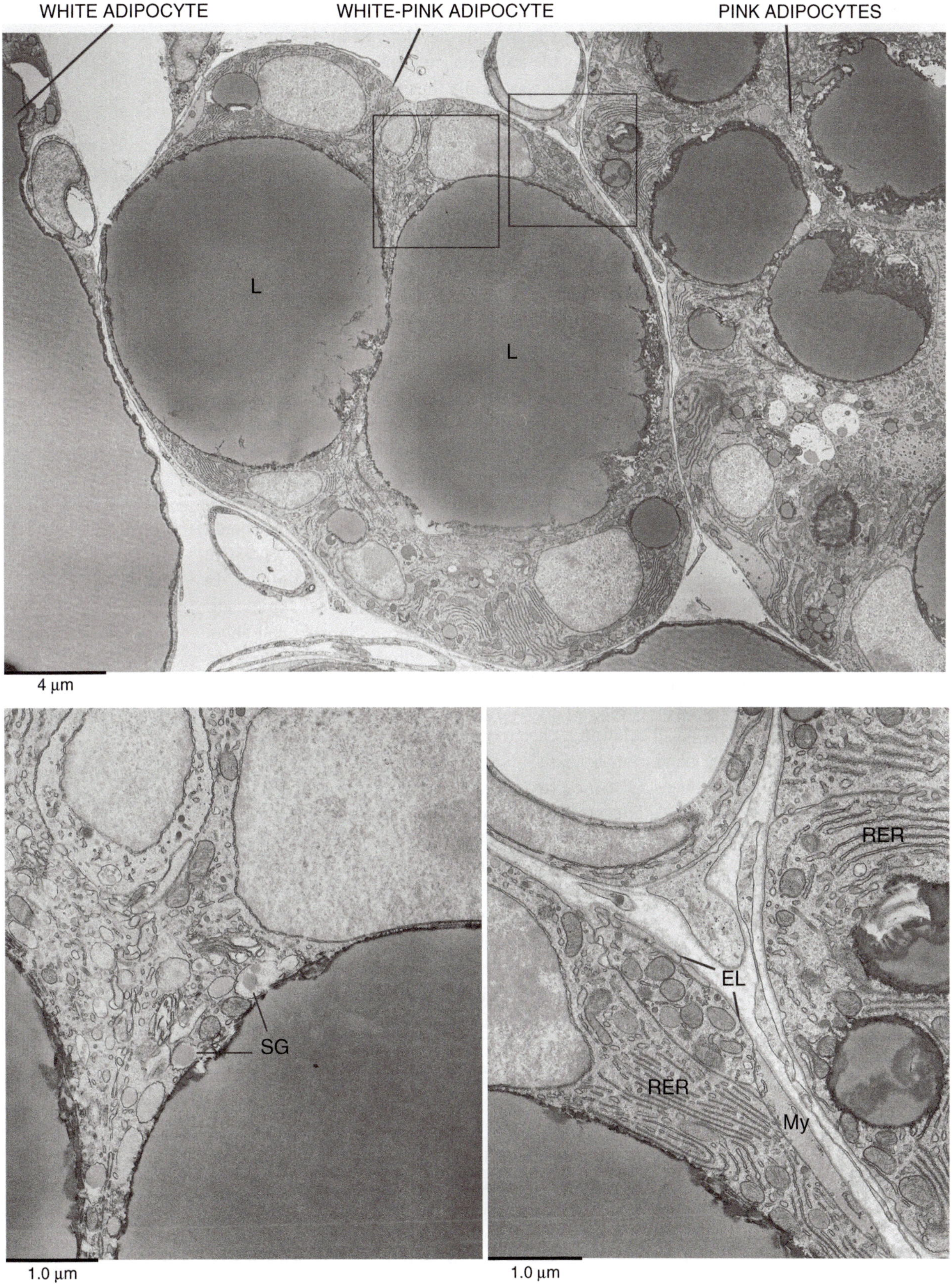

Plate 11.12 Mouse mammary gland at day 18 of pregnancy. Ultrastructure of intermediate structures between white adipocytes and alveoli (white-pink adipocyte). *Lower left*, enlargement of left squared area in the upper panel; *lower right*, enlargement of right squared area in the upper panel. TEM (From Smorlesi A. et al. The adipose organ: white-brown adipocyte plasticity and metabolic inflammation. Obes Rev. 13:83–96, 2012, with permission)

PLATE 11.13

WAT Pinking

Lineage tracing (Cre-loxP DNA recombination system) is a powerful technique useful to follow the developmental destiny of the cells. It is based on double transgenic mice in which the expression of a selected gene marks specifically the cell by beta-galactosidase production (beta-Gal, reporter gene product) detectable by histochemistry (X-Gal). If the chosen gene is expressed specifically from a cell type, the technique is cellular specific. If the selected gene is expressed in a specific period of time, then the technique is also temporally specific.

In order to demonstrate the transdifferentiation of white into epithelial alveolar cells (pink adipocytes), we crossed mice carrying the aP2-Cre transgene, in which expression of the gene for Cre recombinase is controlled by aP2 promoter, with mice carrying the ROSA26 (R26R) reporter transgene, in which the ubiquitous expression of the reporter gene lacZ is blocked by a loxP-flanked stop sequence (see scheme). aP2-Cre mice selectively express Cre recombinase in adipose tissue. Cre-mediated excision is cell heritable, and labeled cells and their progeny should continue to express the reporter gene at later stages even if Cre is no longer expressed. As a consequence, by visualizing the activity of beta-Gal, adipocytes and any other cell type, eventually derived from them, should be labeled. By using X-Gal as a substrate, only beta-Gal-positive adipocytes were detected in the mammary gland of virgin mice. In contrast, at day 18 of pregnancy, epithelial alveolar cells (pink adipocytes) were positive. Morphometric analysis showed that about 70% of epithelial alveolar cells (pink adipocytes) were positive, suggesting that most of them derive from transdifferentiation of white adipocytes.

In the panel below the scheme is shown a X-Gal staining of a mammary gland from aP2-Cre/R26R mouse at day 18 of pregnancy: the most intensely stained structures are lobules of alveolar epithelial cells (pink adipocytes). The bottom panel shows an enlargement of the same tissue showing that both white and pink adipocytes are engulfed by the beta-Gal-derived blue crystals (some indicated in a white adipocyte). The plates are from a pre-embedding preparation that allows detecting the beta-Gal crystals in the thin cytoplasmic rim of adipocytes. This technique allows a better localization of beta-Gal crystals in adipocytes because in this cells routinely prepared (paraffin-embedded material), many beta-Gal crystals can be dislocated into the lipid droplet instead of their cytoplasmic rim.

Suggested Reading

Morroni M, et al. Reversible transdifferentiation of secretory epithelial cells into adipocytes in the mammary gland. Proc Natl Acad Sci U S A. 101:16801–6, 2004.

Prokesch A, et al. Molecular aspects of adipoepithelial transdifferentiation in mouse mammary gland. Stem Cells. 32:2756–66, 2014.

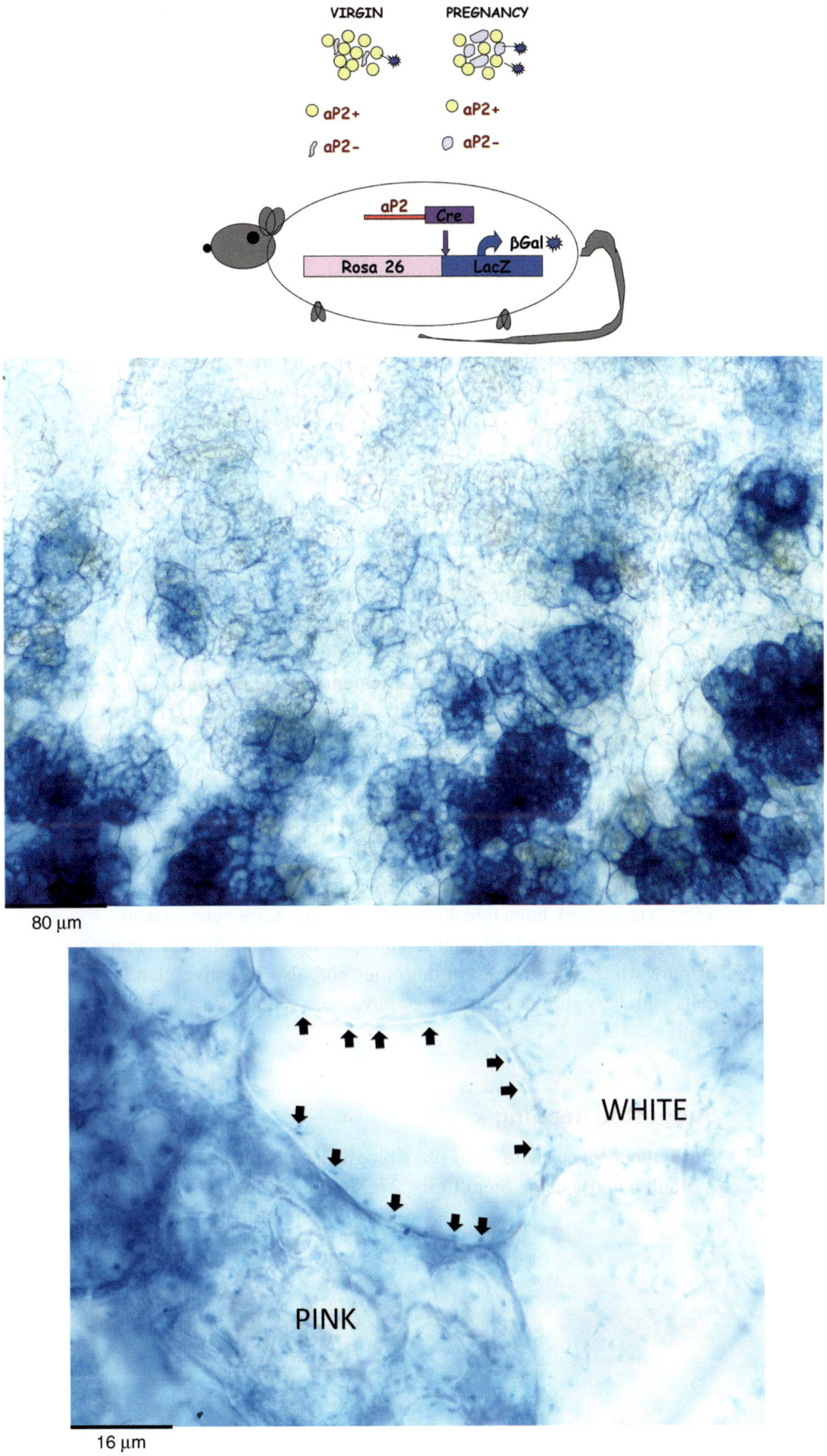

Plate 11.13 Mammary gland of aP2-Cre/R26R double transgenic mouse (see scheme) at day 18 of pregnancy. X-Gal staining. Whole mount preparation. *Lower*: enlargement from the same gland. LM

PLATE 11.14

Explanted Fat Transdifferentiate into Mammary Glands

The experiments shown in previous plates strongly suggest that white adipocytes can convert into epithelial glandular cells (pink adipocytes). In order to confirm this striking result, we performed explant experiments. Grafts of adipose tissue from either subcutaneous or visceral fat of adult male and female Rosa26 mice (in which all cells constitutively express beta-Gal) were able to give rise to milk-secreting epithelial cells when exposed to the microenvironment of the mammary gland in pregnant and lactating mice. We also showed that labeled glands could be obtained by injection of isolated adipocytes. Interestingly, isolated adipocytes, retaining the morphology and protein markers typical of differentiated fat cells, also expressed high levels of stem cell genes and the reprogramming transcription factor Klf4. Altogether these data support the great reprogramming proneness of adult adipocyte genome to direct conversion in a different phenotype: the white-brown-pink triangle (bottom scheme). Recent data seems to support also a reversible brown-pink adipocyte conversion.

In this plate (upper panel) the dotted line delimitates the X-Gal-stained tissue, from pure fat explant (visceral) of the Rosa26 donor, found inside the lactating tissue of the recipient. Both adipocytes and glands of the explant were X-Gal stained. X-Gal-stained glands were immunoreactive for lactating mammary gland-specific proteins such as casein and perilipin2.

The lower left panel shows an enlargement of X-Gal-stained gland from pure fat explant (compare with recipient unstained glands in the lower right panel).

Note that the degree of differentiation of the explant is behind that of the gland of the recipient suggesting that explanted fat is in some way less responsive than the native fat to the pregnancy hormones promoting alveologenesis.

In the gland shown in the bottom left panel, a X-Gal-labeled pink adipocyte (arrow), bona fide derived from white adipocytes explant, is inserted in the gland but retains a morphology very similar to that of pure white adipocytes. On the other end also in native glands, cells with very similar morphology have been found (see also Plate 11.8).

Suggested Reading

De Matteis R, et al. In vivo physiological transdifferentiation of adult adipose cells. Stem Cells. 27:2761–8, 2009.

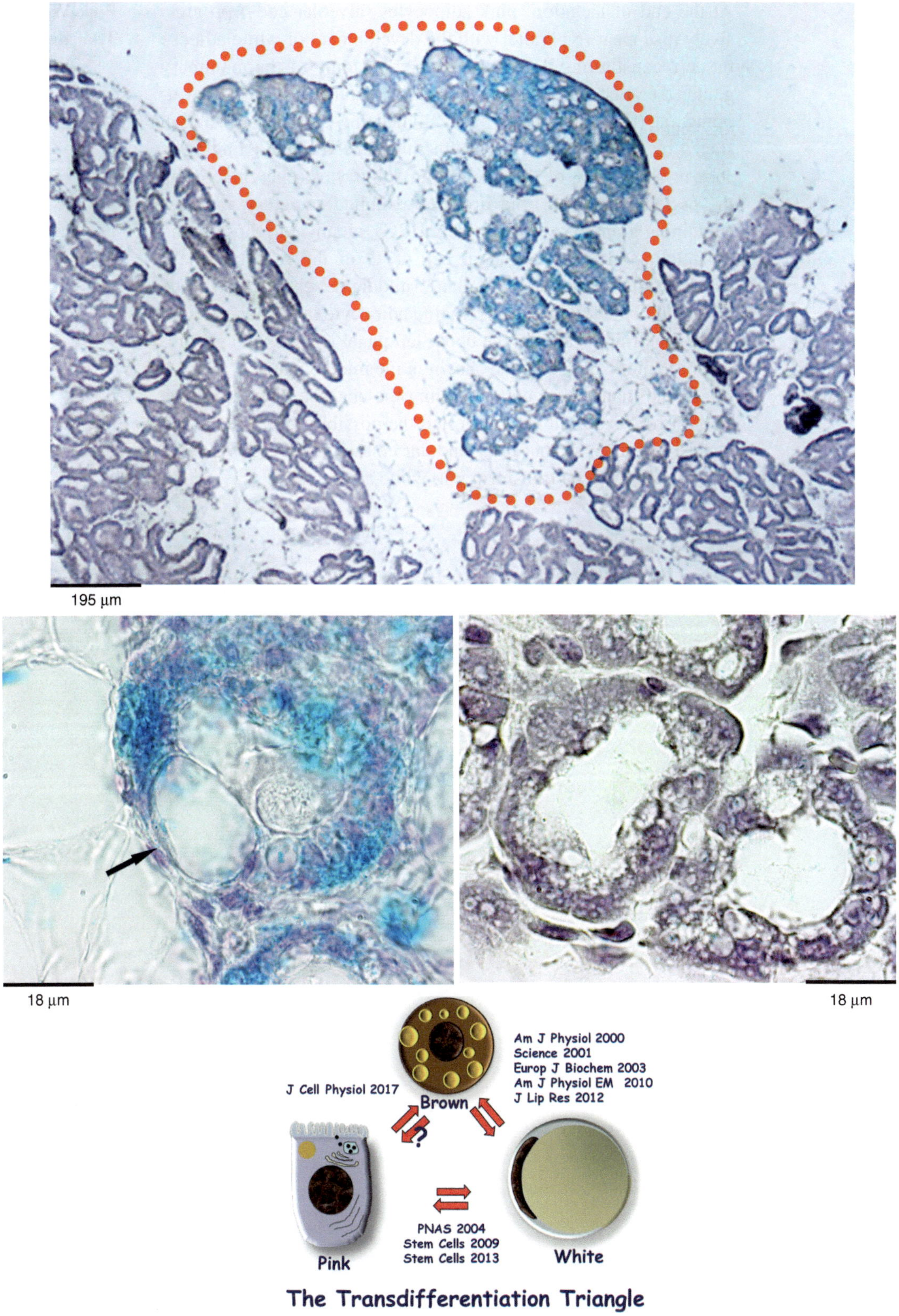

Plate 11.14 Explants of pure WAT from Rosa26 mouse into a mammary gland of wild-type mouse at day 10 of lactation. Explant is transformed into mammary gland. *Lower left*: enlargement of a gland in the explant. *Lower right*: enlargement of glands from recipient mouse. LM. X-Gal staining (From: De Matteis R. et al. In vivo physiological transdifferentiation of adult adipose cells. Stem Cells. 27:2761–8, 2009 with permission)

PLATE 11.15

Pink-White Transdifferentiation I

At the end of lactation, pink adipocytes (alveolar cells) progressively disappear in parallel with the development of white adipose tissue reconstituting the pre-pregnancy anatomy of the mammary glands (see Plate 11.2). In order to understand the origin of developing fat (upper left panel), we studied the early post-lactation stages by electron microscopy. In this plate the main finding is shown: about 15% of the developing adipocytes (one enlarged in the bottom panel; L, lipid droplet) exhibited secretory vacuoles containing granules of milk proteins (SG), identical to those found in lactating alveolar epithelial cells (SG in the middle panel). Compare the epithelium of a gland (middle panel in which some SG are indicated) with the developing adipocyte in the bottom right panel. The framed area in the upper left panel includes the glandular epithelium similar to that shown in the middle panel.
These and many other data including the absence of proliferative signs (BrdU experiments) suggested the possibility, showed in the upper right scheme, that the glandular epithelium at the end of its physiologic role can transform into white adipocytes.

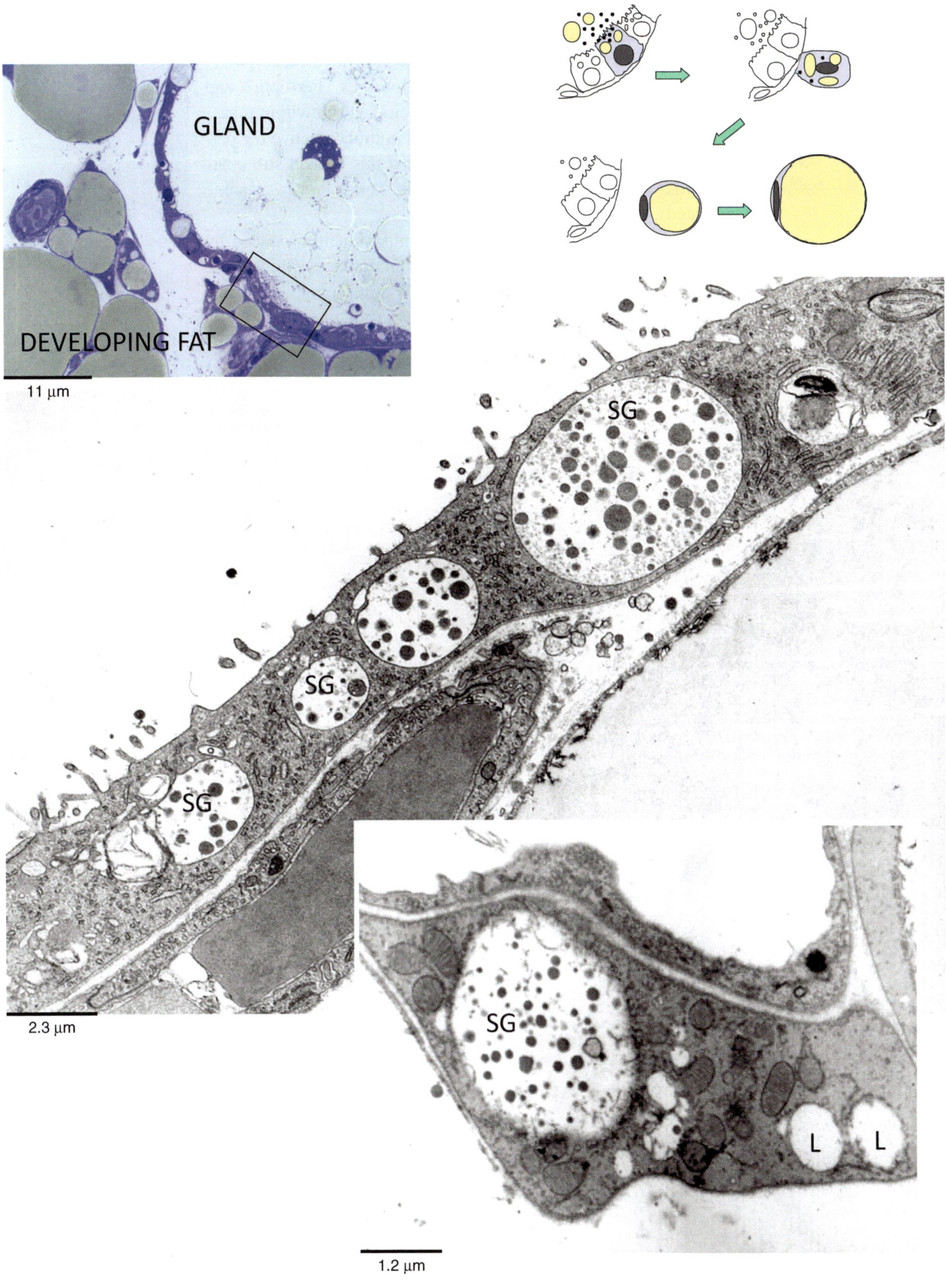

Plate 11.15 Mouse mammary gland at day 1 of post-lactation. Developing adipocytes share specific milk structures (SG) with alveolar cell. TEM (From: Morroni et al. Reversible transdifferentiation of secretory epithelial cells into adipocytes in the mammary gland. Proc Natl Acad Sci U S A. 101:16,801–6, 2004 with permission)

PLATE 11.16

Pink-White Transdifferentiation II

In line with the idea that epithelial alveolar cells at the end of lactation could transdifferentiate into white adipocytes, we found immunohistochemistry evidence of perilipin2 and whey acidic protein (WAP) in post-lactation developing adipocytes. Perilipin2 and WAP are never expressed by mammary adipocytes in virgin mice.
In the upper panel one adipocyte (arrow) immunoreactive for perilipin2 (see Plate 11.8) is visible. Note that this protein still coats the milk lipid droplets in the glands (small arrows, some indicated).
Whey acidic protein is a characteristic milk protein produced by alveolar cells. In the lower panel WAP-immunoreactive milk in the lumen of alveolar glands as well as in developing adipocytes (arrows) is visible.

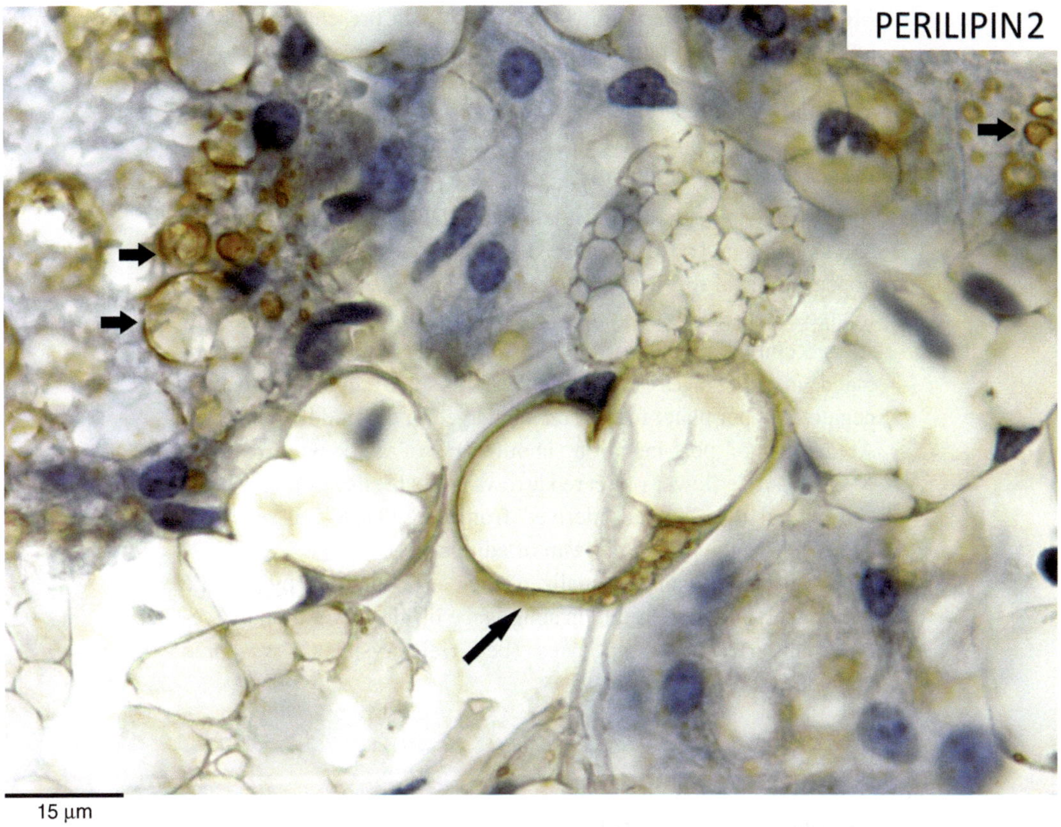

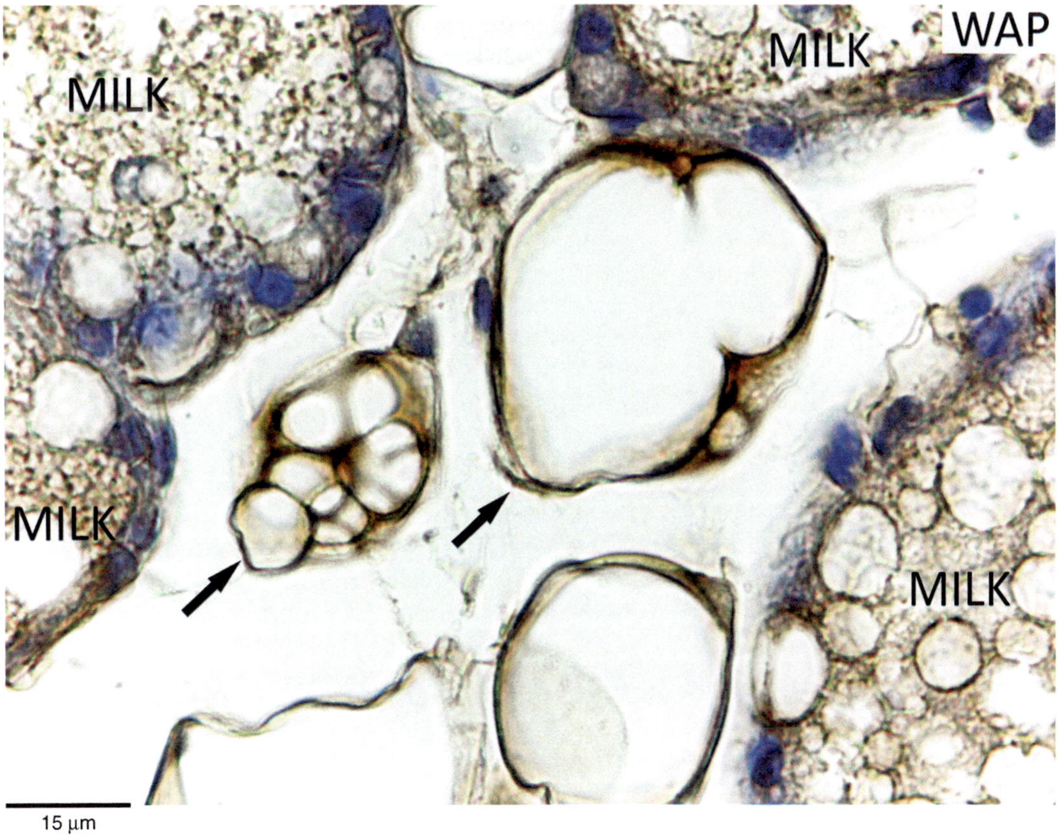

Plate 11.16 Mouse mammary gland at day 1 of post-lactation. LM. IHC ab perilipin2 (1:150), ab WAP (1:400)

PLATE 11.17 Pink-White Transdifferentiation III

Morphologic and immunohistochemistry data presented in previous plates suggest that the white-pink transdifferentiation proved by lineage tracing and explant experiments could be reversible.

Thus we performed lineage tracing experiments using WAP-Cre/R26R mice (see Plate 11.13 for details on this technique).

Whey acidic protein (WAP) is a characteristic milk protein exclusively found in ductal and epithelial alveolar cells during pregnancy and lactation and never expressed by adipocytes (see scheme in the upper left panel for the experimental design).

In agreement with this knowledge, we found intensely X-Gal-stained epithelial cells in the ducts and early alveoli of mammary glands in early stages of pregnancy. At this stage adipocytes resulted negative (upper plate, framed area enlarged in the middle panel).

At day 10 of post-lactation, about 60% of adipocytes resulted X-Gal positive (lower plate: red arrows indicate sites of major beta-Gal crystal (i.e., crystals derived from beta-Gal/X-Gal reaction) deposition in the thin cytoplasm of adipocytes).

Beta-Gal crystals can be visualized by electron microscopy (middle right panel) and were found in abundance inside the epithelial alveolar cells (E) and adipocytes (beta-Gal crystals: Cry, some indicated).

Suggested Reading

Morroni M, et al. Reversible transdifferentiation of secretory epithelial cells into adipocytes in the mammary gland. Proc Natl Acad Sci U S A. 101:16801–6, 2004.

Prokesch A. Molecular aspects of adipoepithelial transdifferentiation in mouse mammary gland. Stem Cells. 32:2756–66, 2014.

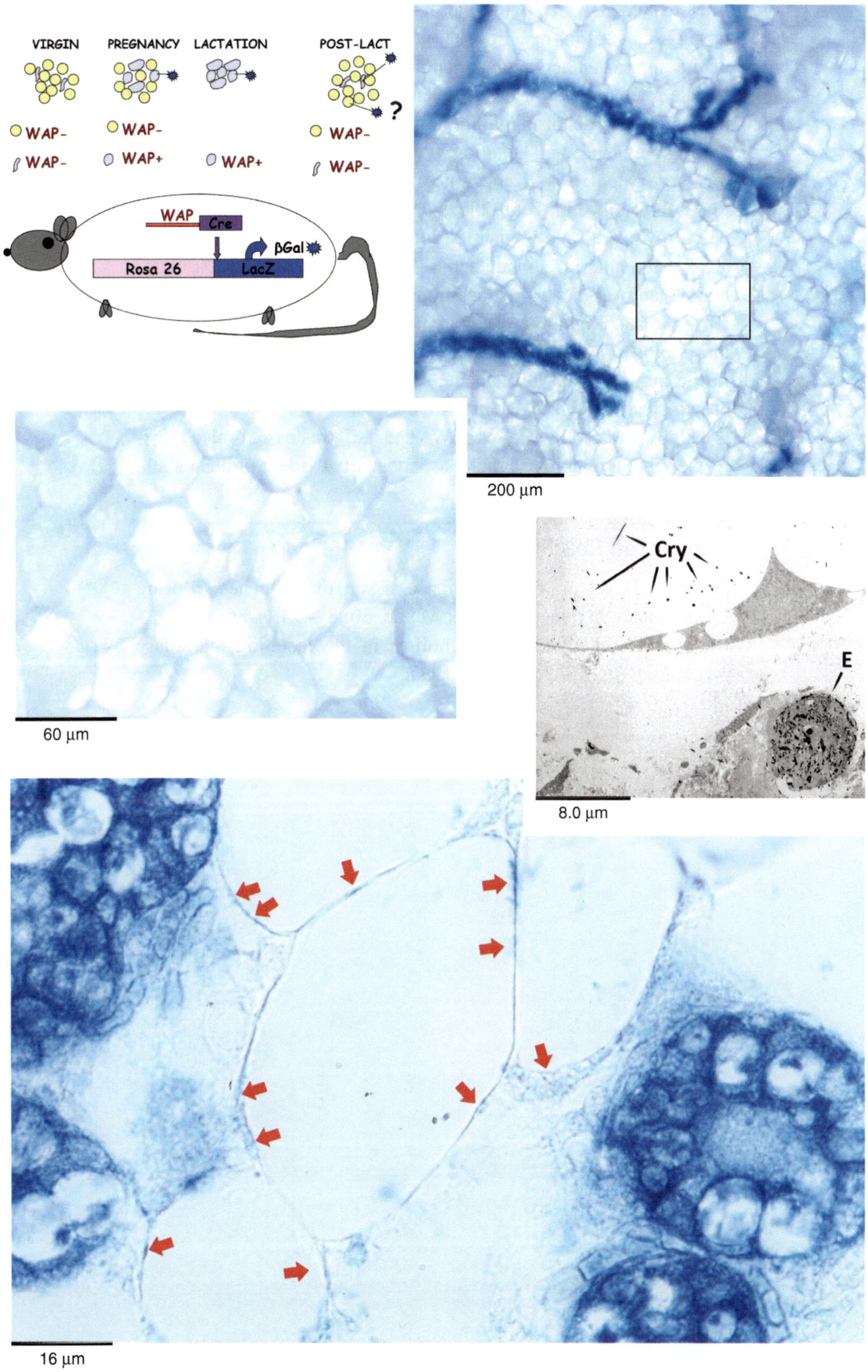

Plate 11.17 *Top* and *middle left*: mouse mammary gland of WAP-Cre/R26R double transgenic mouse at day 11 of pregnancy (only ducts and early alveoli stained). LM. X-Gal staining. *Lower*: mammary gland of WAP-Cre/R26R double transgenic mouse at day 1 post-lactation (adipocytes and alveolar cells stained). LM. X-Gal staining. At electron microscopy (*middle right*) dense crystal derived from the X-Gal reaction is visible in alveoli and adipocytes (*middle panel*; from Morroni et al. Reversible transdifferentiation of secretory epithelial cells into adipocytes in the mammary gland. Proc Natl Acad Sci U S A. 101:16,801–6, 2004 with permission)

PLATE 11.18

IBAT Gross Anatomy

Interscapular BAT (IBAT), one of the most important brown adipose tissue sites in the adipose organ, lies in the interscapular area of the anterior subcutaneous depot (see Chap. 1). In male and in female mice, except during pregnancy and lactation, the remaining portion of this depot is mainly composed of white adipose tissue. During pregnancy and lactation, the anterior subcutaneous depot is, to a large extent, transformed into a mammary gland (this plate and Plates 11.1 and 11.2) with the exception of the IBAT area. Here a pale-brownish tissue is visible (dotted areas) in the middle dorsal area of the anterior subcutaneous depot transformed into a mammary gland (at day 14 of lactation). This area corresponds to the IBAT site, and light microscopy confirmed its brown adipose tissue morphology (see the next plate).

In the mouse of the lower panel (also at day 14 of lactation), the brownish area of IBAT is not evident. It should be noted that IBAT is usually covered by a layer of WAT that, in this case, is also transformed into a mammary gland, as is visually evident in this panel.

Suggested Reading

Andrews JF, et al. Brown adipose tissue thermogenesis during pregnancy in mice. Ann Nutr Metab. 30: 87–93, 1986.

Barber MC, et al. Lipid metabolism in the lactating mammary gland. BBA. 1347: 101–26, 1997.

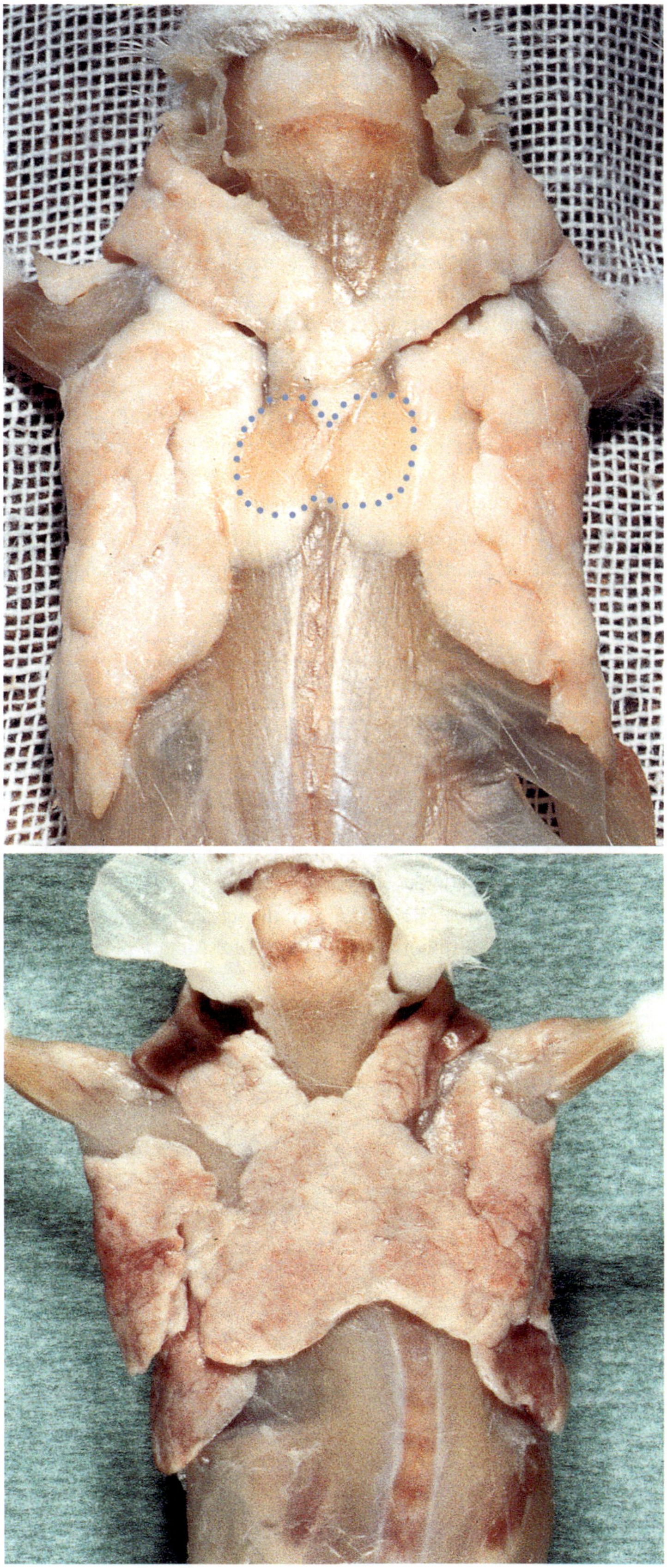

Plate 11.18 Lactating mice (14th day). Dorsal view of the anterior part of the animal after removal of the skin

PLATE 11.19

Interscapular BAT
Histology

Histological appearance of lactating mouse interscapular BAT. Interscapular BAT is composed of small multilocular adipocytes with large lipid vacuoles in the cytoplasm, in line with the well-known reduced activity of BAT during pregnancy and lactation (see also the next plate). It is surrounded by the hypertrophic mammary gland with dilated alveoli and ducts. The glandular parenchyma appears to "infiltrate" the IBAT (framed area, enlarged in the lower panel). This appearance explains the observation of glands at the periphery of post-pregnancy interscapular BAT in early morphological studies in small mammals.

Very recent data from our laboratory seems to suggest that UCP1-immunoreactive adipocytes in interscapular BAT of post-lactation mice derive from direct conversion of pink adipocytes (alveolar cells of pregnancy and lactating mammary glands; see Plates 11.8–11.11) into brown adipocytes. Thus, the reversible ability of white adipocytes to convert into alveolar cells producing milk, under the influence of pregnancy hormones, seems to expand to the brown component of the adipose organ. This could be part of the explanation for the reduced activity of BAT during pregnancy and lactation.

Suggested Reading

Dalquest W, Werner HJ. The interscapular gland of a tropical fruit bat. Anat Rec. 111:345–53, 1951.

Herrera E, et al. Intermediary metabolism in pregnancy. First theme of the Freinkel era. Diabetes. 40:83–88, 1991.

Giordano A, et al. Mammary epithelial alveolar cells convert into brown adipocytes in post-lactating mice. J Cell Physiol. 2017.

Li L, et al. Brown adipocytes can display a mammary basal myoepithelial cell phenotype in vivo. Mol Metab. 6:1198–211, 2017.

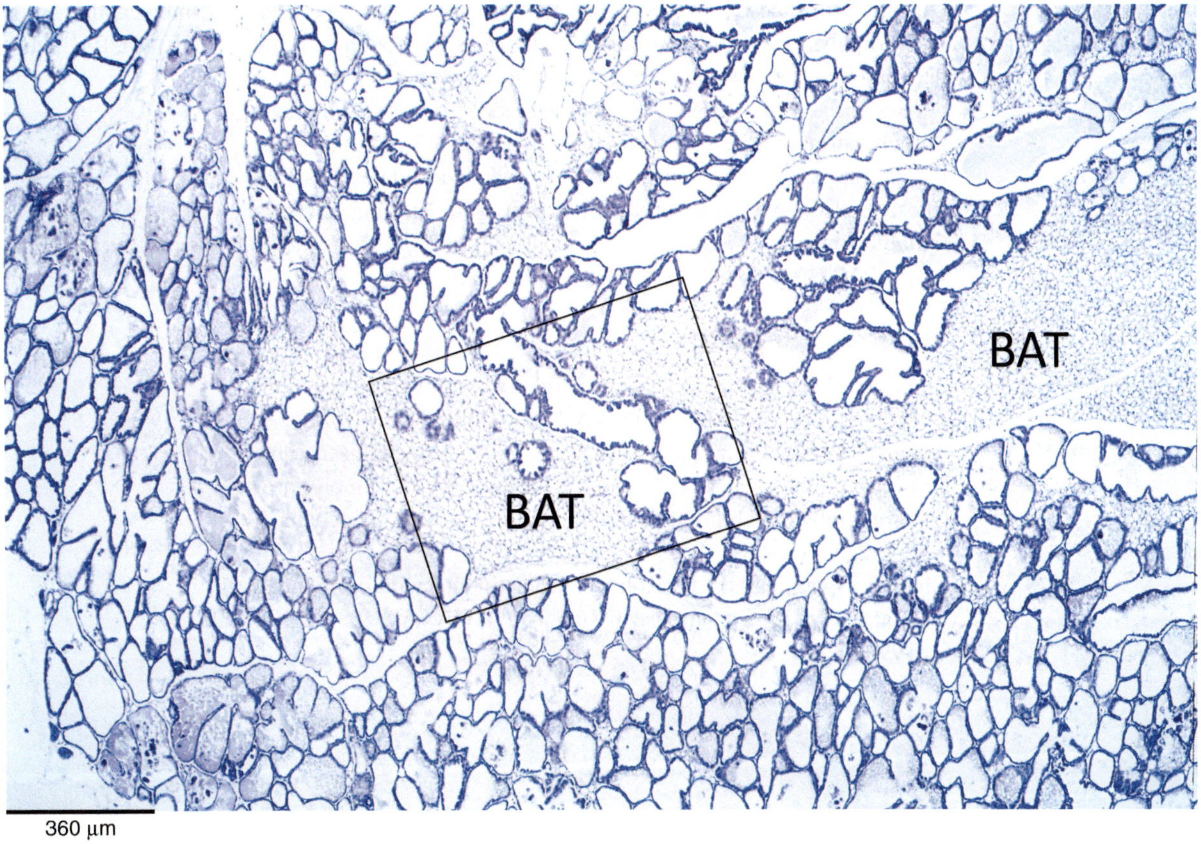

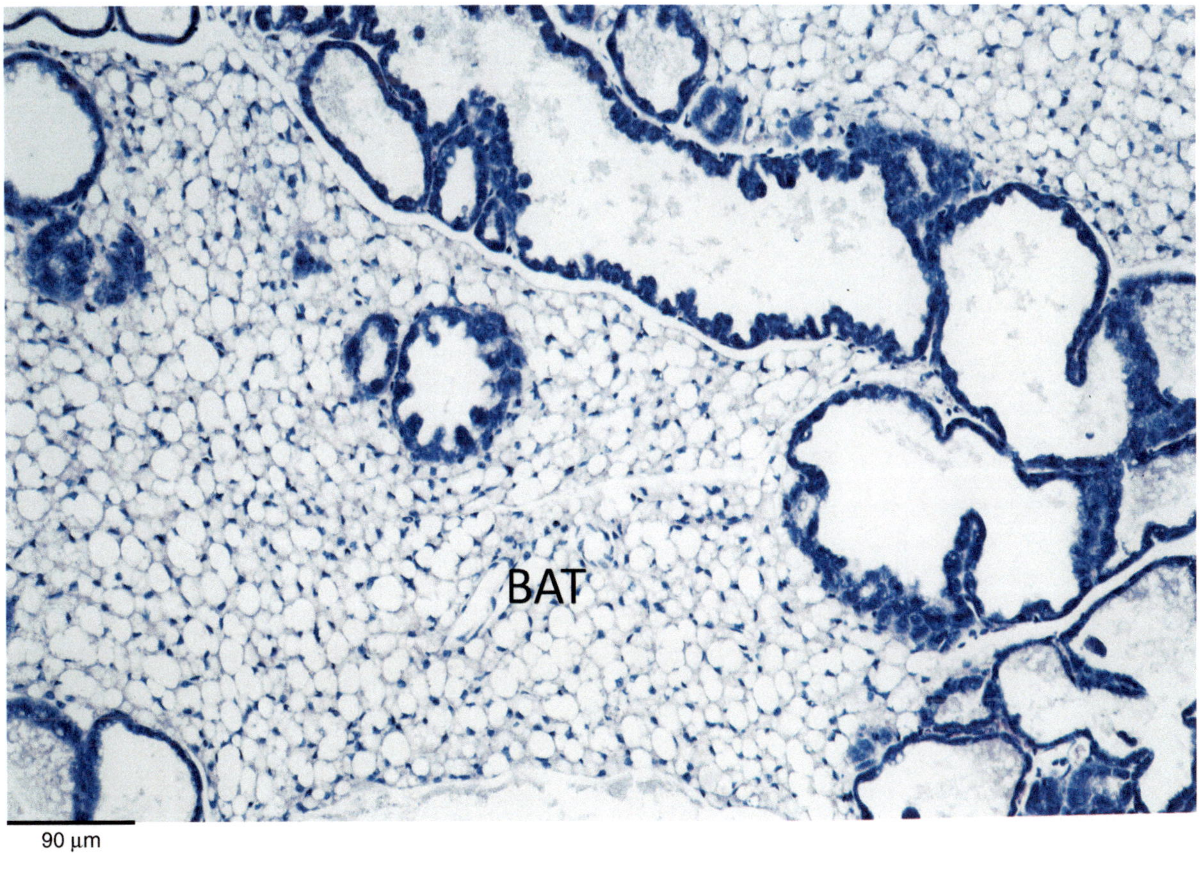

Plate 11.19 IBAT "infiltrated" by mammary gland in lactating (day 14) mouse. *Lower*: enlargement of the framed area. LM. H&E

PLATE 11.20

During pregnancy and lactation, IBAT activity is reduced. Accordingly, immunohistochemical UCP1 expression is not detected in our experimental conditions (upper panel; see technical details in the figure legend). The morphology of brown adipocyte mitochondria and the size of lipid droplets (L) (lower panel) also indicate scarce thermogenic activity (compare with Plates 7.7–7.9). These cells show numerous mitochondria undergoing division (small arrows).

Interscapular BAT
IHC-UCP1, EM

Suggested Reading

Trayhurn P, et al. Brown adipose tissue thermogenesis is 'suppressed' during lactation in mice. Nature. 298:59–60, 1982.

Trayhurn P, et al. Functional atrophy of brown adipose tissue during lactation in mice. Effects of lactation and weaning on mitochondrial GDP binding and uncoupling protein. Biochem J. 248:273–76, 1987.

Chan E, Swaminathan R. Role of prolactin in lactation-induced changes in brown adipose tissue. Am J Physiol. 258:R51–6, 1990.

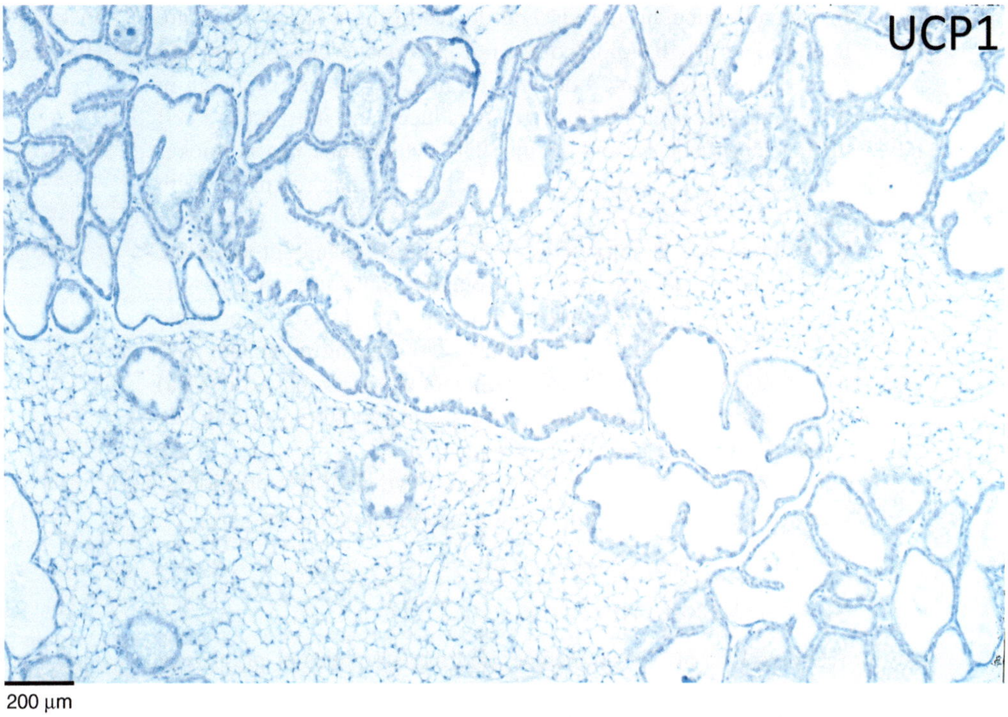

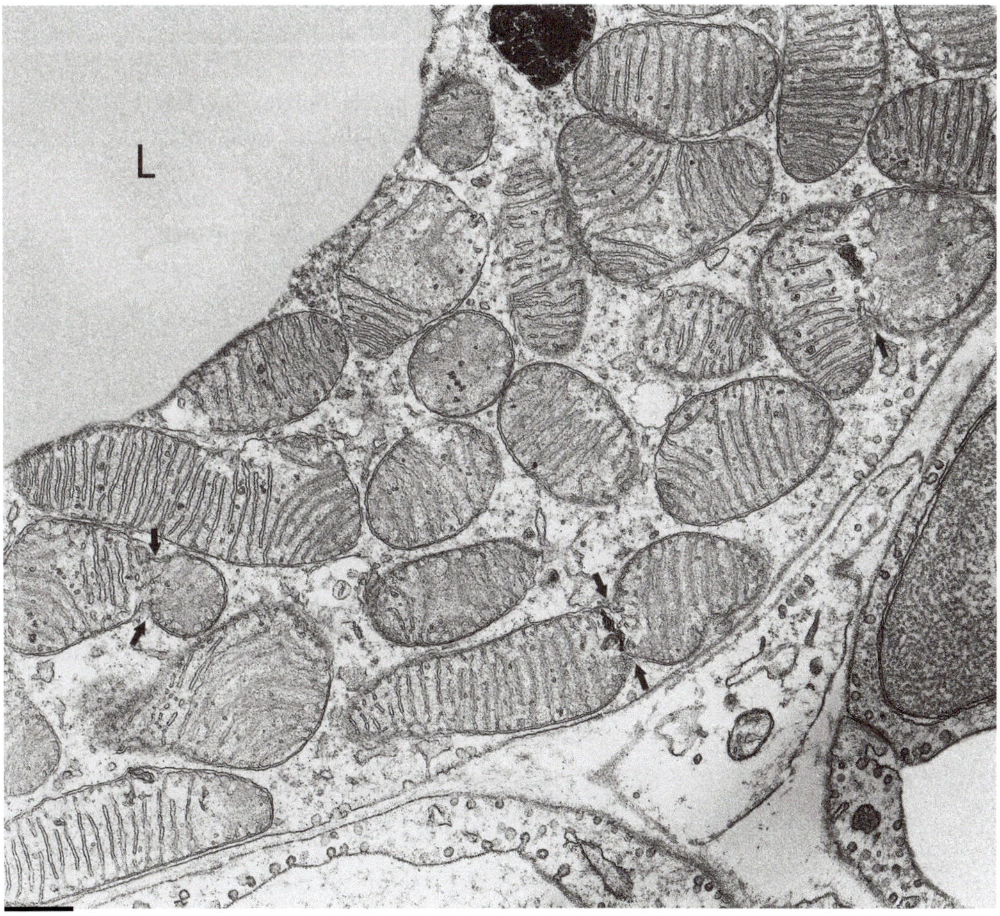

Plate 11.20 IBAT of a lactating mouse (the same of Plate 11.19). Brown adipocytes are UCP1 negative. LM. IHC: UCP1 ab (1:8,000). *Lower*: cytoplasm of a brown adipocyte from the same depot as above. TEM

PLATE 11.21

Visceral WAT
Histology

In lactating mice, all the visceral depots of the adipose organ are hypotrophic. The histology of the retroperitoneal (upper panel) and periovarian (lower panel) depots of a lactating mouse is shown in this plate. The size of adipocytes is reduced and most have a cell diameter between 15 and 25 µm. The cytoplasmic rim is thicker than that of white adipocytes of feeding animals (compare with Plate 4.2).

Interestingly white adipocytes and mammary glands produce the Zn-alfa2-glycoprotein (ZAG), but our IHC data suggest that normal ductal epithelium is not immunoreactive. Thus it is possible that alveolar epithelial cells produce ZAG during pregnancy and lactation. ZAG seems to be responsible for the fat atrophy (cachexia) in several types of cancers; thus the visceral hypotrophy during lactation could be due to ZAG overproduction.

Furthermore the hypothalamic hormone oxytocin that is physiologically overproduced during lactation causes fat reduction.

Suggested Reading

Trahyurn P, et al. Thermogenesis and the energetics of pregnancy and lactation. Can J Physiol. 67:370–75, 1989.

Tada T, et al. Immunohistochemical localization of Zn-alpha 2-glycoprotein in normal human tissues. J Histochem Cytochem. 39:1221–6, 1991.

Bing C, et al. Zinc-alpha2-glycoprotein, a lipid mobilizing factor, is expressed in adipocytes and is up-regulated in mice with cancer cachexia. PNAS. 101:2500–5, 2004.

Altirriba J, et al. Chronic oxytocin administration as a treatment against impaired leptin signaling or leptin resistance in obesity. Front Endocrinol. 6:119, 2015.

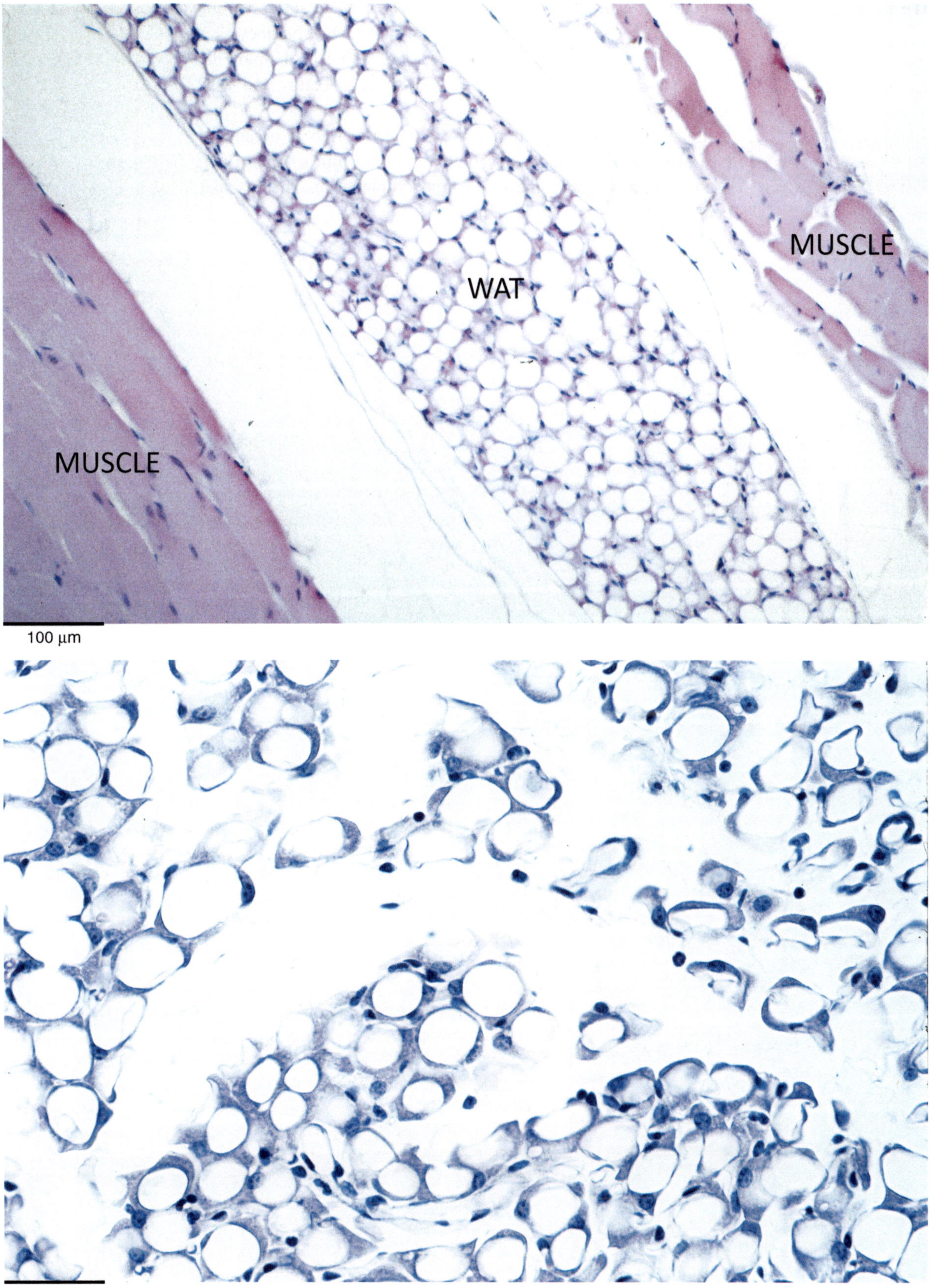

Plate 11.21 Retroperitoneal (*upper*) and periovarian (*lower*) adipose depots of a lactating mouse. LM. H&E

PLATE 11.22

Visceral WAT EM I

In contrast to the hypotrophic appearance of visceral depots, the ultrastructure of visceral (retroperitoneal) WAT white adipocytes is that of hyperfunctioning cells and resembles that of delipidizing adipocytes in cold-acclimated and fasted animals (Plates 7.16–7.18 and 10.6–10.8, respectively).

Unilocular cells show a thick cytoplasmic rim rich in organelles (see also the next plate) and containing many mitochondria (M, some indicated) and some small lipid droplets (L). The vascular bed (CAP) appears well developed.

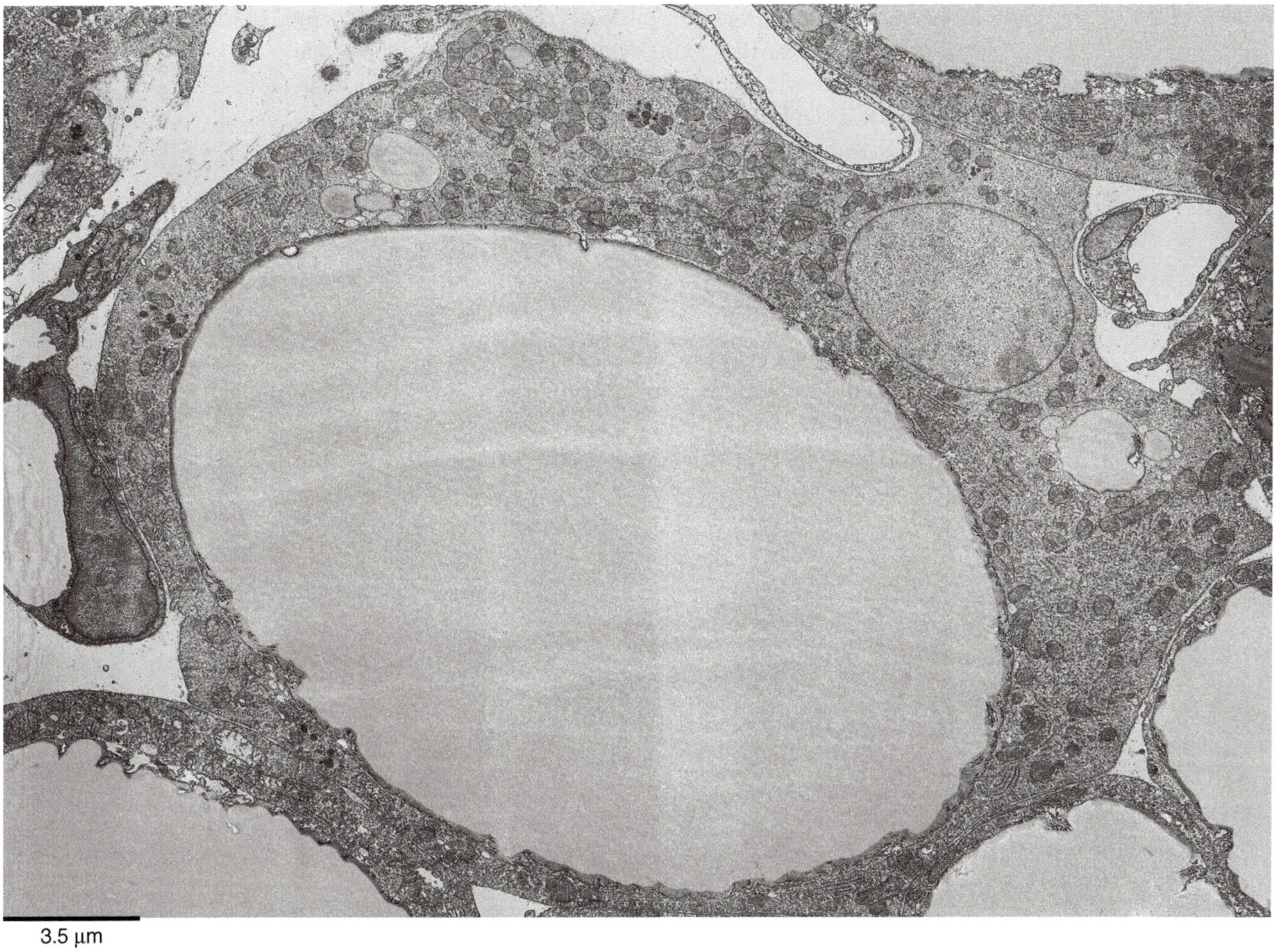

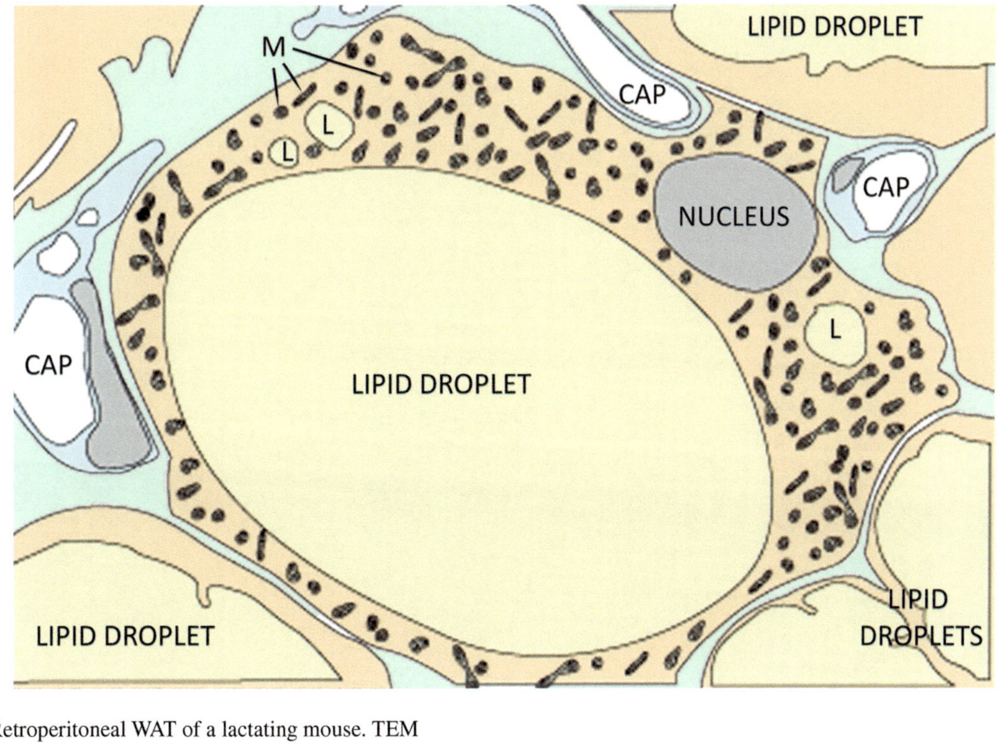

Plate 11.22 Retroperitoneal WAT of a lactating mouse. TEM

PLATE 11.23

Visceral WAT EM II

In lactating mice, retroperitoneal WAT adipocytes exhibit many well-developed organelles in the cytoplasm. The thick cytoplasmic rim of this adipocyte exhibits stacks of rough endoplasmic reticulum (RER), vesicular smooth endoplasmic reticulum (SER), lysosomes (Ly, some indicated), and peroxisomes. A small lipid droplet (L), pinocytotic vesicles (V), and some mitochondria are visible here. Note the signs of mitochondrial division (arrows).

Suggested Reading

Bani-Sacchi T, et al. Ultrastructural studies on white adipocyte differentiation in the mouse mammary gland following estrogen and relaxin. Acta Anat. 129:1–9, 1987.

Trayhurn P, et al. Brown adipose tissue thermogenesis is 'suppressed' during lactation in mice. Nature. 298:59–60, 1982.

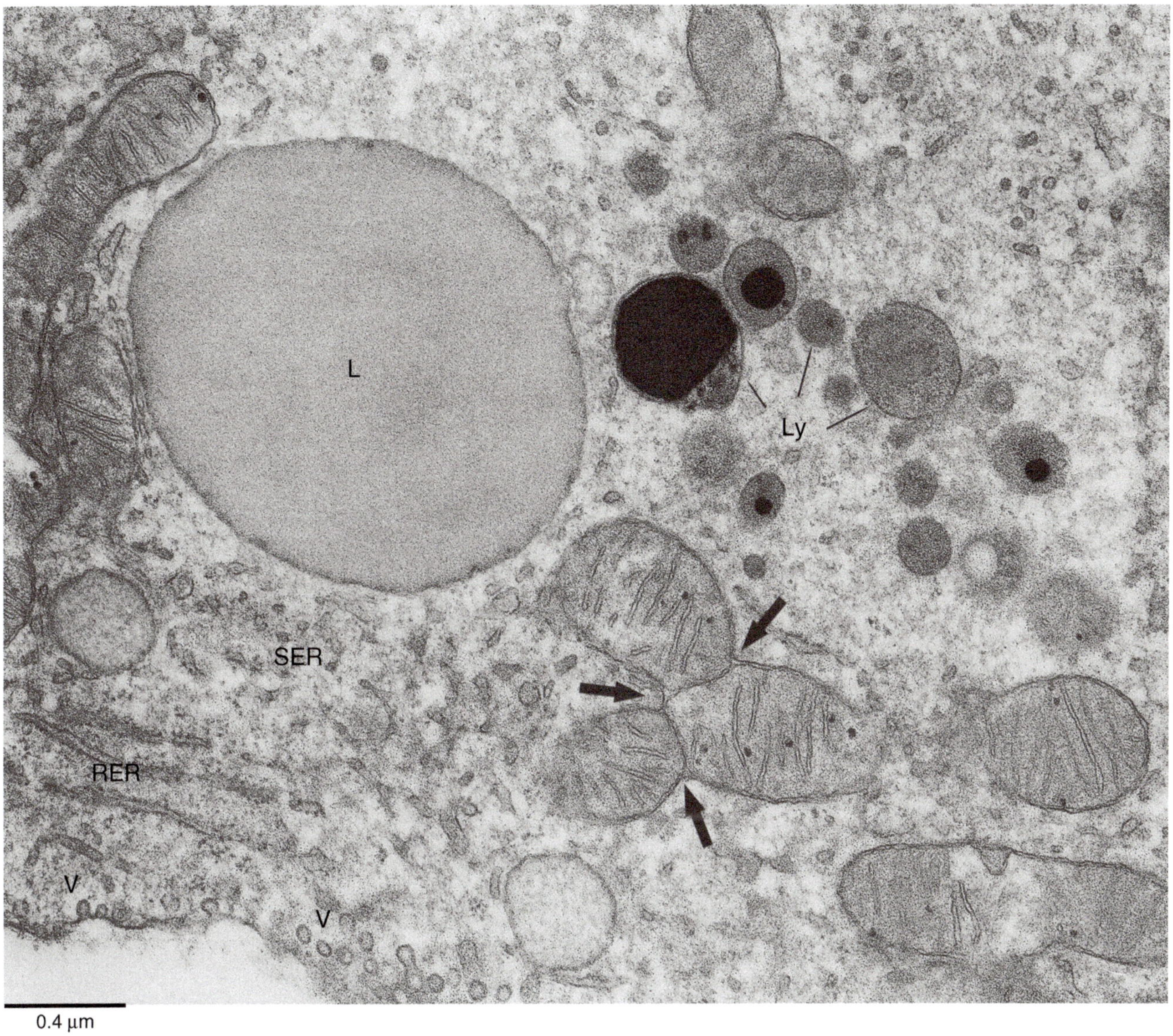

Plate 11.23 Retroperitoneal WAT of a lactating mouse. Cytoplasm of a representative adipocyte. TEM

Murine Adipose Organ Development 12

S. Cinti, *Obesity, Type 2 Diabetes and the Adipose Organ*, https://doi.org/10.1007/978-3-319-40522-3_12

12.1 Murine Adipose Organ Development

PLATE 12.1

Gross Anatomy

The adipose organ of fetal rats is dissectible. In this plate, the fetal adipose organ of a rat at gestational day 20 is shown in the upper panel. It is visually evident that most of the organ is represented by the anterior subcutaneous depot and that all other sites are poorly developed at this gestational stage.

The posterior depot is poorly developed and mainly located in the inguinal area.

Very poorly developed visceral fat is visible in the mesenteric, mediastinal-periaortic, and perirenal sites.

The color of the organ is mainly brown or brownish with the whitest parts represented by the mesenteric fat (see scheme).

These data suggest that the adipose organ development starts with the formation of different independent depots located in subcutaneous and visceral areas of the body. The anatomy of adult murine adipose organ is formed by a unitary structure, likely deriving from a progressive fusion of all different independent depots.

The gross anatomy of progressive enlargement of the organ during the first twelve postnatal days is shown in the lower panel. Development is greatly prevalent in subcutaneous fat where BAT (IS: interscapular, SS: subscapular, DC: deep cervical) is prevalent over WAT (SC: superficial cervical) in the anterior depot and WAT (DL: dorsolumbar, I: inguinal, G: gluteal) is prevalent over BAT in the posterior depot. Visceral depots are poorly developed, but it is visually evident that the most developed is the mediastinal-periaortic (MP) BAT. Mesenteric (M), retroperitoneal (R), and epididymal (E) depots are mainly WAT and inter-renal (IR) mainly BAT.

Note that most of the anterior subcutaneous depot, until postnatal day 2, is formed only by BAT; then (see days 6 and 12) WAT develops into this depot that therefore develops into a mixed depot in adult mice.

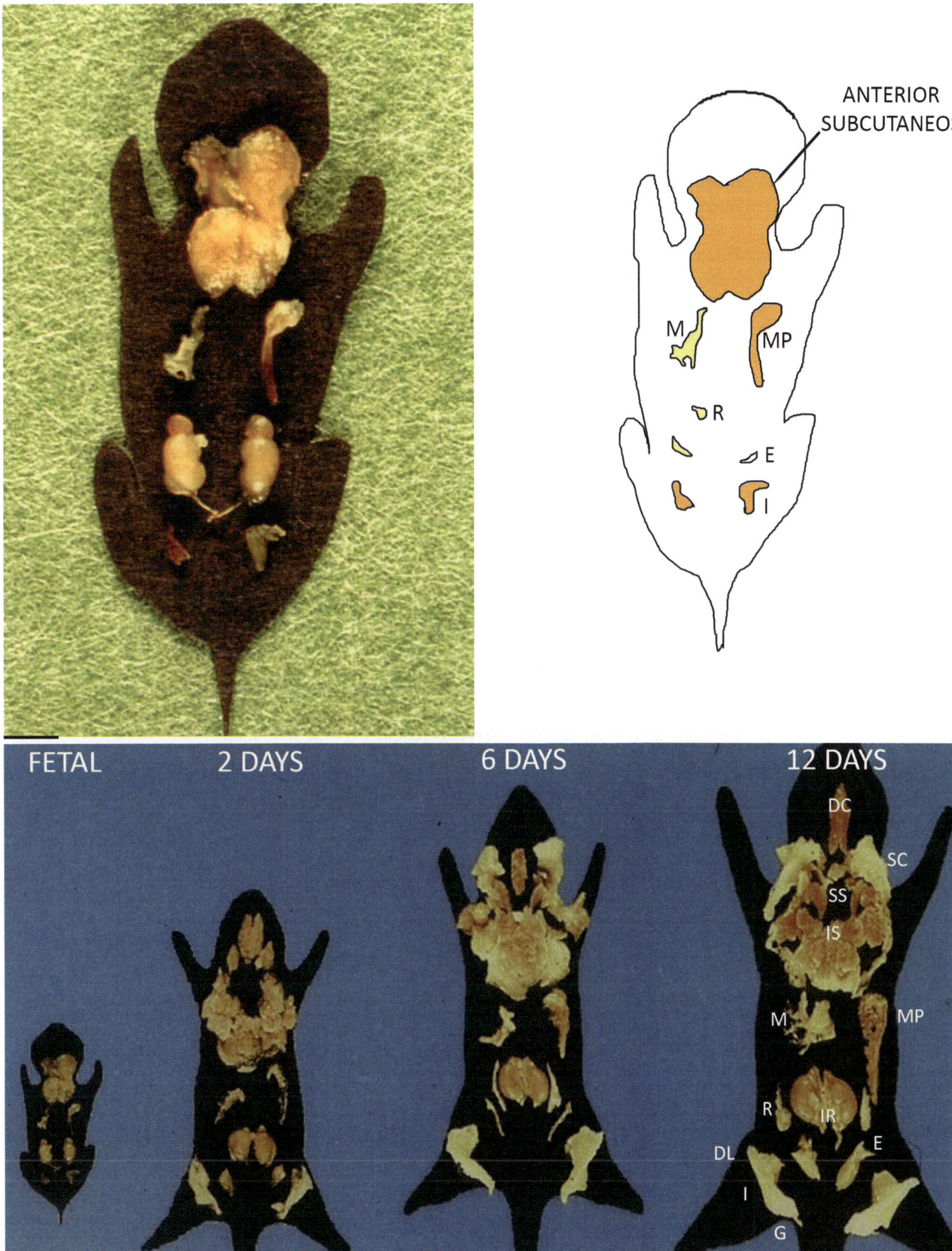

Plate 12.1 Gross anatomy of fetal and newborn rats adipose organ

PLATE 12.2

Early Fetal IBAT

The first signs of development in the adipose organ of fetal rats are observed around the 15th day of intrauterine life in the dorsal upper thoracic region, dorsolaterally to the spinal cord among the dorsal muscles. The anlage of the adipose organ in the perinatal period produces mainly brown adipocytes and has therefore been referred to as brown adipose tissue anlage. Brown adipocytes developing in this area share with muscle cells the transcription factor Myf5, a master regulator of skeletal muscle differentiation and myogenesis. Interestingly retinoblastoma protein (Rb) seems to play an important role determining white versus brown adipocyte differentiation.

Dilated capillaries (CAP) and "mesenchymal" cells in a loose matrix limited by skeletal muscles characterize histologically the anlage at this stage of development (left top panel). "Mesenchymal" cells are tightly connected with capillary walls or scattered in the matrix. Dividing cells (mitosis) are numerous. The ultrastructure of the poorly differentiated cells tightly connected to the capillary walls (pericytic position, all panels) shows very early signs of brown adipoblast differentiation: abundant "pre-typical" mitochondria (bottom panel, arrow). "Pre-typical" mitochondria are described also in Plates 2.26–2.29. Immunogold ultrastructural cytochemistry showed UCP1 immunoreactivity in pre-typical mitochondria.

Suggested Reading

Sidman RL. Histogenesis of brown adipose tissue in vivo and in organ culture. Anat Rec. 124:581–601, 1956.

Nnodim JO. Development of adipose tissues. Anat Rec. 219:331–37, 1987.

Rudnicki MA, et al. MyoD or Myf-5 is required for the formation of skeletal muscle. Cell. 75:1351–9, 1993.

Cinti S, Morroni M. Brown adipocyte precursor cells: a morphological study. Ital J Anat Embryol. 100: 75–81, 1995.

Hansen JB, et al. Retinoblastoma protein functions as a molecular switch determining white versus brown adipocyte differentiation. Proc Natl Acad Sci U S A. 101:4112–7, 2004.

Seale P, et al. PRDM16 controls a brown fat/skeletal muscle switch. Nature. 454: 961–7, 2008.

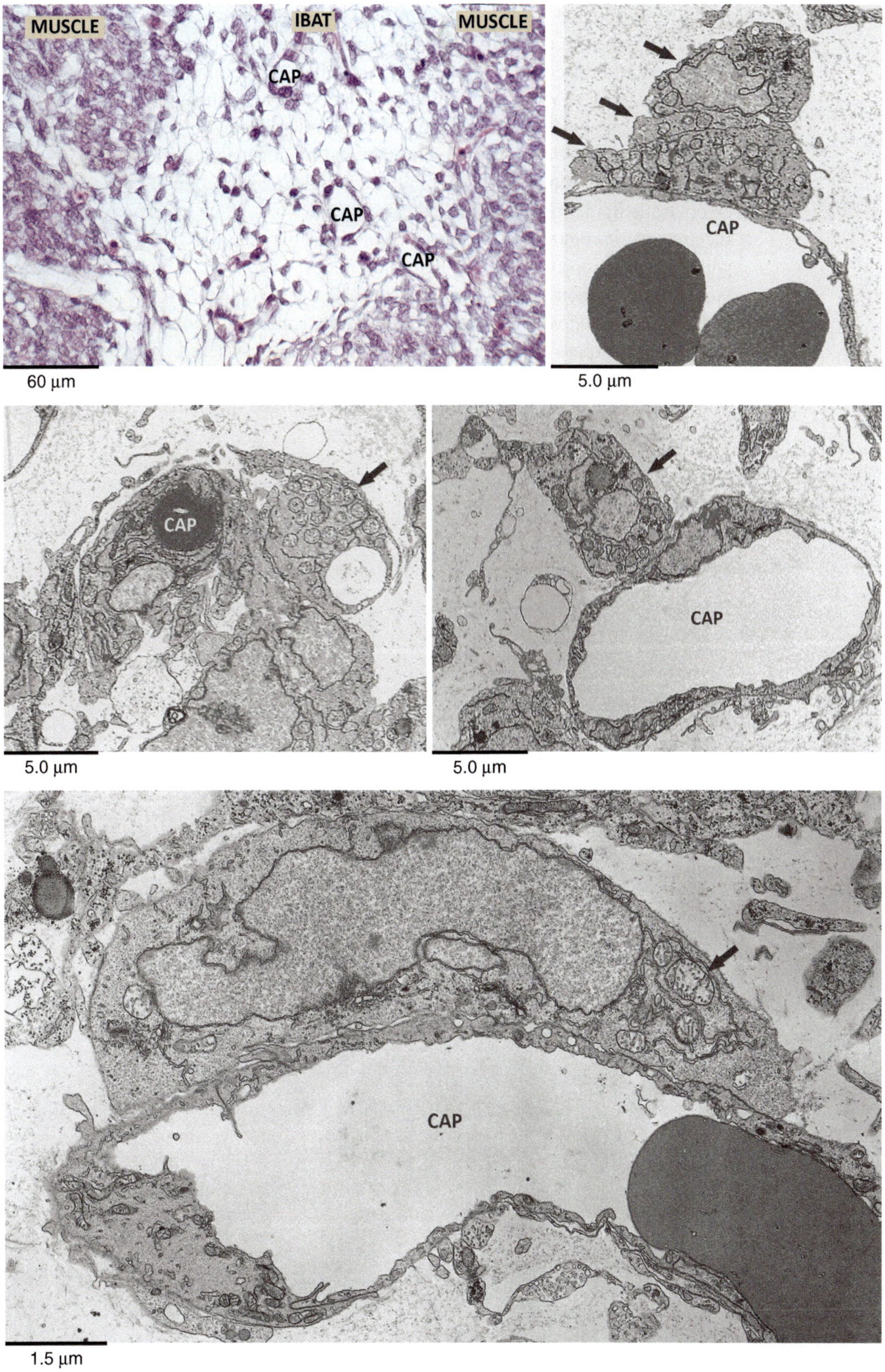

Plate 12.2 IBAT anlage 15th–17th gestational day. *Top left*: LM.E&H. *Top right* and *middle* panels (17th gestational day): pericapillary (CAP) areas with brown precursors (*arrows*). *Bottom*: enlargement of a brown adipocyte precursor (similar to those in top and middle panels) in pericytic position, at early stage of development (15th gestational day). TEM

PLATE 12.3

Late Fetal BAT I

In the fetal adipose organ of a rat at day 18 of intrauterine life, cellularity increases considerably. Most parenchymal cells become rounder and the vascular bed richer (CAP: capillary). aP2 immunoreactivity is present and quite specific for adipoblasts-preadipocytes in the BAT anlage. The morphology of most cells occupying the space between capillaries is quite constant and homogeneous with frequent mitosis. About 20–30% of this cell population shows small cytoplasmic lipid droplets (some indicated by L).

Electron microscopy shows that the vast majority of the cells, together with the lipid droplets visible at light microscopy level, are rich in pre-typical mitochondria and glycogen (see also the next plate).

Interestingly, mice with insulin receptor 80–98% ablation show a lipoatrophic adipose organ, and brown adipocyte ultrastructure is very similar to that of brown preadipocytes shown in this plate.

The framed area in the lower panel is a mitosis enlarged in the next plate.

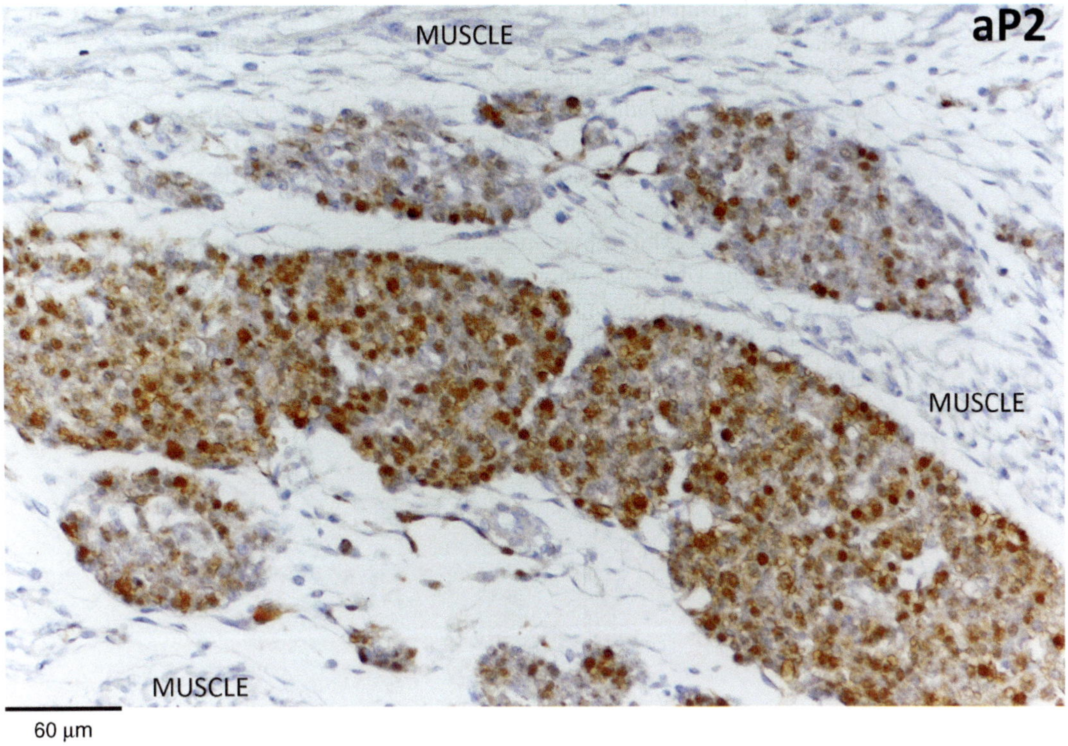

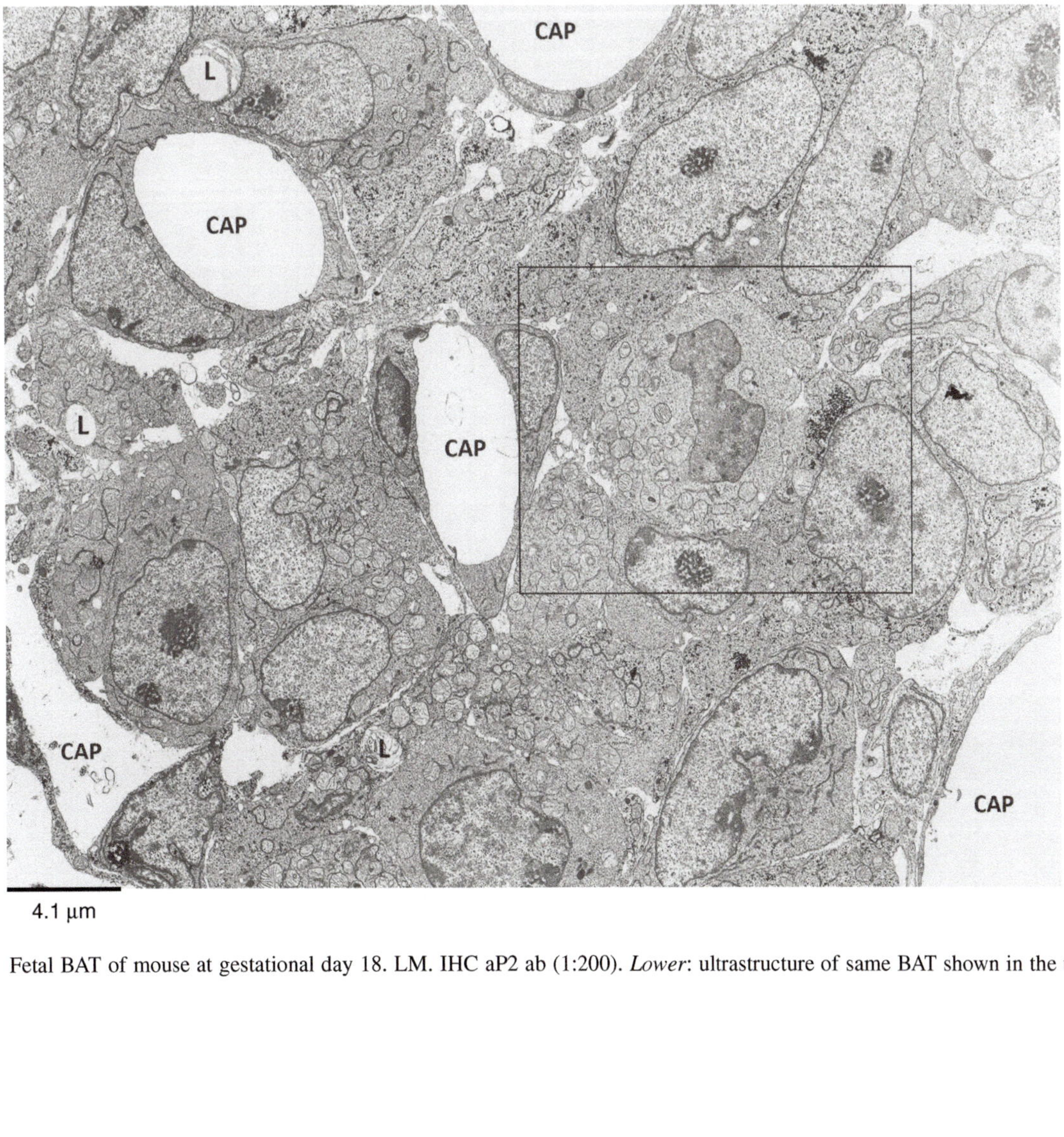

Plate 12.3 Fetal BAT of mouse at gestational day 18. LM. IHC aP2 ab (1:200). *Lower*: ultrastructure of same BAT shown in the upper panel. TEM

PLATE 12.4

Late Fetal BAT II

Most of the cells in the BAT anlage show a tight connection with capillary walls. Almost all the interstitial space among the capillaries is occupied by parenchymal cells with the typical features of brown adipoblasts-preadipocytes (described in detail also in Plates 2.26–2.29). "Pre-typical" mitochondria and glycogen (G) can be seen in these adipoblasts-preadipocytes, in this plate. Most of them are UCP1 immunoreactive (lower right plate).
The cell in mitosis exhibits pre-typical mitochondria (upper panel), in line with the UCP1 immunoreactivity shown in the lower left panel where a UCP1-immunoreactive cell in pericyte position in mitosis is visible (arrow). Of note, we found UCP1-immunogold particles on those "pre-typical" mitochondria.

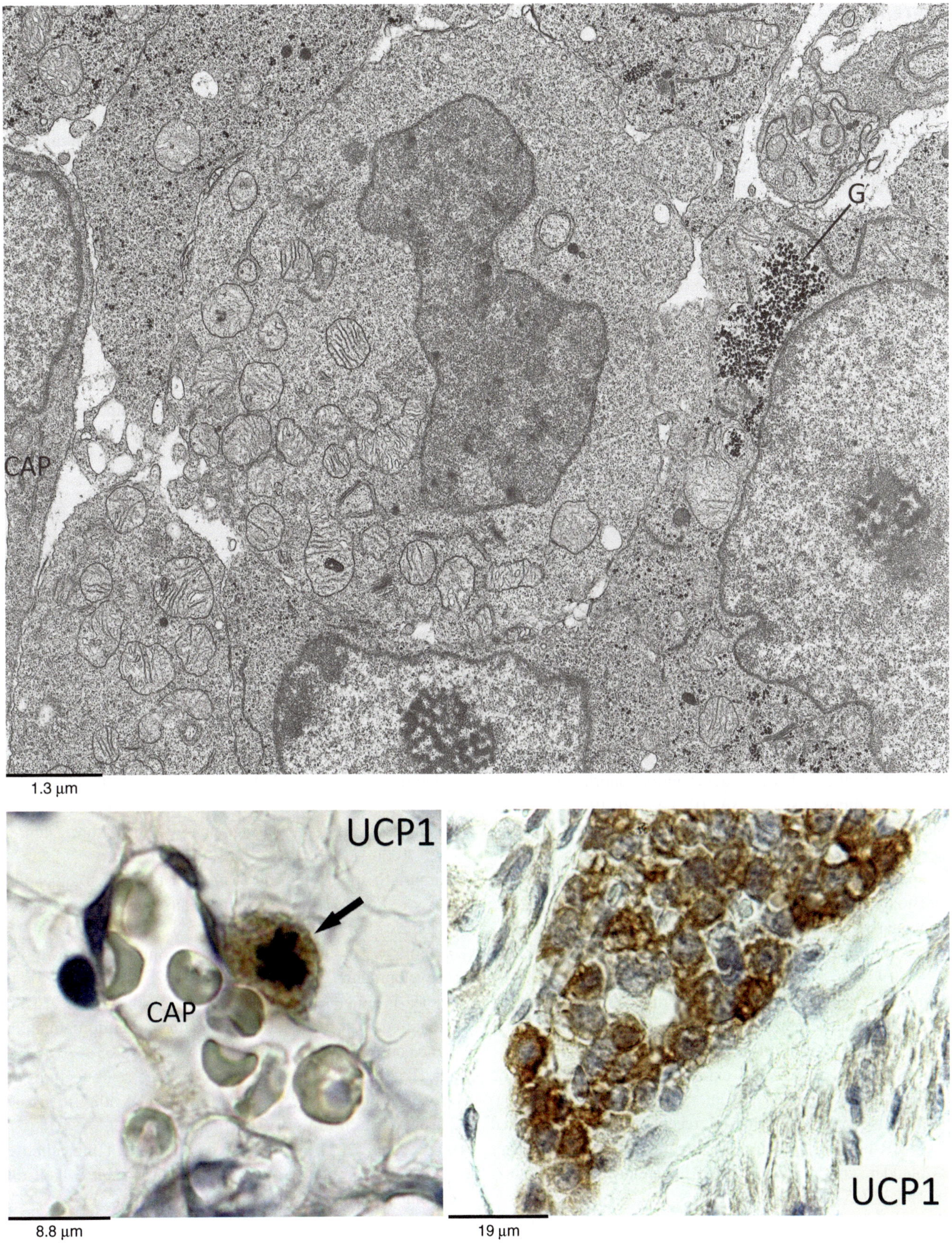

Plate 12.4 *Upper*: enlargement of the framed area in Plate 12.3. Brown adipoblasts show "pre-typical" mitochondria even in mitotic cells. G: glycogen. CAP: capillary. *Lower*: mitotic (*left*) and non-mitotic (*right*) adipoblasts of this BAT anlage are UCP1 immunoreactive

PLATE 12.5

Late Fetal III

In this rat anlage at day 21 of fetal life, brown adipocytes are in a stage of differentiation similar to that of brown preadipocytes described in Plate 2.28: abundant cytoplasm rich in mitochondria, lipid droplets (L), and a variable amount of glycogen. Some cells, like the one shown in this plate, contain a considerable amount of glycogen (G). The mitochondrial morphology is less typical than that observed in brown adipoblasts of mice, but the number of mitochondria is impressive. In the lower panel S-100B-immunohistochemistry demonstrates that brown adipocyte precursors are not immunoreactive to this protein. In the lower left part of the panel, S-100B-immunoreactive chondrocytes (internal positive control) are visible. Interestingly, white adipocyte precursors and mature adipocytes of WAT are intensely S100B immunoreactive (see Plate 4.5); thus this protein could play a role in the specific white phenotype determination.

A cascade of transcription factors that is in large part shared by both white and brown adipocytes controls adipogenesis. An early step is the up regulation of the CCAAT/Enhancer Binding Proteins β and δ (C/EBP β and δ), which induce the expression of C/EBP α and Ppar γ (see also Plate 12.9). Other transcription factors are able to induce the development of the specific characteristics of either type of adipocytes. It has been shown that differentiation of brown fat cells is enhanced by expression of the zinc finger protein Prdm16, and interestingly, transduction of both C/EBP β and Prdm16 into murine or human fibroblasts is sufficient to induce brown fat differentiation.

Recently bone morphogenetic protein 7 and Plac 8 have been suggested as upstream regulators of C/EBP β and PRDM16. MicroRNA-26 seems also required for adipogenesis and drives characteristics of brown adipocytes.

Suggested Reading

Suter ER. The fine structure of brown adipose tissue. II. Perinatal development in the rat. Lab Invest. 21: 246–58, 1969.

Barnard T. The ultrastructural differentiation of brown adipose tissue in the rat. J Ultrastruct Res. 29:311–33, 1969.

Houstek J, et al. Uncoupling protein in embryonic brown adipose tissue—existence of nonthermogenic and thermogenic mitochondria. BBA. 935:19–25, 1988.

Houstek J, et al. Postnatal appearance of uncoupling protein and formation of thermogenic mitochondria in hamster brown adipose tissue. BBA. 1015:441–9, 1990.

Manchado C, et al. CCAAT/enhancer-binding proteins alpha and beta in brown adipose tissue: evidence for a tissue-specific pattern of expression during development. Biochem J. 302:695–700, 1994.

Zancanaro C, et al. An ultrastructural study of brown adipose tissue in pre-term human new-borns. Tiss Cell. 27:339–48, 1995.

Teruel T, et al. Differentiation of rat brown adipocytes during late foetal development: role of insulin-like growth factor I. Biochem J. 310:771–6, 1995.

Jain S, et al. Differential expression of the peroxisome proliferator-activated receptor gamma (PPARgamma) and its coactivators steroid receptor coactivator-1 and PPAR-binding protein PBP in the brown fat, urinary bladder, colon, and breast of the mouse. Am J Pathol. 153:349–54, 1998.

Braissant O, Wahli W. Differential expression of peroxisome proliferator-activated receptor-alpha, -beta, and -gamma during rat embryonic development. Endocrinology. 139:2748–54, 1998.

Donato R. Functional roles of S100 proteins, calcium-binding proteins of the EF-hand type. Biochim Biophys Acta. 1450:191–231, 1999.

Donato R. Intracellular and extracellular roles of S100 proteins. Microsc Res Tech. 60:540–51, 2003.

Kitamura T, et al. Mosaic analysis of insulin receptor function. J Clin Invest. 113:209–19, 2004.

Farmer SR. Transcriptional control of adipocyte formation. Cell Metab. 4:263–73, 2006.

Rosen ED, MacDougald OA. Adipocyte differentiation from the inside out. Nat Rev Mol Cell Biol. 7:885–96, 2006.

Seale P, et al. Transcriptional control of brown fat determination by PRDM16. Cell Metab. 6:38–54, 2007.

Tseng YH, et al. New role of bone morphogenetic protein 7 in brown adipogenesis and energy expenditure. Nature. 454:1000–4, 2008.

Kajimura S, et al. Initiation of myoblast to brown fat switch by a PRDM16-C/EBP-beta transcriptional complex. Nature. 460:1154–8, 2009.

Kajimura S, et al. Transcriptional control of brown fat development. Cell Metab. 11: 257–62, 2010.

Jimenez-Preitner M, et al. Plac8 is an inducer of C/EBPβ required for brown fat differentiation, thermoregulation, and control of body weight. Cell Metab. 14:658–70, 2011.

Taga H, et al. Cellular and molecular large-scale features of fetal adipose tissue: is bovine perirenal adipose tissue brown? J Cell Physiol. 227:1688–700, 2012.

Tran KV, et al. The vascular endothelium of the adipose tissue gives rise to both white and brown fat cells. Cell Metab. 15:222–9, 2012.

Karbiener M, et al. MicroRNA-26 family is required for human adipogenesis and drives characteristics of brown adipocytes. Stem Cells. 32:1578–90, 2014.

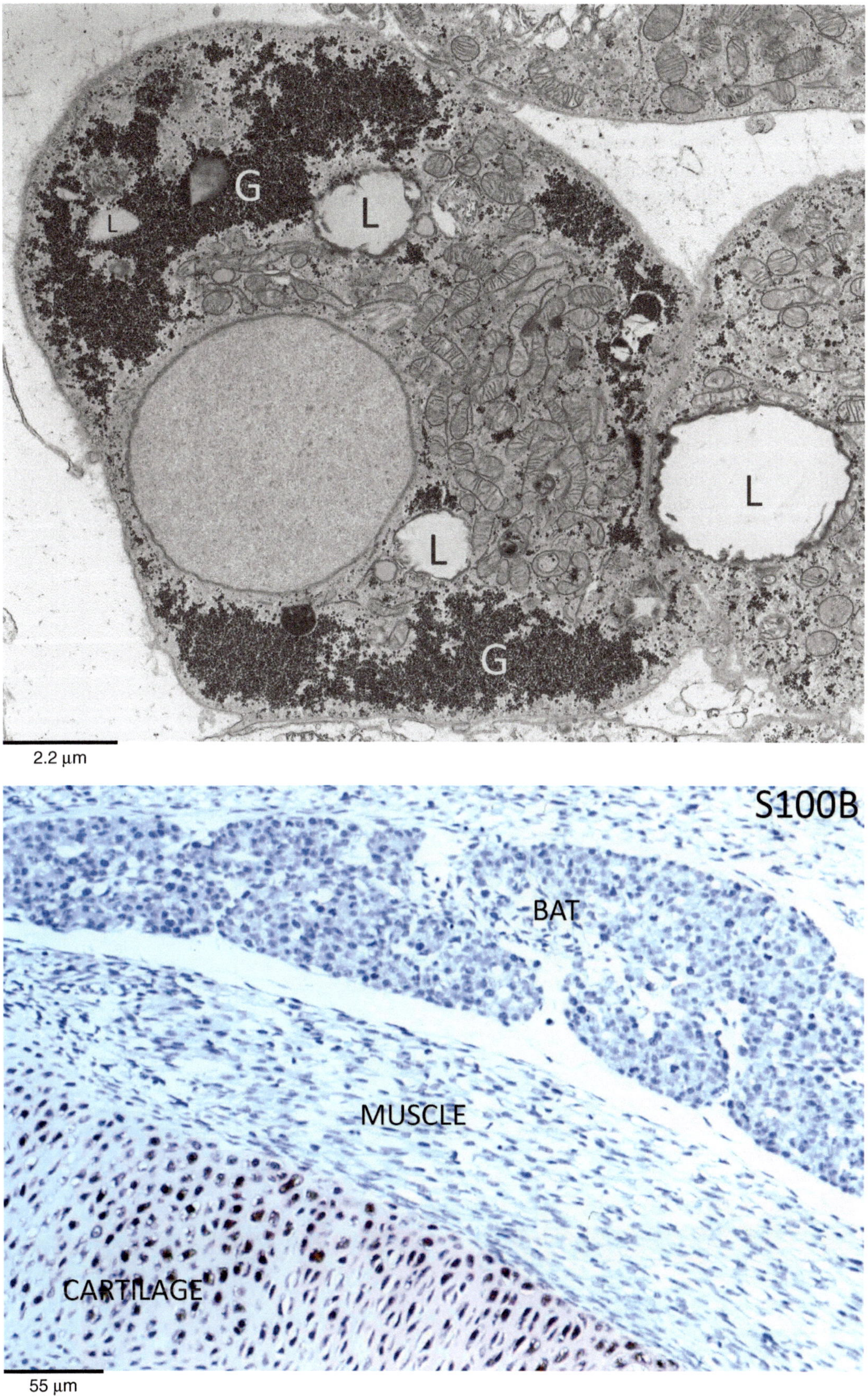

Plate 12.5 Rat BAT anlage 21st gestational day. *Lower*: Mouse BAT anlage at gestational day 18. LM. IHC ab S100B (1:300)

PLATE 12.6

Newborn IBAT TEM

In IBAT of newborn rat, mature brown adipocytes reach a maximum level of organelles development and differentiation. Note the impressive number of cytoplasmic mitochondria, their regular spherical shape, and the regular small size of numerous lipid droplets.
In the lower panel, mitochondria are enlarged and show the typical laminar cristae. Note the numerous secretory endocrine granules visible among the mitochondria (S, some indicated).

Suggested Reading

Cannon B, et al. In "The Endocrine Control of the Fetus", Kunzel and Jensen Eds, Springer, 1988.
Obregon MJ, et al. Postnatal recruitment of brown adipose tissue is induced by the cold stress experienced by the pups. An analysis of mRNA levels for thermogenin and lipoprotein lipase. Biochem J. 259:341–6, 1989.
Finn D, et al. An immunohistochemical and in situ hybridisation study of the postnatal development of uncoupling protein-1 and uncoupling protein-1 mRNA in lamb perirenal adipose tissue. Cell Tiss Res. 294:461–6, 1988.

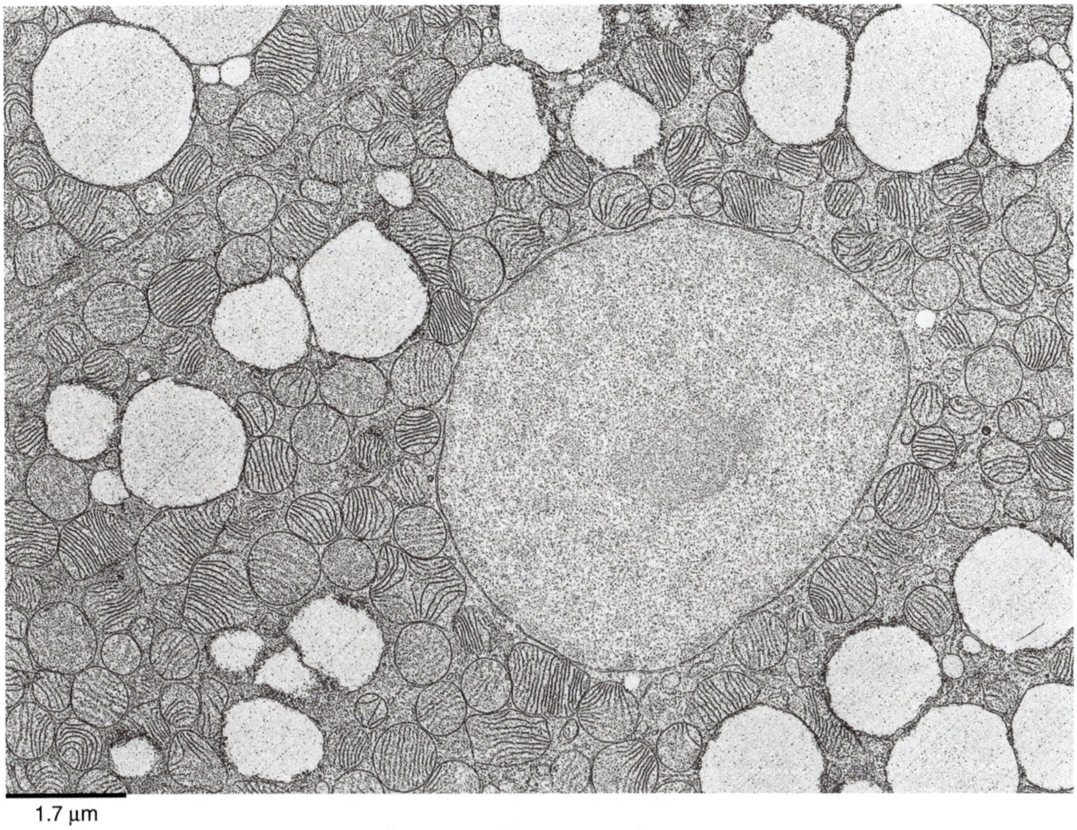

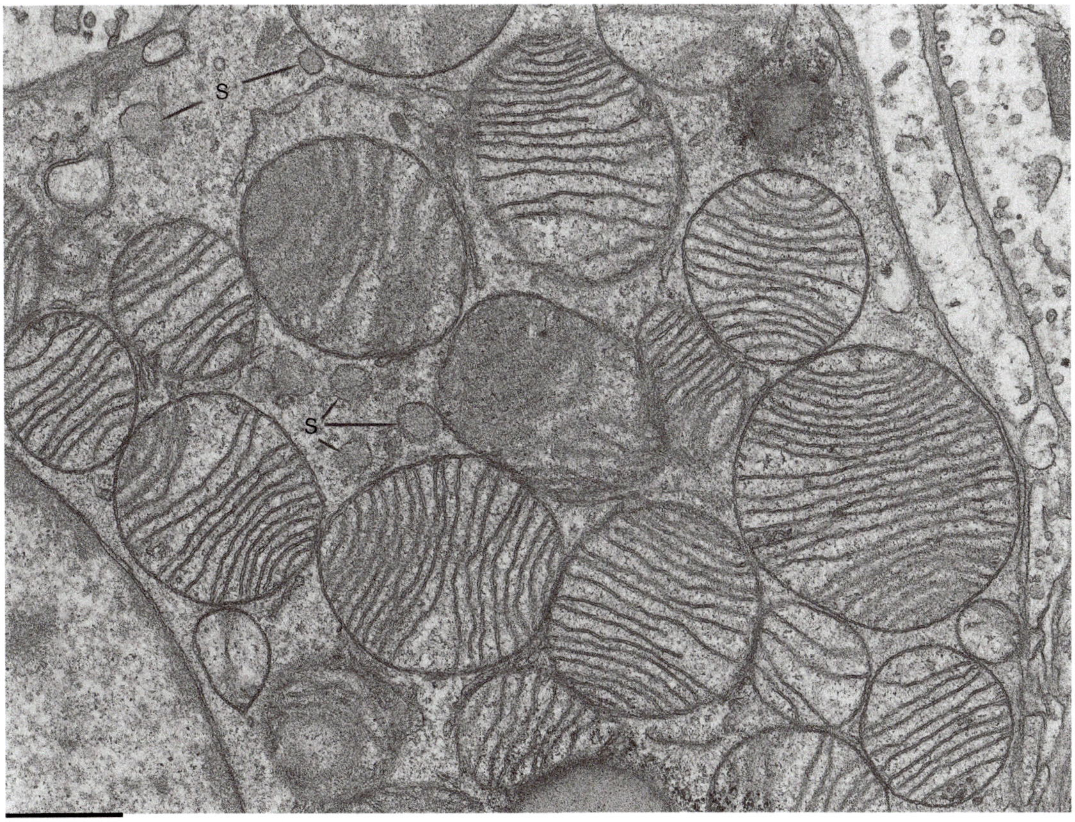

Plate 12.6 Newborn rat (9 days old) IBAT. Brown adipocytes TEM

PLATE 12.7

Parenchymal Nerves in IBAT of Newborn Rat

Together with cellular signs of hyperactivity (see the previous plate), IBAT of newborn rats and mice is very rich in parenchymal nerve fibers. In this plate, a large nerve (evidenced by dotted line) running among brown adipocytes is well visible. It is composed of unmyelinated fibers. Nucleus of Schwann cell is indicated (N). Note the high density of capillaries (CAP).

Suggested Reading

Bartness TJ, et al. Brain-adipose tissue cross talk. Proc Nutr Soc. 64:53–64, 2005.

Bartness TJ, Song CK. Thematic review series: adipocyte biology. Sympathetic and sensory innervation of white adipose tissue. J Lipid Res. 48:1655–72, 2007.

Bartness TJ, Song CK. Brain-adipose tissue neural crosstalk. Physiol Behav. 91:343–51, 2007.

Bartness TJ, et al. Sensory and sympathetic nervous system control of white adipose tissue lipolysis. Mol Cell Endocrinol. 318:34–43, 2010.

Bartness TJ, et al. Sympathetic and sensory innervation of brown adipose tissue. Int J Obes. 34(Suppl 1):S36–42, 2010.

Bartness TJ, et al. Neural and hormonal control of food hoarding. Am J Physiol Regul Integr Comp Physiol. 301:R641–55, 2011.

Bartness TJ, et al. Neural innervation of white adipose tissue and the control of lipolysis. Front Neuroendocrinol. 35(4):473–93, 2014.

Labbé SM, et al. Hypothalamic control of brown adipose tissue thermogenesis. Front Syst Neurosci. 9:150, 2015.

Bartness TJ, Ryu V. Neural control of white, beige and brown adipocytes. Int J Obes Suppl. 5(Suppl 1):S35–9, 2015.

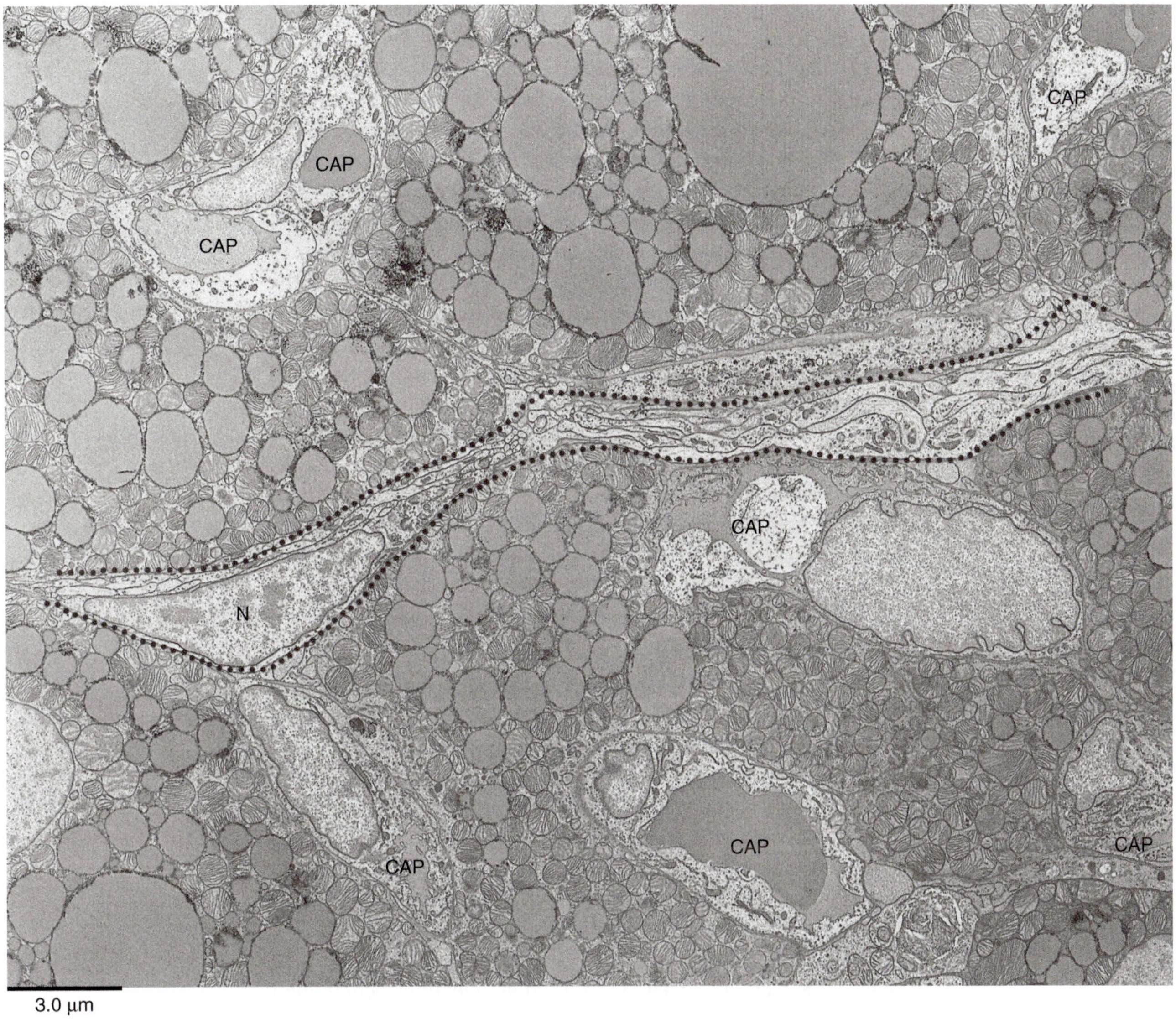

Plate 12.7 Newborn rat (9 day old) IBAT. Parenchymal nerve. TEM

PLATE 12.8

Origin of Brown Adipoblasts

In order to try to detect the cell of origin of brown adipoblasts, we used the lineage tracing technique described in detail on Plate 11.13. Morphology data presented in previous plates strongly pointed to the capillary wall as the niche for brown adipoblasts stem cells. We found similarities between the endothelial cells of BAT anlage and some brown adipoblasts. In particular, mitochondria of some endothelial cell were similar to the characteristic "pre-typical" mitochondria. The morphology of endothelial cell mitochondria is usually quite different from that of brown adipoblasts; thus, the similarity found in some endothelial cells suggested that only some endothelial cells could be able to differentiate into adipoblasts.
Therefore, we used Ve-Cadherin-Cre/R26R double transgenic mice to support our theory (scheme). In these mice, beta-Gal is expressed only in hematopoietic cells of the bone marrow and in all endothelial cells or the organism. In line with these data, we found X-Gal-stained endothelial cells in skeletal muscles surrounding the BAT anlage of fetal mice and in the vast majority of brown adipoblasts-preadipocytes and in postnatal brown adipocytes (lower panel).

Suggested Reading

Alva JA, et al. VE-Cadherin-Cre-recombinase transgenic mouse: a tool for lineage analysis and gene deletion in endothelial cells. Dev Dyn. 235:759–67, 2006.

Cinti S, Morroni M. Brown adipocyte precursor cells: a morphological study. Ital J Anat Embryol. 100: 75–81, 1995.

Gupta RK, et al. Transcriptional control of preadipocyte determination by Zfp423. Nature. 464:619–23, 2010.

Tran KV, et al. The vascular endothelium of the adipose tissue gives rise to both white and brown fat cells. Cell Metab. 15:222–9, 2012.

Gupta RK, et al. Zfp423 expression identifies committed preadipocytes and localizes to adipose endothelial and perivascular cells. Cell Metab. 15:230–9, 2012.

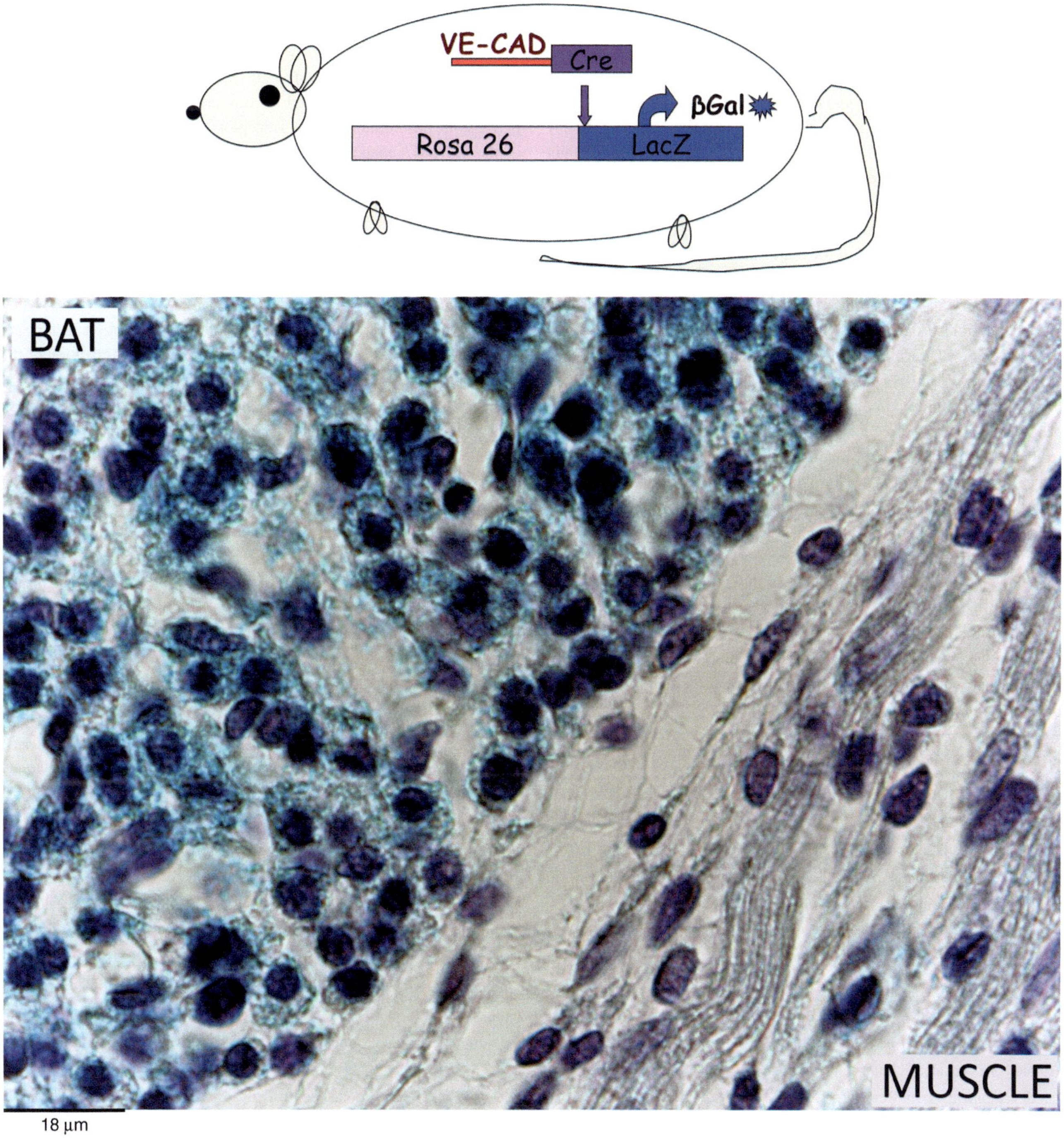

Plate 12.8 Fetal IBAT (gestational day 18) of double transgenic mouse Ve-Cad-Cre/R26R. LM. X-Gal staining

PLATE 12.9

Both in rats and mice, WAT development occurs mainly postnatally with very similar aspects. The most pure WAT depot (i.e., composed exclusively of white adipocytes) in rats and mice is the epididymal fat. Prenatally peri-epididymal tissue is present, but we never observed any sign of adipoblasts differentiation in this developmental stage. At light microscopy level, it is formed mainly by capillaries surrounded by mesenchymal cells, and the general histology is quite similar to that of early BAT anlage presented in Plate 12.2.

Postnatally, usually at day 4–6 for both rats and mice, the histology of peri-epididymal WAT is quite characteristic and presented in this plate. Large and very abundant capillaries together with cells with a variable amount of lipid droplets in their cytoplasm (adipocyte precursors at various stages of development) and other cell types are delimited by elongated fibroblast-like cells (see also Plate 12.19) into islets that we denominate vasculo-adipocytic islets (upper panel, yellow: lipid droplets in adipocyte precursors).

In the scheme, the fibroblast-like cells are indicated in black (see also Plate 12.19 for their ultrastructure). Capillaries in green and adipocytes and preadipocytes are outlined in orange. Note the different amounts of lipid droplets (yellow) in the developing adipocytes. Outside the vasculo-adipocytic islets, macrophages (violet) are visible.

Most of the cells with lipid droplets in the cytoplasm contained into vasculo-adipocytic islets resulted immunoreactive for aP2 antibodies at immunohistochemistry (right lower panel).

Of note, no adipocytes at any stage of differentiation were found outside the islets, strongly suggesting that the islets are preferential sites for the development of adipocytes.

WAT Development

The molecular mechanisms of white adipocytes development have been studied mainly in preadipocyte cell lines and embryonic fibroblasts. These studies have described a transcriptional cascade involving peroxisome proliferator-activated receptor γ (PPARγ) and three members of the CCAAT/enhancer-binding protein (C/EBP) family, C/EBPδ, C/EBPβ, and C/EBPα, that are activated sequentially during adipogenesis. C/EBPβ and C/EBPδ are induced early and transiently during differentiation and are considered to play key roles during the initiation of the adipogenic program. Their activation leads to the induction of C/EBPα and PPARγ expression promoting terminal adipocyte differentiation.

Besides PPARγ and the three C/EBPs, other transcription factors are reported to be necessary for adipocyte differentiation. Activation of the cAMP regulatory element-binding protein (CREB) at the onset of adipocyte differentiation is critical for adipogenesis. The recent cloning and characterization of a CREB cofactor family, denoted as CREB-regulated transcription coactivator (Crtc/TORC), have revealed how CREB can induce expression of distinct target genes dependent on different stimuli.

The murine double minute 2 (Mdm2) is an E3 ubiquitin ligase with oncogenic properties.

Interestingly, mdm2 is amplified in nearly all liposarcomas and in the widely used preadipocyte cell line, 3T3-L1. It has been recently shown that Mdm2 regulates adipogenesis by promoting cAMP-mediated transcriptional activation of CREB and induction of C/EBPδ expression, thus suggesting that Mdm2 is a player in the network of factors that regulate CREB-dependent transactivation and adipocyte differentiation.

Suggested Reading

Iyama K, et al. Electron microscopical studies on the genesis of white adipocytes: differentiation of immature pericytes into adipocytes in transplanted preadipose tissue. Virch Arch B. 31: 143–55, 1979.

Hausman GJ, Richardson RL. Cellular and vascular development in immature rat adipose tissue. J Lipid Res. 24: 522–32, 1983.

Cinti S, et al. A morphological study of the adipocyte precursor. J Submicrosc Cytol. 16:243–51, 1984.

Hauner H, Loffler G. Adipose tissue development: the role of precursor cells and adipogenic factors. Part I: adipose tissue development and the role of precursor cells. Klin Wochenschr. 65:803–11, 1987.

Ailhaud G, et al. Cellular and molecular aspects of adipose tissue development. Annu Rev Nutr. 12:207–33, 1992.

Spiegelman BM, Flier JS. Adipogenesis and obesity: rounding out the big picture. Cell. 87:377–89, 1996.

Spiegelman BM, et al. PPAR gamma and the control of adipogenesis. Biochimie. 79:111–2, 1997.

Gregoire FM, et al. Understanding adipocyte differentiation. Physiol Rev. 78:783–809, 1998.

Rosen ED, Spiegelman BM. Molecular regulation of adipogenesis. Annu Rev Cell Dev Biol. 16:145–71, 2000.

Reusch JE, et al. CREB activation induces adipogenesis in 3T3-L1 cells. Mol Cell Biol. 20:1008–20, 2000.

Rodeheffer MS, et al. Identification of white adipocyte progenitor cells in vivo. Cell. 135:240–9, 2008.

Tang W, et al. White fat progenitor cells reside in the adipose vasculature. Science. 322:583–6, 2008.

Lefterova MI, et al. PPARgamma and C/EBP factors orchestrate adipocyte biology via adjacent binding on a genome-wide scale. Genes Dev. 22:2941–52, 2008.

Cao Y. Adipose tissue angiogenesis as a therapeutic target for obesity and metabolic diseases. Nat Rev Drug Discov. 9:107–15, 2010.

Rydén M, et al. Transplanted bone marrow-derived cells contribute to human adipogenesis. Cell Metab. 22:408–17, 2015.

Crossno JT Jr., et al. Rosiglitazone promotes development of a novel adipocyte population from bone marrow-derived circulating progenitor cells. J Clin Invest. 116:3220–28, 2006.

Farmer SR. Transcriptional control of adipocyte formation. Cell Metab. 4:263–73, 2006.

Lijnen HR, et al. Impaired adipose tissue development in mice with inactivation of placental growth factor function. Diabetes. 55:2698–704, 2006.

Gupta RK, et al. Transcriptional control of preadipocyte determination by Zfp423. Nature. 464:619–23, 2010.

Han J, et al. The spatiotemporal development of adipose tissue. Development. 138:5027–37, 2011.

Gupta RK, et al. Zfp423 expression identifies committed preadipocytes and localizes to adipose endothelial and perivascular cells. Cell Metab. 15:230–9, 2012.

Hallenborg P, et al. Mdm2 controls CREB-dependent transactivation and initiation of adipocyte differentiation. Cell Death Differ. 19:1381–9, 2012.

Shao M, et al. Zfp423 maintains white adipocyte identity through suppression of the beige cell thermogenic gene program. Cell Metab. 23:1167–84, 2016.

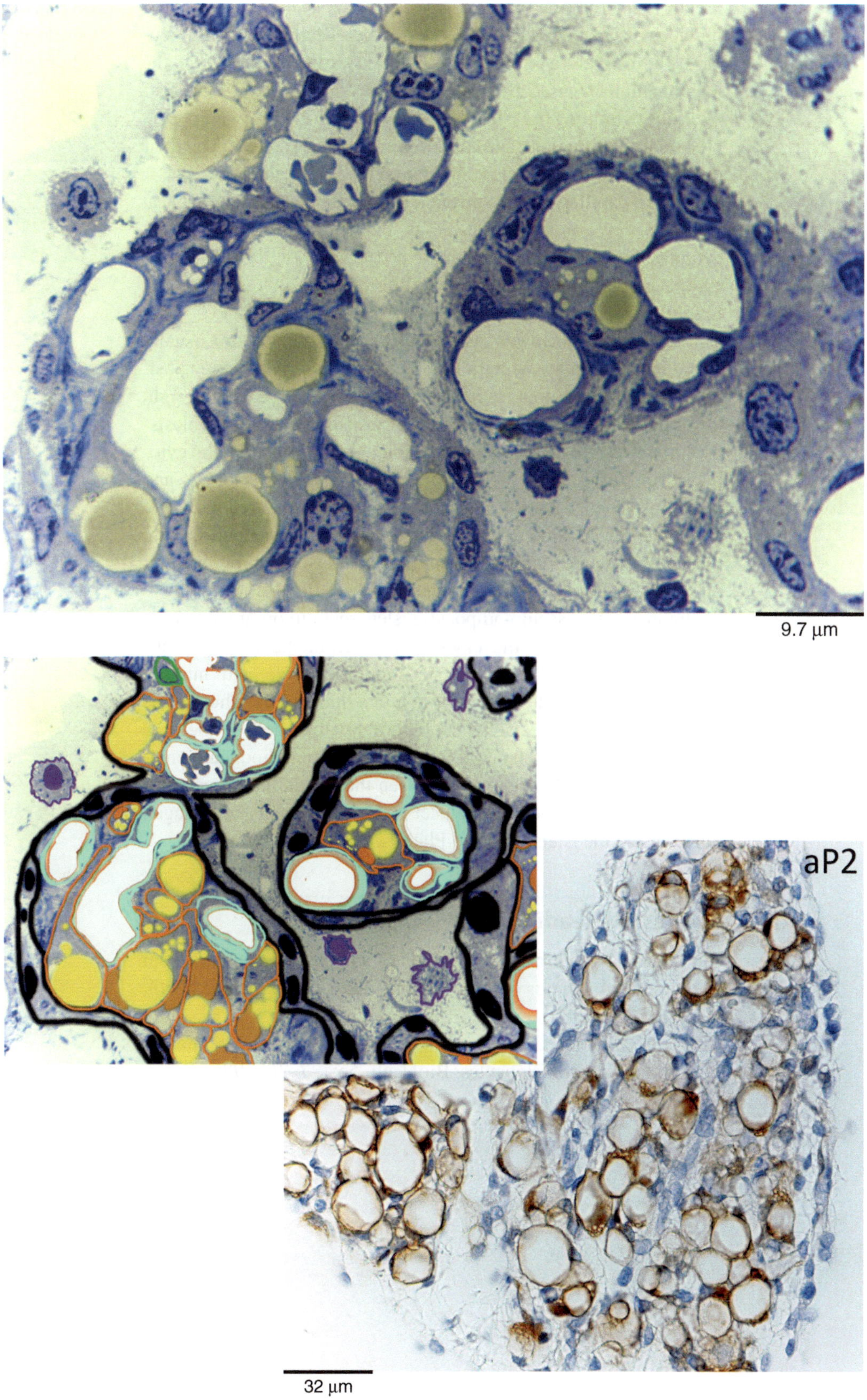

Plate 12.9 Epididymal WAT of newborn rat (postnatal day 6). *Top*: resin-embedded tissue. Vasculo-adipocytic islets. LM. Toluidine blue. *Bottom*: epididymal WAT of newborn mouse (postnatal day 6). Vasculo-adipocytic islets. LM. IHC aP2 ab (1.300)

PLATE 12.10

Ultrastructure of Developing Visceral Adipocytes

Electron microscopy of vasculo-adipocytic islets shown in the previous plate showed the presence of several cell types. In particular the ultrastructure of the cells present inside the islets allowed the identification of mast cells (see Plate 12.18), macrophage, fibroblast-like cells delimiting the islets (see Plate 12.19), and many adipocyte precursors at different stages of differentiation as suggested by their different amounts of lipid accumulation (L, some indicated).

The large capillaries are surrounded by adipocyte precursors at different developmental stages as denoted by their different cytoplasmic lipids (L, some indicated). Most of the cells with cytoplasmic lipid droplets of different sizes resulted aP2 immunoreactive (lower left panel).

The cells with the lower amount of cytoplasmic fat are usually found in tight contact with the capillary wall (also in pericytic position). The squared area in the upper panel is enlarged in the right lower panel and shows part of two poorly differentiated adipoblasts-preadipocytes. Together with small amounts of lipids (L), the cytoplasm of these cells is occupied mainly by ribosomes and polyribosomes (*, a generic sign of poorly differentiated cells; see also Plate 2.27). Among organelles, few small mitochondria with random cristae are also visible (m). Long and isolated rough endoplasmic reticulum cisternae are also visible (RER).

In summary, the vasculo-adipocytic islets seem to organize a well-delimited area where the environment favors the adipogenesis. Capillaries are essential elements, and their size and number strongly suggest a relevant active role in adipogenesis. The precise delimitation by a special kind of fibroblast-like cell of the area seems also very important for the creation of an adipogenic environment. A striking difference between the interstitial space composition inside and outside the islet is the high density of collagen fibrils inside the islets (see also Plate 12.19).

Suggested Reading

Cinti S, et al. An ultrastructural study of adipocyte precursors from epididymal fat pads of adult rats in culture. J Submicrosc Cytol. 17:115–22, 1985.

Gregoire F, et al. Ultrastructural analysis of the in vitro differentiation of female rat preadipocytes. Biol Cell. 56:127–36, 1986.

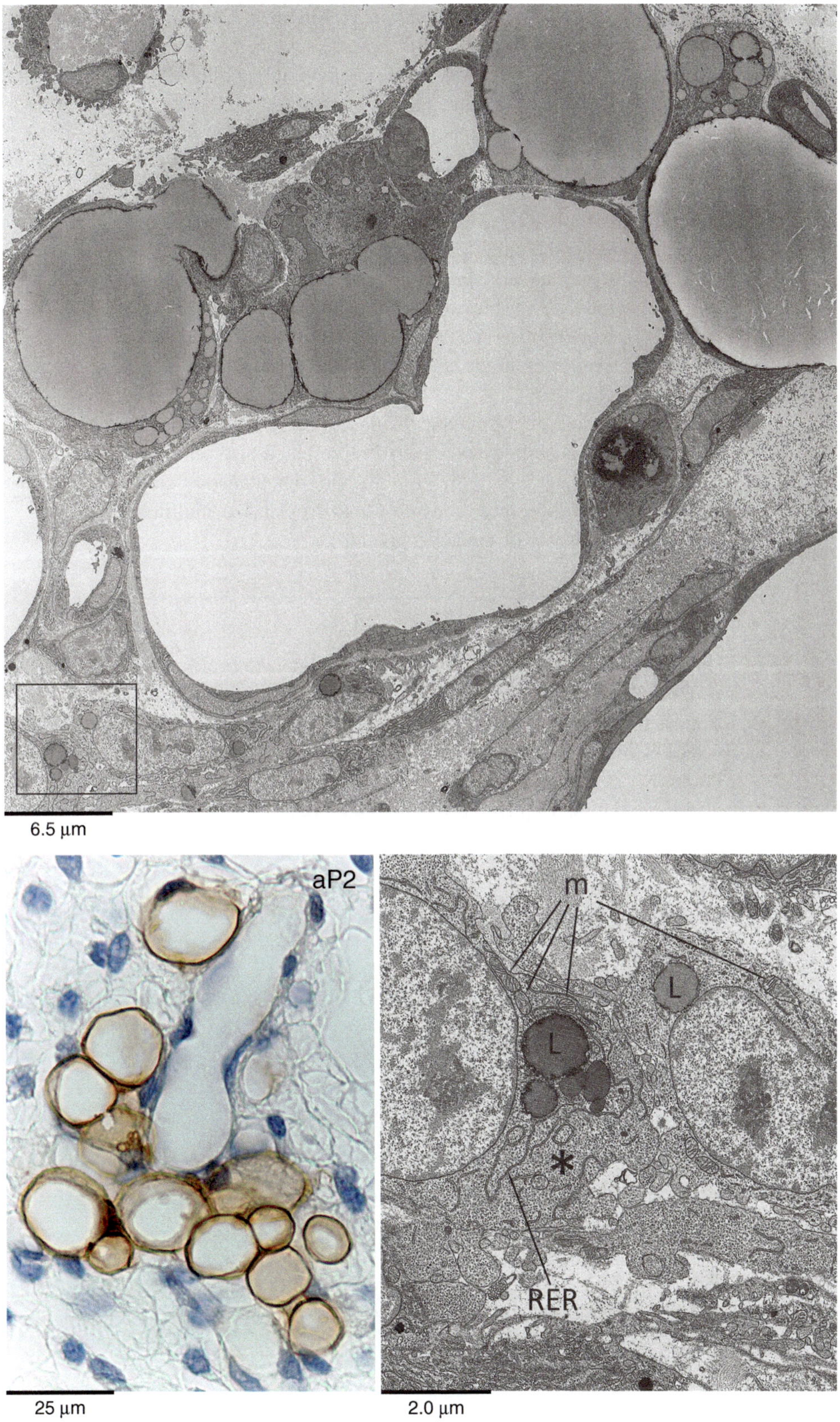

Plate 12.10 Epididymal WAT of newborn rat (postnatal day 6). Vasculo-adipocytic islet. *Upper* and *lower right*: TEM. *Lower left*: LM. IHC aP2 ab (1: 300)

PLATE 12.11

Ultrastructure of Developing Subcutaneous Adipocytes

The fine structure of developing adipocytes in subcutaneous fat is quite similar to that described for visceral fat. In this plate, the ultrastructure of developing adipocytes in inguinal fat of a 12 h old mouse is shown. Note the tight connection with the capillary (CAP) wall of these developing adipocytes. The cell in pericyte position is rich in glycogen (G), and no lipid vacuoles are visible in its cytoplasm. Developing adipocytes are multilocular with a predominant central lipid droplet (L). Mitochondria (lower panel, enlargement of framed area in the upper panel) are mainly small elongated and with randomly oriented cristae. Short rough endoplasmic reticulum (RER) cisternae are visible among mitochondria. Glycogen particles (G) are often observed. Numerous pinocytotic vesicles are present at plasma membrane, and a distinct external lamina (EL) is always visible.

In summary, most of the organelles described in mature visceral and subcutaneous adipocytes are well represented also during the developmental stages of both visceral and subcutaneous adipocytes. The major differences consist of lipid droplet size, multilocularity, and persistence of glycogen granules.

Suggested Reading

Hausman DB, et al. The biology of white adipocyte proliferation. Obes Rev. 2: 239–54, 2001.

Hausman GJ, Richardson RL. Adipose tissue angiogenesis. J Anim Sci. 82, 925–34, 2004.

Poulos SP, et al. The increasingly complex regulation of adipocyte differentiation. Exp Biol Med. 241:449–56, 2016.

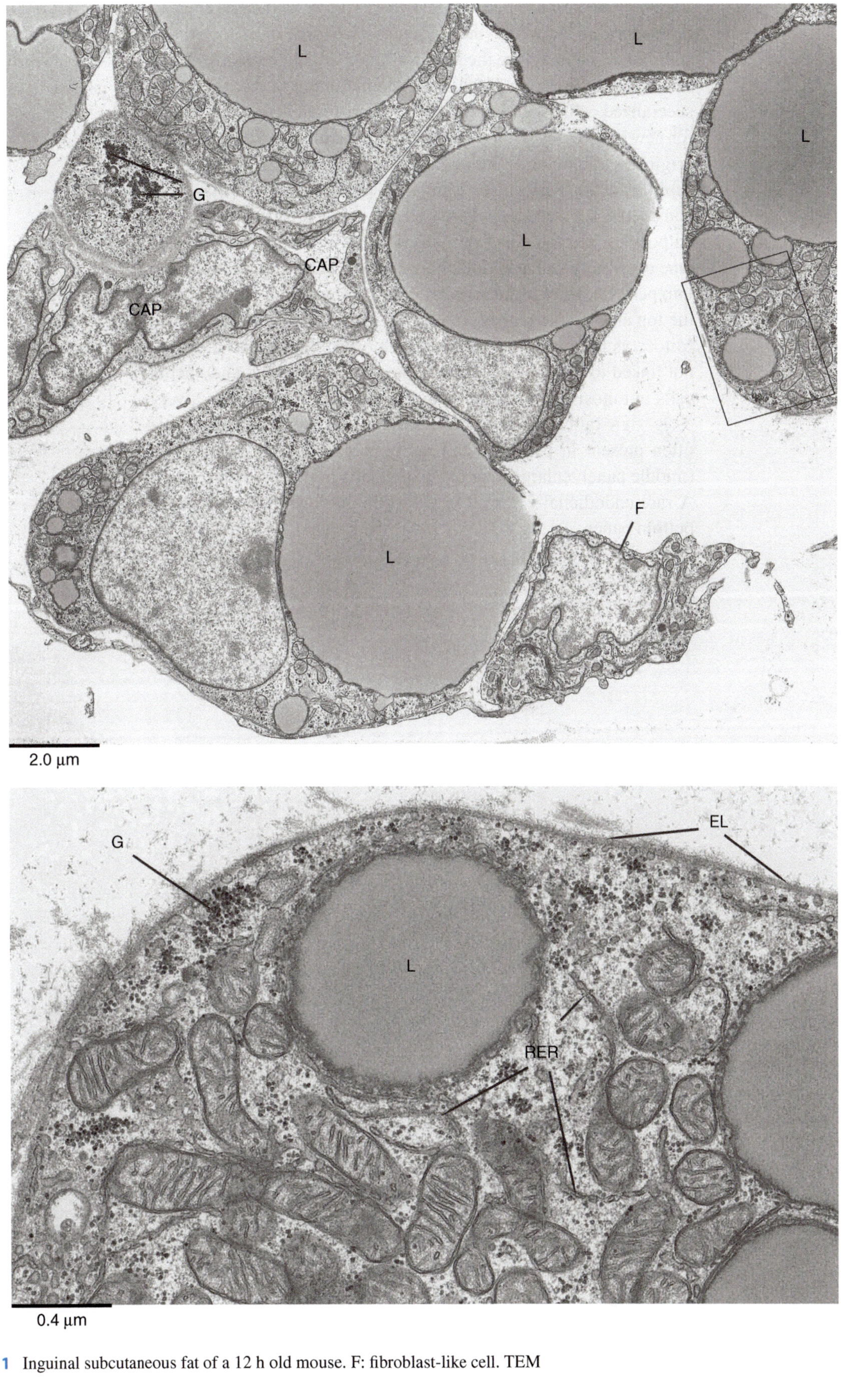

Plate 12.11 Inguinal subcutaneous fat of a 12 h old mouse. F: fibroblast-like cell. TEM

PLATE 12.12

Ultrastructure of Endothelial Cells in Vasculo-Adipocytic Islets I

Capillary of vasculo-adipocytic islets is large and numerous. A disproportion between the vascular network and the tissue cellularity and therefore the need for blood of this tissue is evident. This disproportion and the clear delimitation of the islets by specialized cells (see Plate 12.19) of a tissue that is the only source for new adipocytes strongly point to the vascular wall as a possible origin for adipoblasts. Endothelial cells and pericyte make up the capillary wall. Pericyte of capillaries in adipose tissue has been considered for decades where cells are able to differentiate into adipocytes, but the cell from which pericyte derives is unknown. One possibility is that endothelial cells themselves could transform into pericyte. Here some aspects of the capillary wall are shown. In the top and middle panels, an endothelial cell in mitosis is shown. Mitosis is frequent even in the middle of capillaries and therefore not linked to the capillary development itself. Of note, endothelial cells in mitosis are often rich in glycogen (G). Glycogen is a very early sign (although not specific) of adipocyte phenotype, very often present in pericytes and rarely present in endothelial cells (middle panel, enlargement of squared area in the top panel).
A rare endothelial cell rich in glycogen particles is shown in the bottom panel.

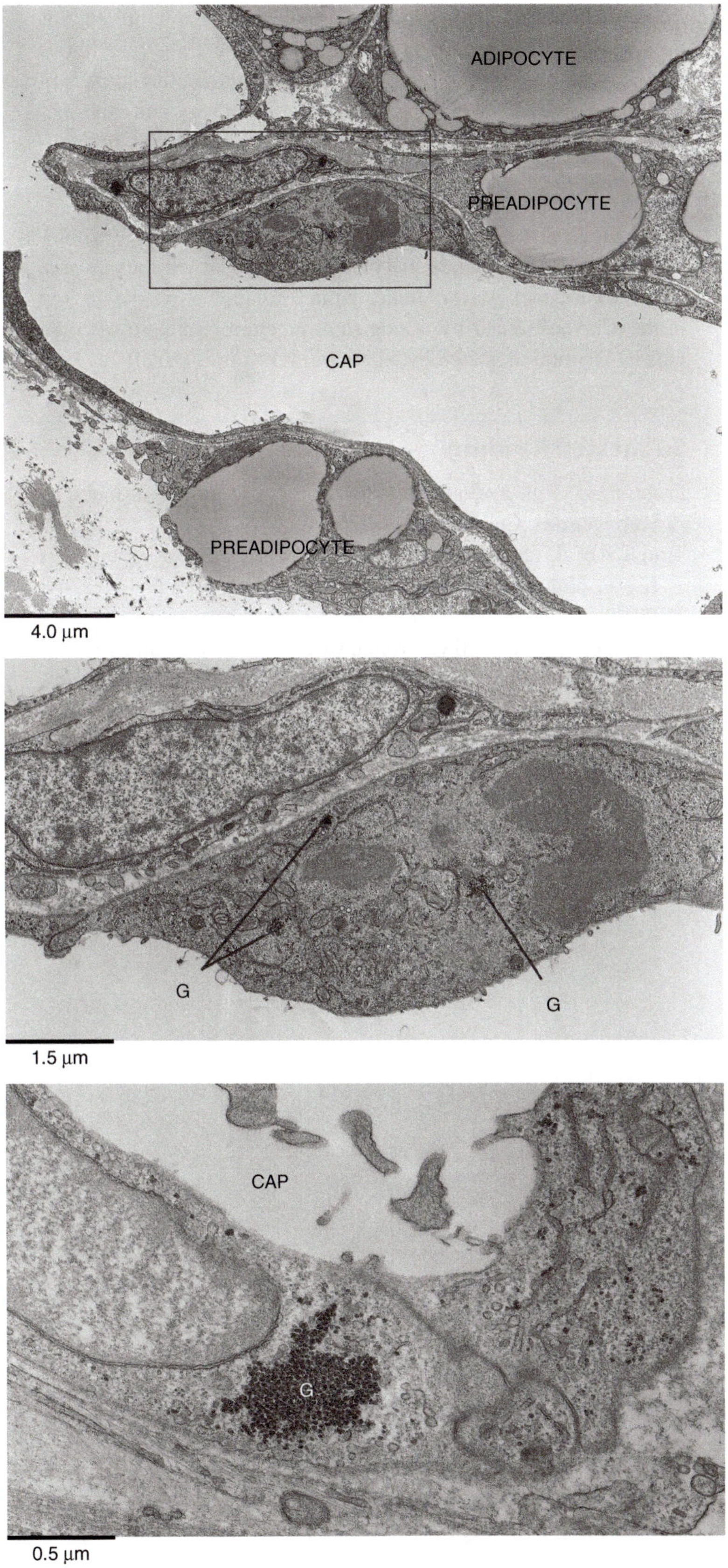

Plate 12.12 Epididymal WAT of newborn rat (postnatal day 6). Vasculo-adipocytic islet. Endothelial cells. TEM

PLATE 12.13

Ultrastructure of Endothelial Cells in Vasculo-Adipocytic Islets II

Tight junctions extending on overlapping cytoplasmic projections of neighboring cells usually join endothelial cells of capillaries (arrow). The overlapping projections in normal endothelial cells of capillaries in fat are usually short, but we found very unusual junctions in long overlapping projections of endothelial cells in capillaries of vasculo-adipocytic islets (squared area, enlarged in the lower panel).

An example of these long junctions in a capillary of rat vasculo-adipocytic islet is shown in this plate. See the enlarged squared area in the lower panel. Arrows indicate the overlapping cytoplasm (red in the scheme) joined by a long tight junction (compare with the normal junction indicated by an arrow in the upper panel).

Suggested Reading

Frontini A, et al. Endothelial cells of adipose tissues: a niche of adipogenesis. Cell Cycle. 11:2765–6, 2012.

Tran KV, et al. The vascular endothelium of the adipose tissue gives rise to both white and brown fat cells. Cell Metab. 15:222–9, 2012.

Hausman GJ, Dodson MV. Stromal vascular cells and adipogenesis: cells within adipose depots regulate adipogenesis. J Genomics. 1:56–66, 2013.

Poloni A, et al. Plasticity of human dedifferentiated adipocytes toward endothelial cells. Exp Hematol. 43:137–46, 2015.

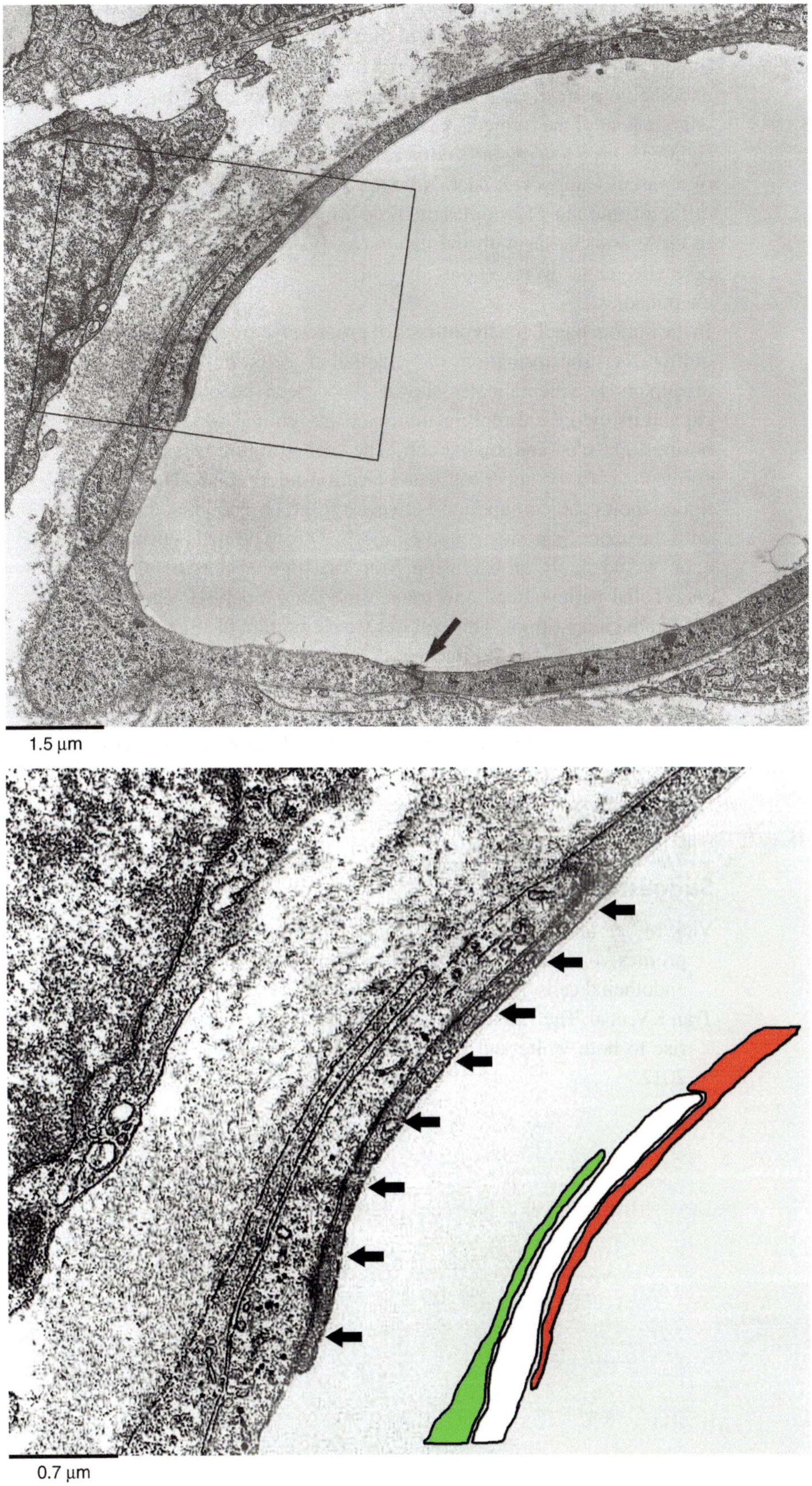

Plate 12.13 Epididymal WAT of newborn rat (postnatal day 6). Vasculo-adipocytic islet. Special overlapping projections and junctions between endothelial cells. Scheme: *green*: pericyte, *white* overlapped endothelial cell, *red*: endothelial cell with overlapping projection. TEM

PLATE 12.14

Endothelial-Pericytes

In these vasculo-adipocytic islets, we found rare endothelial-pericytic cells, i.e., cells in part in direct contact with the capillary lumen and in part adopting a pericytic position. In this plate, an endothelial-pericytic cell is shown in the left upper panel that is an enlargement of the framed area in the right middle panel. The upper right panel is a low magnification of the classic enlarged capillaries of a vasculo-adipocytic islet. Note the developing adipocytes with different amounts of cytoplasmic lipid droplets (L, some indicated) in close association with the capillaries (CAP). The endothelial-pericytic cells were about 3% of all endothelial cells we examined.

In the bottom panel, the hypothesis of progressive staging occurring during the transformation of endothelial cells into adipocyte precursors is schematically shown. The green endothelial cells expand its cytoplasmic projection over the luminal part of neighboring light blue endothelial cell. The second figure in the panel corresponds to the upper left panel electron micrograph. The third figure shows the conjunction between the green endothelial cells with the upper light blue endothelial cell. This hypothetic phenomenon would imply an exclusion from the luminal contact of the endothelial-pericytic cell now transformed into a pericyte abutting toward the interstitium. This cell has two important distinctive features of early adipose cell lineage: delimitation by a distinct external lamina and cytoplasmic glycogen. Of note, we observed this type of pericytic cells abutting into the interstitial space (see Plate 4.17) in these vasculo-adipocytic islets. The development of pericapillary preadipocytes with progressive lipid droplets enlargement is a step well known and widely accepted.

Suggested Reading

Vici M, et al. Electron microscopic and immunocytochemical profiles of human subcutaneous fat tissue microvascular endothelial cells. Ann Vasc Surg. 7:541–8, 1993.

Tran KV, et al. The vascular endothelium of the adipose tissue gives rise to both white and brown fat cells. Cell Metab. 15:222–9, 2012.

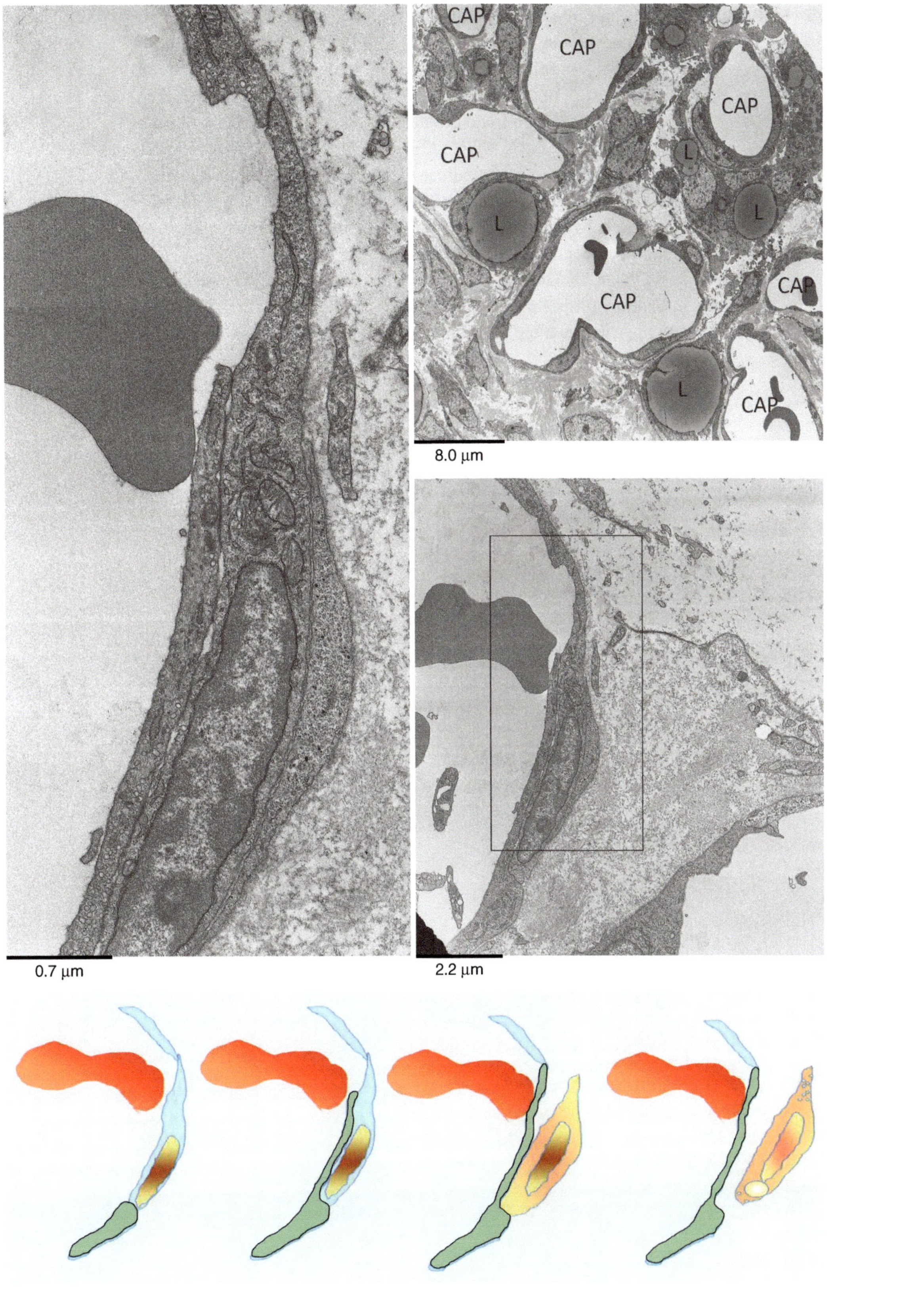

Plate 12.14 Endothelial-pericytic cell in a capillary of vasculo-adipocytic islet. TEM Scheme of proposed differentiative steps from endothelium to preadipocyte. From: Tran KV et al. The vascular endothelium of the adipose tissue gives rise to both white and brown fat cells. Cell Metab. 15:222–9, 2012, with permission

PLATE 12.15

Ve-Cad Lineage Tracing I

All data presented in previous plates seem to suggest that endothelial cells in developing BAT and WAT could play an important role as stem cells for adipogenesis. Lineage tracing technique is quite appropriate to this end. Thus, we used double transgenic mice Ve-Cad-Cre/R26R to trace the destiny of endothelial cells in both developing BAT and WAT. Ve-Cad is never expressed in other cells than endothelial cells and hematopoietic cells in the bone marrow.
We found X-Gal-stained capillaries in all organs studied, but the only parenchymal cells that resulted positive were brown and white preadipocytes and adipocytes (see also Plate 12.8 and the next plate).
In this plate, X-Gal-positive unilocular white adipocytes are shown in anterior (upper panel) subcutaneous fat. Note the negative skeletal muscle in which X-Gal-positive capillaries are visible (arrows, some indicated).
In the inguinal fetal subcutaneous tissue of a Ve-Cad-Cre/R26R mouse, clusters of poorly differentiated cells resulted intensely X-Gal positive. Electron microscopy revealed that these cells are adipocyte precursors in close contact with stained capillaries (see arrow in the lower right panel, enlargement of squared area in the lower left panel).

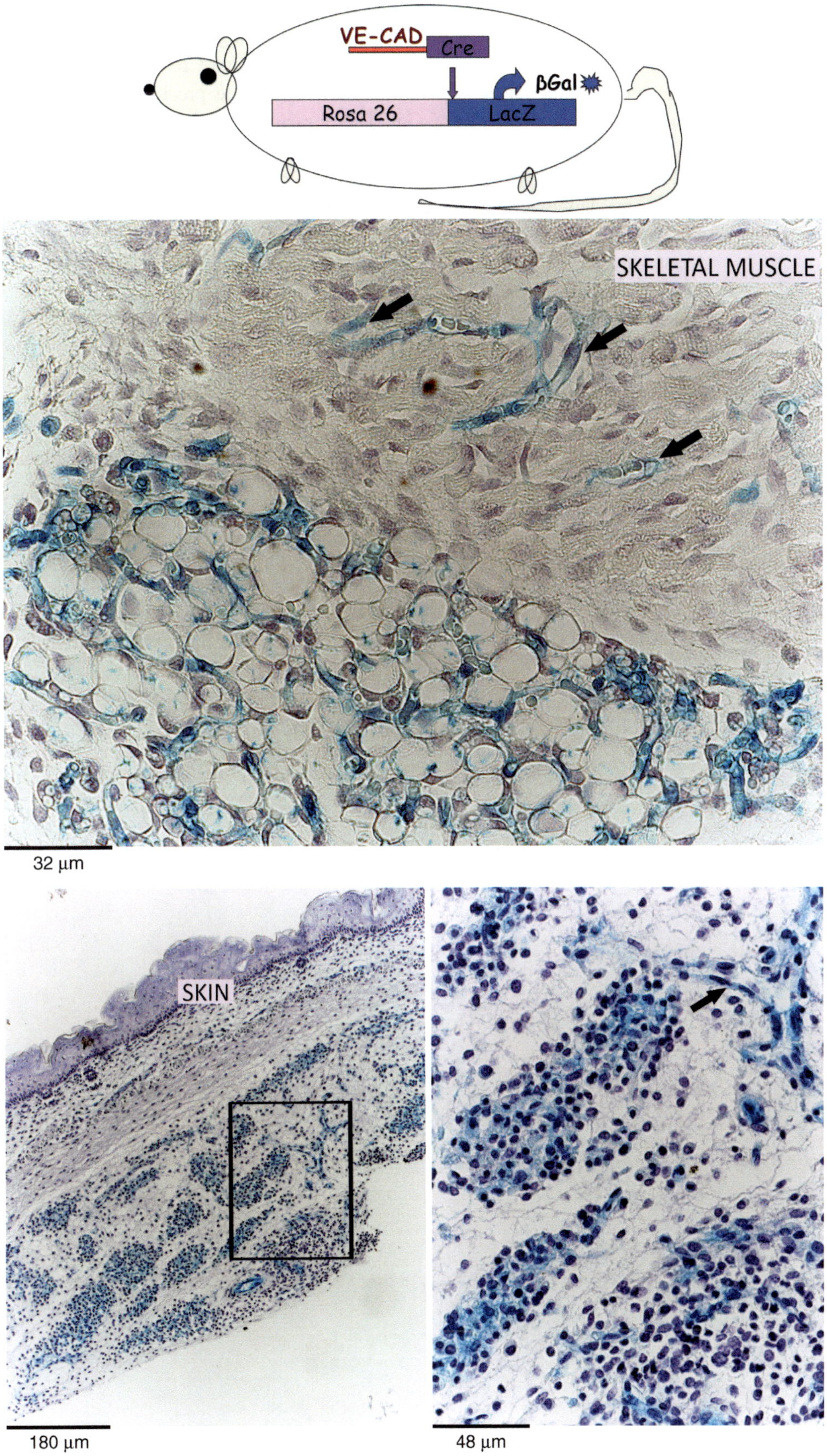

Plate 12.15 Anterior subcutaneous WAT of newborn Ve-Cad-Cre/R26R mouse. *Lower*: inguinal fetal (day 18) fat anlage of Ve-Cad-Cre/R26R mouse. LM. X-Gal staining

PLATE 12.16

Ve-Cad Lineage Tracing II

Inguinal fat of young mice is composed by a mixture of white and brown adipocytes. In the upper panel, the morphology of poorly differentiated cells of inguinal fat anlage of fetal Ve-Cad-Cre/R26R is shown. Endothelial cells of vessels and adipocyte precursors resulted intensely stained by X-Gal. The ultrastructure of inguinal adipocyte precursors is shown in the next plate.

Endothelial cells of vessels (arrows) and mature white adipocytes of the same depot were also intensely stained in their cytoplasm.

All our lineage tracing data from brown, white, and mixed fat depots of fetal and adult Ve-Cad-Cre/R26R mice strongly suggest the endothelial origin of both white and brown adipocytes (see also Plates 12.8 and 12.15).

Suggested Reading

Tran KV, et al. The vascular endothelium of the adipose tissue gives rise to both white and brown fat cells. Cell Metab. 15:222–9, 2012.

Min SY, et al. Human 'brite/beige' adipocytes develop from capillary networks, and their implantation improves metabolic homeostasis in mice. Nat Med. 22:312–8, 2016.

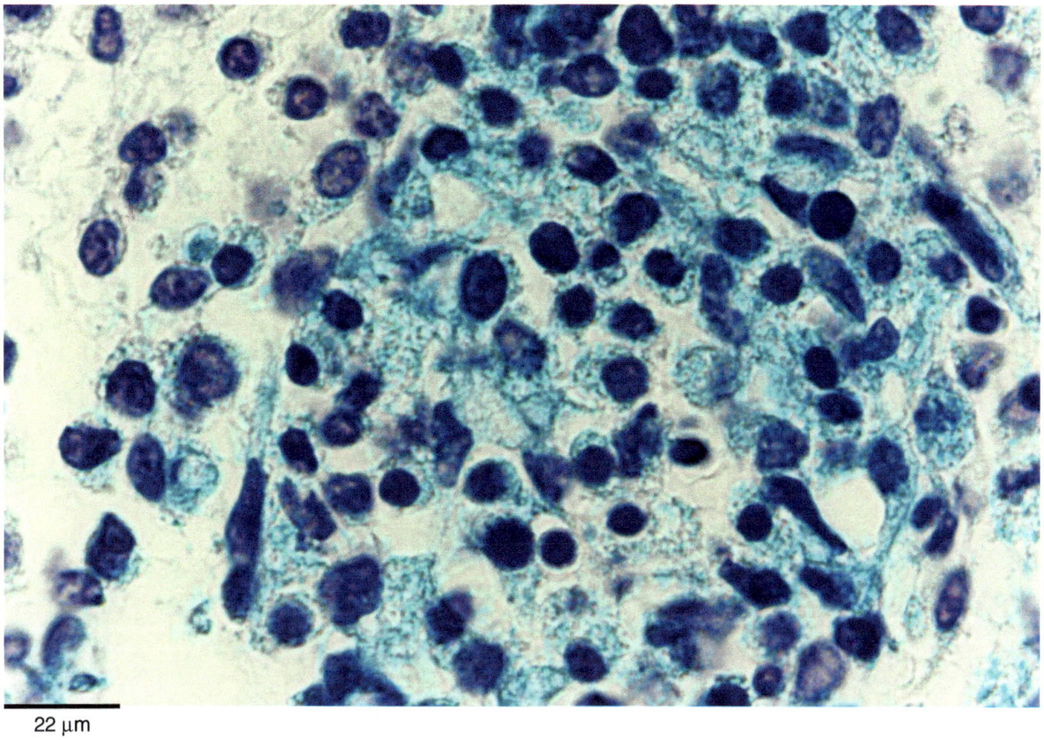

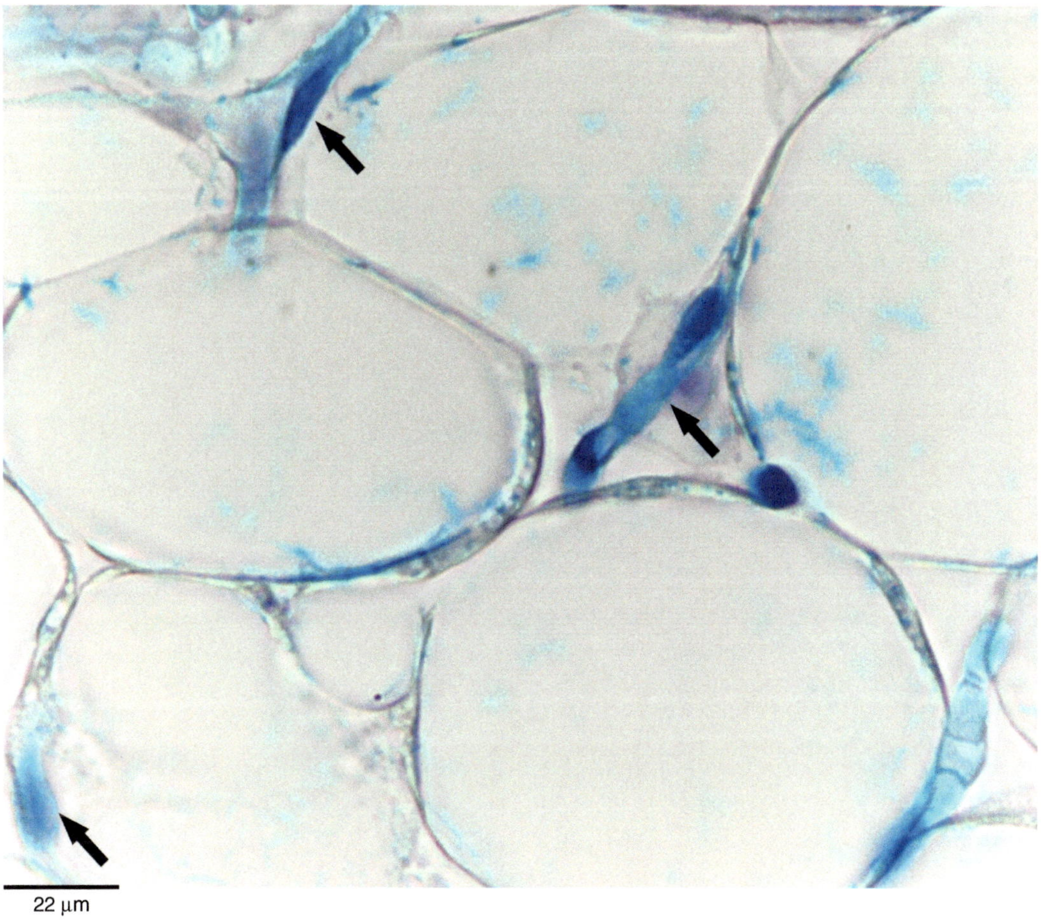

Plate 12.16 *Upper*: inguinal fetal (day 18) fat anlage of Ve-Cad-Cre/R26R mouse. Enlargment of a cluster of preadipocytes shown in the lower panels of Plate 12.15. LM. X-Gal staining. *Lower*: inguinal adipocytes of adult Ve-Cad-Cre/R26R. LM. X-Gal staining

PLATE 12.17

Inguinal Adipocyte Precursors TEM

The ultrastructure of adipocyte precursors in fetal inguinal subcutaneous fat is shown in this plate.

Clusters of poorly differentiated cell with euchromatin-rich roundish nuclei with hypertrophic nucleoli (typical of poorly differentiated cells) are closely apposed to capillaries (CAP). These cells show minimal signs of adipocyte differentiation (glycogen, G, and lipid droplets, L, some indicated).

At higher magnification (lower panel), numerous large mitochondria (m, some indicated) are visible in a cytoplasm full of ribosomes and polyribosomes (sign of poor differentiation).

Overall these adipocyte precursors are very similar to those described in fetal interscapular brown adipose tissue (see Plate 12.3).

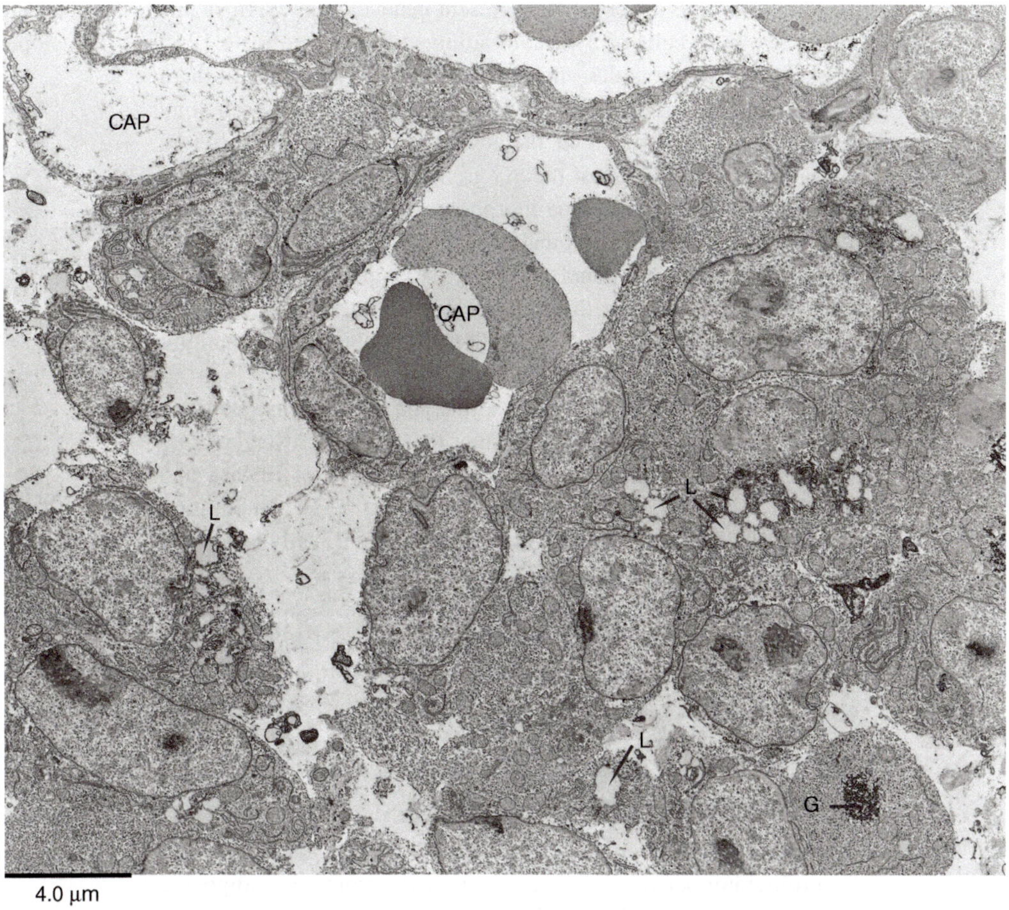

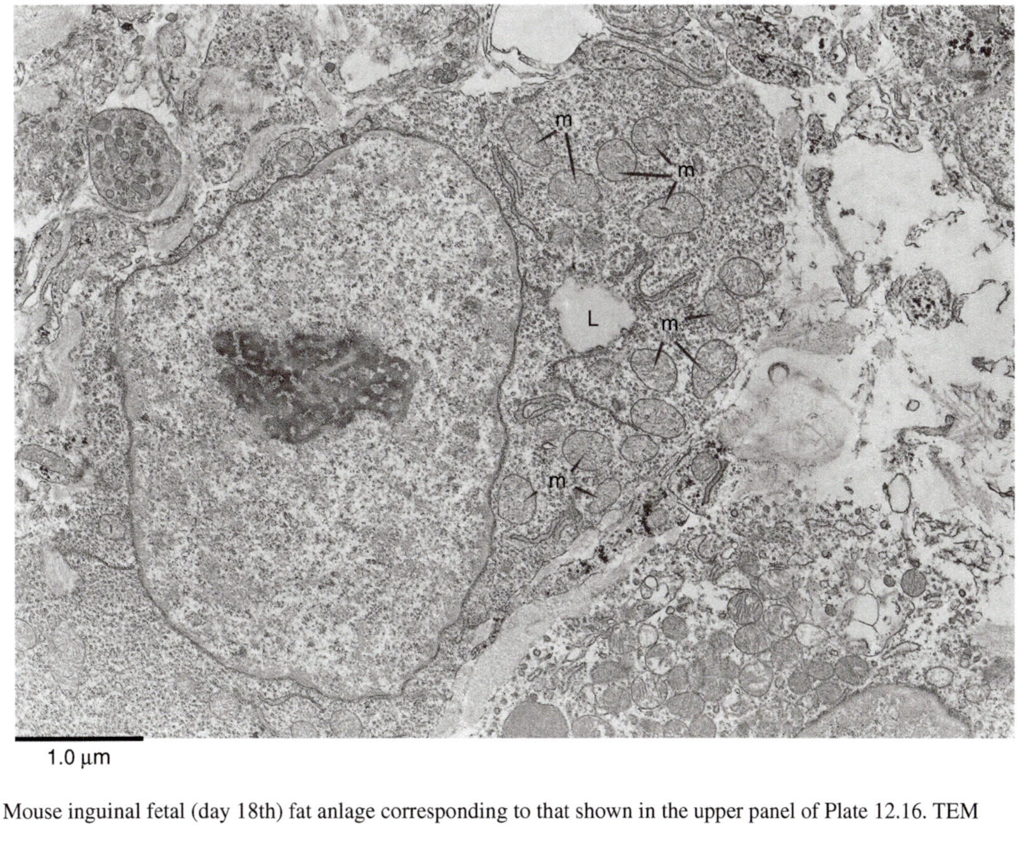

Plate 12.17 Mouse inguinal fetal (day 18th) fat anlage corresponding to that shown in the upper panel of Plate 12.16. TEM

PLATE 12.18

Mast Cells in Developing WAT

Several mast cells are constantly present in developing WAT. In this plate, two mast cells of a vasculo-adipocytic islet (see Plate 12.9) are shown. Their granules, morphology suggests that some of them (SG) are actively secreting their content. Compare the morphology of granules of mast cell in the lower panel. Note the different density and morphology of the SG granules in the upper panel and those in the lower panel. The morphology of SG granules in mast cell in the lower panel is typical of secretory stage.

In the upper and lower panels, pericytes (P) with glycogen granules (G, early sign of adipose differentiation; see Plates 4.17 and 12.11) and a fibroblast (F) rich in dilated rough endoplasmic reticulum (RER) near a collagen fiber (COL) are visible.

The role of mast cells in vasculo-adipocytic islets is unknown, but a role for the cyclooxygenase product PGD_2 (PG: prostaglandins) and its PGJ_2 derivatives as efficacious activators of PPARa and PPARγ has been proven. Furthermore, the PGJ dehydration product, 15-deoxy-$\Delta^{12,14}$-PGJ_2, is shown to bind directly to PPARγ and to promote adipogenesis of cultured fibroblasts.

These data suggest that the J_2 series of PGs may exert their biological effects in part through activation of the PPARγ signaling pathways. Interestingly, mast cells are a natural source of prostaglandins.

Suggested Reading

Kliewer SA, et al. A prostaglandin J2 metabolite binds peroxisome proliferator-activated receptor γ and promotes adipocyte differentiation. Cell, 83:813–9, 1995.

Forman BM, et al. 15Deoxy-$\Delta^{12,14}$-Prostaglandin J_2 is a ligand for the adipocyte determination factor PPARγ. Cell. 83:803–12, 1995.

Nosjean O, Jean A. Boutin natural ligands of PPARgamma: are prostaglandin J2 derivatives really playing the part? Cell Signal. 14:573–83, 2002.

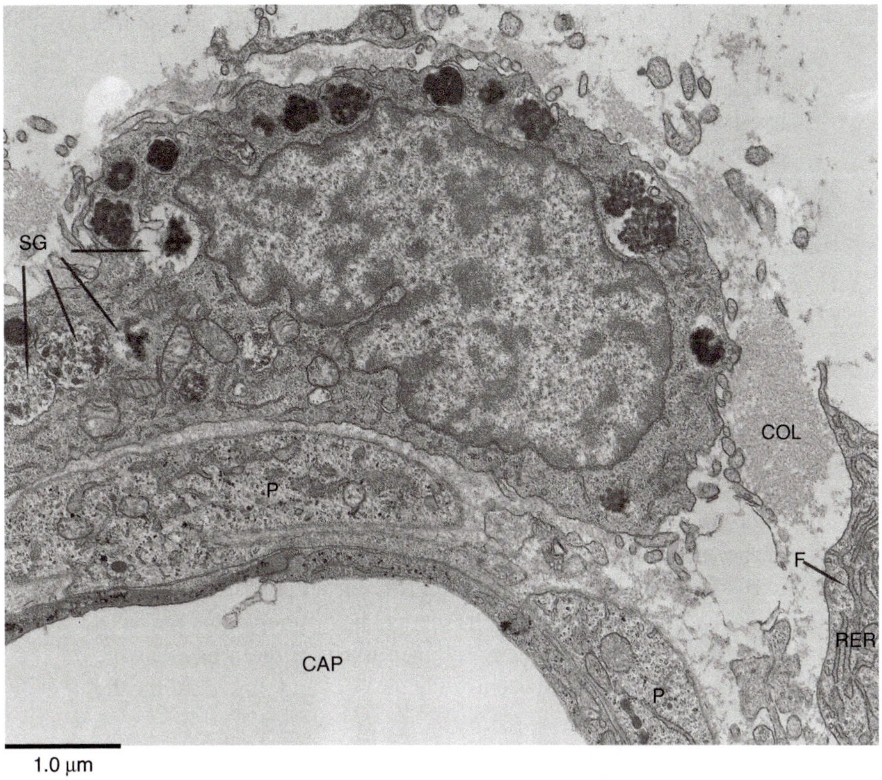

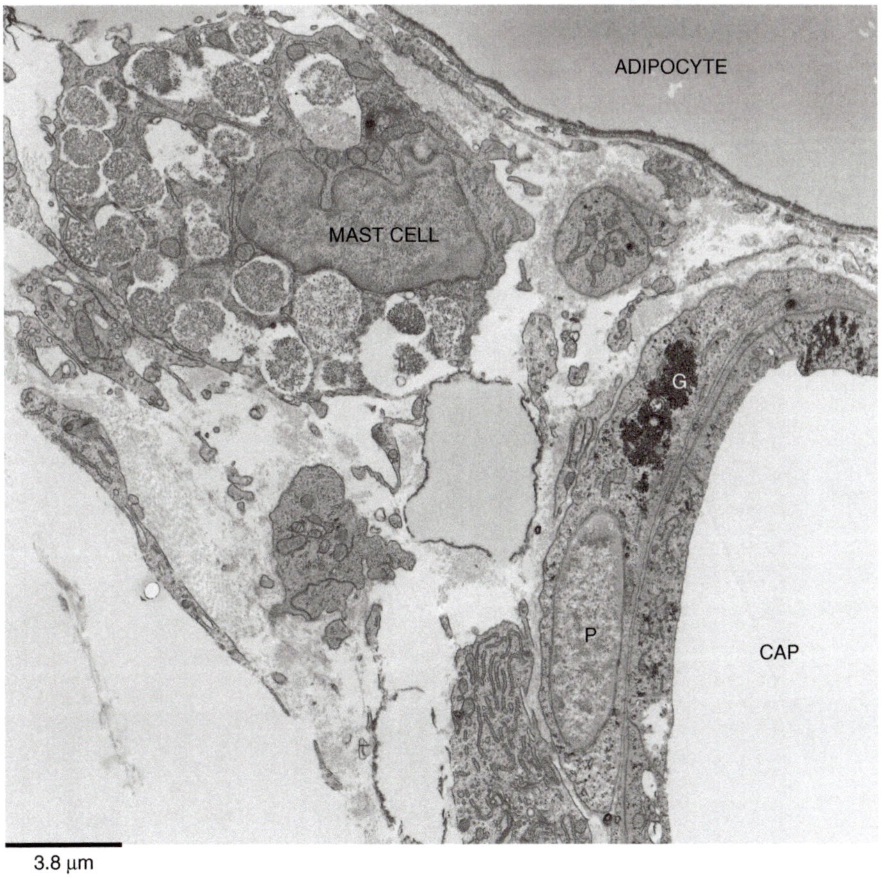

Plate 12.18 Partially degranulated mast cells in developing WAT (vasculo-adipocytic islet). CAP: capillary. TEM

PLATE 12.19

Polarized Fibroblasts

The epididymal WAT anlage is formed by specific structures denominated vasculo-adipocytic islets (see Plate 12.9). The islets are delimitated by a cellular boundary represented by fibroblast-like cells. Adipocytes develop only inside the islets delimited by this boundary. In this plate, the ultrastructure of the fibroblast-like cells is shown. The most developed organelle of these elements is the rough endoplasmic reticulum stacked in dilated cisternae. This feature is quite a characteristic of active fibroblasts producing collagen fibrils. In line with this aspect, a very dense collagen is present inside the islets (see the squared area enlarged in the lower panel). The outward side of fibroblast-like cells is very different from the inward side because of the presence of several irregular villi-like projections. This evident difference between the outward and inward sides of the cell parallels the matrix content difference: dense collagen inside and loose matrix outside the fibroblast-like cells. Our interpretation of these ultrastructural data is that the fibroblast-like elements delimit an area specifically rich in collagen fibrils that could play an important role for adipose cells development. These fibroblast-like cells seem to be different from the common fibroblast that produces collagen fibrils without any specific polarization that instead seems to be present and important for the cells shown here.

Suggested Reading

Prager-Khoutorsky M, et al. Fibroblast polarization is a matrix-rigidity-dependent process controlled by focal adhesion mechanosensing. Nat Cell Biol. 13:1457–65, 2011.

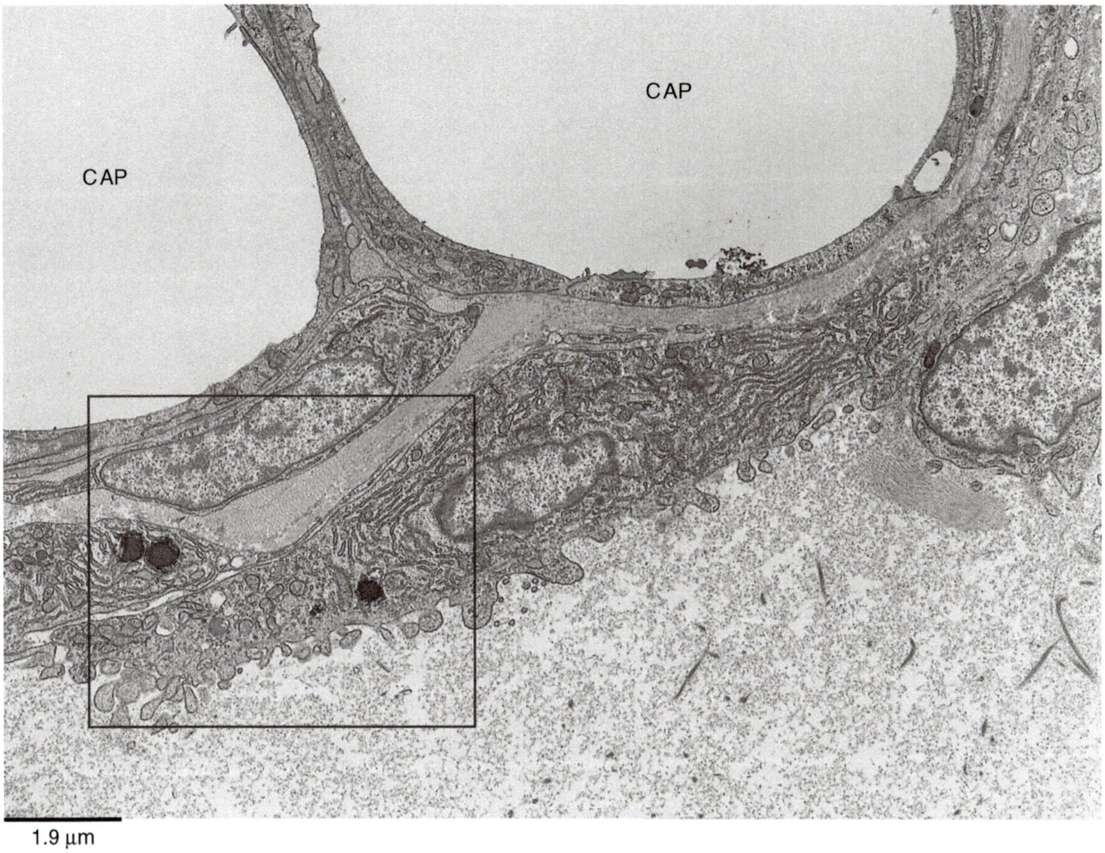

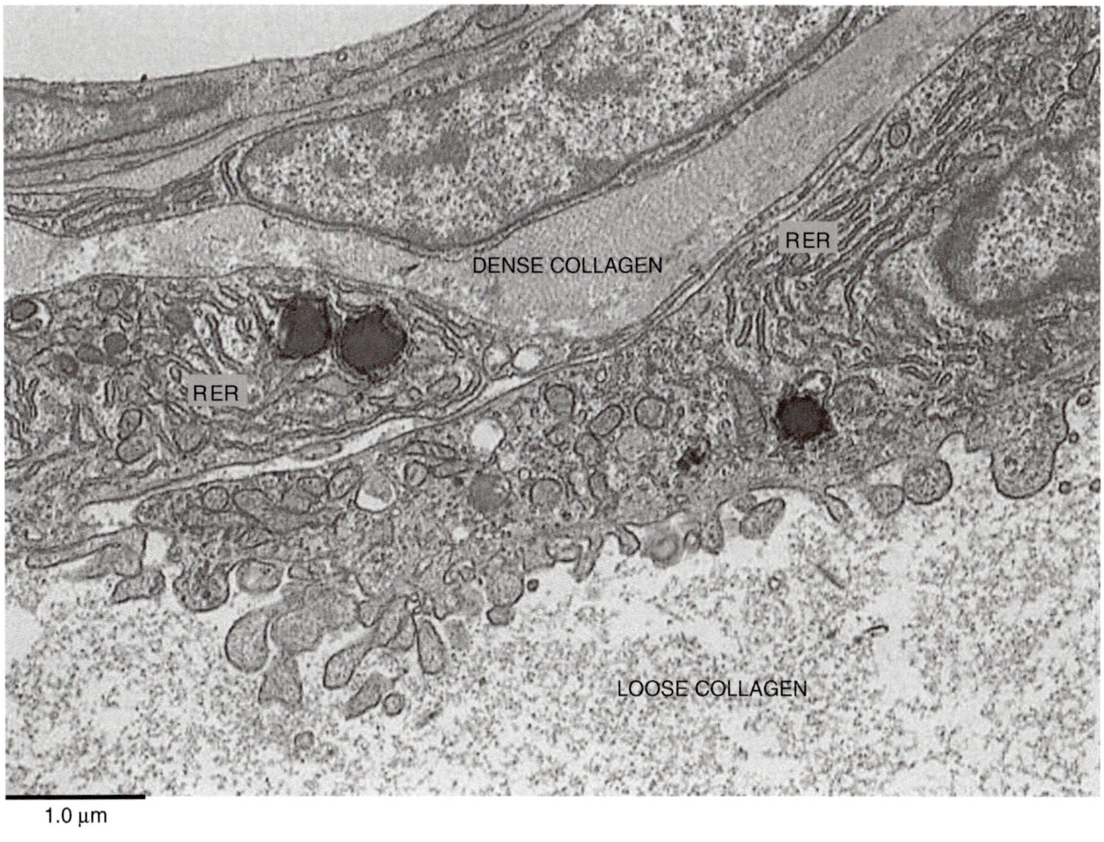

Plate 12.19 Polarized fibroblast-like cells delimiting vasculo-adipocytic islets. TEM

13 Development in Humans

S. Cinti, *Obesity, Type 2 Diabetes and the Adipose Organ*, https://doi.org/10.1007/978-3-319-40522-3_13

13.1 Development in Humans

PLATE 13.1

Vasculo-adipocytic Islets

Stellate mesenchymal-like cells (M) dispersed in a loose extracellular matrix (top left panel) formed the subcutaneous tissue in very early fetuses (10–12 gestational weeks). Capillaries of this tissue were rich in pericyte-like cells (P in the top right panel, enlargement of squared area in the top left panel).

We found the first signs of fat development below the skin of the upper body in early human fetuses (16–20 gestational weeks).

Distinct roundish islets of variable size were visible to the naked eye after skin removal (middle left panel). A dense vascular (capillaries) network (signed by red blood cells in bottom panels) and a variable amount of parenchymal cells with or without signs of adipocyte differentiation characterize the islets. Each islet is separated from the loose embryonic matrix by fibroblast-like cells (F) forming a net boundary (middle and bottom panels). Thus, the islets' histology was reminiscent of that described for vasculo-adipocytic structures in the murine fat development (see Plates 12.9 and 12.18). Together with the vascular network, the content of each islet was quite variable in dependence of the degree of adipocyte differentiation: from the absence of adipogenesis (nude islets: bottom right panel, enlargement of islet in the lower right corner in the middle right panel) to very rich in fully differentiated adipocytes (parenchymal islets: bottom left panel, enlargement of the islet in the upper left corner of the right middle panel). Partially differentiated islets were also present. Nude islets were more frequent in early and intermediate fetal ages (23–27 gestational weeks), but a progressively reduced number of them were found in all fetal ages studied.

Parenchymal and partially differentiated islets were occupied by multilocular UCP1-immunoreactive adipocytes (bottom left panel and the next plate). Small islets coalesce progressively during development to form larger structures that are quite common in intermediate fetuses. In late fetuses (36–39 gestational weeks), coalesced islets form a continuous layer of fat derived from both lateral and multilayered fusion processes as indicated by the presence of intermediate features. Strands of collagen persist and separate lobules of fat in late fetuses, and in some areas, such as the lower part of abdomen, a net fibrous strand divides the superficial part from the deep part.

Suggested Reading

Poissonnet CM, et al. Growth and development of human adipose tissue during early gestation. Early Hum Dev. 8:1–11, 1983.

Tran KV, et al. The vascular endothelium of the adipose tissue gives rise to both white and brown fat cells. Cell Metab. 15:222–9, 2012.

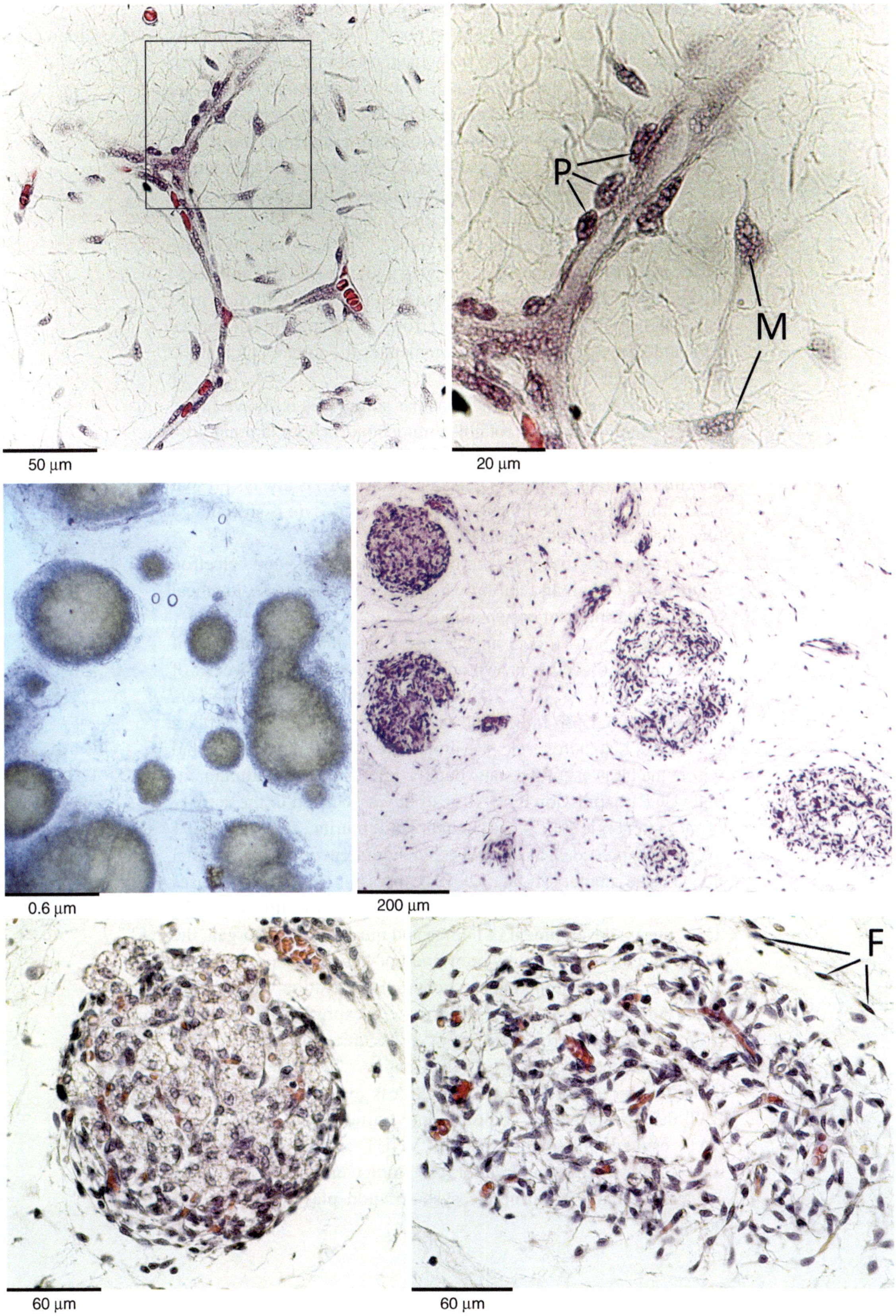

Plate 13.1 *Top panels*: subcutaneous tissue of a human fetus at gestational age of 12 weeks. *Middle* and *bottom panels*: vasculo-adipocytic islets forming the subcutaneous fat of human fetus at 17 weeks. LM. H&E. *Middle left*: whole mount

PLATE 13.2

Adipocyte Development in Islets I

Light microscopy, electron microscopy, and immunohistochemistry show that the parenchymal adipocytes of fetal subcutaneous islets in the upper part of the body have predominantly the brown phenotype. In the left top panel, low magnification of several UCP1-immunoreactive islets is visible. The top right panel shows the low magnification morphology of resin-embedded tissue that allows the maximal cytological details. The sharp delimitation of the islets and the abundance of multilocular adipocytes (lipids stain yellow-green in this type of preparation) are evident. Middle panels are enlargements of islets in resin-embedded tissue. Note the tight relationship of multilocular adipocytes with the wall of capillaries. Some poorly differentiated multilocular cells (small with tiny lipid vacuoles) are in pericyte position (arrows in the middle left panel). The middle right panel is an enlargement of the squared area in the top right panel.

The ultrastructure of these multilocular adipocytes is shown in the bottom panel. Numerous roundish mitochondria with laminar cristae are visible. Glycogen granules are frequently observed in close proximity to lipid droplets (G). A dense line (DL) is always present at the lipid droplets periphery. Each single adipocyte is surrounded by a distinct external lamina (EL).

Thus, light microscopy, immunohistochemistry, and electron microscopy of human fetal brown adipocytes seem to be identical to that of murine fetal brown adipocytes.

Parenchymal nerve fibers appear in the fat anlages composed of UCP1-immunoreactive brown adipocytes around 24–26 weeks of gestation. We first (16th–21st week) detected constitutive markers of the fibers (CD56) in cervical fat and interscapular BAT. After a few weeks also adrenergic TH-immunoreactive fibers were found within the fat islets of the same depots. Interestingly, in adult mammals UCP1 expression by BAT is strictly associated to the activity of noradrenergic fibers. In human and murine fetuses, UCP1 expression precedes the presence of noradrenergic parenchymal fibers: as a matter of fact UCP1 expression in human fetuses appears around 20–22 gestational weeks (see the upper panel). Thus, during development of human and murine adipose organ, the UCP1 protein expression by brown adipocytes seems to be dissociated from the noradrenergic parenchymal innervation. We recently found another example of UCP1 protein expression dissociated from the noradrenergic activity in β-less mice (lacking all beta adrenergic receptors). Several data support the hypothesis that under chronic subordination stress, β-less mice express UCP1 in BAT due to purinergic stimulus. Interestingly nerves of human BAT resulted immunoreactive for VNUT (vesicular nucleotide transporter, which is required for ATP storage in secretory vesicles) suggesting that the purinergic system could play a role also in humans.

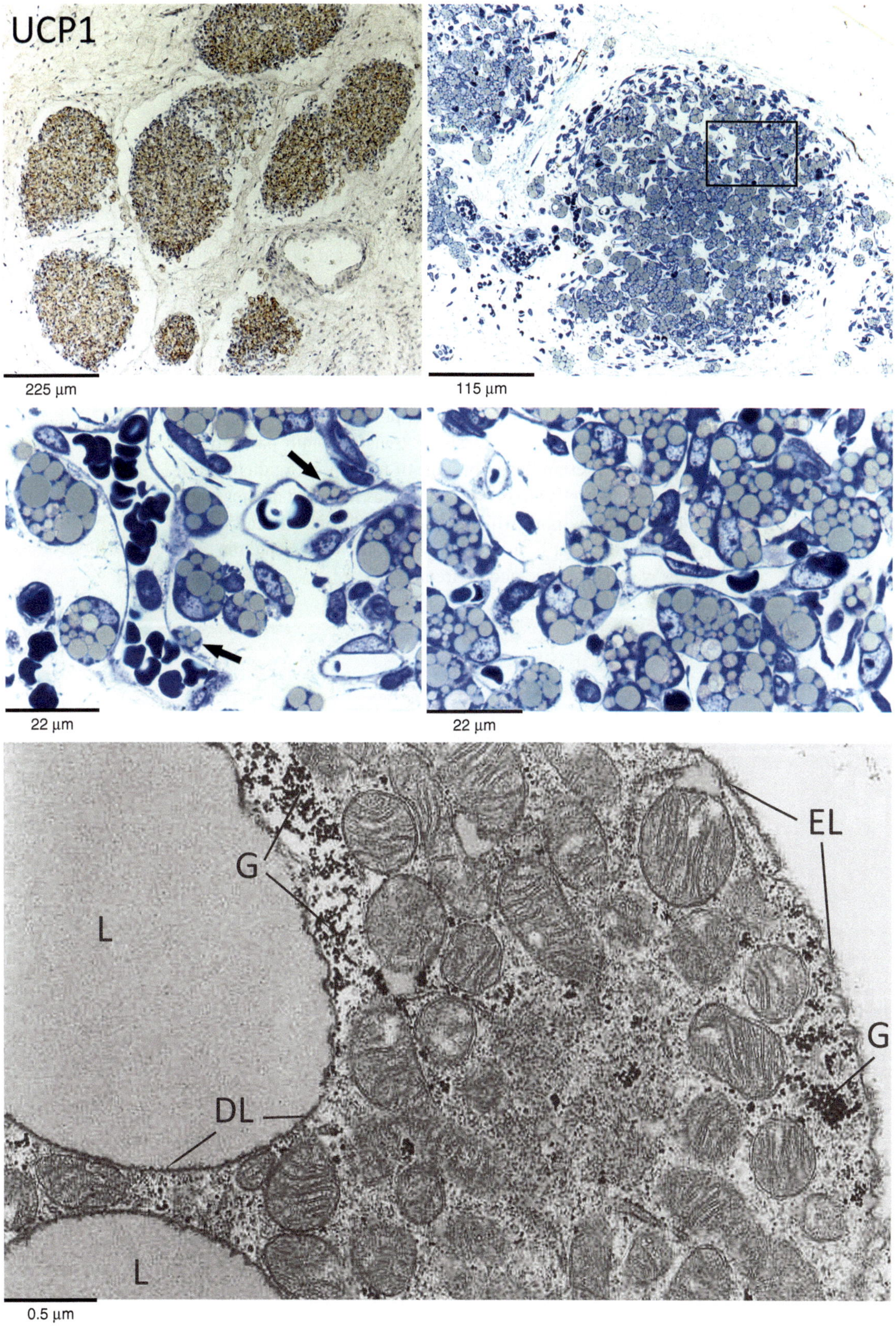

Plate 13.2 *Top left*: cervical subcutaneous vasculo-adipocytic islets of a human fetus at gestational age of 20 weeks. LM. IHC UCP1 ab (1:4,000). *Top right* and *middle*: cervical subcutaneous vasculo-adipocytic islets of a human fetus at gestational age of 17 weeks. Resin-embedded tissue. Toluidine blue staining. LM. *Bottom*: same tissue of middle panels. TEM

PLATE 13.3

Adipocyte Development in Islets II

In the lower part of the trunk since the early gestational age of fetuses, a mixture of multilocular, paucilocular, and unilocular adipocytes forms subcutaneous parenchymal vasculo-adipocytic islets (upper panel).
Interestingly, immunohistochemistry revealed UCP1 immunoreactivity in both multilocular and paucilocular adipocytes (lower panel) suggesting a whitening phenomenon.
Electron microscopy showed typical intermediate features similar to those described for paucilocular adipocytes in Plates 6.7–6.8.
Mixed islets or islets formed by paucilocular and unilocular adipocytes or only by unilocular cells were progressively more frequent in intermediate and late fetuses even in the upper part of the body.
The composition of multilayered areas in the upper part of the body showed that the deeper lobules were formed mainly by brown adipocytes even in late fetuses.
Visceral fat develops by a very similar process.
Single nude islets that progressively transform into parenchymal islets always represent the early stage of formation. Again the earliest parenchymal cells are brown adipocytes followed at later stages by a mixture or by pure white cells composition. The earliest age we found visceral fat is around 23 gestational weeks, and the earliest sites were peri aortic and perirenal.

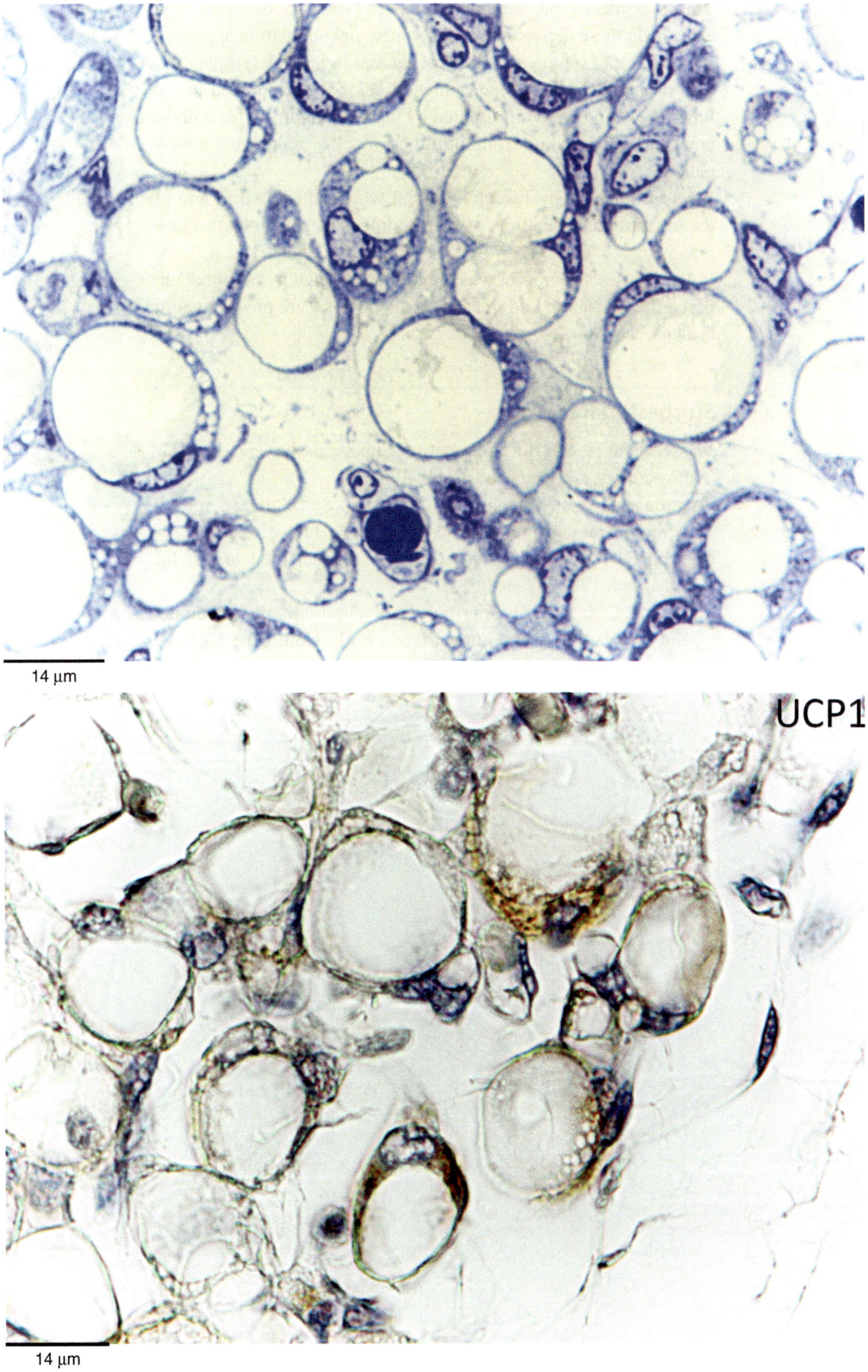

Plate 13.3 Vasculo-adipocytic islet of abdominal subcutaneous tissue of a human fetus at gestational age of 20 weeks. *Upper*: resin-embedded tissue. LM. Toluidine blue. *Lower*: LM. IHC UCP1 ab (1:4,000)

PLATE 13.4

Adipocyte Development in Islets III

The mesentery and omentum showed specific developmental aspects. In these depots the first parenchymal population appears at 23 weeks of gestation and was mainly represented by lymphocytes (top panels). Mesenteric and omental adipocytes appeared in late fetal period and were represented by unilocular adipocytes without any signs of whitening from multilocular cells (middle and bottom panels).

Electron microscopy revealed typical white mitochondria and all the ultrastructural features of white adipocytes described in Plates 5.5–5.7.

In late fetuses visceral fat was mainly represented by perirenal and periaortic fat, and in both locations adipocytes were predominantly brown.

Suggested Reading

Wassermann F. The development of adipose tissue. Handbook of Physiology, Chapter 10:87–100, 1965.

Ponrartana S, et al. Changes in brown adipose tissue and muscle development during infancy. J Pediatr. 173:116–21, 2016.

Merklin RJ. Growth and distribution of human fetal brown fat. Anat Rec. 178. 637–46, 1973.

Poissonnet CM, et al. The chronology of adipose tissue appearance and distribution in the human fetus. Early Hum Dev. 10:1–11, 1984.

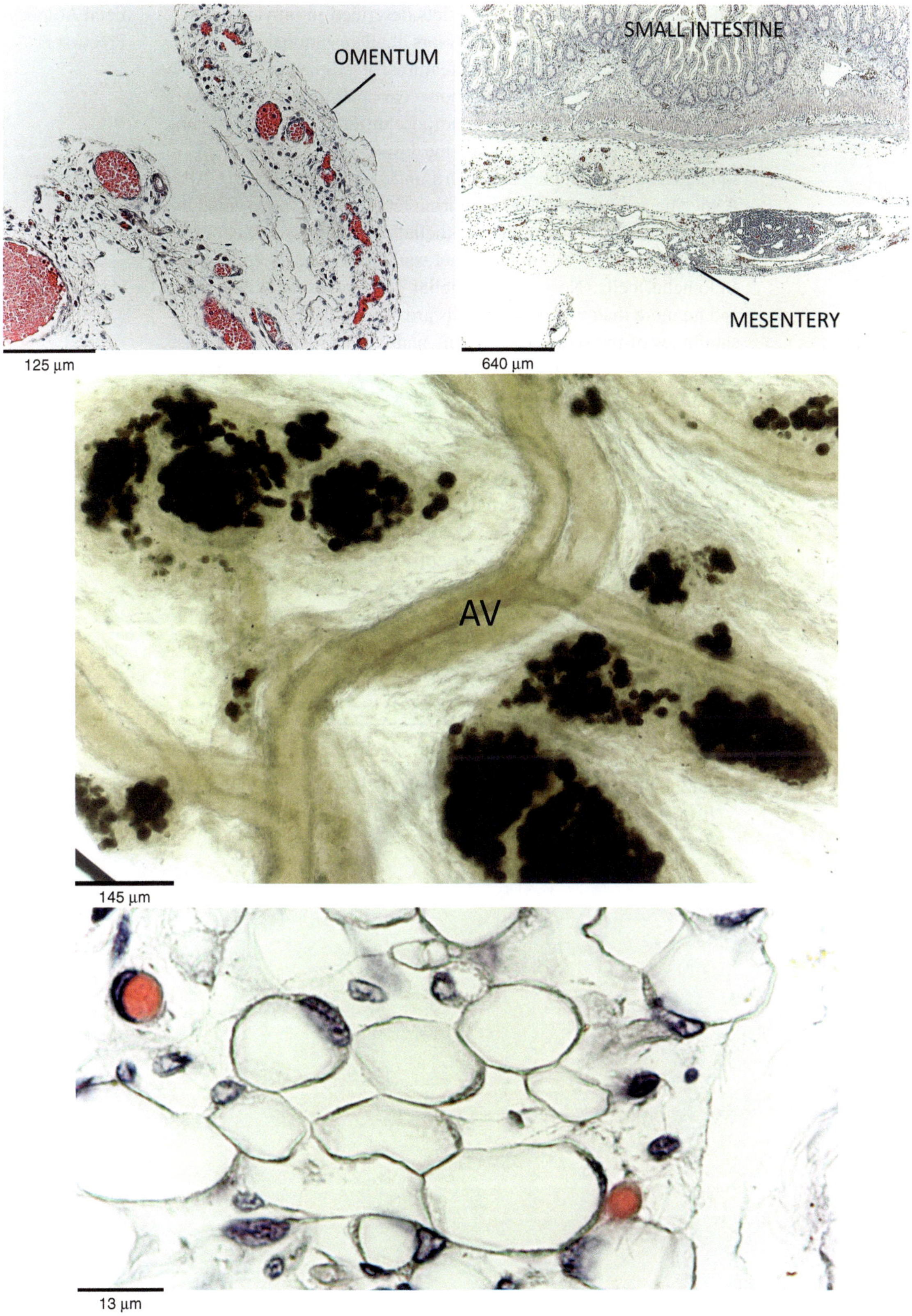

Plate 13.4 *Top left*: omental tissue of a human fetus at gestational age of 23 weeks. Only dispersed lymphocytes and dilated capillaries containing red blood cells are visible. LM. *Top right*: mesenteric tissue of a human fetus at gestational age of 24 weeks. Only dispersed lymphocytes and a lymph node are visible. LM. *Middle*: omentum of human fetus at gestational age of 36 weeks. Islets containing spherical adipocytes stained in black by osmium-tetroxide are visible. Note the vasculature branching toward the islets. Whole mount preparation of glutaraldehyde/osmium-tetroxide fixed pre-embedded tissue. LM. *Bottom*: histology of one of the islet shown in middle panel. LM. H&E staining

PLATE 13.5

Fetal Adipocyte Precursors

All types of vasculo-adipocytic islets described in previous plates were very rich in adipocyte precursors at all gestational ages.
In this plate the ultrastructural features of adipocyte precursors found in the islet in subcutaneous cervical tissue are shown. Pericytes (P) with early signs of adipose differentiation (glycogen, G, and external lamina, EL; see the lower panel, enlargement of squared area in the upper panel) surrounded most capillaries (CAP). A specific aspect, not found in murine fetal fat, was represented by the unusual ultrastructure of endothelial cells lining some capillaries (upper panel). The lumen in fact was surrounded by epithelioid endothelial cells. Normal endothelial cells are usually flattened, and no more than two or three cells are present in cross sections of capillaries of the size shown in this plate. In this capillary at least ten endothelial cells line the lumen (CAP). Note the unusual thickness of each endothelial cell. This aspect could be in relationship with the role of endothelial cells as origin for both white and brown adipocyte precursors suggested by experimental data in murine adipose organ (see Plates 12.8 and 12.15–12.16). The abundance of pericytes with early signs of adipogenesis very similar to those found in murine adipose organ during development (see Chap. 12) confirms the importance of the vascular wall as a niche for adipose stem cells. The recent data supporting a bone marrow origin of adipocyte precursors do not contrast the vascular origin. The vascular phenotype could in fact represent a tissue-specific step before the final adipose phenotype development.

Suggested Reading

Schulz TJ, Tseng YH. Brown adipose tissue: development, metabolism and beyond. Biochem J. 453:167–78, 2013.

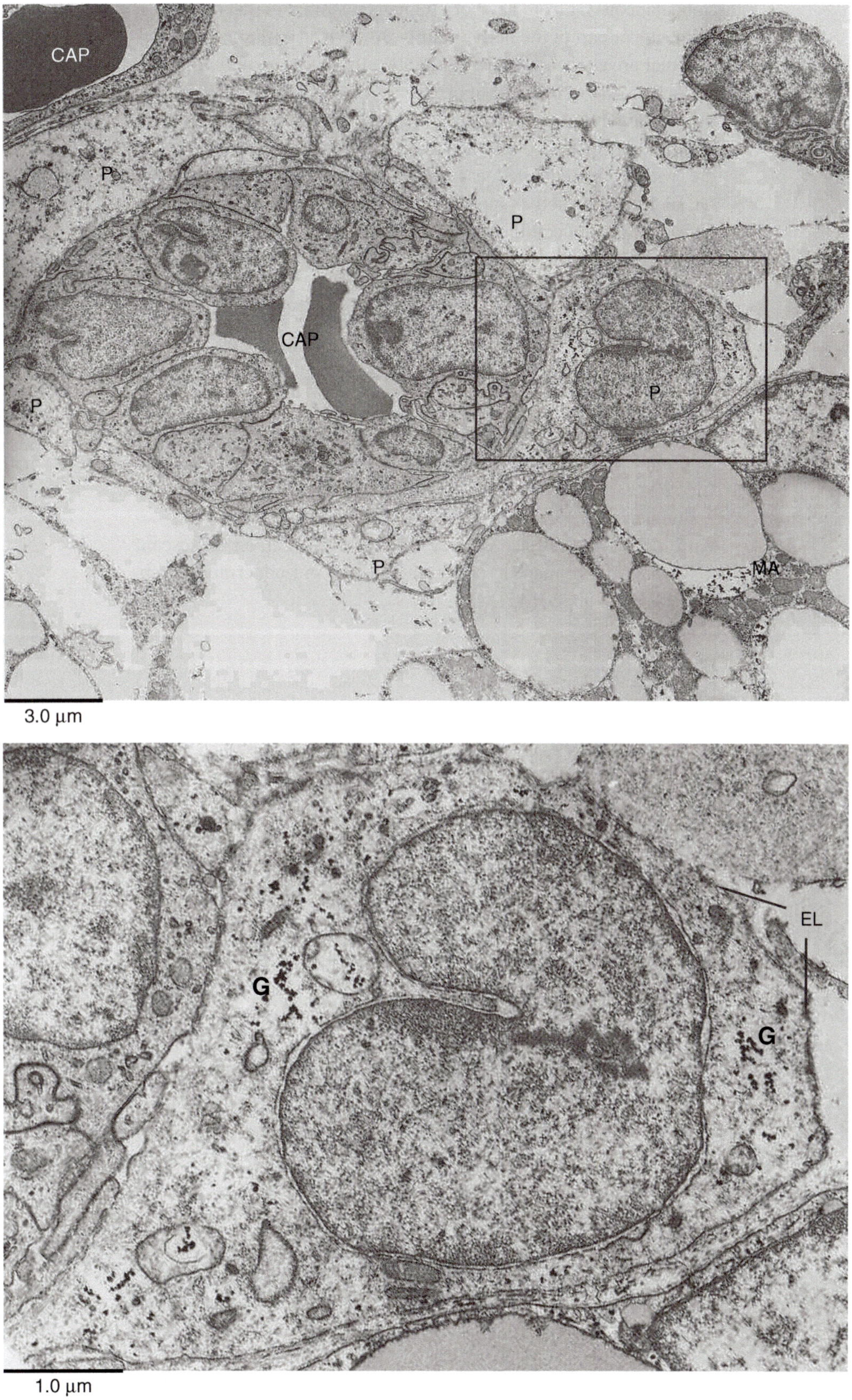

Plate 13.5 Ultrastructure of a vasculo-adipocytic islet of human fetal cervical subcutaneous tissue at gestational age of 16–17 weeks. MA: mature brown adipocyte

PLATE 13.6

Subcutaneous BAT of Newborns

Subcutaneous fat from newborn humans is similar to that of fetuses. In the upper part of the body (mainly in cervical, axillary, and interscapular areas), it shows the histology, ultrastructure, and immunohistochemistry of brown adipose tissue. Islets are still recognizable, but are larger and clustered, although a clear boundary of connective tissue is often present; see the upper panel. These larger islets are widely denominated as lobules. Lobules were engulfed by UCP1-immunoreactive multilocular adipocytes (lower panel). A dense network of capillaries was also present in all areas of lobules (arrows, some indicated).

Suggested Reading

Enerback S. Brown adipose tissue in humans. Int J Obesity. 34:S43–6, 2010.

Lecoultre V, Ravussin E. Brown adipose tissue and aging. Curr Opin Clin Nutr Metab Care. 14:1–6, 2011.

Lidell ME, et al. Evidence for two types of brown adipose tissue in humans. Nat Med. 19:631–4, 2013.

Kim MS, et al. Presence of brown adipose tissue in an adolescent with severe primary hypothyroidism. J Clin Endocrinol Metab. 99:E1686–90, 2014.

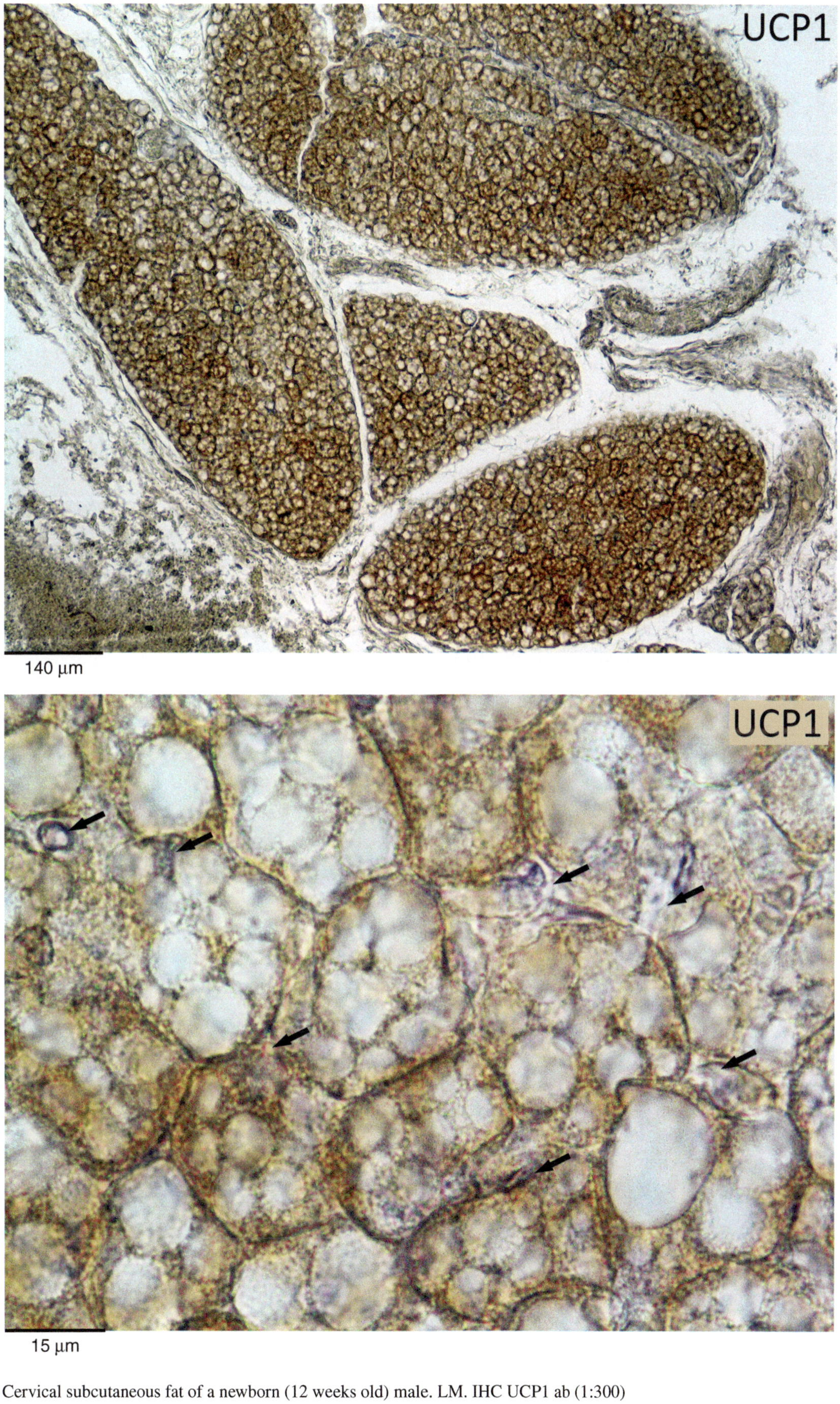

Plate 13.6 Cervical subcutaneous fat of a newborn (12 weeks old) male. LM. IHC UCP1 ab (1:300)

PLATE 13.7

Visceral BAT in Newborns

Perirenal (abdominal) and periaortic (mediastinal) fat is composed of lobules very similar to those described in the previous plate (upper panel). Multilocular UCP1-immunoreactive adipocytes in a dense network of capillaries (CAP, some indicated) are visible at higher magnification in the lower panel. Note the Harlequin phenomenon (see Plate 7.4): intensely UCP1-immunoreactive brown adipocytes are close to UCP1-negative multilocular adipocytes suggesting a strong functional activation of BAT in human newborns (unpublished data in collaboration with Prof Daniel Ricquier Université Paris Descartes, Paris).

Suggested Reading

Cinti S, et al. CL316,243 and cold stress induce heterogeneous expression of UCP1 mRNA and protein in rodent brown adipocytes. J Histochem Cytochem. 50:21–31, 2002.

Poulos SP, et al. The development and endocrine functions of adipose tissue. Mol Cell Endocrinol. 323:20–34, 2010.

Scheele C, et al. Novel nuances of human brown fat. Adipocyte. 3:54–7, 2013.

Tchkonia T, et al. Mechanisms and metabolic implications of regional differences among fat depots. Cell Metab. 17:644–56, 2013.

Rogers NH. Brown adipose tissue during puberty and with aging. Ann Med. 47:142–9, 2015.

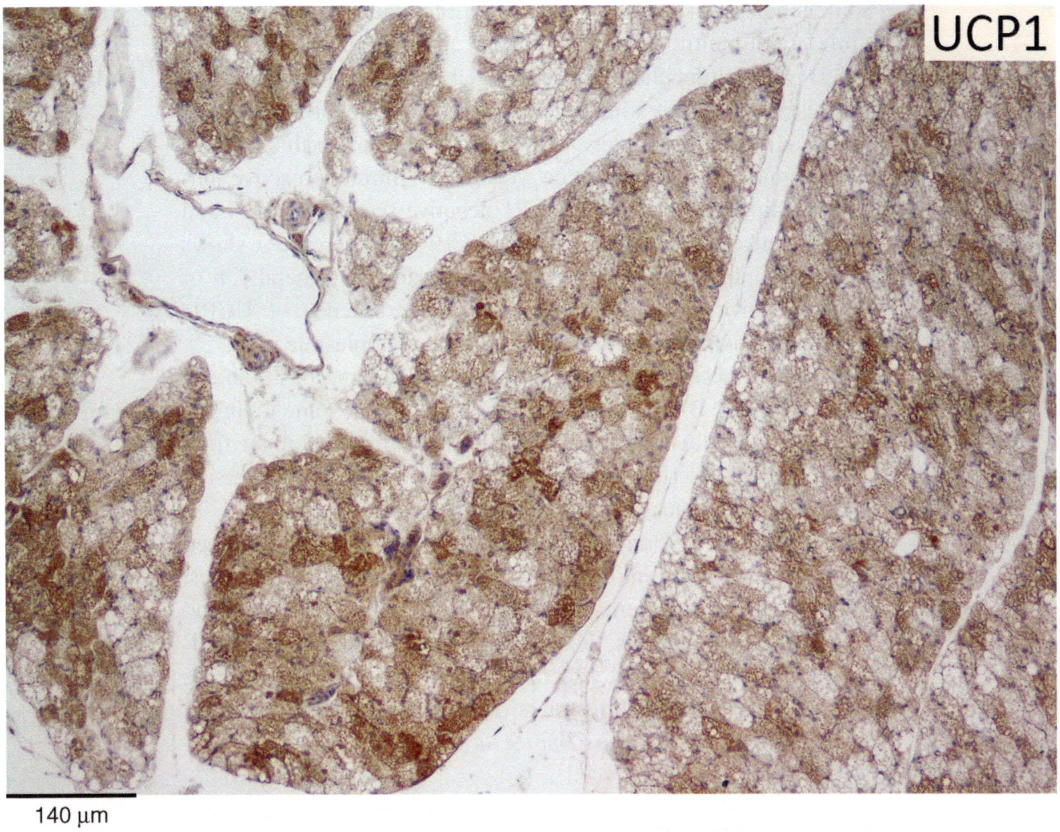

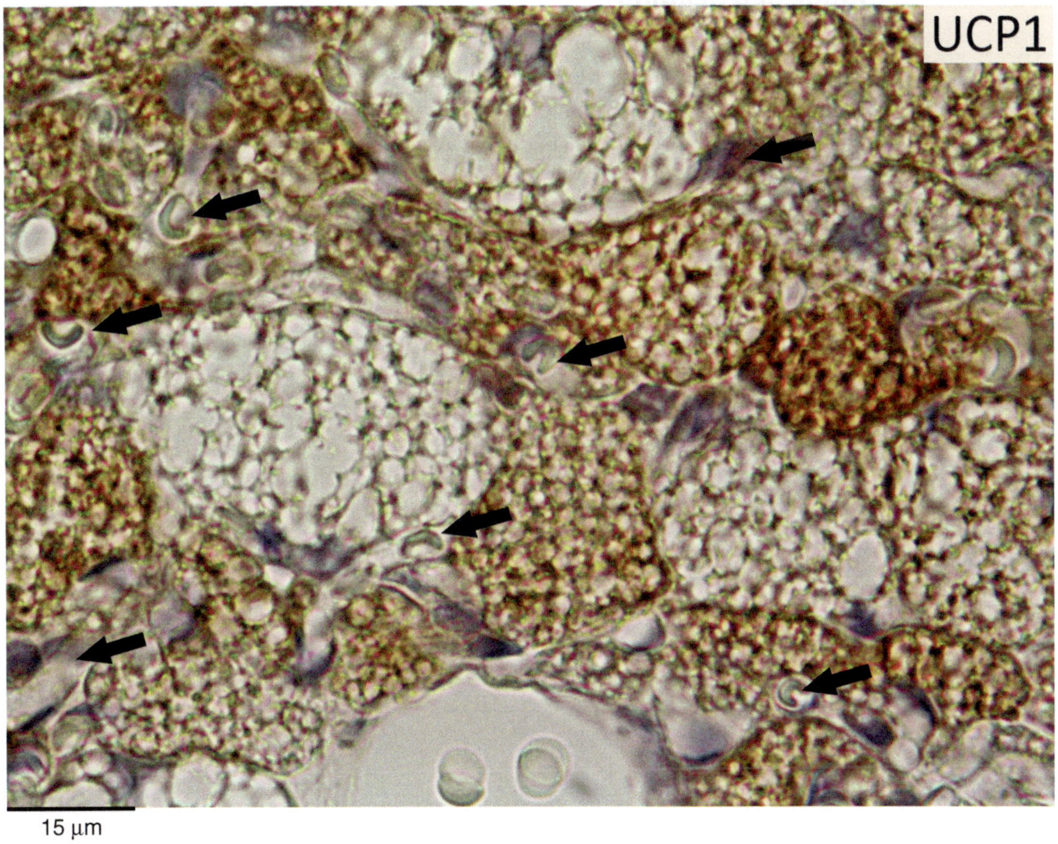

Plate 13.7 Perirenal BAT of a newborn (5-month-old) male. LM. IHC UCP1 ab (1:300)

PLATE 13.8

Unilocular UCP1-Immunoreactive Adipocytes in BAT of Newborns

Some lobules, in some individuals, in visceral areas are formed by a mixture of multilocular, paucilocular, and unilocular cells (upper panel). All multilocular and paucilocular and some unilocular adipocytes resulted UCP1 immunoreactive (enlargement in the lower panel) in newborn samples. A clear difference in the thickness of cytoplasmic rim was evident between UCP1-immunoreactive unilocular adipocytes and those UCP1 negative (compare THIN and THICK cells in the lower panel). The UCP1 immunoreactive shows a thick peripheral rim in contrast with the thin peripheral rim of UCP1-negative adipocytes, suggesting a persistence of UCP1-immunoreactive large mitochondria in thick cytoplasmic rims.

All together these data suggest that for unknown reasons (genetic, environmental), BAT in some visceral areas and in some individuals undergo a whitening process with the appearance of all the transition forms described for murine BAT to WAT conversion (whitening phenomenon; see Plates 8.2, 9.4, and 10.2).

Whitening of BAT is an important phenomenon because whitened brown adipocytes are more prone to death than white adipocytes. Death of adipocytes seems to play a role in insulin resistance and T2 diabetes pathogenesis, thus offering an explanation to the well-known clinical notion that visceral obesity is much more dangerous for metabolic-associated disorders (mainly T2 diabetes) than subcutaneous obesity (see also Chap. 9 for further details).

Suggested Reading

Aherne W, Hull D. The site of heat production in the newborn infant. Proc Royal Soc Med. 57:1172–3, 1964.

Emery JL, Dinsdale F. Structure of periadrenal brown fat in childhood in both expected and cot deaths. Arch Dis Child. 53:154–8, 1978.

Symonds ME, et al. Adipose tissue development e impact of the early life environment. Prog Biophys Mol Biol. 106:300–6, 2011.

Vijgen GHEJ, et al. Increase in brown adipose tissue activity after weight loss in morbidly obese subjects. J Clin Endocrinol Metab. 97:E1229–33, 2012.

Sacks H, Symonds MA. Anatomical locations of human brown adipose tissue. Diabetes. 62:1783–90, 2013.

Graja A, Schulz TJ. Mechanisms of aging-related impairment of brown adipocyte development and function. Gerontology. 61:211–7, 2015.

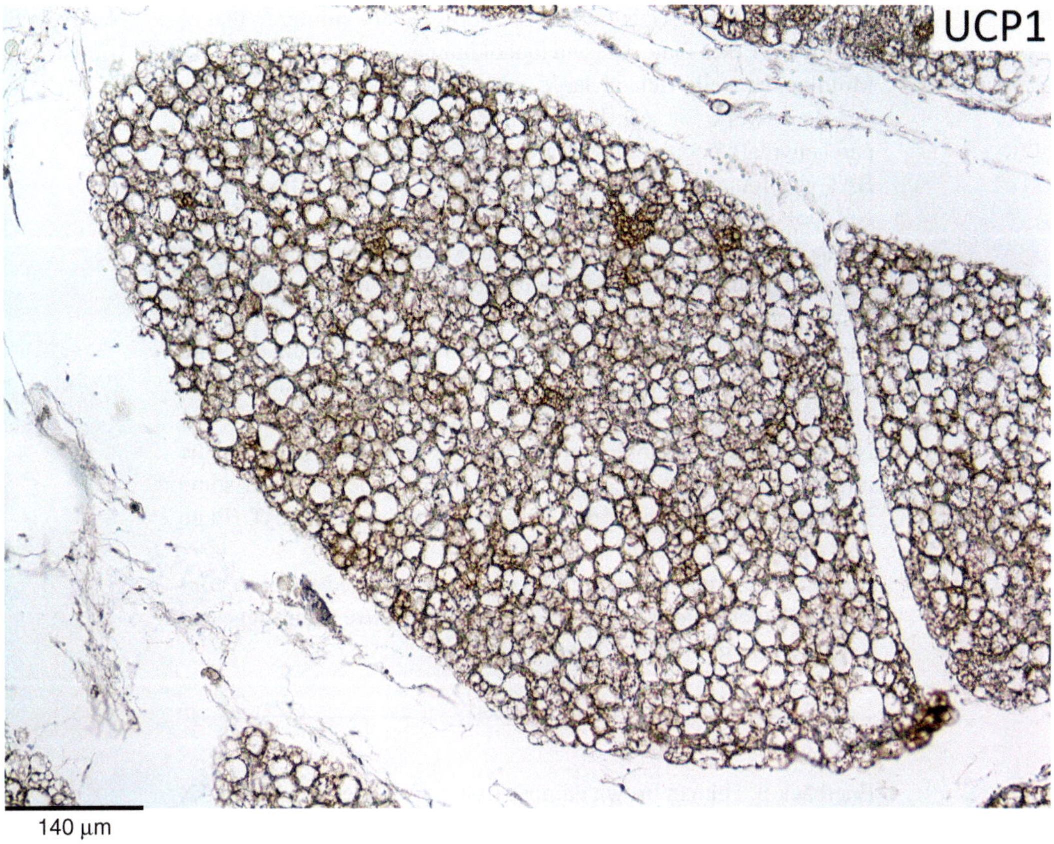

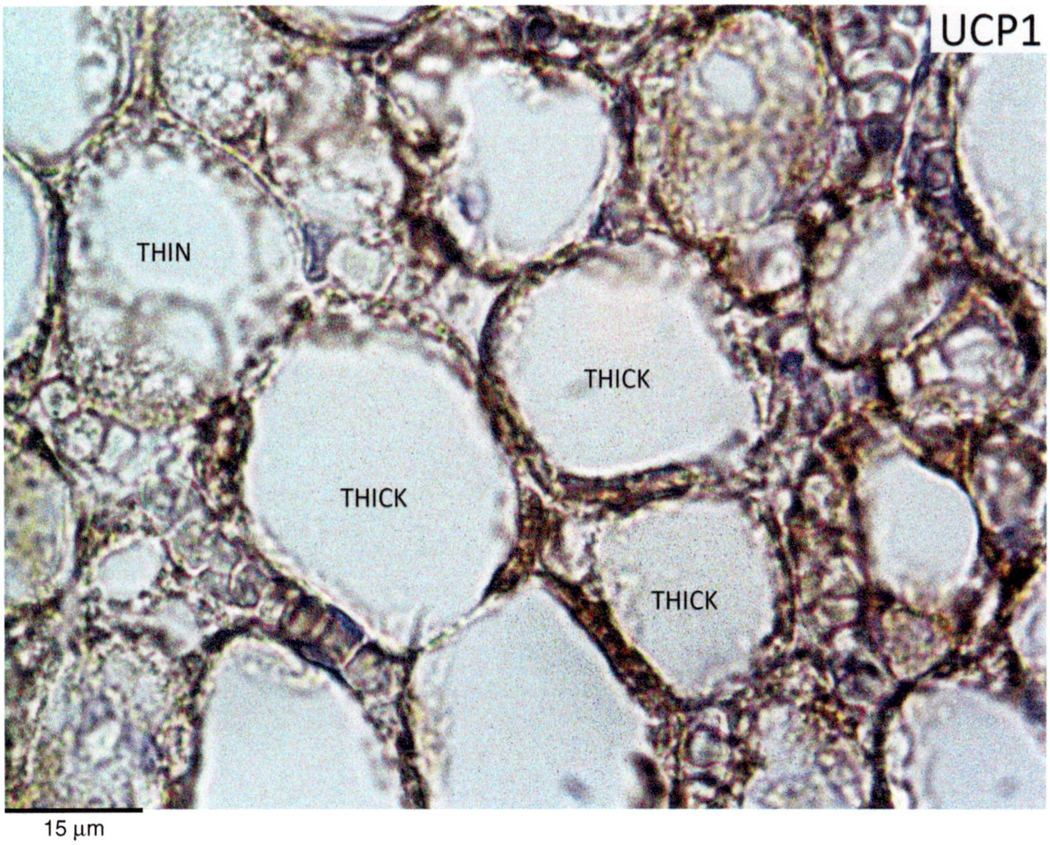

Plate 13.8 Perirenal BAT of a newborn (25-day-old) male. LM. IHC UCP1 ab (1:300)

PLATE 13.9

Newborn BAT Ultrastructure

Ultrastructure of BAT in human newborns is very similar to that of murine BAT (see Plate 2.2) and that of human adults (see Plate 3.3). Multilocular cells rich in large mitochondria are immersed in a dense network of capillaries (upper panel). All side (non-parenchymal) population described in murine and adult humans BAT was found in newborns. In this panel a poorly differentiated cell (possibly a preadipocyte) is visible (arrow).

All the organelles typical of brown adipocytes are visible at higher magnification (middle panel). Here typical large mitochondria with laminar cristae, pinocytotic vesicles (PV), a short cisterna of rough endoplasmic reticulum (RER), and a thin external lamina (EL) are visible. Note the dense line at the periphery of the small lipid droplet (L).

Numerous dense granules are present among the cristae in the mitochondria matrix (enlarged in the lower panel, arrows: some indicated). This aspect is present also in murine fetal BAT (Plate 12.4) and absent in adult murine and human BAT.

These dense granules seem to be closely associated to areas containing mitochondrial DNA (see Plate 7.8) and have been suggested to play a role in the development of cristae.

Suggested Reading

Enerbäck S. Human brown adipose tissue. Cell Metab. 11:248–52, 2010.

Nedergaard J, Cannon B. How brown is brown fat? It depends where you look. Nat Med. 19:540–1, 2013.

Betz MJ, Enerbäck S. Human brown adipose tissue: what we have learned so far. Diabetes. 64:2352–60, 2015.

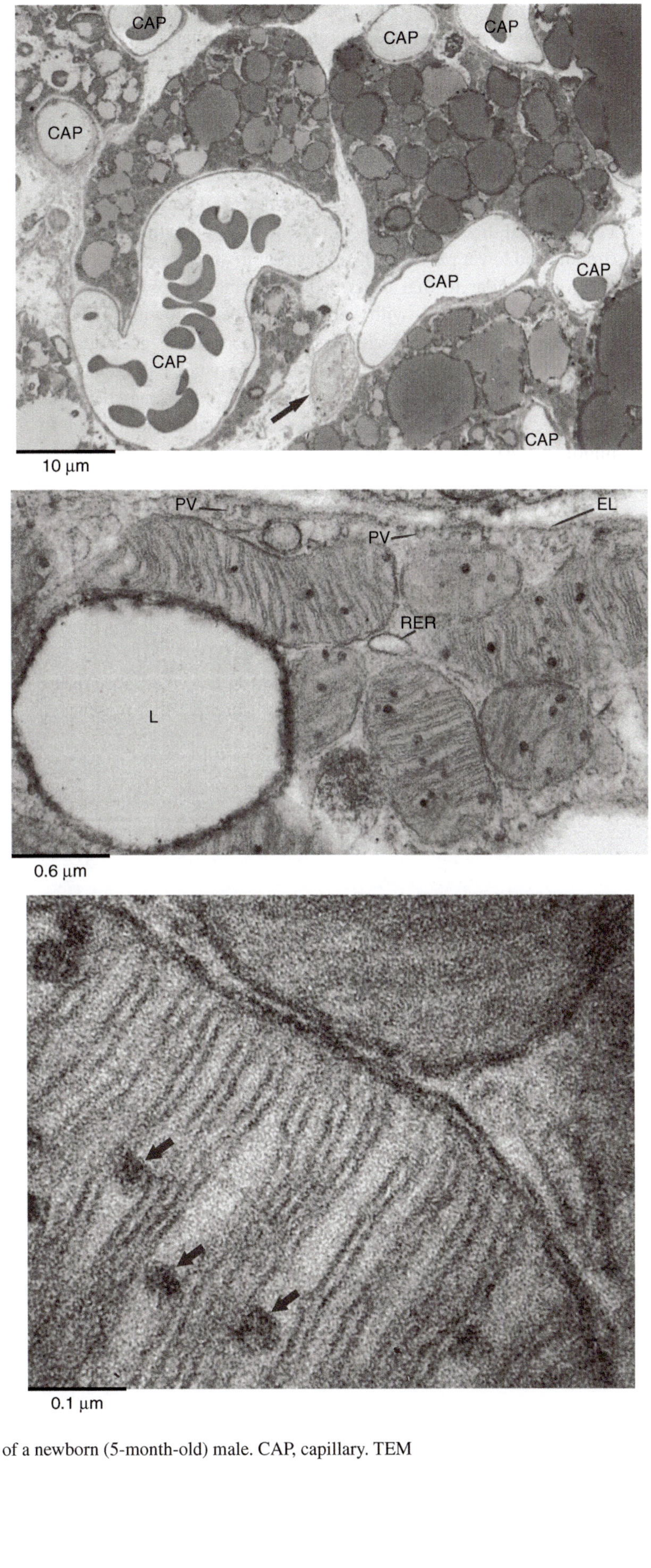

Plate 13.9 Perirenal BAT of a newborn (5-month-old) male. CAP, capillary. TEM

PLATE 13.10

Nerves

Newborn BAT lobules contain a dense network of parenchymal TH-immunoreactive (noradrenergic) fibers (upper panel), similar to those found in adult humans (see Plate 3.2). Synaptic enlargements are also well visible (arrows). Thus noradrenergic parenchymal innervation of BAT in human adipose organ seems to start as early as 22–23 weeks during the fetal life, increase its density during the last part of the fetal period, and is very high in newborns in line with the thermogenic needs of the perinatal period.

Parenchymal fibers resulted visible also at ultrastructural level (middle and lower panels). The ultrastructure of parenchymal fibers was very similar to that described in murine adipose organ (see Plates 2.22 and 2.23) with very small fibers showing synaptic enlargements. Empty vesicles and rare dense-core granules are present in synaptic enlargements (lower right panel, enlargement of squared area in the lower left panel). Small unmyelinated nerves running close to brown adipocytes are also visible (dotted line in middle panel).

Suggested Reading

Himms-Hagen J. Brown adipose tissue thermogenesis: interdisciplinary studies. FASEB J. 4:2890–8, 1990.

Cypess AM, et al. Cold but not sympathomimetics activates human brown adipose tissue in vivo. PNAS. 19:1001–5, 2012.

Razzoli M, et al. Stress-induced activation of brown adipose tissue prevents obesity in conditions of low adaptive thermogenesis. Mol Metab. 5:19–33, 2015.

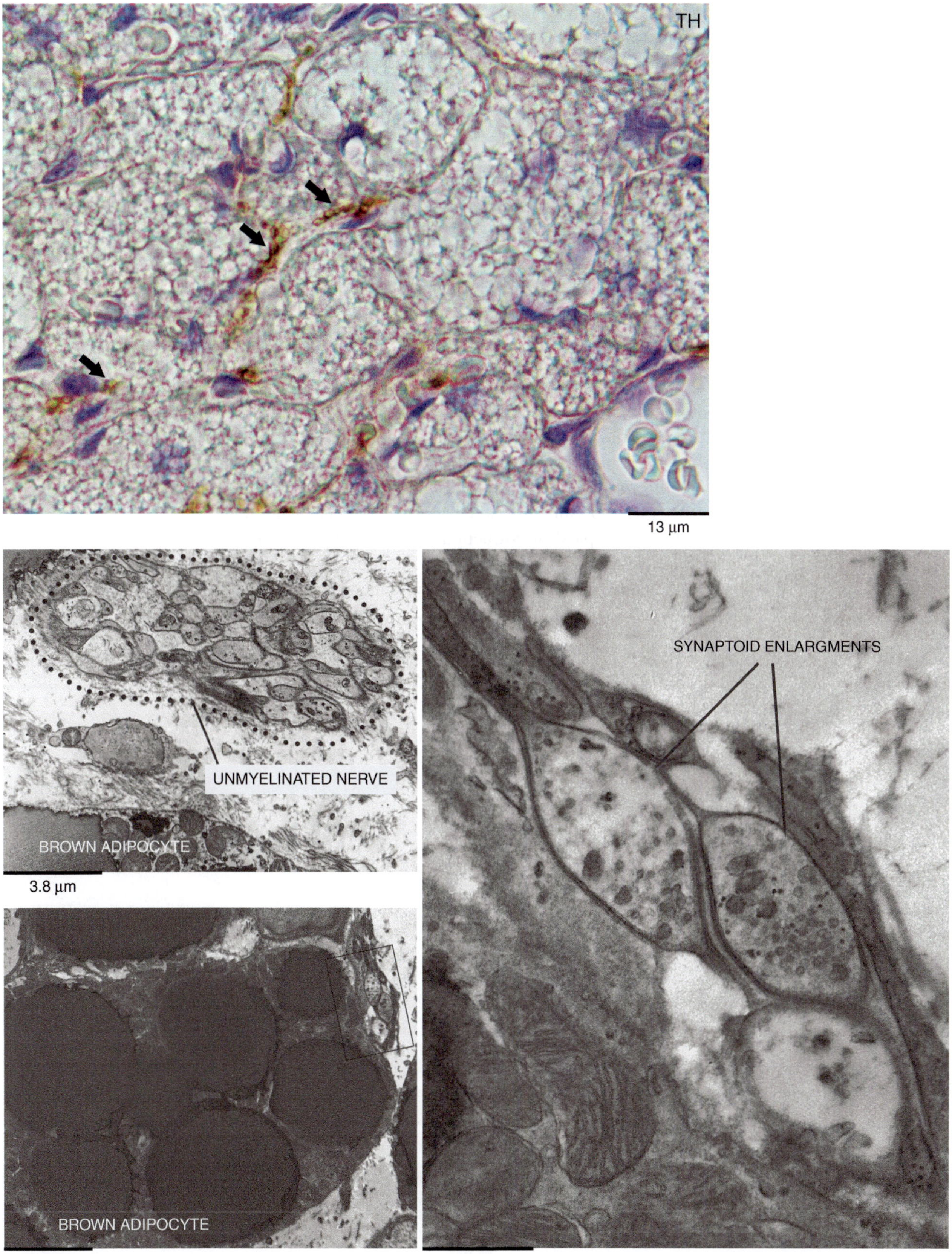

Plate 13.10 Parenchymal nerves and nerve fibers in perirenal BAT of a newborn (5-month-old) male. *Upper*: LM. IHC TH ab (1:300). *Middle* and *lower* panels: TEM

PLATE 13.11

Pericyte-Preadipocyte Ultrastructure I

During development of murine and human adipose organ, a constant feature is the observation that capillaries are very rich in large pericytes. For decades this cell has been proposed as the earliest step of preadipocyte development. Several plates in this book (mainly 4.16–4.17, 5.10–5.11, and 13.5) show the ultrastructural characteristics of these cells with some features supporting this idea.

In line with data supporting the progressive increase in the number of adipocytes until puberty, the adipose organ of human newborns is rich in capillaries enriched with pericytes having some ultrastructural features consistent with the idea that they could represent an early stage of preadipocyte development.

This plate shows perirenal fat from a 5-month-old male. A capillary (CAP) with two pericytes (P) rich in cytoplasmic glycogen (G) is visible. Of note, a poorly differentiated cell very close to this capillary is also visible. The ultrastructural features of this poorly differentiated cell and those of pericytes are very similar suggesting that the poorly developed cell close to the capillary could represent an early developmental step of pericytes into preadipocytes. The typical ultrastructure of a poorly developed cell is identified by the high nucleus/cytoplasm ratio and by poorly developed cytoplasmic organelles. The typical ultrastructural features uniquely found in poorly differentiated preadipocytes are identified by its distinct external lamina (EL) and abundant cytoplasmic glycogen (G). All together these data further support the vascular nature of this cell type.

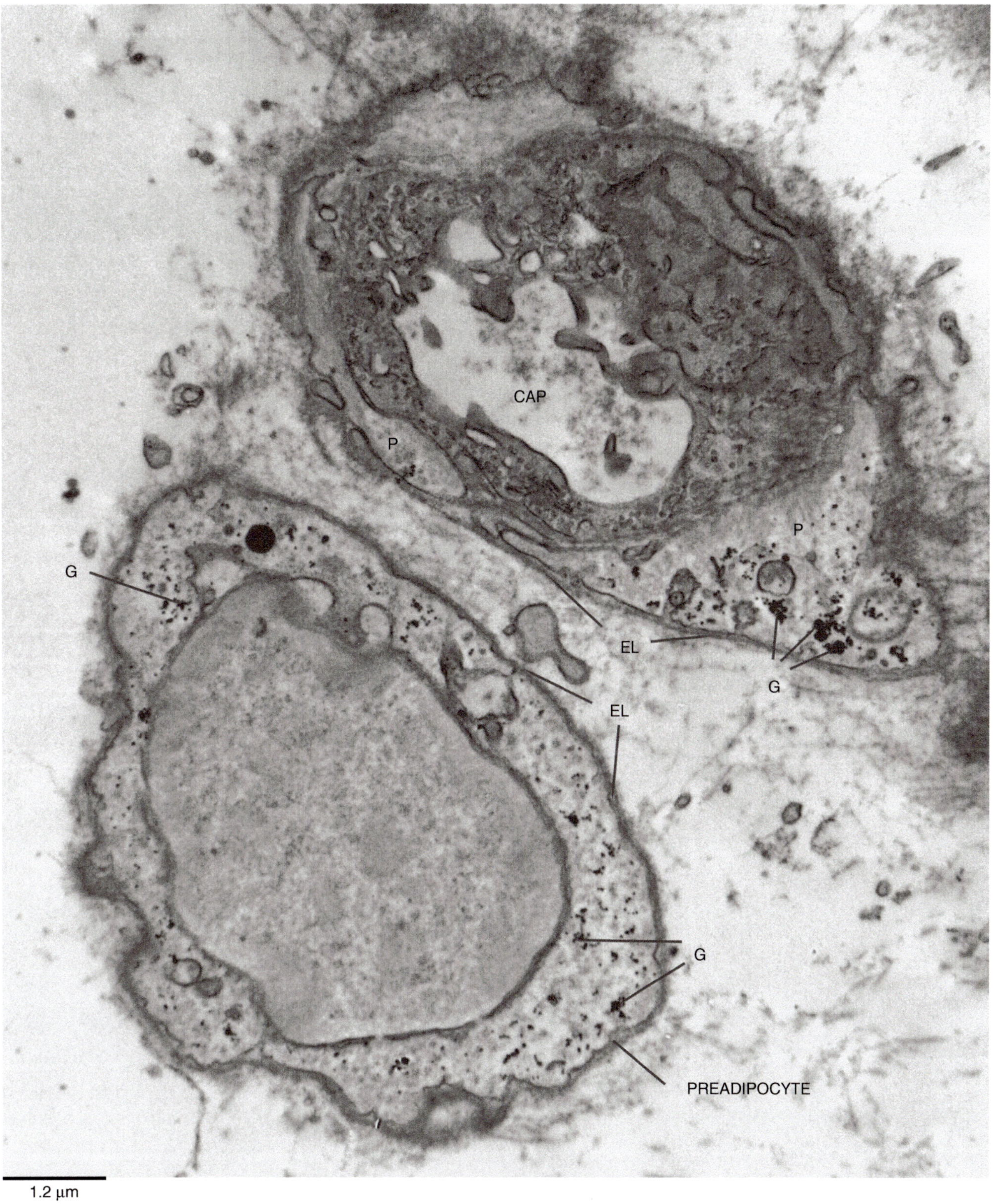

Plate 13.11 Perirenal BAT of a newborn (5-month-old) male. Pericytes and preadipocyte. TEM

PLATE 13.12

Pericyte-Preadipocyte Ultrastructure II

Pericytes in the wall of capillaries could represent the early step of adipocyte precursors (see the previous plate); thus an abundance of this cell type is expected as a characteristic feature of capillaries in developing fat depots such as those of human newborns.

This plate shows a representative aspect of BAT capillary (CAP), between two mature brown adipocytes (BA), with numerous pericytes (P) in their wall.

One important feature supporting the preadipocyte role of pericytes is the identification of their "detaching position," i.e., pericytes with part of the cell in contact with an endothelial cell and a part abutting into the interstitial space. In the lower panel (enlargement of the squared area in the upper panel), a pericyte in "detaching position" is visible. The arrow points to the cytoplasmic segment connecting the part in contact with the endothelial cell (E, nucleus; EL, external lamina) and the roundish part abutting toward the interstitial space (IS). Similar aspects of the developmental stages of murine adipose organ were also found (see Plate 4.17).

Suggested Reading

Zuk PA. Multilineage cells from human adipose tissue: implications for cell-based therapies. Tissue Eng. 7:211–28, 2001.

Traktuev DO, et al. A population of multipotent CD34-positive adipose stromal cells share pericyte and mesenchymal surface markers, reside in a periendothelial location, and stabilize endothelial networks. Circ Res. 102:77–85, 2008.

Lin G, et al. Defining stem and progenitor cells within adipose tissue. Stem Cells Dev. 17:1053–63, 2008.

Tang W, et al. White fat progenitor cells reside in the adipose vasculature. Science. 322:583–6, 2008.

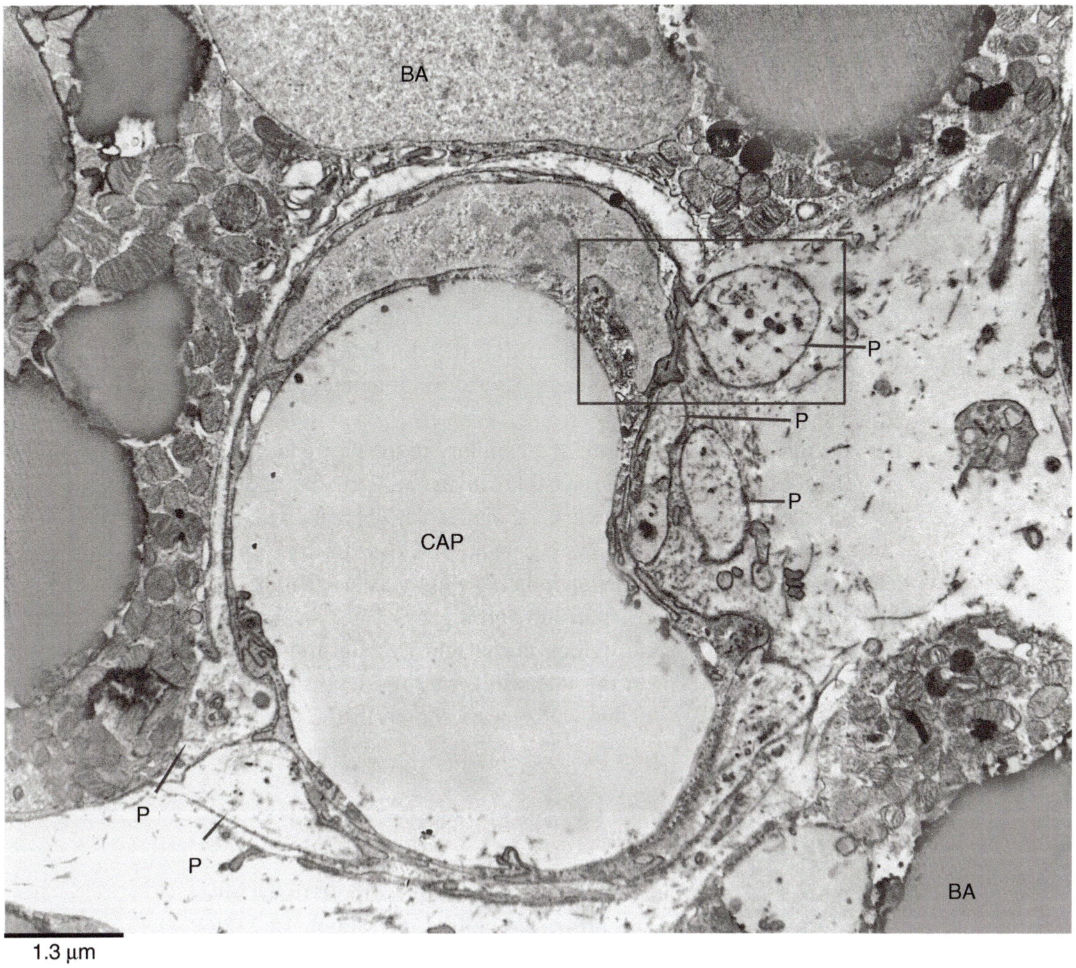

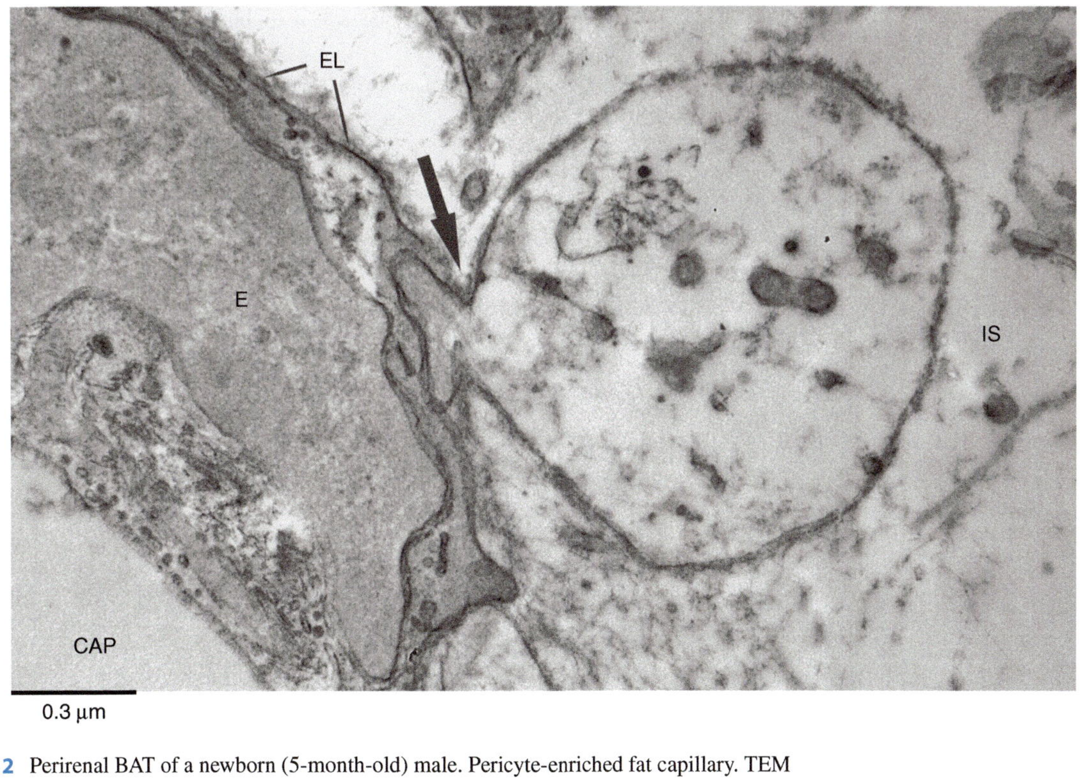

Plate 13.12 Perirenal BAT of a newborn (5-month-old) male. Pericyte-enriched fat capillary. TEM

PLATE 13.13

Endothelial-Pericyte

The origin of preadipocytes is still a controversial field in literature. Our morphologic and lineage tracing data support the idea that some endothelial cells of capillaries in the adipose organ can give rise to pericytes to develop into both white and brown preadipocytes depending on environmental conditions and anatomical area occupied in the adipose organ (see Chap. 12). One aspect supporting this hypothesis is the morphologic observation that unique cells in endothelial-pericyte position can be observed in murine developing adipose organ (see Plate 12.14). These endothelial-pericytes could represent a stage of endothelial cell conversion into a pericyte. Pericytes of adipose organ during development are widely considered an early step of preadipocyte development (see previous plates).

In this plate the ultrastructure of a capillary in the perirenal fat of a 5-month-old male human is visible. In the wall of the capillary (CAP), an endothelial-pericyte is recognizable. This elongated thin cell (red in the scheme) shows a part in contact with the capillary lumen and joined to another endothelial cell by a classic tight junction (TJ) (endothelial part: arrow) and a part located in the space between the endothelium (green in the scheme) and the capillary external lamina (EL) on the interstitial side (pericytic part). The hypothetic evolution of this cell type is shown in the scheme of Plate 12.4.

Suggested Reading

Tran KV, et al. The vascular endothelium of the adipose tissue gives rise to both white and brown fat cells. Cell Metab. 15:222–9, 2012.

Frontini A, et al. Endothelial cells of adipose tissues: a niche of adipogenesis. Cell Cycle. 11:2765–6, 2012.

Symonds ME, et al. The ontogeny of brown adipose tissue. Annu Rev Nutr. 35:295–320, 2015.

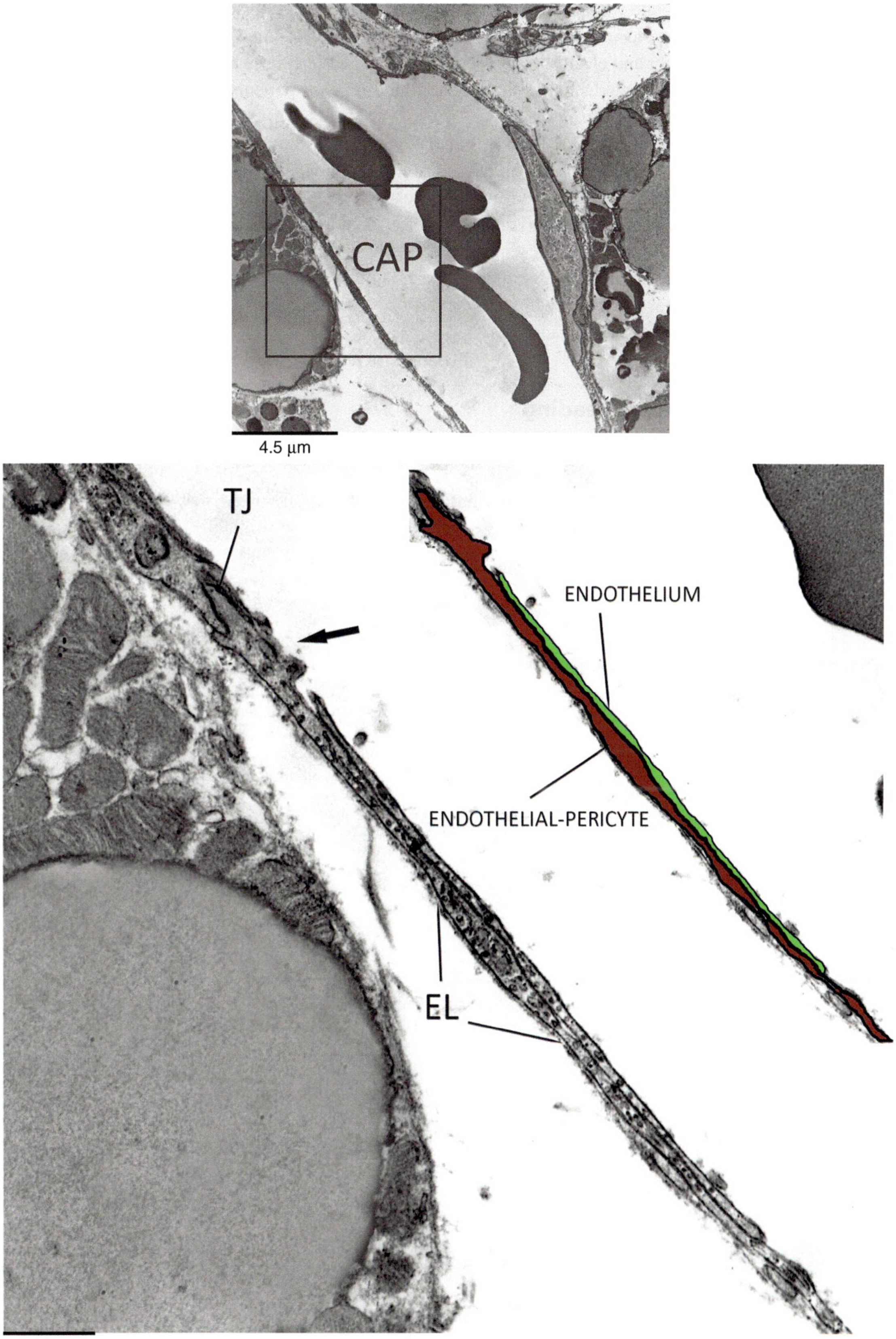

Plate 13.13 Perirenal BAT of a newborn (5-month-old) male. Ultrastructure of an endothelial-pericyte. TEM

PLATE 13.14

WAT from an Infant

In this plate white adipocytes of subcutaneous WAT biopsied from a 4-year-old male patient are shown. The tissue resulted normal after light and electron microscopy analysis. Unilocular white adipocytes resulted smaller than those found in adult patients (about 35–40% smaller).

Electron microscopy (lower panels) revealed a surprising high number of mitochondria (m in the lower right plate, enlargement of squared area in the lower middle panel) and well-developed cytoplasmic organelles. Short cisternae of rough endoplasmic reticulum (RER) are diffusely present together with glycogen particles (G). All other organelles, including external lamina (EL), are very similar to those found in white adipocytes of adolescent humans (compare with Plates 5.5 and 5.6).

Suggested Reading

Baker GL. Human adipose tissue and age. Am J Clin Nutr. 22:829–35, 1969.

Harrington TAM, et al. Distribution of adipose tissue in the newborn. Pediatric Res. 55:437–41, 2004.

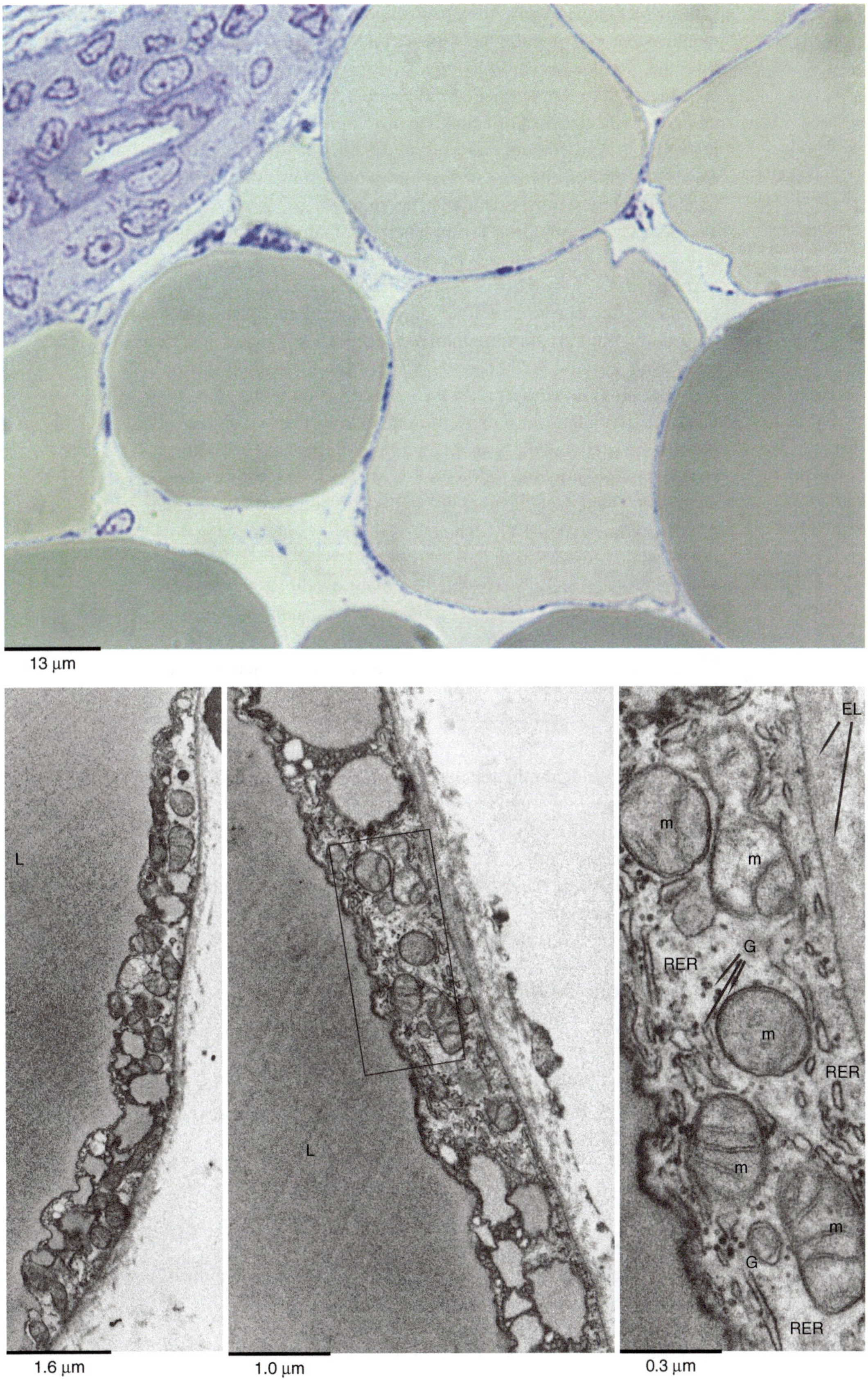

Plate 13.14 Subcutaneous WAT from a 4-year-old boy. *Upper*: LM of resin-embedded tissue. In the upper left corner, a duct of a sweat gland is visible. Toluidine blue staining. *Lower*: cytoplasm of two different adipocytes from the same subject. TEM

PLATE 13.15

Rainbow Adipocyte

Murine and human isolated mature adipocytes maintained in vitro exhibit stem cell phenotypic aspects and properties. These cells lose their unilocular morphology to convert into fibroblast-like cells lacking the characteristic lipid vacuole. Lipid droplet enlargement is a typical aspect of adipocyte development; thus adipocytes losing their lipid content were often classified as dedifferentiated cells. Their multi-lineage differentiative properties reinforced the concept of their stemness and dedifferentiation.

The dedifferentiation process implies that a mature cell undergoes a backward differentiative process ending into a phenotype corresponding to the early differentiative stage of that specific cell type. Thus the absence of lipid droplet is widely considered as typical for the early differentiative stage of adipocytes. On the other hand, it is also well known that the physiologic lipolysis (due, e.g., to fasting) induces a progressive modification of the adipocyte morphology ending into a specific phenotype (that we defined as the slimmed cells) without significant lipid droplet and exhibiting a specific morphology that allows an easy identification by electron microscopy and well distinct from that of poorly differentiated cells (see Plates 10.6–10.8). Thus, loss of lipid vacuole per se does not mean dedifferentiation.

The delipidated cells derived from mature adipocytes in vitro undergoes a process of liposecretion (upper panels) that can be visualized also by time-lapse movies.

Electron microscopy of these post-liposecretion cells demonstrates their fully differentiated organelles typical of a mature state (lower panel). Thus, the post-liposecretion phenotype of a mature adipocyte in vitro is a specific mature phenotype rather than a dedifferentiation state. We denominated this type of cell as rainbow adipocyte because this cell derived from direct conversion of a white adipocyte is able to differentiate into several lineages under appropriate stimuli, strongly reinforcing the concept widely showed and discussed in this book, the extraordinary plasticity and multifunctionality of adipose cells.

Suggested Reading

Poloni A, et al. Human dedifferentiated adipocytes show similar properties to bone marrow-derived mesenchymal stem cells. Stem Cells. 30:965–74, 2012.

Poloni A, et al. Biosafety evidence for human dedifferentiated adipocytes. J Cell Physiol. 230:1525–33, 2015.

Poloni A, et al. Plasticity of human dedifferentiated adipocytes toward endothelial cells. Exp Hematol. 43:137–46, 2014.

Poloni A, et al. Glial-like differentiation potential of human mature adipocytes. J Mol Neurosci. 55:91–8, 2015.

Maurizi G, et al. Human white adipocytes convert into "rainbow" adipocytes in vitro. J Cell Physiol. 232:2887–2899, 2017.

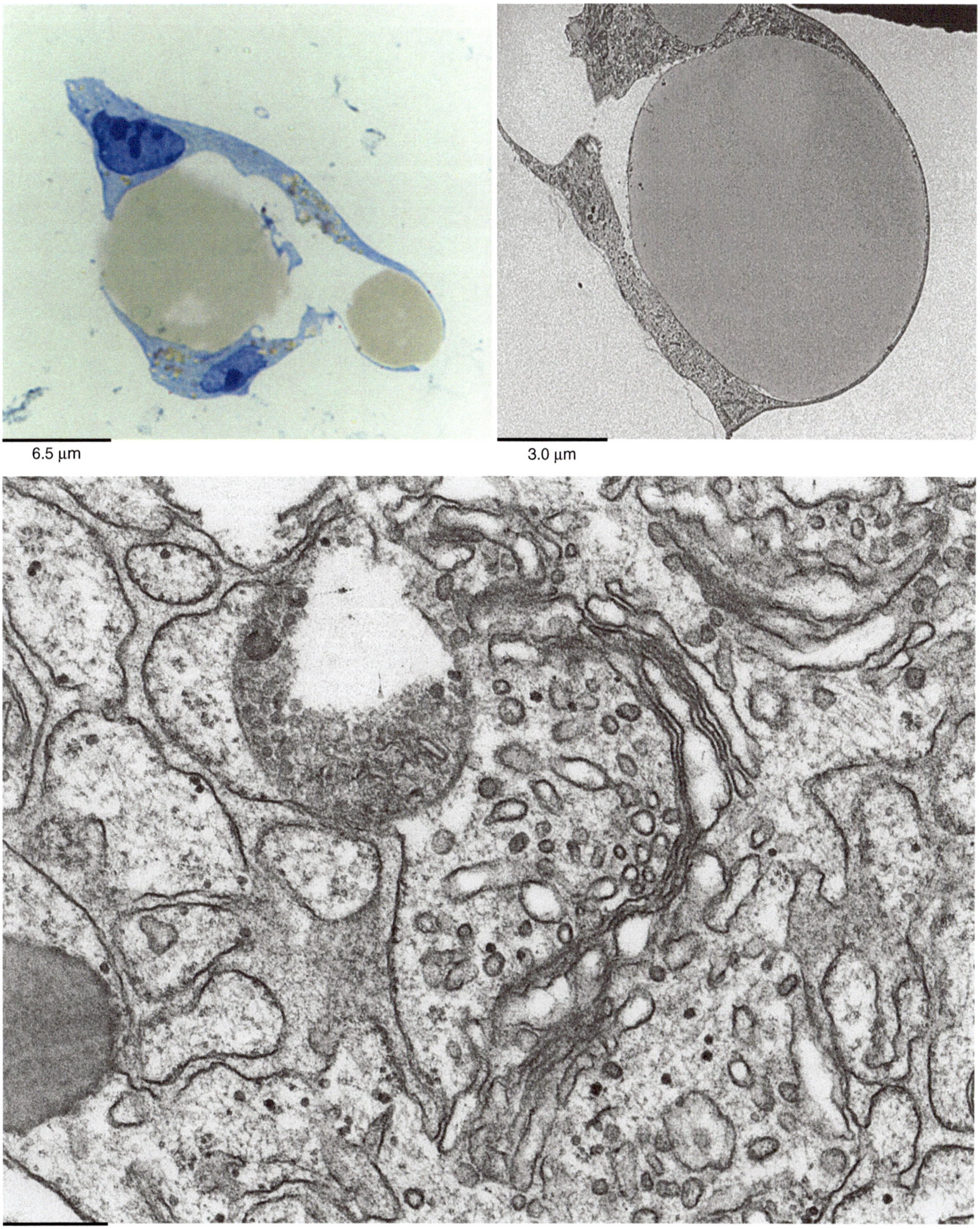

Plate 13.15 Human omental mature adipocytes in vitro. *Upper*: aspects of liposecretion. Resin-embedded tissue. Toluidine blue staining. LM (*left*). TEM (*right*). *Lower*: well-developed organelles of a rainbow adipocyte. TEM (Panels from: Maurizi G et al. Human white adipocytes convert into "rainbow" adipocytes in vitro. J. Cell. Physiol. 10:2887–99, 2017 with permission)

GPSR Compliance

The European Union's (EU) General Product Safety Regulation (GPSR) is a set of rules that requires consumer products to be safe and our obligations to ensure this.

If you have any concerns about our products, you can contact us on ProductSafety@springernature.com

In case Publisher is established outside the EU, the EU authorized representative is:

Springer Nature Customer Service Center GmbH
Europaplatz 3
69115 Heidelberg, Germany

Batch number: 10684834

Printed by Printforce, the Netherlands